Degenerative Cervical Myelopathy and Radiculopathy

Michael G. Kaiser • Regis W. Haid
Christopher I. Shaffrey
Michael G. Fehlings
Editors

Degenerative Cervical Myelopathy and Radiculopathy

Treatment Approaches and Options

Springer

Editors
Michael G. Kaiser
Columbia University Medical Center
New York, NY
USA

Regis W. Haid
Atlanta Brain and Spine Care
Atlanta, GA
USA

Christopher I. Shaffrey
Duke University Health System
Durham, NC
USA

Michael G. Fehlings
Toronto Western Hospital
University of Toronto
Toronto, ON
Canada

ISBN 978-3-319-97951-9 ISBN 978-3-319-97952-6 (eBook)
https://doi.org/10.1007/978-3-319-97952-6

Library of Congress Control Number: 2018957703

This Springer imprint is published by the registered company Springer Nature Switzerland AG
The registered company address is: Gewerbestrasse 11, 6330 Cham, Switzerland

Contents

Part III Surgical Decision-Making

Part IV Motion Preservation Surgery for Cervical Degenerative Disorders

Part V Fusion Techniques for Cervical Degenerative Disorders

Contributors

Nitin Agarwal, MD Department of Neurological Surgery, University of Pittsburgh Medical Center, Pittsburgh, PA, USA

Mohanad Alazzeh, BS University of California, San Francisco, CA, USA

Todd J. Albert, MD Hospital for Special Surgery, New York, NY, USA

Christopher P. Ames, MD Department of Neurological Surgery, University of California, San Francisco, CA, USA

Peter D. Angevine, MD Department of Neurological Surgery, Columbia University Medical Center, New York, NY, USA

Grigoriy Arutyunyan, MD Department of Orthopedic Surgery, UCSF Medical Center, San Francisco, CA, USA

Azam Basheer, MD Department of Neurosurgery, Neuroscience Institute, Henry Ford Health System, Detroit, MI, USA

Edward C. Benzel, MD Department of Neurosurgery, Center for Spine Health, Neurological Institute, Cleveland Clinic Foundation, Cleveland, OH, USA

Maxwell Boakye, MD, MPH, MBA, FACS Department of Neurosurgery, University of Louisville, Louisville, KY, USA

Scott D. Boden, MD Department of Orthopaedic Surgery, Emory University School of Medicine, Atlanta, GA, USA

Avery L. Buchholz, MD, MPH Department of Neurological Surgery, Medical University of South Carolina, Charleston, SC, USA

Hsuan-Kan Chang, MD Department of Neurological Surgery and Rehabilitation Medicine, University of Miami Miller School of Medicine, Miami, FL, USA

Randy S. D'Amico, MD Department of Neurological Surgery, Columbia University Medical Center, New York, NY, USA

Harel Deutsch, MD Department of Neurologic Surgery, Rush University Medical Center, Chicago, IL, USA

Anthony M. DiGiorgio, DO, MHA Department of Neurological Surgery, University of California, San Francisco, CA, USA

Department of Neurological Surgery, Louisiana State University Health Sciences Center, New Orleans, LA, USA

Kurt M. Eichholz, MD, FACS, FAANS St. Louis Minimally Invasive Spine Center, St. Louis, MO, USA

Michael G. Fehlings, MD, PhD, FRCSC, FACS Division of Neurosurgery and Spine Program, Toronto Western Hospital, University of Toronto, Toronto, ON, Canada

Richard G. Fessler, MD Department of Neurosurgery, Rush University, Chicago, IL, USA

Mario Ganau, MD, PhD Division of Neurosurgery and Spine Program, Toronto Western Hospital, University of Toronto, Toronto, ON, Canada

Matthew F. Gary, MD Department of Orthopaedic Surgery, Emory University School of Medicine, Atlanta, GA, USA

Zoher Ghogawala, MD, FACS Department of Neurosurgery, Lahey Hospital and Medical Center, Burlington, MA, USA

Department of Neurosurgery, Tufts University School of Medicine, Boston, MA, USA

John L. Gillick, MD Department of Neurosurgery, Thomas Jefferson University, Philadelphia, PA, USA

Department of Neurosurgery, Rutgers-New Jersey Medical School, Newark, NJ, USA

Jian Guan, MD Department of Neurosurgery, University of Utah, Salt Lake City, UT, USA

Alan L. and Jacqueline Stuart Spine Center, Department of Neurosurgery, Lahey Hospital and Medical Center, Burlington, MA, USA

Regis W. Haid, MD Atlanta Brain and Spine Care, Atlanta, GA, USA

James S. Harrop, MD, FACS Department of Neurological and Orthopedic Surgery, Division of Spine and Peripheral Nerve Surgery, Delaware Valley SCI Center, Thomas Jefferson University, Philadelphia, PA, USA

Cory J. Hartman, MD Department of Neurosurgery, University of Florida, Gainesville, FL, USA

Robert F. Heary, MD Department of Neurological Surgery, Rutgers New Jersey Medical School, Newark, NJ, USA

Dominque M. O. Higgins, MD, PhD Department of Neurological Surgery, Columbia University Medical Center, New York, NY, USA

Daniel J. Hoh, MD Department of Neurosurgery, University of Florida, Gainesville, FL, USA

Langston T. Holly, MD Department of Neurosurgery, University of California-Los Angeles, Los Angeles, CA, USA

Ming-Hsiao Hu, MD Institute of Biomedical Engineering, College of Medicine and College of Engineering, National Taiwan University, Taipei, Taiwan

Department of Orthopedics, National Taiwan University College of Medicine and National Taiwan University Hospital, Taipei, Taiwan

Deeptee Jain, MD Department of Orthopedic Surgery, UCSF Medical Center, San Francisco, CA, USA

Jacob Januszewski, MD Department of Neurosurgery and Brain Repair, University of South Florida, Tampa, FL, USA

Michael G. Kaiser, MD, FACS, FAANS Department of Neurological Surgery, Columbia University Medical Center, New York, NY, USA

Mena G. Kerolus, MD Department of Neurosurgery, Rush University Medical Center, Chicago, IL, USA

Jerry Ku, MD Division of Neurosurgery, St. Michael's Hospital, University of Toronto, Toronto, ON, Canada

Shekar N. Kurpad, MD, PhD Department of Neurosurgery, Medical College of Wisconsin, Milwaukee, WI, USA

Frank LaMarca, MD Department of Neurosurgery, Henry Ford Health System, Detroit, MI, USA

Anthony C. Lau, MD Department of Neurological Surgery, University of Miami Miller School of Medicine, Miami, FL, USA

Bryan S. Lee, MD Department of Neurosurgery, Center for Spine Health, Neurological Institute, Cleveland Clinic Foundation, Cleveland, OH, USA

Allan D. Levi, MD Department of Neurological Surgery, University of Miami Miller School of Medicine, Miami, FL, USA

Mohammed Macki, MD Department of Neurosurgery, Henry Ford Hospital, Detroit, MI, USA

Hani R. Malone, MD Department of Neurological Surgery, Columbia University Medical Center, New York, NY, USA

David McCarthy, BS Department of Neurological Surgery and Rehabilitation Medicine, University of Miami Miller School of Medicine, Miami, FL, USA

Mark R. McLaughlin, MD, FACS, FAANS Princeton Brain and Spine Care, LLC, Princeton, NJ, USA

Lionel N. Metz, MD Department of Orthopedic Surgery, UCSF Medical Center, San Francisco, CA, USA

Joseph E. Molenda, MD Department of Neurosurgery, Rush University Medical Center, Chicago, IL, USA

Praveen V. Mummaneni, MD Department of Neurological Surgery, University of California, San Francisco, CA, USA

Hamadi Murphy, MD, MS Department of Orthopaedics, Rothman Institute at Thomas Jefferson University Hospital, Philadelphia, PA, USA

Jean-Christophe Murray, MD, FRCSC Division of Neurosurgery and Spine Program, Toronto Western Hospital, University of Toronto, Toronto, ON, Canada

Daniel T. Nagasawa, MD Department of Neurosurgery, University of California-Los Angeles, Los Angeles, CA, USA

Ha Son Nguyen, MD Department of Neurosurgery, Medical College of Wisconsin, Milwaukee, WI, USA

Tianyi Niu, MD Department of Neurosurgery, University of California-Los Angeles, Los Angeles, CA, USA

Aria Nouri, MD, MSc Department of Neurosurgery, Yale University and University of Cincinnati, Cincinnati, OH, USA

John E. O'Toole, MD Department of Neurosurgery, Rush University Medical Center, Chicago, IL, USA

Joseph A. Osorio, MD, PhD Department of Neurological Surgery, University of California, San Francisco, CA, USA

John C. Quinn, MD Department of Neurosurgery, University of Virginia Health System, Charlottesville, VA, USA

K. Daniel Riew, MD The Spine Hospital, Columbia University Medical Center, New York, NY, USA

Justin K. Scheer, MD Department of Neurosurgery, University of Illinois at Chicago, Chicago, IL, USA

Christopher I. Shaffrey, MD Departments of Orthopaedic and Neurological Surgery, Duke University Health System, Durham, NC, USA

Stephen Silva, BA Department of Orthopaedics, Rothman Institute at Thomas Jefferson University Hospital, Philadelphia, PA, USA

Justin S. Smith, MD, PhD Department of Neurological Surgery, University of Virginia Health System, Charlottesville, VA, USA

Derek G. Southwell, MD, PhD Department of Neurological Surgery, University of California, San Francisco, CA, USA

Blake N. Staub, MD Texas Back Institute, Plano, TX, USA

Lee A. Tan, MD The Spine Hospital, Columbia University Medical Center, New York, NY, USA

Meena Thatikunta, MD Department of Neurosurgery, University of Louisville, Louisville, KY, USA

Santan Thottempudi University of California, San Francisco, CA, USA

Matthew J. Tormenti, MD, FACS, FAANS Princeton Brain and Spine, Langhorne, PA, USA

Vincent Traynelis, MD Department of Neurosurgery, Rush University Medical Center, Chicago, IL, USA

Alexander Tuchman, MD Department of Neurological Surgery, Columbia University Medical Center, New York, NY, USA

Alexander Tucker, MD Department of Neurosurgery, University of California-Los Angeles, Los Angeles, CA, USA

Luis M. Tumialán, MD Department of Neurosurgery, Barrow Neurological Institute, St. Joseph's Hospital and Medical Center, Phoenix, AZ, USA

Juan S. Uribe, MD Department of Neurosurgery and Brain Repair, University of South Florida, Tampa, FL, USA

Alex Vaccaro, MD, PhD, MBA Department of Orthopaedics, Rothman Institute at Thomas Jefferson University Hospital, Philadelphia, PA, USA

Michael S. Virk, MD, PhD Department of Neurosurgery, University of California, San Francisco, CA, USA

Scott C. Wagner, MD Department of Orthopaedics, Rothman Institute at Thomas Jefferson University Hospital, Philadelphia, PA, USA

Michael Y. Wang, MD, FACS Department of Neurological Surgery and Rehabilitation Medicine, University of Miami Miller School of Medicine, Miami, FL, USA

Jefferson R. Wilson, MD, PhD, FRCSC Division of Neurosurgery, St. Michael's Hospital, University of Toronto, Toronto, ON, Canada

Jau-Ching Wu, MD, PhD Department of Neurosurgery, Taipei Veteran's General Hospital, Taipei, Taiwan

School of Medicine, National Yang-Ming University, Taipei, Taiwan

Rahel Zewude, BSc Division of Neurosurgery and Spine Program, Toronto Western Hospital, University of Toronto, Toronto, ON, Canada

Part I

The Basics

Functional Anatomy of the Spinal Cord

1

Mario Ganau, Rahel Zewude, and Michael G. Fehlings

Basic Anatomy of the Spinal Cord

Located in the upper two-thirds of the spinal canal, within the hollow portion of a multiarticulated flexible structure called the vertebral column, the SC has a length of approximately 45 cm in humans. The vertebral column is divided into cervical, thoracic or dorsal, lumbar, and sacrococcygeal vertebral segments. Each vertebral segment is formed by bony and cartilaginous components, known as a functional spinal unit (FSU). The FSU can be defined as the smallest physiological motion segment of the vertebral column capable of motion that exhibits biomechanical characteristics similar to those of the entire spine [18]. The SC extends from the foramen magnum at the base of the skull to a cone-shaped termination, the conus medullaris, which is anchored caudally to the coccyx through a non-neural filament known as the filum terminale. Nerve fibers emerge from the SC in an uninterrupted series of dorsal and ventral roots, which join to form 31 spinal nerves: 8 cervical, 12 thoracic or dorsal, 5 lumbar, 5 sacral, and 1 coccygeal. The thoracic, lumbar, and sacral nerves are numbered after the vertebra just rostral to the respective foramen through which they pass (i.e., T12 nerves are caudal to the T12 vertebral body). Conversely, the cervical nerves are numbered for the vertebral body just caudal (i.e., the C1 nerve roots are rostral to the C1 vertebral body, while the C8 nerves are rostral to the body of T1). This distribution explains the different lengths and orientation of each pair of nerve roots: in fact, since the SC is shorter than the vertebral column, the lumbar and sacral nerves develop long roots running caudally below the conus medullaris in the spinal cistern to form the cauda equina.

The three meningeal layers surrounding the SC are a continuation of those found around the brain. The most external layer, the dura mater, does not adhere to the vertebral bone, contrary to the dura of the brain. The spinal dura terminates with a cul-de-sac at the sacral level (S1–S2) forming the dural sac. Overlying the dura is the epidural space, containing fat and vessels, and underlying the dura is the arachnoid space, containing the cerebrospinal fluid (CSF). The third meningeal layer, the pia mater, follows the contours of the SC as well as the arteries and veins supplying the SC; of note, the pia is firmly attached to the dura by a series of 22 denticulate ligaments. These ligaments begin at the foramen magnum and are located on each side of the cord in the interval between two adjacent spinal nerve roots, being attached to the SC roughly halfway between the dorsal and ventral nerve root entry

M. Ganau · R. Zewude · M. G. Fehlings (✉)
Division of Neurosurgery and Spine Program, Toronto Western Hospital, University of Toronto, Toronto, ON, Canada
e-mail: Michael.Fehlings@uhn.ca

M. G. Kaiser et al. (eds.), *Degenerative Cervical Myelopathy and Radiculopathy*,
https://doi.org/10.1007/978-3-319-97952-6_1

zones. The meningeal layers and the compartments they create represent important anatomical regions: the epidural space is where anesthetic drugs are injected to induce local anesthesia during surgical procedures or childbirth; and the arachnoid space in the lumbar cistern, extending from L2 to S2, is the ideal place for CSF collection and injection of drugs or contrast medium through lumbar puncture (ideally performed at the L3/4, L4/5 or L5/S1 interlaminar spaces).

Embryology

The neural tube is the primordial structure for the CNS, with the neural crest appearing at approximately 20 days of gestation and giving rise to a number of neural and nonneural derivatives (including neurons, meningeal cells, etc.). During the third week of gestation, mesenchymal tissue from the mesoderm differentiates into segmented somites. The segmented somites are bilateral structures that develop on either side of the notochord while distending the overlying ectoderm. These somites differentiate into the sclerotome and myodermatome during the fourth week of gestation. The genes regulating the direction and order of the craniocaudal axis development and differentiation are known as Hox genes: spinal congenital anomalies may result from their mutations [15]. Adjacent to the neural tube are 31 pairs of somites; those embryonic segmental structures differentiate into muscles as well as bony and connective tissues, which are arranged in sequence from the first cervical through the coccygeal levels. Each pair of nerves develops in association with each pair of somites. The apparent segmentation of the SC is dependent upon the development of paired segmental spinal nerves and radicular vessels on both sides of the midline. The bilateral neural crest in fact becomes segmented into paired units, one pair for each future sensory dorsal root ganglion of each spinal nerve.

Up to the third fetal month, the SC extends throughout the entire length of the developing vertebral column. The growth of the SC over the subsequent months leads to the elongation of the roots of the spinal nerves between the SC and the intervertebral foramina, so that at birth the caudal end of the SC is located at the level of L3. As a result of canalization and retrogressive differentiation, an ependymal lined space known as the central canal forms at the innermost portion of the SC and terminates at the conus medullaris with the ventriculus terminalis, or fifth ventricle [5]. This structure, which is filled with CSF, is described in the literature as a normal developmental phenomenon, especially in newborns and during childhood, with regression in the adult life. Persistence of this structure may in fact lead to a pathological condition called dilatation of the ventriculus terminalis [9].

Functional Spinal Segments

Each portion of the SC where the corresponding pairs of ventral and dorsal roots attach is called a spinal segment. As such, each spinal segment (except the upper cervical segments) is located slightly higher than the respective FSU. The rootlets forming each nerve root enter the root sleeve after passing obliquely, laterally, and caudally within the vertebral canal. The sleeve contains motor and sensory roots separated by the interradicular septum. The dorsal and ventral roots come together and form the spinal nerve root. Before forming the spinal nerve root, the dorsal root contains an oval enlargement called the dorsal root ganglion.

The cell bodies of motor neurons and interneurons are located in an area of gray matter within the SC, characterized by a butterfly-like shape. The white matter surrounding this gray matter structure is made of the nerve fibers and glia of ascending and descending tracts, as shown in Fig. 1.1. As a result, the nerve fibers of the gray matter are oriented in the transverse plane, whereas those of the white matter are oriented in the longitudinal plane parallel to the neuraxis. The gray matter has been parceled anatomically, primarily on the basis of the microscopic appearance, into nuclei and laminae. This organization is often referred to as being composed of ten laminae, named after the anatomist Rexed, resulting in a posterior horn (laminae I through VI), an intermediate zone (lamina VII), an anterior horn (laminae VIII to IX), and a region surrounding the central canal (lamina X) [19]. Figure 1.1 and Table 1.1 provide details regarding the anatomical organization of the ten Rexed laminae and their specific functions.

The horns of the gray matter contain different classes of functional neurons: second-order interneurons in the dorsal horn process sensory information from the first-order sensory afferents; this may eventually result in di-, tri-, or polysynaptic pathways [6, 7]. Ventral horns contain motoneurons of various types: fundamentally, α-motoneurons innervating skeletal muscle fibers and γ-motoneurons innervating extrafusal motor fibers in muscle spindles.

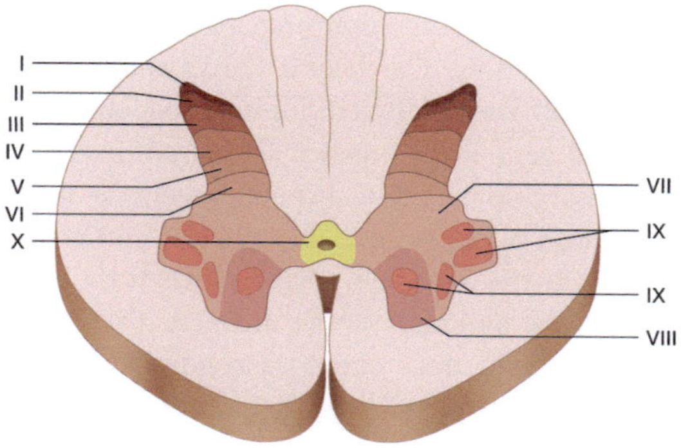

Fig. 1.1 Anatomical distribution of Rexed laminae

As the rostrocaudal distribution of motor neurons follows the body scheme, with more rostral segments innervating muscles of more proximal joints and vice versa, the SC shows two enlarged segments innervating the upper (cervical or brachial enlargement; C5–T1) and lower extremities (lumbosacral enlargement; L3–S2). Also, the spatial distribution of motoneurons within the ventral horn is structurally organized with those innervating axial or proximal muscles located more medially, and those innervating distal muscles in upper and lower extremities located more laterally. Finally, the lateral horn is found at the thoracic and upper lumbar segments only and contains preganglionic sympathetic neurons whose axons reach the sympathetic ganglia adjacent to the vertebral bodies through white communicating rami from the ventral roots. Preganglionic

Table 1.1 Anatomy and function of Rexed laminae

Lamina	Anatomical location	Fibers	Function of fibers
I	Posteromarginal nucleus	Aδ	Sensation of temperature and fast pain
II	Substantia gelatinosa	C	Sensation of slow pain
III	Nucleus proprius	A-b	Mechanoreceptors for touch and proprioception
IV	Nucleus proprius	A-b	Mechanoreceptors for touch and proprioception
V	Nucleus dorsalis	Aδ, C	Receives information on pain sensation and movement
VI	Nucleus dorsalis	Ia/A-alpha Ib/A-alpha/Golgi	Spinal reflexes, integration of somatic motor function
VII	Intermediolateral (IML) cell column, intermediate gray, intermediomedial (IMM) cell column	Spinocerebellar tract C8–L3: nucleus dorsalis T1–L2: IML S2–S4 preganglionic sacral autonomic nucleus	Preganglionic parasympathetic neurons
VIII	Anterior fasciculus	Descending tracts	Modulate muscular tone and movement
IX	Anterior horn	Somatic α- and γ-motor neurons	Innervation of extrafusal fibers of skeletal muscle Innervation of intrafusal fibers of neuromuscular spindles
X	Perimeter of the central canal	Anterior commissure tracts	Decussation of axons

parasympathetic neurons are located similarly at the S2–S4 levels for visceral innervations [21].

Different classes of spinal interneurons are involved in the process of sensory-motor integration, typically being localized in Rexed laminae VII and VIII. Experimental studies have documented how this integration of motor commands and sensory feedback signals is used to control muscle activity during movement. The sum of convergent inputs from sensory neurons and from the central pattern generator (CPG), neural networks that produce rhythmic patterned outputs without sensory feedback, gives rise to the activity of the interneurons. During locomotion, the firing level of interneurons is modulated via excitation or inhibition depending on the reflex pathways, so that different patterns of interneuronal activity determine which pathways are open, blocked, or modulated at any given moment [20].

Spinal Pathways

The white matter is organized within the SC into the following three columns: posterior, lateral, and anterior. Those fibers form tracts that eventually represent the components of sensory, motor, propriospinal, and autonomic pathways; Fig. 1.2 provides further anatomical details of these tracts.

The posterior column is found between the posterior horns of the gray matter, and it is divided by the posterior median septum in the midline. The posterior column contains the fasciculus cuneatus laterally and the fasciculus gracilis medially. These tracts carry ascending information of proprioception, vibration, and light touch sensation. Fasciculus gracilis carries information from lower limbs while fasciculus cuneatus carries information from upper limbs.

The lateral column lies between the dorsal and ventral root entry zones. It is composed of the lateral corticospinal tract and the lateral spinothalamic tract. The lateral corticospinal tract carries descending information regarding voluntary motor function. The lateral corticospinal tract, along with the small anterior corticospinal tract, and the very small anterior lateral corticospinal tract make up the cortical spinal system. With the exception of axons from the anterior corticospinal tract, the axons in corticospinal tract cross over at the pyramids of the medulla. The lateral spinothalamic tract carries ascending information for pain and thermal sensation. This tract decussates upon entry to the spinal cord and as a result carries the impulses from the contralateral side of the body. In the posterior lateral periphery of the spinal cord, the posterior spinocerebellar tract is found. This tract is an uncrossed tract that carries ascending information regarding fine coordination of limb movement and posture.

The anterior column of the white matter is found between the anterior median fissure and the

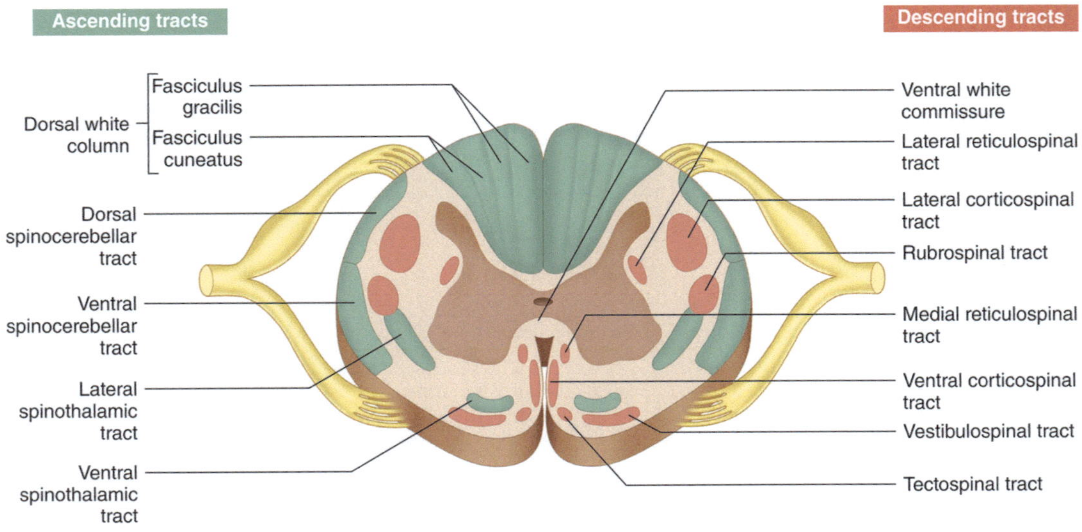

Fig. 1.2 Cross-sectional diagram of the spinal cord with details of ascending and descending tracts

anterior root entry zone. This column contains the anterior corticospinal tract and the anterior spinothalamic tract. The ascending fibers of the anterior spinothalamic tract convey impulses associated with light touch. The anterior corticospinal tract is a descending uncrossed tract responsible for fine motor skills.

Fibers and Spinal Nerves

The fibers contained within each spinal nerve can be responsible for general somatic (innervating the outer body and extremities) or general visceral (innervating the internal organs) functions and therefore can be either afferent or efferent depending on their primarily sensory or motor role.

The dorsal roots are sensory stations consisting of afferent fibers that convey input via spinal nerves from the sensory receptors in the body to the SC. The dorsal root ganglion described above contains the unipolar cell bodies of those neurons. The sensory afferents with their cell bodies and central axon are called first-order neurons. The central axon enters the SC at the level of the posterolateral sulcus, whereas the peripheral axons reach the related receptor in the peripheral tissues. As anticipated, the skin segment supplied by each spinal nerve is called a dermatome. Dermatomes tend to functionally overlap; thus, the loss of one dorsal root usually results in hypesthesia (reduced sensation) rather than anesthesia (complete loss of sensation). The afferent fibers responsible for general somatic and general visceral sensation can be classified according to their conduction velocity into groups I to IV. The fibers of groups I, II, and III are myelinated which allow for faster conduction velocity, while those of group IV are unmyelinated. As described above, the ventral roots are predominantly embodied into the motor pathways, while the lateral horns are autonomic relays. Of note, some sensory fibers have been identified as well within ventral roots [7].

Each α-motor neuron and the muscle fibers it innervates constitute a motor unit; given the specific focus of this book on the pathologies of the cervical spine, a schematic representation of the spinal nerves radiating in the upper limbs is

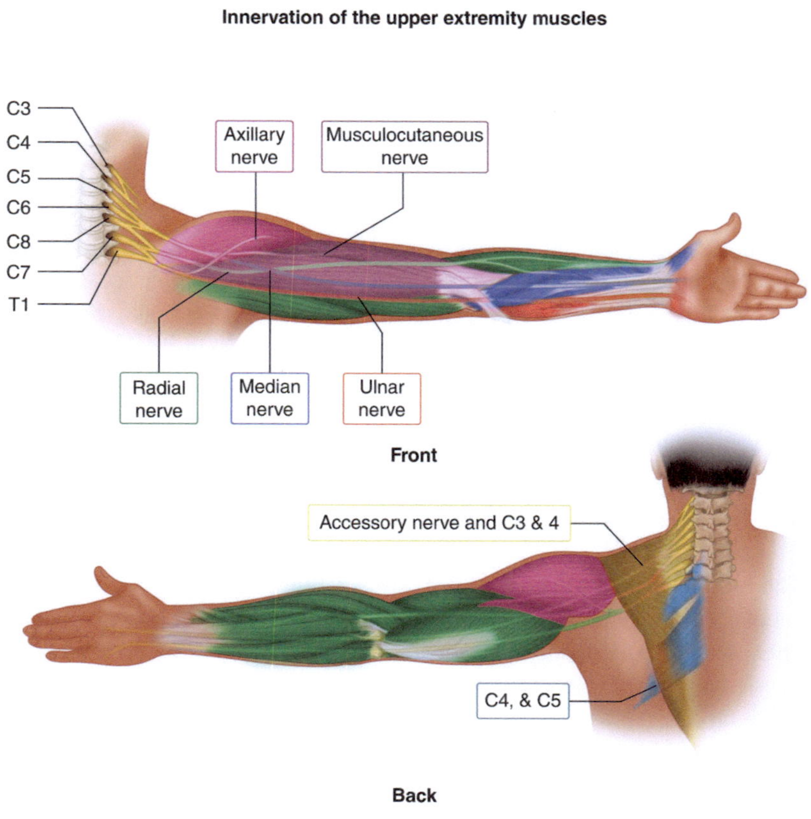

Fig. 1.3 Spinal nerves radiating into the upper limb

Table 1.2 Characteristics and functions of motor neurons as well as autonomic and sensory fibers

Fiber type and innervation	Role	Conduction velocity (m/s)	Diameter (μm)
Motor neurons Anterior horns – ventral roots			
Alpha (A-α) Impulses to end plates of voluntary muscle fibers	Voluntary muscle contraction	15–120 Myelinated	12–20
Gamma (A-γ) Impulses to motor endings of intrafusal fibers of muscle spindle	Fine adjustment of muscle tone	10–45 Myelinated	2–10
Autonomic fibers	*Thoracolumbar intermediate zone (T1–L2) sympathetic system – ventral roots* *Sacral (S3–S4) parasympathetic system – ventral roots*		
Preganglionic fibers (B) Impulses to sympathetic/parasympathetic ganglions	Regulating Heart rate Gastrointestinal and bladder activities	3–15 Myelinated	>3
Postganglionic fibers (C) Impulses to visceral organs		2 Unmyelinated	1
Sensory fibers Dorsal root ganglion – dorsal roots			
Ia (A-α) Impulses from the muscle spindles	Muscle tone	70–120 Myelinated	12–20
Ib (A-α) Impulses from the Golgi tendon organs	Light touch and pressure	70–120 Myelinated	12–20
II (A-β) Impulses from encapsulated skin and joint (Meissner's and Pacinian) receptors	Touch, pressure, and vibratory sense	30–70 Myelinated	5–14
III (A-δ) Impulses from non-encapsulated skin endings	Pain and temperature	12–30 Myelinated	2–7
IV(C) Impulses from non-encapsulated skin endings	Pain and temperature	0.5–2 Unmyelinated	0.5–1

shown in Fig. 1.3. The number of muscle fibers in each motor unit ranges from just 3–8 muscle fibers in small, finely controlled, extraocular muscles of the eye to as many as 2000 muscle fibers in postural muscles of the legs [10]. Regardless of their motor or sensory nature, fibers are also classified based on their conduction velocity into A, B, and C. A fibers are further classified depending on their size into α, β, γ, and δ [13]. Table 1.2 provides a summary of nerve fiber classification.

Vascularization of the Spinal Cord

The blood supply to the SC is provided craniocaudally by one anterior and two posterior spinal arteries and horizontally by several radicular arteries originating at various levels, whereas the radicular arteries vascularize the ventral and dorsal roots [2]. A graphical representation of the horizontal vascularization of the SC is provided in Fig. 1.4. A precise description of the spinal vascular territories aids understanding of many pathologic conditions, especially those referring to spinal syndromes, as well as relatively safe surgical entry zones [8].

Originating from the fusion of the vertebral arteries, the anterior spinal artery is located within the pia mater in the median sulcus. The anterior spinal artery descends in front of the SC continuing as a slender twig on the filum terminale and gives off, along its course, to central branches supplying the anterior third of the SC. The anterior vertebral artery also receives several small branches, known as anterior segmental medullary arteries, which enter the vertebral canal through the intervertebral foramina. These feeders originate from the ascending cervical artery (a branch of the inferior thyroid artery) in the neck, the intercostal arteries in the thorax, and the lumbar artery, iliolumbar artery,

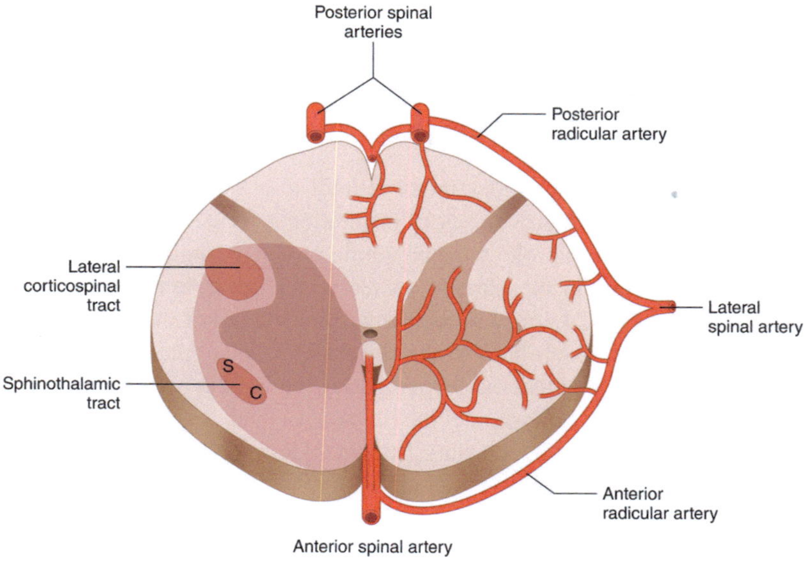

Fig. 1.4 Anatomical distribution of anterior and posterior vertebral arteries to the spinal cord

and lateral sacral arteries in the abdomen and pelvis. Of note, the artery of Adamkiewicz, usually originating from an intercostal artery at the level of the 8th to 12th vertebral body (roughly in 75% of the cases), is the largest anterior segmental medullary artery and the major supply to the lower two-thirds of the spinal cord [14].

The posterior spinal arteries irrigate the posterior third of the cord; they arise from the vertebral arteries in 25% of the cases and from the posterior inferior cerebellar arteries in the remaining 75%. Unlike the anterior spinal artery, the posterior spinal arteries are rather discontinuous in the tract between the subaxial cervical and thoracic spine, showing instead a tendency to create anastomoses and a characteristic basket which angiographically defines the caudal portion of the SC and its transition to the cauda equine. Beside the fasciculus gracilis and cuneatus, the lateral columns of the SC depend on the posterior spinal arteries for their arterial supply.

The venous drainage from the SC largely follows its arterial supply: it is in fact characterized longitudinally by two median veins, one located in the anterior fissure and the other behind the posterior sulcus of the SC with four lateral veins running behind the ventral and dorsal roots. The spinal veins form a minute, tortuous venous plexus situated in the pia mater and freely communicate with the internal vertebral plexus in the epidural space. The internal and external vertebral plexuses eventually drain into the intervertebral veins, which once out of the intervertebral foramina drain toward the vertebral vein in the neck, the intercostal veins in the thorax, and the lumbar and lateral sacral veins in the lumbosacral region. Of note, contrary to the intervertebral veins, the spinal veins are valveless.

Spinal Cord and the Respiratory Drive

Although respiratory drive centers lie in the brainstem, further integration is provided by anterior horn cells of the upper cervical SC. The main respiratory muscles are under both voluntary and involuntary control. Voluntary control arises from the motor and premotor cortex and descends through the corticospinal tract, while involuntary control is mediated by both rhythmic and nonrhythmic systems including the pneumotaxic and apneustic centers in the pons, as well as the ventral and dorsal respiratory groups in the medulla. The pneumotaxic and apneustic centers regulate the speed of inhalation and exhalation by inhibitory and stimulatory impulses, located in the rostral lateral pons and lower pons/medulla oblongata, respectively. The ventral and dorsal respiratory groups regulate the rhythm of inhalation and exhalation. The groups are located in the reticular formation of the medulla and include the following nuclei: the nucleus ambiguous and nucleus of the tractus solitarius [16].

The phrenic nerve provides motor stimuli to the diaphragm, the primary muscle of inspiration, and thus plays a central role in the breathing process. Contributions to the phrenic nerves originate from the C3, C4, and C5 segments. Many accessory muscles contribute to the inspiratory (I) and expiratory (E) processes by regulating the elevation of the ribs, expansion of the rib cage, or compression of the abdominal wall. They include the following:

(a) The intercostal muscles (innervations T2 to T11), which are arranged as three layers: external layer (I), internal layer, and an incomplete innermost layer (E).
(b) The posterior thoracic muscles which include the serratus posterior (E, innervations T1–T5) but also the levatores costarum brevis and longus (I, innervations T2–T12).
(c) The pectoralis muscles, major and minor (I, innervations C4–T1).
(d) The trapezius, scalene, and sternocleidomastoid muscles (I, innervations C2–C6).
(e) The serratus anterior (I, innervations C5–C7) and levator scapulae (I, innervations C1–C4).
(f) The abdominal muscles, including the rectus abdominis, transverse abdominis, and external and internal oblique muscles (E, innervation T7–L1).

Because of the association of cervical spinal cord injury with respiratory dysfunction, the neurologic examination of cervical spinal cord injury includes a respiratory functional assessment. Given the above, a complete transection of the SC at the C1 to C3 levels is almost always fatal unless immediate respiratory support is provided. In the case of complete C4 injuries, the C3 segment may be preserved providing innervation to the diaphragm and allowing it to provide adequate function to support respiration. In this scenario, the respiratory rate is increased, and the patient uses accessory breathing muscles such as the sternocleidomastoid and trapezius to compensate. Due to the limited functioning of the diaphragm, the patient is unable to cough effectively and requires frequent suctioning. In the management of C1 to C4 injuries, artificial ventilation and tracheostomy are often necessary. Impaired diaphragmatic function is also seen in the initial stages of complete C5 injuries; however, in this case, diaphragmatic function may be fully restored once the spinal shock wears off. C5 also partially innervates levator scapulae and other accessory muscles of respiration mentioned above, thus providing a better vital capacity of the lung when compared with C1 to C4 lesions. On the other hand, patients with a complete C6 injury have intact diaphragmatic function and sufficiently strong respiration, and although intensive monitoring is required, tracheostomy and ventilation support are likely not necessary [23].

Aside from respiratory dysfunction as a result of cervical spine impairment on respiratory musculature, direct injury to the brainstem structures can cause a cervicomedullary syndrome, also referred as cruciate paralysis. The injuries in this syndrome may extend from the pons to C4 or even lower in the cord. The more rostral the lesion, the more severe the clinical manifestations that include respiratory arrest, hypotension, and tetraparesis.

Understanding the Functional Anatomy of the Spinal Cord: Spinal Syndromes and Pain

A deep knowledge of the pathways and vascular supplies described in this chapter is fundamental to clinical practice when it comes to diagnosing myelopathies, spinal cord syndromes, and radiculopathies.

The Brown-Sequard syndrome refers to hemisection of the SC, which may result from intradural or extradural tumors, disk herniation, or epidural hematomas. One of the manifestations of this syndrome is loss of contralateral pain and temperature sensation. This deficit is the result of destruction of decussating spinothalamic tracts.

The motor impairment associated with this condition is due to the destruction of the corticospinal tract. At the level of the spinal cord lesion, the motor impairments manifest with lower motor neuron signals, while distal to the lesion, impairments manifest as upper motor neuron lesions. In this syndrome, deficits with ipsilateral vibration and proprioceptive sensation present due to damage to the dorsal column.

Central cord syndrome, usually resulting from hyperextension cervical traumas, is characterized by damage to the decussating spinothalamic fibers at the center of the SC. This syndrome will cause bilateral pain and loss of temperature sensation from upper extremities, leaving the lower extremities unaffected. Also, the sensation of vibration, tactile and proprioception modalities is spared in this syndrome, creating a dissociated sensory loss. The motor deficits observed in this syndrome are typically prominent in the upper extremities and manifest with lower motor signs [1]. Bladder dysfunction is another common presentation of central cord syndrome [3]. Neurogenic atrophy and paresis can occur in this syndrome if there is involvement of ventral SC. Spastic paralysis can result if there is damage to the corticospinal tract due to involvement of the lateral spinal cord. Involvement of the lateral SC can also affect other structures such as the dorsomedian and ventromedian motor nuclei and the ciliospinal center of Budge at C8–T2 and result in kyphoscoliosis and ipsilateral Horner's syndrome. If the involvement extends to the dorsal columns, loss of vibration and proprioception may take place [11].

Anterior cord syndrome can result from damage to the anterior spinal artery, traumas, and epidural hematomas. Spinal traumas such as dorsally displaced osseous fragments or cervical disk herniations can result in this syndrome, as well as any ischemic event resulting from the blockage of the anterior spinal artery or its various branches. This syndrome is characterized by a bilateral loss of pain and temperature sensation due to destruction of the bilateral spinothalamic tracts. Pressure and light touch sensation are also affected to varying degrees in this syndrome. Flaccid paralysis distal to the lesion results from damage to the anterior horn cells and corticospinal tracts. This flaccid paralysis often progresses to spasticity. Dorsal column function is typically spared with anterior cord syndrome, resulting in dissociation of sensory loss, as vibration and proprioceptive sensations distal to the lesion remain preserved with the loss of pain and temperature sensation. In the initial stages of this syndrome, urinary retention and constipation may be observed. Typically, patients with anterior cord syndrome are areflexic.

Posterior cord syndrome is characterized by a loss of vibration, proprioception, and light touch sensation distal to the lesion. Any mechanism damaging the dorsal columns and affecting their function, such as traumas, infections, or vascular injuries, can result in posterior cord syndrome. The main clinical features are paresthesias and bladder and bowel dysfunction. The paresthesias in posterior cord syndrome can include Lhermitte's sign and lancinating pains on neck flexion. Sensory ataxia may also be present in this syndrome. Motor function, pain, and temperature sensation are often spared in posterior cord syndrome, as there is no involvement of spinothalamic or corticospinal tracts [17].

Pain syndromes can result from any pathology affecting the SC segments that innervate peripheral dermatomes or specific nerve roots resulting in peripheral radiculopathies. They are usually characterized by positive neurological findings such as weakness, areflexia, paresthesia, and numbness in the segmental distribution of the affected spinal nerve; musculature also plays a role in existing loading and painful conditions [12]. Unmyelinated Aδ- and C-type fibers and half of the neural units in the skeletal muscle have been shown to have nociceptive function. The dura mater also contains nociceptive nerve fibers that express calcitonin gene-regulated peptide (CGRP) and substance P; however, the role of the spinal dura mater in the pathogenesis of pain syndromes may be limited to modulation of pain through releasing proinflammatory cytokines [22]. Furthermore, pain syndromes can also result from direct injury to vascular structures (i.e., the vertebral arteries in cervical traumas resulting in a compromise of blood supply to the brain and pressure gradients around the spinal cord which can potentially lead to nociceptive responses). Finally, myofascial pain syndromes refer to chronic musculoskeletal neck pain that is associated with painful muscular "trigger points" within bands of muscle that replicate symptoms in predictable referral patterns. This condition usually presents without neurologic deficits but is associated with a remarkably decreased range of motion [4].

References

1. Anderson KK, Tetreault L, Shamji MF, Singh A, Vukas RR, Harrop JS, Fehlings MG, Vaccaro AR, Hilibrand AS, Arnold PM. Optimal timing of surgical decompression for acute traumatic central cord syndrome: a systematic review of the literature. Neurosurgery. 2015;77(Suppl 4):S15–32.
2. Bosmia AN, Hogan E, Loukas M, Tubbs RS, Cohen-Gadol AA. Blood supply to the human spinal cord: part I. Anatomy and hemodynamics. Clin Anat. 2015;28(1):52–64. https://doi.org/10.1002/ca.22281. Epub 2013 Jun 27.
3. Brooks NP. Central cord syndrome. Neurosurg Clin N Am. 2017;28(1):41–7.
4. Chiarotto A, Clijsen R, Fernandez-de-Las-Penas C, Barbero M. Prevalence of myofascial trigger points in spinal disorders: a systematic review and meta-analysis. Arch Phys Med Rehabil. 2016;97(2):316–37.
5. Choi BH, Kim RC, Suzuki M, Choe W. The ventriculus terminalis and filum terminale of the human spinal cord. Hum Pathol. 1992;23(8):916–20.
6. Christensen BN, Perl ER. Spinal neurons specifically excited by noxious or thermal stimuli: marginal zone of the dorsal horn. J Neurophysiol. 1970;33(2):293–307.
7. Coggeshall RE, Carlton SM. Receptor localization in the mammalian dorsal horn and primary afferent neurons. Brain Res Brain Res Rev. 1997;24(1):28–66.
8. Colman MW, Hornicek FJ, Schwab JH. Spinal cord blood supply and its surgical implications. J Am Acad Orthop Surg. 2015;23(10):581–91.
9. Ganau M, Talacchi A, Cecchi PC, Ghimenton C, Gerosa M, Faccioli F. Cystic dilation of the ventriculus terminalis. J Neurosurg Spine. 2012;17(1):86–92.
10. Ijkema-Paassen J, Gramsbergen A. Development of postural muscles and their innervation. Neural Plast. 2005;12(2–3):141–51. discussion 263-72.
11. Kanagalingam S, Miller NR. Horner syndrome: clinical perspectives. Eye Brain. 2015;7:35–46.
12. Kerstman E, Ahn S, Battu S, Tariq S, Grabois M. Neuropathic pain. Handb Clin Neurol. 2013;110:175–87. https://doi.org/10.1016/B978-0-444-52901-5.00015-0.
13. Lawson SN. Phenotype and function of somatic primary afferent nociceptive neurones with C-Adelta- or Aalpha/beta-fibres. Exp Physiol. 2002;87(2):239–44.
14. Lazorthes G, Gouaze A, Zadeh JO, Santini JJ, Lazorthes Y, Burdin P. Arterial vascularization of the spinal cord. Recent studies of the anastomotic substitution pathways. J Neurosurg. 1971;35(3):253–62.
15. Mavilio F, Simeone A, Giampaolo A, Faiella A, Zappavigna V, Acampora D, Poiana G, Russo G, Peschle C, Boncinelli E. Differential and stage-related expression in embryonic tissues of a new human homoeobox gene. Nature. 1986;324(6098):664–8.
16. Mitchell RA, Berger AJ. Neural regulation of respiration. Am Rev Respir Dis. 1975;111(2):206–24.
17. Novy J. Spinal cord syndromes. Front Neurol Neurosci. 2012;30:195–8.
18. Panjabi MM, White AA 3rd. Basic biomechanics of the spine. Neurosurgery. 1980;7(1):76–93.
19. Rexed B. Some aspects of the cytoarchitectonics and synaptology of the spinal cord. Prog Brain Res. 1964;11:58–92.
20. Rossignol S, Dubuc R, Gossard JP. Dynamic sensorimotor interactions in locomotion. Physiol Rev. 2006;86(1):89–154.
21. Saper CB. The central autonomic nervous system: conscious visceral perception and autonomic pattern generation. Annu Rev Neurosci. 2002;25:433–69. Epub 2002 Mar 25.
22. Tomlinson DR, Fernyhough P, Diemel LT. Neurotrophins and peripheral neuropathy. Philos Trans R Soc Lond Ser B Biol Sci. 1996;351(1338):455–62.
23. Zimmer MB, Nantwi K, Goshgarian HG. Effect of spinal cord injury on the respiratory system: basic research and current clinical treatment options. J Spinal Cord Med. 2007;30(4):319–30.

Cervical Spine Biomechanics

2

Bryan S. Lee and Edward C. Benzel

Key Points

- There are multiple structures in the upper and subaxial cervical spine, including the discoligamentous complex, which contribute to spinal stability. The unique contributions of these structures have been evaluated via cadaveric studies.
- Changes in cervical biomechanics can be determined, either by clinical means or via the assessment of imaging.
- Cervical spondylotic myelopathy is the direct result of repetitive trauma to the spinal cord, thus resulting in abnormal motor and sensory findings. Such trauma can take the form of stretching/distraction, compression, and angular distortion.
- Significant increases in motions in all three planes are observed in the setting of multilevel laminectomies. The performance of medial facetectomies exaggerates such motion.
- One of the primary objectives of surgical stabilization should be to halt the progression of spine deformation, particularly kyphotic deformation, and to restore the normal lordotic curvature via spinal fixation and fusion when appropriate.
- In the upper cervical region, solid arthrodesis is difficult to achieve due to the complex anatomy and motions in multiple planes that must be restricted by the implant.
- Rigid fixation via Magerl or Goel-Harms techniques of C1–C2 enhances biomechanical stability and facilitates successful fusion in the upper cervical spine.
- In clinical settings in which poor bone quality is present, either very rigid fixation or axially dynamic fixation may be required. In the case of the former, pedicle screw-rod construct in the subaxial cervical spine may be more advantageous than the lateral mass screw-rod construct despite the higher risks. In the case of the latter, ventral axially dynamic fixation constructs can minimize the stress shielding seen with more rigid systems that inhibit load sharing across

B. S. Lee · E. C. Benzel (✉)
Department of Neurosurgery, Center for Spine Health, Neurological Institute, Cleveland Clinic Foundation, Cleveland, OH, USA
e-mail: benzele@ccf.org

M. G. Kaiser et al. (eds.), *Degenerative Cervical Myelopathy and Radiculopathy*,
https://doi.org/10.1007/978-3-319-97952-6_2

the bone graft/end plate interface, which to some degree can promote successful fusion.

- The proper placement and fixation of the anterior cervical plate also help to achieve the optimal stabilization and restoration of the lordotic curve, thus maximizing fusion rate and decreasing the risk of adjacent segment disease.
- A long construct extended to C7 significantly increases the stress placed at the cervicothoracic junction. This junction is vulnerable to injury and instability, and thus an extended construct ending at C7 increases the risk of junctional instability.
- In long anterior cervical constructs, stability can be improved by the addition of intermediate fixation points – thus, providing the addition of a three-point bending fixation mechanism. The application of supplemental posterior fixation can add extra stability and should be considered when attempting a lengthy anterior cervical construct.

Introduction of Spine Biomechanical Concepts and Fundamental Anatomy

The biomechanics of spine and the determination of spinal stability involve topics that are controversial and difficult to define. In 1990, White and Panjabi defined spinal clinical instability as "the loss of the ability of the spine, under physiologic loads to maintain relationships between vertebrae in such a way that there is neither initial nor subsequent damage to the spinal cord or nerve roots, and in addition, there is neither development of incapacitating deformity nor severe pain" [34]. Such spinal instability can be induced by many etiologies, including degenerative changes, trauma, infection, or tumor.

The spinal column consists of various complex anatomical structures, and it is essential to fully understand the biomechanically relevant anatomy and its mechanical properties. The vertebral bodies and intervertebral discs comprise the anterior vertebral column and provide for the majority of the axial load bearing of the spine. The pedicle connects the vertebral body to the posterior components of the spine; the lamina extends from the pedicle to complete the vertebral arch dorsally and fuses to form the spinous process at its junction; the facet joints allow limited rotation, flexion/extension, lateral bending, and translation. The facet joints assume the axial load-bearing capacity primarily when the spine is in a lordotic posture [2]. Forces acting on the spinal segments act on a lever arm, which results in a bending moment. When this bending moment is applied, rotation occurs. The instantaneous axis of rotation (IAR) is the axis around which a vertebral segment rotates. The facet joint surfaces in the subaxial spine face the IAR. The IAR, which can be viewed as a fulcrum, is dynamic and therefore moves along with the movement of the involved spinal segment [18]. Due to the coronal plane orientation, the facet joints in the cervical spine substantially allow flexion/extension, lateral bending, and rotation, in contrast to the lumbar spine where the facet joints are oriented in a sagittal plane, which diminishes the ability to rotate but substantially allows flexion/extension.

Spinal instability can be fundamentally categorized into *acute* and *chronic*. In this chapter we will focus on the chronic nature of spinal instability, secondary to degenerative changes in the spine. With the definition of stability/instability stated and the fundamental concepts of biomechanics in relation to the basic spinal anatomy outlined, the goals of this chapter are set to explain and recapitulate the basics of cervical spine biomechanics, which have been investigated in numerous in vivo and in vitro studies, as well as clinical applications of such principles including the stabilization process provided by various surgical procedures.

Biomechanics and Stability of the Upper Cervical Spine

The upper cervical spine is composed of occiput, C1 (atlas), and C2 (axis). These segments are unique anatomically and, thus, contribute to the stability of the upper and overall cervical spine in distinctive ways. Each of the various ligamentous structures, such as the anterior and posterior atlanto-occipital membrane, the atlantoaxial membrane, the transverse ligament, the apical ligament, and the alar ligaments, contributes to the stability of the occipitocervical junction (OCJ) and the upper cervical spine. Their biomechanical properties have been extensively studied from cadaveric in vitro studies, and the mean load to failure, which was used to determine the failure strength of different spinal ligaments, was evaluated (Table 2.1). Normally, the occiput-C1 joint is associated with 25° of flexion/extension and 5° of lateral bending and axial rotation to one side. The C1–C2 joint is associated with 20° of flexion/extension, 5° of lateral bending, and 40° of axial rotation to one side [2].

The complex anatomical relationships of the OCJ allow the most motion of any cervical spine segment, as the majority of the spine's rotation and flexion-extension occur at this junction [26]. The occipital condyles are turned laterally and form inferior convexities, which allow articulation with the superomedially facing C1 joints. This unique articulation allows a great degree of flexion-extension at the occiput-C1 segment. The atlas lacks a vertebral body and articulates with the dens of the axis. This joint segment, along with the horizontal facets, allows rotational motion. The transverse ligament borders the dens posteriorly and thereby constrains the dens within 3 mm of the anterior ring of the atlas [25]. The transverse ligament forms the cruciate ligament with the superior and inferior crural ligaments crossing the dens and attaching to anterior foramen magnum and the body of the axis. This ligament contributes substantial stability across the OCJ by preventing the dens from folding into and compressing the brainstem during flexion [21]. The alar ligaments, which arise from the anterolateral aspect of the dens and attach to the medial aspect of the occipital condyles, restrict rotation of the cranium and also help to maintain stability of the OCJ [21]. Other ligamentous and membranous structures, such as the tectorial membrane and apical ligament, do not add as much biomechanical stability to the OCJ. Due to the chronic degenerative changes occurring at the joints and ligaments, physiological motion of the OCJ and upper cervical spine decreases. The instability of the OCJ resulting from chronic degenerative changes is rare but can lead to increased mobility, requiring surgical stabilization involving screw fixation and implants in order to achieve the restoration of lordosis and biomechanically appropriate instrumented fusion.

Biomechanics and Stability of the Subaxial Spine

Uniquely, in the subaxial cervical spine, the structures contributing to overall stability, including the disc, the facet joints and the facet capsule, and the ligamentous structures, are collectively called the discoligamentous complex. From the multiple biomechanical studies, the average load to failure strengths of the various ligaments of the subaxial spine have been determined (Table 2.2).

In a cadaveric study, anterior structural instability was induced when an injury resulted in greater than 3.3 mm displacement or greater than 3.8° of rotation, and posterior instability was induced when greater than 27 mm of interspinous distance or greater than 30° of angulation was observed [26]. Such posterior elements as the supraspinous and interspinous ligaments and the ligamentum flavum add stability to the cervical spine; and removal of those structures is known to cause instability. Instability was demonstrated in cadaveric studies when a 10%

Table 2.1 The average loads to failure in various elements of the upper cervical spine ligamentous complex

	Ligaments							
	AAOM	PAOM	ALL	AAM	TAL	AL	Alar	TM
Average load to failure (N)	233	83	281	113	354–692[a]	214	286	76

AOM anterior atlanto-occipital membrane, *POM* posterior atlanto-occipital membrane, *ALL* anterior longitudinal ligament, *AAM* atlantoaxial membrane, *TAL* transverse ligament, *AL* apical ligament, *TM* tectorial membrane
[a]Heller et al. [14]; Panjabi

Table 2.2 The average loads to failure in various elements of the subaxial cervical spine ligamentous complex (Panjabi)

	Ligaments			
	ALL	PLL	LF	CL
Average load to failure (N)	111.5	74.5	138.5	204

ALL anterior longitudinal ligament, *PLL* posterior longitudinal ligament, *LF* ligamentum flavum, *CL* capsular ligament

increase in flexion-extension motion was reported after a multilevel cervical laminectomy [10]; and significant increases in all motions were shown when multilevel laminectomies were performed with medial facetectomies [24]. Cervical facet joints and their capsule contribute significantly to overall cervical spine stability, as demonstrated in multiple cadaveric studies. More than 50% resection of the combined facet complex, either bilateral facet joints or joint capsules, created instability [37]. Anterior elements, including the disc, have also been found to play a significant role in providing stability. This is demonstrated by the instability induced with increased ranges of motions in all three planes (>66% increase in flexion/extension, >40% increase in lateral bending and axial rotation), when anterior cervical discectomy is performed without fusion [31].

Segmental motions in different planes allowed in the cervical spine vary at each level. The range of motion (ROM) of combined flexion and extension is the greatest at the OC junction with up to 25° of motion and then changes incrementally from 10° at the level of C2–C3 to 20° at the levels of C5–C6 and C6–C7. Unilateral axial rotation has the greatest ROM of more than 40° at C1–C2 and is similar across all remaining levels with approximately 5°. Unilateral bending does not vary as much and is steady throughout the cervical spine with ROM of 5–10° at each level [34]. Spondylotic changes tend to occur more frequently at the subaxial levels where greater ROM is allowed, C5–C6 and C6–C7 in particular.

Coupling is defined as the phenomenon in which a movement of the spine along one axis in the Cartesian coordinate system obligates a movement of the spine along another axis [2]. As such, motion between different vertebral segments can be coupled, and this coupled motion refers to the simultaneous motion in different planes. For example, due to the presence of the uncovertebral joints in the subaxial spine and the coronal orientation of the cervical facet joints, lateral bending results in rotation of the spinous processes away from the concave side. The average ratio of the coupled lateral bending to the axial rotation in the cervical spine is 0.51 [23]. In contrast, coupled motion associated with lateral bending occurs in the opposite direction in the lumbar spine, with the spinous processes rotating toward the concave side of the curvature, and this coupling phenomenon explains the rotatory subluxation associated with the degenerative scoliosis [2].

Biomechanics of Cervical Spondylotic Myelopathy

Cervical spondylosis is a common manifestation of progressive degeneration of the cervical spine. It is one of the most common causes of acquired spinal cord dysfunction [36], and such a degenerative process can result in spinal deformity, as well as myelopathy and/or radiculopathy. *Spondylosis*, often preceded by mild segmental instability, is defined as "vertebral osteophytosis secondary to degenerative disc disease," and it is associated with the arthritic inflammatory process involving the facet joints and osteophyte formation [33]. Due to degenerative changes, the disc desiccates resulting in disc height loss and potential disc herniation due to continuous application of various motions, which then alters the load transmission across and along the cervical spine (Figs. 2.1 and 2.2). Cervical spondylotic myelopathy (CSM) is the direct result of repetitive trauma to the spinal cord, thus resulting in abnormal motor and sensory findings, and ultimately cervical spondylosis can lead to chronic kyphotic deformation. Such trauma can take the form of stretch/distraction, compression, and angular distortion [15].

Degeneration of the spine involves the intervertebral disc, disc interspace, facet joints, and paraspinal and intraspinal tissues. The degenerative changes in the intervertebral disc typically involve the loss of disc and disc interspace height, end plate changes, sclerosis of the disc interspace, and osteophyte formation [2]. The disc degeneration process is initiated by disc desiccation due to the loss of water, protein, and mucopolysaccharide and an increased content of keratin/chondroitin sulfate. As a result, the nucleus pulposus becomes fibrotic. Its subsequent obligatory loss of elasticity leads to a decreased size of the nucleus pulposus [7]. Due to the dorsal weakness of the annulus fibrosus relative to the ventral and lateral aspects, the disc is prone to the bulge in the dorsal direction. When disc bulging occurs, the periosteum over the end plates becomes elevated, leading to subperiosteal osteophyte formation causing central and neuroforaminal stenosis.

The disc space in the cervical spine is thicker ventrally than dorsally, and this formation contributes to the normal cervical lordosis. The process of disc bulging/herniation in the dorsal direction combined with the loss of internal integrity causes greater loss of anterior as opposed to posterior disc space height, inducing the development of kyphosis. Moreover, the loading forces placed on the ventral aspect of the vertebral bodies increase due to the straightening or loss of lordosis of the cervical spine. Because eccentric loading causes stress concentration, increased length of the moment arm increases the stress on the ventral aspects of the vertebral bodies with a higher tendency toward compression; the vertebral bodies tend to lose more height in the ventral aspect than the dorsal

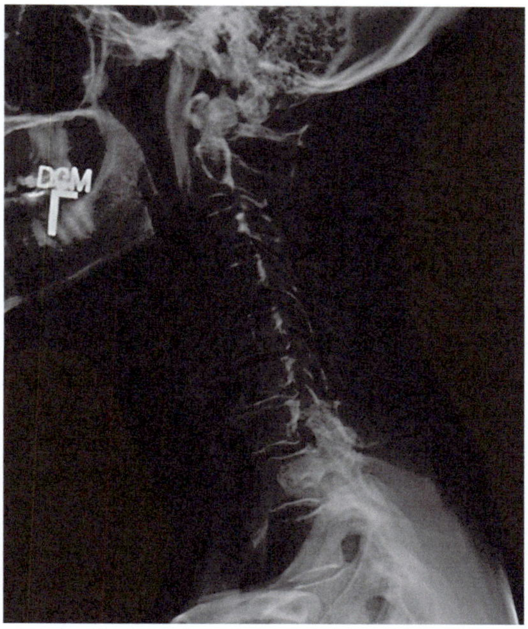

Fig. 2.2 Lateral X-ray of the cervical spine demonstrating severe spondylosis at the levels of C5/C6 and C6/C7 with the loss of height of the disc space and osteophyte formation

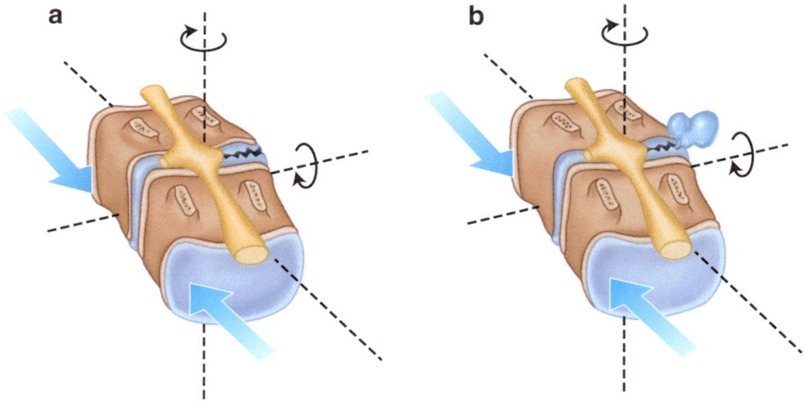

Fig. 2.1 Demonstration of the application of various motions, including axial loading, lateral bending, and flexion, causing herniation of the degenerated disc. (**a**) Annular tear with the application of multiple motions; (**b**) migration of nucleus pulposus leading to disc herniation as a result. (Permission from Thieme has been granted. Adapted from Benzel's Biomechanics of Spine Stabilization, 2015 (third edition); Fig. 5.9, page 51)

aspect, accentuating the kyphotic deformity [2]. When axial loads are applied, kyphotic deformity elongates the moment arm at the point of rotation, which induces further progression of the deformity (Fig. 2.3). This constellation of degenerative changes creates a negative feedback loop further propagating the kyphotic deformity, "kyphosis begets kyphosis."

CSM is typically associated with cervical sagittal imbalance, and therefore, surgical intervention to correct such a deformity is warranted. The role of sagittal balance and imbalance in the cervical spine has focused on the prediction of clinical outcomes of CSM, as cervical sagittal imbalance has been correlated with the severity of CSM [6]. The main objectives of surgical interventions should therefore be to decompress the neural elements, halt the progression of kyphotic deformity, and restore the lordotic curvature. A loss of cervical lordosis is known to indicate neck pathology and is directly associated with high risk of soft tissue injuries to the neck and therefore poor clinical outcomes. When stabilization is achieved in the anterior column, a much-improved resistance to axial loading is achieved, along with the transmission of the majority of axially applied loads to the anterior column. This minimizes the risk for progression of deformity and enhances the chance of restoring the natural lordotic posture [2]. Adequate decompression combined with solid arthrodesis must be achieved when kyphotic deformity is corrected, as the restoration of lordosis without solid fusion can shift the load-bearing capacity to the posterior half of the vertebral body and facet joints. Patients with CSM show significant clinical improvements when decompression is performed. However, there are no established guidelines to dictate the surgical approach (ventral versus dorsal), and, therefore, the optimal approach for surgical decompression and instrumented fusion has not been clearly defined [9]. A prospective observational multicenter study, however, demonstrated that patients treated with the ventral approach were younger, had less neurological impairment,

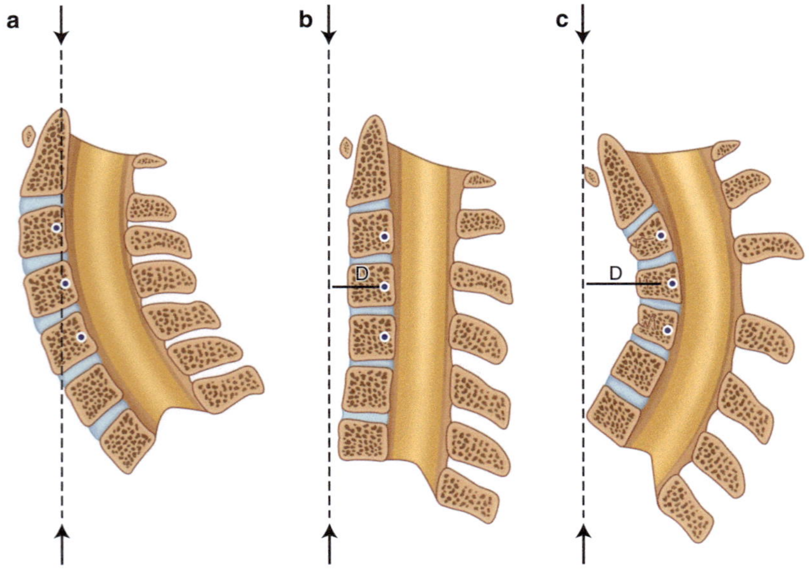

Fig. 2.3 (**a**) Physiological situation with the axial loading applied in arrows; (**b**) loss of lordosis due to the disc desiccation and height loss in multiple levels, leading to the mild elongation of moment arm applied to the spine (D); (**c**) kyphotic deformity with further elongation of the moment arm exaggerating the pathological deformity. (Permission from Thieme has been granted. Adapted from Benzel's Biomechanics of Spine Stabilization, 2015 (third edition); Fig. 5.14, page 56)

and had more of a focal pathology, in comparison to the dorsal approach cohort [6].

Biomechanics and Stability of Cervical Spine Instrumentation

Operative treatment options should involve the elimination of repetitive trauma and deformity correction via decompression and spinal fixation and fusion in a normal or relatively normal lordotic posture [19]. More complicated deformities require a combined anterior and posterior approach in order to optimize the biomechanical stabilization by providing both anterior and posterior column support [9].

Certain patient-specific characteristics should be considered that may compromise or impact biomechanical considerations. Osteoporosis is the most known and studied degenerative human bone disease, and osteoporotic patients might present as a challenging surgical cohort, as the bone quality and bone healing process are compromised in osteoporosis and fixation techniques via implants heavily depend on these two characteristics [13]. A retrospective analysis by Guzman et al. demonstrated that osteoporotic patients were more likely to undergo posterior cervical fusion, circumferential fusion, and revision surgeries and therefore had all the associated complications and more complex and longer postoperative hospital course and recovery process, compared to non-osteoporotic patients [13]. When performing fusion on osteoporotic patients with such higher risk of implant failures and complications, it is essential for the surgeon to plan the procedure accordingly to achieve a solid fixation and to utilize appropriate intraoperative implants and grafts, along with perioperative medical therapy that can optimize the fusion rate and quality.

Instrumentation in the Upper Cervical Region

When achieving occipitocervical fixation, it may prove difficult to couple C1 screw fixation to the rod. The addition of C1 screw fixation, however, is known to reduce the range of motion in all directions and is associated with lower occipital screw and superior rod stresses in all loading conditions. Therefore, the addition of supplemental C1 screw fixation when attempting to achieve O-C2 arthrodesis optimizes stability by more evenly distributing the stress and reducing the risk of occipital screw pullout and rod fractures [20]. The utilization of bicortical purchase of screws can be an option to achieve the optimal fixation and clinical outcomes in osteoporotic patients.

Occipitocervical fixation is complicated if the intent is to incorporate the subaxial spine, requiring long posterior fixation lever arms. With excessively rigid fixation achieved through the OCJ, the lower end of the construct at the subaxial levels can potentially become the weakest link, inducing instrumentation failure and pseudarthrosis [2]. Wire or cable-rod fixation, which allows some dynamic motion through the OCJ, can be considered to avoid such instrumentation failure (Fig. 2.4). The occiput provides few options for instrumentation and implant fixation. Due to a short depth of the occipital bone, screws have a limited depth of purchase, except in the middle keel. Therefore, the midline screw fixation technique is a commonly practiced option. However, the midline fixation does not resist rotation optimally as the screw is situated in a single row (Fig. 2.5). Another option is the lateral placement of occipital screws. However, as these screws do not provide as much fixation as the midline screws, cross fixation with a connector can be placed to compensate for the weakness of lateral fixation [2] (Fig. 2.6).

In the upper cervical region, a solid arthrodesis is difficult to achieve due to the presence of multiple motions that must be restricted by the implant and instrumentation and the complex characteristics of the discoligamentous complex of the subaxial spine [2]. Initially, this was a challenge, as the accomplishment of dorsal fixation at C1–C2 with wiring techniques could not restrict rotation and translation well, interfering with the fusion process. The more modern techniques of rigid fixation, including the Magerl technique of transarticular screws and the Goel-Harms technique of

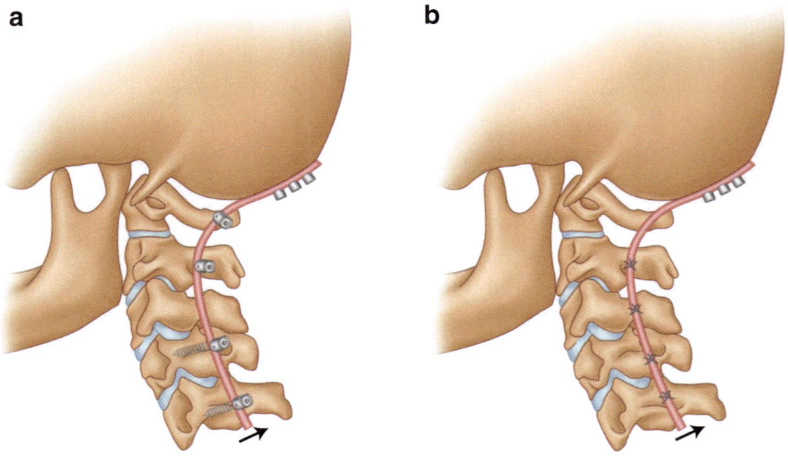

Fig. 2.4 (**a**) If excessively rigid fixation is achieved at the occiput, the occipitocervical fixation may fail at the lower end of the construct due to the relatively weaker subaxial fixation. (**b**) Wire or cable-rod fixation can be considered to permit dynamic motion to minimize the risk of such instrumentation failure. (Permission from Thieme has been granted. Adapted from Benzel's Biomechanics of Spine Stabilization, 2015 (third Fig. 17.27AB, page 233)

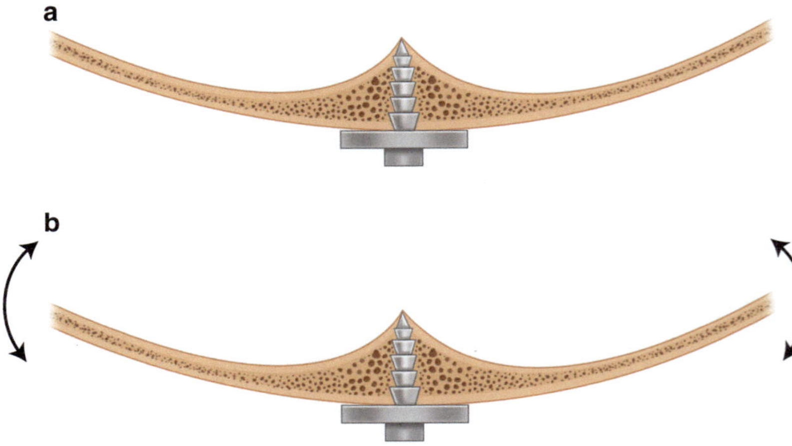

Fig. 2.5 (**a**) Midline occipital bone screw through the keel has the optimal screw penetration through the relatively dense bone. (**b**) It, however, does not resist rotation optimally as the screw is situated in a single row. (Permission from Thieme has been granted. Adapted from Benzel's Biomechanics of Spine Stabilization, 2015 (third edition) Fig. 28.3AB, page 396)

C1 lateral mass/C2 pars screw constructs, achieved greater stability with improved fusion rates than had been previously achieved (Fig. 2.7) [12, 22]. The Magerl technique of transarticular C1-C2 screws achieved a tenfold increase in rotational stiffness, in comparison to the dorsal wiring techniques, and the Goel-Harms technique of C1-C2 screw fixation yielded a much improved biomechanical stability, especially in achieving resistance to lateral bending and axial rotation [12, 22]. The newly popularized placement of translaminar screws achieves equivalent biomechanical stabilization, compared to the traditional C2 screw fixation, and without the risk of vertebral artery injury [11]. Moreover, translaminar screw placement can be an effective bailout or an alternative option for patients with suboptimal fixation or failed placement of C2 pars/pedicle screws.

Instrumentation in the Subaxial Cervical Spine

In the subaxial cervical spine, instrumentation with the placement of lateral mass screws has

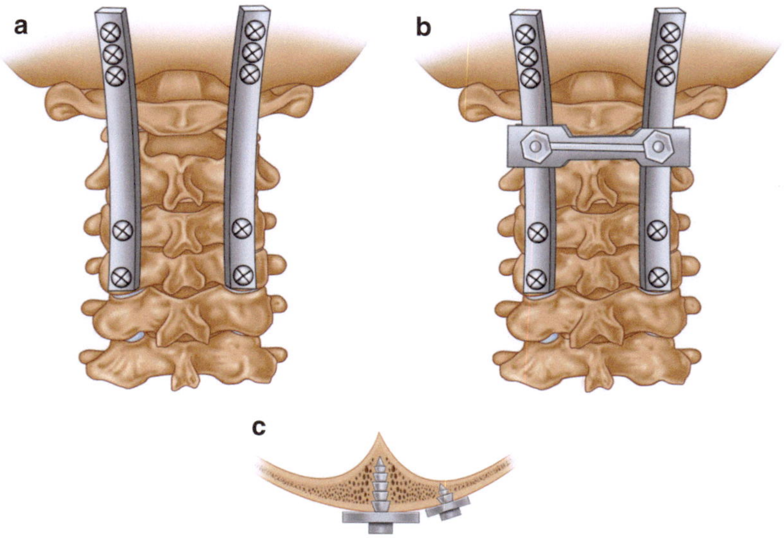

Fig. 2.6 (**a**) Occipitocervical fixation with laterally placed occipital screws, which minimize rotation. (**b**) Cross fixation can be incorporated to provide more rigid fixation to compensate for the shallow depth of lateral screw penetration. (**c**) Depth of screw penetration is optimal in the midline keel. (Permission from Thieme has been granted. Adapted from Benzel's Biomechanics of Spine Stabilization, 2015 (third edition) Fig. 28.4ABC, page 397)

become the widely accepted and popularized technique, as the placement of pedicle screws is associated with a greater risk of neurovascular injury. In vitro studies have demonstrated that pedicle screws have stronger biomechanical properties, with the mean pullout strength of the pedicle screws to be nearly four times greater than that of the lateral mass screws [16], and significantly higher stability in lateral bending [17]. Moreover, pedicle screws can achieve a greater reduction in axial load transfer through the intervertebral disc, as compared to the lateral mass screw-rod construct. Therefore, in clinical settings when bone fixation is compromised due to poor bone quality, in the presence of the need for multisegmental dorsal fixation, pedicle screw-rod constructs in the subaxial cervical spine may provide an advantage despite the associated higher risks [5].

The determination of the length of the upper cervical spine constructs remains controversial in regard to the placement of the caudal extent of the construct. As a general rule, solid fixation to the occiput to C2 is sufficient regarding rostral fixation. Such constructs can be extended caudally, when necessary, to C5 or C6 [2]. However, when the construct is extended to C7 due to the need for longer multisegmental fixation and stabilization, significantly increased stress is placed at the cervicothoracic junction (CTJ), thus increasing the risk of pseudarthrosis, hardware failure, and junctional instability (Fig. 2.8) [2].

The CTJ, which involves the C7 and T1 vertebrae, the C7/T1 intervertebral disc, and all the associated muscular and ligamentous structures, is prone to injury and instability, as it bears the high-stress mechanical loading forces between the mobile cervical spine and the relatively fixed thoracic spine supported by the rigid rib cage, particularly in the trauma population [32]. In degenerative spine pathologies, these factors also play a role, though. Moreover, the transition from the cervical lordosis to the thoracic kyphosis at this region is another stress riser, accentuating the high biomechanical stresses at the junction. It is therefore essential to understand the associated principal characteristics of the CTJ that pose special considerations to surgical instrumentation, in order to avoid achieving an unstable construct that leads to

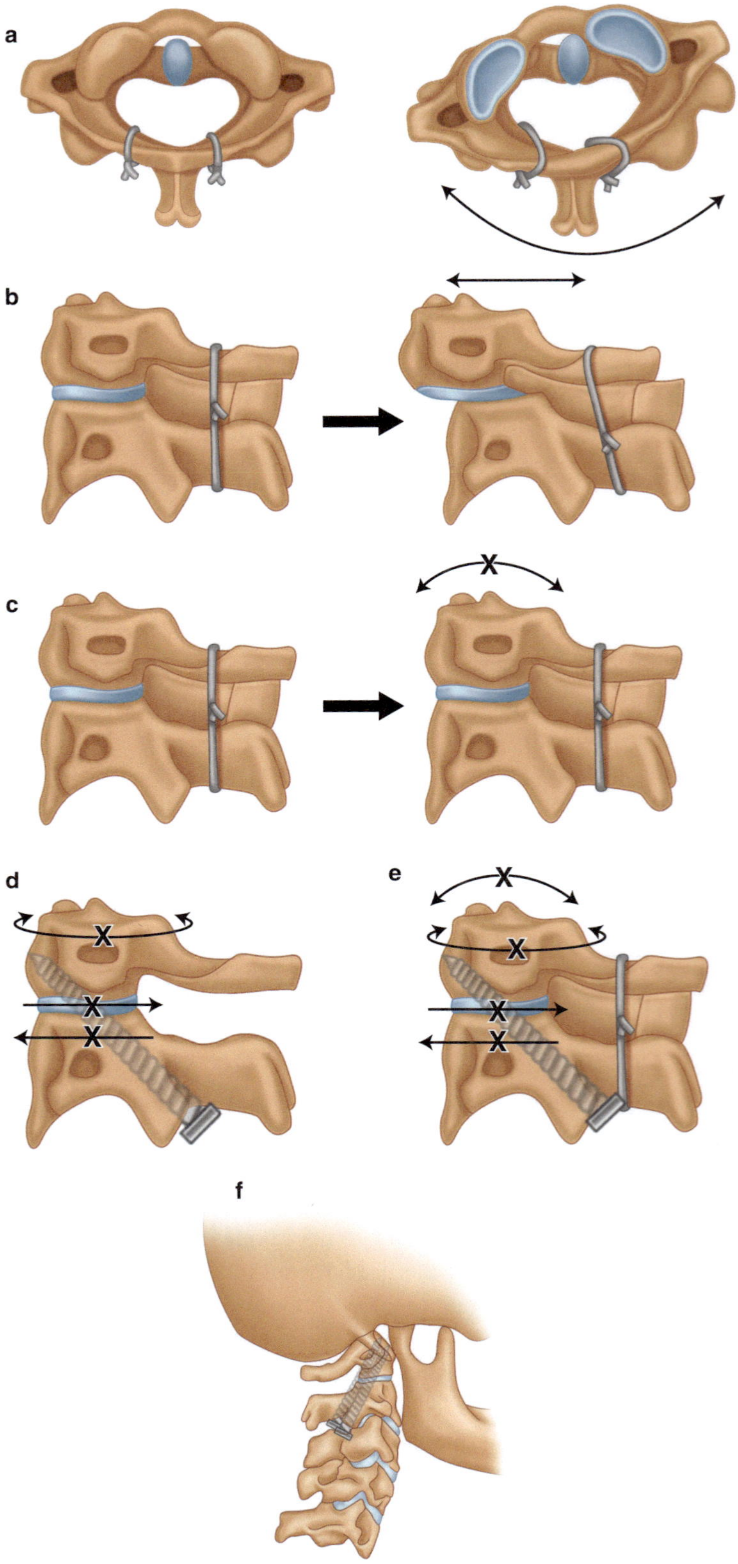

Fig. 2.7 Comparison of the wiring technique with the screw fixation technique in the upper cervical region and demonstration of the improved resistance of various motions achieved by the screw fixation technique. (**a**, **b**) Dorsal wiring fixation restricting the flexion/extension motion only, while the axial rotation and translation motions are still allowed; (**c**) the addition of a dorsal bone graft in the construct to further enhance the resistance of extension; (**d**, **e**) C1–C2 screw fixation, resisting motions in all three planes. (**f**) Postoperative plain film depicting such a construct. (Permission from Thieme has been granted. Adapted from Benzel's Biomechanics of Spine Stabilization, 2015 (third edition); Fig. 20.2, page 231)

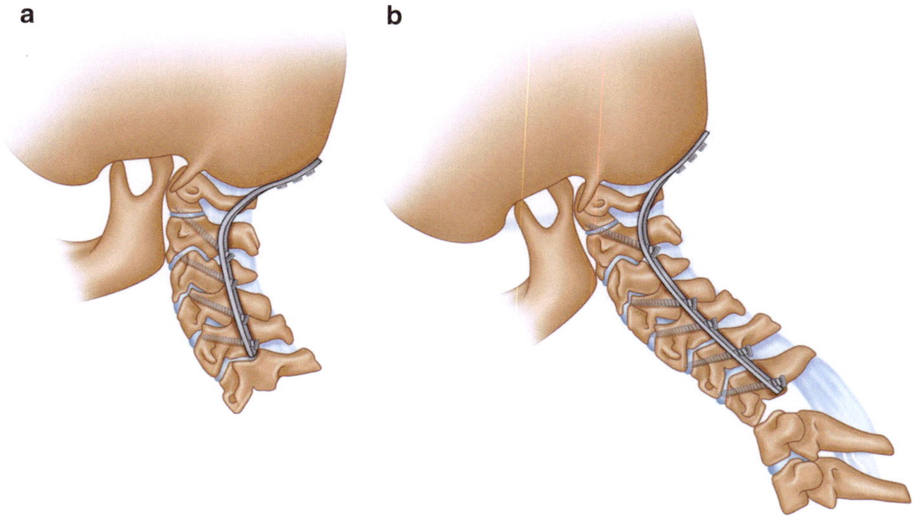

Fig. 2.8 Complication from a short occipitocervical construct. (**a**) Construct with caudal extent to C5; (**b**) construct with extension to C7 placing a significantly increased stress on the cervicothoracic junction. (Permission from Thieme has been granted. Adapted from Benzel's Biomechanics of Spine Stabilization, 2015 (third edition); Fig. 20.33, page 247 – A and B only)

instrumentation failure and adjacent segment disease (ASD). The risk of clinical ASD is not low, when performing a fusion to eliminate motion, which increases the intradiscal pressure and expedites the degenerative process at the adjacent levels, particularly when the normal lordotic posture is not maintained or restored. The risk becomes higher at the CTJ, as the fixation construct to C7 and the rigid thoracic spine with the intact rib cage create an iatrogenic lever arm at this transition zone. A potential solution is extending the instrumentation and fusion across the CTJ down to the upper thoracic levels. A biomechanical, cadaveric study by Cheng et al. performed an exploratory analysis comparing changes in the intradiscal pressures at various levels when long cervical or cervicothoracic fusions are achieved and concluded that it might be advantageous to extend the construct down to T2, as a significant decrease in pressures from all directions of bending was shown at this level [4].

Anterior procedures, including anterior cervical discectomy and fusion (ACDF), are commonly performed for single- or multilevel disc pathologies and kyphotic deformities. Decompression, stabilization, and restoration of lordosis and sagittal balance in the cervical spine are the goals of surgical intervention. The restoration of a lordotic posture can be maximized with the placement of lordotic-shaped interbody cages, with Caspar pin placement in a divergent fashion to facilitate the distraction in a convergent manner, and with maintenance of PLL during distraction. The placement of screws via a plate results in the creation of a cantilever beam construct. Such a cantilever beam construct can either be a fixed or non-fixed moment arm construct. Fixed moment arm cantilever beam constructs include screws that are rigidly fixed to the plate and that do not permit toggling of the screws. Non-fixed moment arm cantilever beam constructs allow toggling of the screws that are not completely locked into the plate. They, thus, allow screw toggling and facilitate subsidence [3]. Fusion is impeded by excessive motion, and such motion is prevented by the fixed moment arm cantilever beam system. However, the complete elimination of motion and the associated reduction of stresses and loading effect on the graft-bone interface can inhibit bone growth and healing – according to Wolff's law [1, 35]. The rigidity of the plating system can decrease the loading effect on the bone graft, as demonstrated in cadaveric studies; 23% of the load was borne by rigid plates placed for a C5 corpectomy, in contrast to only 9% with dynamic plates [28]. Such dynamic plates minimize stress shielding and excessive plate rigidity that inhibits compressive forces across the bone graft and therefore fusion. However, it remains controversial, particularly when undergoing a one- or two-level ACDF. A systematic review demonstrated that there is no significant difference in the fusion or complication rate between fully constrained (rigid) and semiconstrained (dynamic) plates [30].

The proper placement and fixation of the anterior cervical plate also help to achieve the optimal stabilization, restoration of the lordotic curve, maximization of the fusion rate, and decreased risk of the ASD. A positive correlation has been achieved between adjacent-level ossification with shorter plate-to-disc distance, and the placement of plate away from the adjacent segment disc space can help to decrease the incidence of adjacent-level ossification and ASD [27]. The utilization of aforementioned dynamic plates provides comparable fusion rates to rigid plates [30], but subsidence of the interbody graft can result, leading to the potential impingement of the plate on the adjacent segment disc space, along with local loss of lordosis. However, a retrospective cohort study has demonstrated that there is no significant association between the changes in local cervical alignment from subsidence and the clinical outcomes [8].

Anterior cervical implants/instrumentations are associated with variable responses to different loading conditions (Fig. 2.9). For example, the implants act as distraction devices by resisting flexion forces and compression under axial loading conditions and, conversely, function as compression devices when an extension moment is applied [2]. With longer constructs, stability can also improve by the addition of an extra, intermediate point of fixation, allowing the resistance of translation deformation through a three-point bending force application (Fig. 2.10). In addition, the placement of bicortical screws has been shown to improve the holding strength of anterior cervical plating system, in comparison to the placement of unicortical screws, and should be considered in the setting of osteoporosis and other associated risk factors for instrumentation failure [29].

The concept of subsidence, which refers to the vertical height loss, is important in achieving the proper spine construct to avoid further deformities and accomplish appropriate stabilization. Angular deformation along the sagittal axis is associated with the loss of the height of the vertebral body and/or intervertebral disc, and it leads to the progression of kyphotic deformity. When ventral approach is taken for cervical spine stabilization and correction of kyphotic deformity, one has to fully understand the concept of subsidence to avoid pseudarthrosis, instrumentation failure, further kyphotic deformity, and iatrogenic instability. This subsidence process involves a combination of pistoning of the strut graft into the vertebral body, collapse or shortening of the strut graft, and poor surgical techniques, which all result in creating persistent gaps between the graft and the end plates that induce subsidence [2]. The incidence and extent of subsidence and suboptimal stabilization are affected by the fit of the bone graft in the vertebral body, the contact surface area between the graft and the body, and the quality and quantity of the contact surfaces [2]. The maximal contact surface area is achieved by optimizing the closeness of fit between the graft and the body, which minimizes the stress concentration and thereby minimizes the rate of pseudarthrosis or subsidence. Moreover, when the contact surface area is larger (which occurs when the bone graft is nearly the same size as the vertebral body end plate), a greater biomechanical advantage is achieved, since contact on the vertebral end plate periphery engages more dense cortical bone and helps to buttress an axial load [2] (Fig. 2.11).

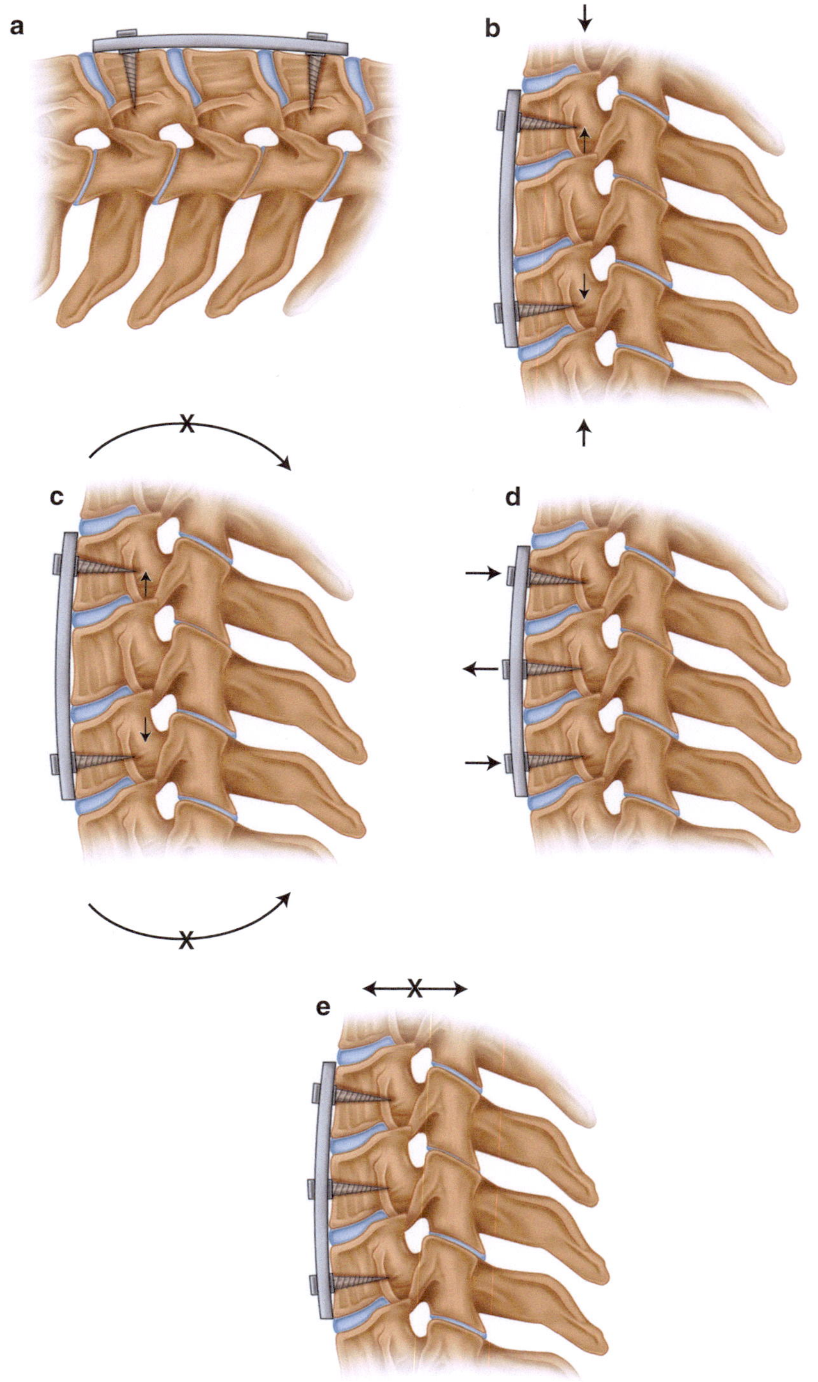

Fig. 2.9 Response of anterior cervical implants to various loading conditions. (**a**) Fixed moment arm cantilever beam construct placed on the anterior cervical spine; (**b**) application of axial loads in an upright position; (**c**) implant functioning as a tension-band fixation device via compression when the extension moment is applied; (**d**) three-point bending forces resisted by the multisegmental implant; (**e**) translation resisted by the multisegmental implant. (Permission from Thieme has been granted. Adapted from Benzel's Biomechanics of Spine Stabilization, 2015 (third edition); Fig. 21.2, page 252)

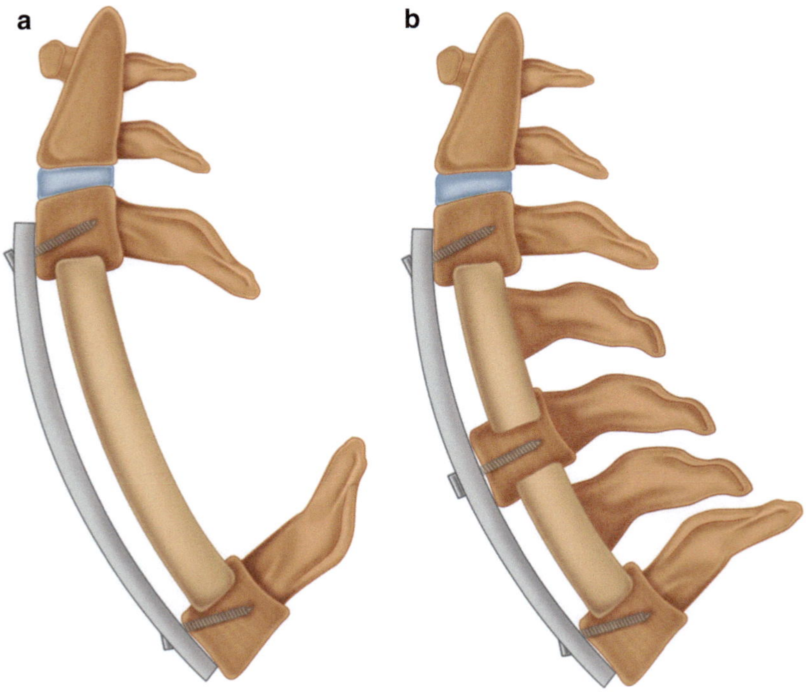

Fig. 2.10 Enhanced stability by the addition of an intermediate fixation point in a cantilever beam construct in the anterior cervical spine. (**a**) Anterior cervical construct with a long strut graft after a multilevel corpectomy; (**b**) the intermediate fixation point providing increased axial load bearing, thus increasing the resistance to deformation and implant failure. (Permission from Thieme has been granted. Adapted from Benzel's Biomechanics of Spine Stabilization, 2015 (third edition); Fig. 21.14, page 260)

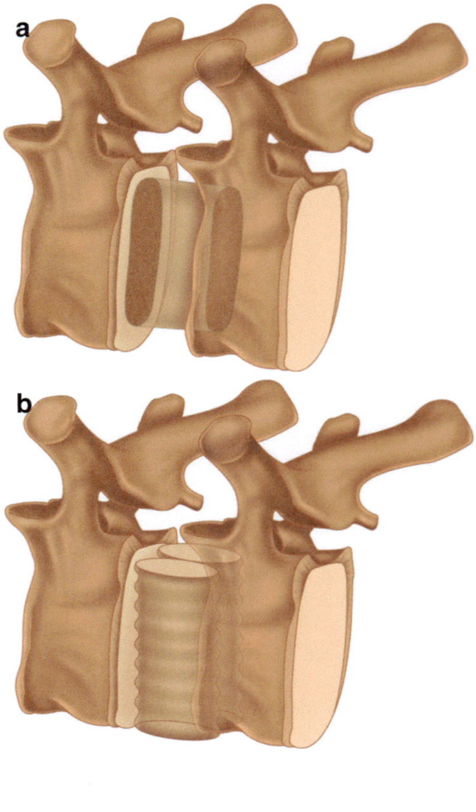

Fig. 2.11 The contact surface area between the bone graft and the vertebral body is inversely proportional to the extent of subsidence. For example, flat-faced cages (**a**) provide a greater surface area of contact, compared to round-faced cages (**b**). (Permission from Thieme has been granted. Adapted from Benzel's Biomechanics of Spine Stabilization, 2015 (third edition) Fig. 20.19AB, page 184)

Conclusions

Due to the complex anatomy of the cervical spine, which incorporates the OCJ, upper cervical, and subaxial spine, the clinical application of biomechanical principles is essential. In order to properly manage the degenerative cervical spine, one must fully understand the complexity of the degenerative process and appreciate and account for the cervical spinal anatomy along with the various treatment modalities. Biomechanical principles are an adjunct to the surgical decision-making process. They also contribute to the establishment of guidelines for the management of the degenerative cervical spine and therefore the decision-making process in selection of the optimal spine stabilization strategy.

References

1. Anand N. Overview of biologics. Spine (Phila Pa 1976). 2016;41(S)7:S10.
2. Benzel EC. Biomechanics of spine stabilization. Rolling Meadows: American Association of Neurological Surgeons Publications; 2001.
3. Brodke DS, Gollogly S, Alexander Mohr R, et al. Dynamic cervical plates: biomechanical evaluation of load sharing and stiffness. Spine (Phila Pa 1976). 2001;26:1324–9.
4. Cheng I, Sundberg EB, Iezza A, Lindsey DP, Riew KD. Biomechanical determination of distal level for fusions across the cervicothoracic junction. Global Spine J. 2015;5(4):282–6.
5. Dunlap BJ, Karaikovic EE, Park HS, Sokolowski MJ, Zhang LQ. Load sharing properties of cervical pedicle screw-rod constructs versus lateral mass screw-rod constructs. Eur Spine J. 2010;19(5):803–8.
6. Fehlings MG, Gray R. Importance of sagittal balance in determining the outcome of anterior versus posterior decompressive surgery for cervical spondylotic myelopathy. J Neurosurg Spine. 2009;11:518–519; discussion 9-20.
7. Ferrara LA. The biomechanics of cervical spondylosis. Adv Orthop. 2012;493605 .
8. Ghahreman A, Rao PJ, Ferch RD. Dynamic plates in anterior cervical fusion surgery: graft settling and cervical alignment. Spine (Phila Pa 1976). 2009;34(15):1567–71.
9. Ghogawala Z, Martin B, Benzel EC, et al. Comparative effectiveness of ventral vs dorsal surgery for cervical spondylotic myelopathy. Neurosurgery. 2011;68(3):622–30.
10. Goel VK, Clark CR, Harris KG, et al. Kinematics of the cervical spine: effects of multiple total laminectomy and facet wiring. J Orthop Res. 1988;6:611–9.
11. Gorek J, Acaroglu E, Berven S, et al. Constructs incorporating intralaminar C2 screws provide rigid stability for atlantoaxial fixation. Spine (Phila Pa 1976). 2005;30:1513.
12. Grob D, Crisco JJ 3rd, Panjabi MM, et al. Biomechanical evaluation of four different posterior atlantoaxial fixation techniques. Spine (Phila Pa 1976). 1992;17:480–90.
13. Guzman JZ, Feldman ZM, McAnany S, Hecht AC, Qureshi SA, Cho SK. Osteoporosis in cervical spine surgery. Spine (Phila Pa 1976). 2016;41(8):662–8.
14. Heller JG, Amrani J, Hutton WC. Transverse ligament failure: a biomechanical study. J Spinal Disord. 1993;6:162–5.
15. Henderson FC, Geddes JF, Vaccaro AR, Woodard E, Berry KJ, Benzel EC. Stretch-associated injury in cervical spondylotic myelopathy: new concept and review. Neurosurgery. 2005;56(5):1101–13.
16. Ito Z, Higashino K, Kato S, Kim SS, Wong E, Yoshioka K, Hutton WC. Pedicle screws can be 4 times stronger than lateral mass screws for insertion in the midcervical spine: a biomechanical study on strength of fixation. J Spinal Disord Tech. 2014;27(2):80–5.
17. Kothe R, Rüther W, Schneider E, Linke B. Biomechanical analysis of transpedicular screw fixation in the subaxial cervical spine. Spine (Phila Pa 1976). 2004;29(17):1869–75.
18. Kowalski RJ, Ferrera LA, Benzel EC. Biomechanics of the spine. Neurosurg Q. 2005;15(1).
19. Lee BS, Ghogawala Z, Benzel EC. Cervical spondylotic myelopathy and sagittal deformity. World Spinal Column J. 2014;5:119–23.
20. Liu H, Zhang B, Lei J, Cai X, Li Z, Wang Z. Biomechanical role of the C1 lateral mass screws in occipitoatlantoaxial fixation: a finite element analysis. Spine (Phila Pa 1976). 2016;41(22):E1312–8.
21. Lopez AJ, Scheer JK, Leibl KE, Smith ZA, Dlouhy BJ, Dahdaleh NS. Anatomy and biomechanics of the craniovertebral junction. Neurosurg Focus. 2015;38(4):E2.
22. Montesano PX, Juach EC, Anderson PA, et al. Biomechanics of cervical spine internal fixation. Spine (Phila Pa 1976). 1991;16(Suppl):S10–6.
23. Moroney SP, Schultz AB, Miller JA, et al. Load-displacement properties of lower cervical spine motion segments. J Biomech. 1988;21:769–79.
24. Nowinski GP, Visarius H, Nolte LP, et al. A biomechanical com- parison of cervical laminaplasty and cervical laminectomy with progressive facetectomy. Spine (Phila Pa 1976). 1993;18:1995–2004.
25. Oda T, Panjabi MM, Crisco JJ III, Oxland TR, Katz L, Nolte LP. Experimental study of atlas injuries. II. Relevance to clinical diagnosis and treatment. Spine (Phila Pa 1976). 1991;16(10 Suppl): S466–73.

26. Panjabi MM, White AA, Keller D, et al. Stability of the cervical spine under tension. J Biomech. 1978;11:189–97.
27. Park JB, Cho YS, Riew KD. Development of adjacent-level ossification in patients with an anterior cervical plate. J Bone Joint Surg Am. 2005;87(3):558–63.
28. Reidy D, Finkelstein J, Nagpurkar A, et al. Cervical spine loading characteristics in a cadaveric C5 corpectomy model using a static and dynamic plate. J Spinal Disord Tech. 2004;17:117–22.
29. Ryken TC, Clausen JD, Traynelis VC, Goel VK. Biomechanical analysis of bone mineral density, insertion technique, screw torque, and holding strength of anterior cervical plate screws. J Neurosurg. 1995;83(2):324–9.
30. Schroeder GD, Kepler CK, Hollern DA, Rodrigues-Pinto R, Kurd MF, Wilson JR, Maltenfort MG, Paul JT, Fleischman AN, Dwight K, Millhouse PW, Vaccaro AR. The effect of dynamic versus static plating systems on fusion rates and complications in 1-level and/or 2-level anterior cervical discectomy and fusion: a systematic review. Clin Spine Surg. 2017;30(1):20–6.
31. Schulte K, Clark CR, Goel VK. Kinematics of the cervical spine following discectomy and stabilization. Spine (Phila Pa 1976). 1989;14(10):1116–21.
32. Techy F, Benzel EC. Stabilization of the cervicothoracic junction: part I. Cont Spine Surg. 2011;12(5):1–5.
33. Weinstein PR, Ehni G, Wilson CB. Lumbar spondylosis: diagnosis, management and surgical treatment. Chicago: Year Book; 1977. p. 13–87.
34. White AA, Panjabi MM. Clinical biomechanics of the spine. 2nd ed. Philadelphia: Lippincott; 1990.
35. Wolff J. The law of bone remodeling. Berlin/Heidelberg/New York: Springer; 1986. (translation of the German 1892 edition).
36. Young WF. Cervical spondylotic myelopathy: a common cause of spinal cord dysfunction in older persons. Am Fam Physician. 2000;62:1064–70 and 73.
37. Zdeblick TA, Abitbol JJ, Kunz DN. Cervical stability after sequential capsule resection. Spine (Phila Pa 1976). 1993;18:2005–8.

Cervical Alignment and Sagittal Balance

3

Alexander Tuchman and Dominque M. O. Higgins

Pitfalls and Pearls

(a) Cervical sagittal alignment is qualified as lordosis or kyphosis and can be measured utilizing Cobb angles, Harrison posterior tangent, and Jackson physiologic stress lines.
(b) Studies demonstrate a correlation between cervical kyphosis and myelopathy.
(c) Chin brow angle is used to assess horizontal gaze.
(d) Abnormalities of horizontal gaze have been shown to have negative impact on ADLs and quality of life.
(e) Cervical sagittal balance can be measured with C2–C7 SVA.
(f) Abnormal cervical sagittal balance has been associated with poor quality of life and disability.
(g) Deviations of thoracolumbar alignment can lead to compensatory changes of cervical alignment.
(h) Thoracolumbar deformity surgery should incorporate the potential impact on cervical alignment.

Introduction

In patients with cervical spine pathologies, surgical consideration of alignment and balance is critical for obtaining optimal outcomes [1]. Preoperative evaluation of these patients must therefore take into account baseline deformity, as well as potential risk of progression. As such, reliable methods of describing cervical alignment and balance and awareness of their surgical implications are of the utmost importance. Here, we describe standard parameters utilized in classification of cervical spine alignment, deformity, and their key clinical associations.

Cervical Alignment

Spinal alignment refers to the local relationship of the vertebrae to one another. Spondylolisthesis describes translation of one vertebral body in

A. Tuchman (✉) · D. M. O. Higgins
Department of Neurological Surgery, Columbia University Medical Center, New York, NY, USA
e-mail: Alexander.tuchman@cshs.org

M. G. Kaiser et al. (eds.), *Degenerative Cervical Myelopathy and Radiculopathy*,
https://doi.org/10.1007/978-3-319-97952-6_3

relation to the next most distal vertebra. Angular relationships in the sagittal plane are measured in terms of lordosis and kyphosis, while coronal angularity is described as scoliosis. By convention lordosis is described as a negative value while kyphosis is positive. A variety of techniques can be used to determine the angular alignment of the cervical spine on upright anteroposterior and lateral radiographs, including Cobb angles, Harrison posterior tangent, and the Jackson physiologic stress lines. The Cobb angle is one of the most commonly used technique to determine the alignment in the sagittal or coronal plane [2]. The Cobb angles for assessing cervical sagittal alignment from C2 to C7 can be determined by first drawing a line parallel to the inferior end plate of C2 and a second line parallel to the inferior end plate of C7, and then perpendicular lines are drawn from each of the two (Fig. 3.1a). The Cobb angle is the angle subtended between the crossing of the perpendicular lines. Some studies refer to cervical alignment over the C1–C7 segments. In this case, a line extending from the anterior tubercle of C1 to the posterior margin of the spinous process may be used rather than the C2 inferior end plate line [2]. C1–C7 tends to overestimate cervical lordosis, and C2–C7 underestimates lordosis. Coronal deformity may also be analyzed on anteroposterior radiograph using the Cobb method. In this case, the initial two lines are drawn parallel to the two most angled vertebrae, and the degree of scoliosis is determined by the angle subtended by the two intersecting lines perpendicular to the end plates. A coronal Cobb angle of greater than 10° indicates cervical scoliosis.

Harrison posterior tangent provides an estimate of overall cervical curvature in the sagittal plane by the summation of parallel lines to the posterior surface of cervical vertebral bodies from C2 to C7 (Fig. 3.1b). Similarly, the Jackson physiologic stress line utilizes parallel lines to posterior vertebral body of C2 and C7, and measuring the angle between them (Fig. 3.1c).

Mean cervical alignment from C2 to C7 in normal controls is −17° of lordosis with a range within two standard deviations between −45° of lordosis and 11° of kyphosis [3]. The mean angle between O and C1 is 2.1° ± 5.0° and C1 and C2 is −32.2° ± 7.0°, and the subaxial levels range between −0.6° and −4.5° [4, 5].

Despite increased cervical kyphosis being recognized as a form of cervical deformity [3, 6], there is not a strong relationship between increasing cervical kyphosis and neck pain or disability. This is likely related to the fact that cervical alignment has a large physiologic normal range to compensate for the variable sagittal alignment and angulation of the proximal thoracic spine while maintaining cranial balance and horizontal gaze. In fact cervical lordosis tends to increase with age [4, 5]. Grob et al. found no relationship

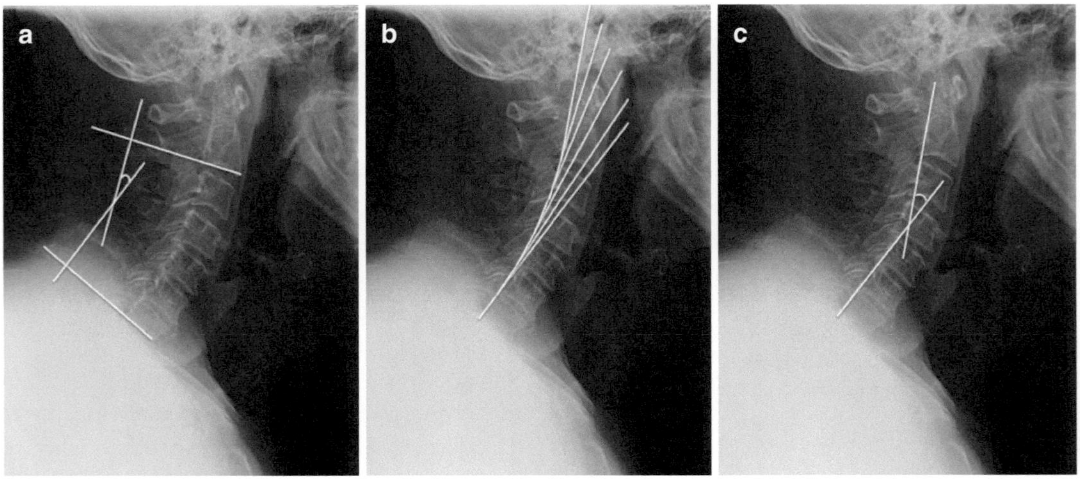

Fig. 3.1 (**a**) Cobb angle. (**b**) Harrison posterior tangent line. (**c**) Jackson physiologic stress line

between neck pain and global or segmental cervical angles [7]. Le Huec et al. likewise found that 1/3 of the asymptomatic patients have cervical kyphosis [8].

On the contrary, multiple studies have demonstrated a relationship between cervical kyphosis and myelopathy. Mechanistically, this is hypothesized to be due to impaired blood supply due to anterior cord flattening and compression of arterial feeders [9]. Longitudinal cord tension resulting in tethering may also play a role, causing increased intramedullary cord pressure leading to demyelination and neuronal apoptosis [10]. Oshima et al. found segmental kyphosis to be predictive of neurologic worsening in patients with mild cervical myelopathy [11]. Furthermore, patients with preoperative lordotic alignment have greater improvement in myelopathy postoperatively compared to kyphotic counterparts [12]. Kyphotic patients, though, demonstrate greater improvement with regard to myelopathy when treated with anterior approaches versus posterior [12].

There is evidence to suggest, though, that correcting segmental alignment postoperatively rather than global alignment does improve neck pain [13].

Horizontal Gaze

Chin-brow vertical angle (CBVA) is used to assess horizontal gaze, measured by the angle subtended by a vertical line intersecting a second line from the forehead to the chin [2, 14, 15]. CBVA can be measured on clinical photos or relevant anatomy radiographs (Fig. 3.2). Mean neutral angle range is estimated to be -1 ± 3 [3]. Loss of horizontal gaze has a significant impact on activities of daily living (ADLs) and quality of life [16]. CBVA of $<-4.8°$ or $>17.7°$ correlates with severe disability [16]. Surgical correction of CBVA ($\pm$ 10°) is associated with improved gaze, ambulation, and ADLs [14, 15, 17]. Slope of line of sight, measuring from the inferior margin of the orbit to the top of the external auditory canal (EAC), and McGregor slope, measuring from the posterior margin of the hard palate to the

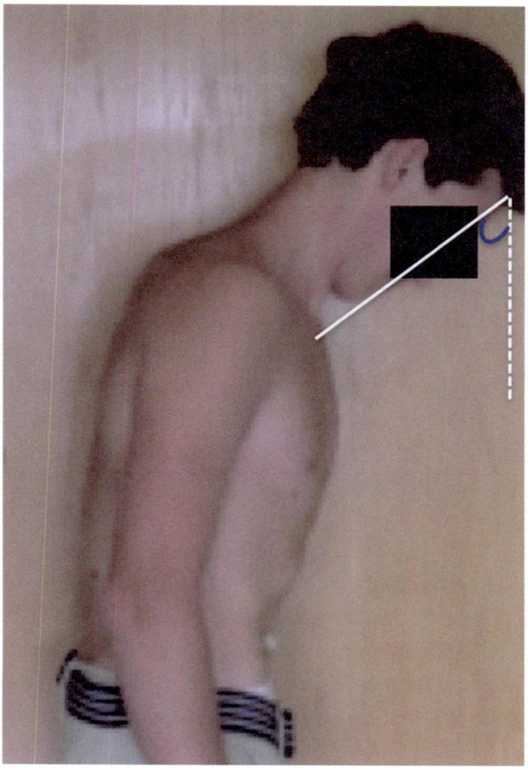

Fig. 3.2 Chin-brow vertical angle (*blue*)

opisthion, are also similar metrics for assessing gaze, the former of which has been shown to independently predict quality of life [16]. These can be helpful when X-rays do not allow for the measurement of CBVA and can be converted to the equivalence of CBVA with mathematical equations [16].

In patients undergoing occipital cervical (O-C) fusion, the fixed head position is of great importance not only to optimize horizontal gaze but also to minimize potential for dysphagia, which is associated with cervical immobility, mid-cervical hyperextension, and flexed position of the O-C junction resulting in reduced O-C2 angle [18–21]. Furthermore, reduction of atlanto-occipital (AO) subluxation is associated with a reduction in oropharyngeal airway space [22]. Radiographically, measuring the pharyngeal inlet angle (PIA) may help predict the risk of dysphagia, because it encompasses most of these risk factors within its calculation

[23, 24]. PIA is determined by measuring the angle intersecting McGregor's line and a vertical line from the center of the C1 anterior arch through the apex of cervical sagittal curvature. Patients with a PIA of <90° are at an increased risk of postoperative dysphagia [23, 24]. Keeping the O-C2 angle the same or slightly greater than preoperatively is also recommended, as dysphagia is associated with flexed position of the O-C junction and reduced O-C2 angle [18, 20]. Some groups advocate preoperative halo immobilization prior to fusion to help predict potential postoperative issues with dysphagia; however this too is not entirely reliable in preventing such complications [23–26].

Sagittal Balance

Global measurements of alignment, as the name implies, take into account additional factors in the neuraxis that will ultimately influence the cervical spine [2]. Sagittal vertical axis (SVA) is a useful method that takes into account alignment with respect to the sacrum [2]. Techniques for measurement include drawing a vertical line from C7, the plumb line, and measuring the distance from it to the posterior superior corner of S1. This measures thoracolumbar balance but ignores the cervical spine. Newer methods incorporate the cervical spine using C2 or the anterior EAC as a starting point to determine the cranial center of gravity (CCOG) and give a more complete assessment of global spine balance. A more focused assessment of cervical sagittal axis can be made with a C2–C7 SVA with a plumb line from the centroid of C2 (or dens) and the posterosuperior aspect of C7 (Fig. 3.3a) [6, 27–29]. A C2–C7 SVA of >4 cm suggests cervical deformity [6, 29] (Fig. 3.3b). A retrospective analysis of 56 patients prior to surgery demonstrated that higher C2–C7 SVA correlated with worse myelopathy as measured by the modified Japanese orthopedic scale [28].

In addition to the aforementioned neurologic sequelae from abnormal cervical alignment, patients have also been shown to suffer poor health-related quality of life (HRQoL) and increased disability, as measured by validated measures such as the Neck Disability index (NDI) and the Short Form 36 (SF-36) [27, 29–31].

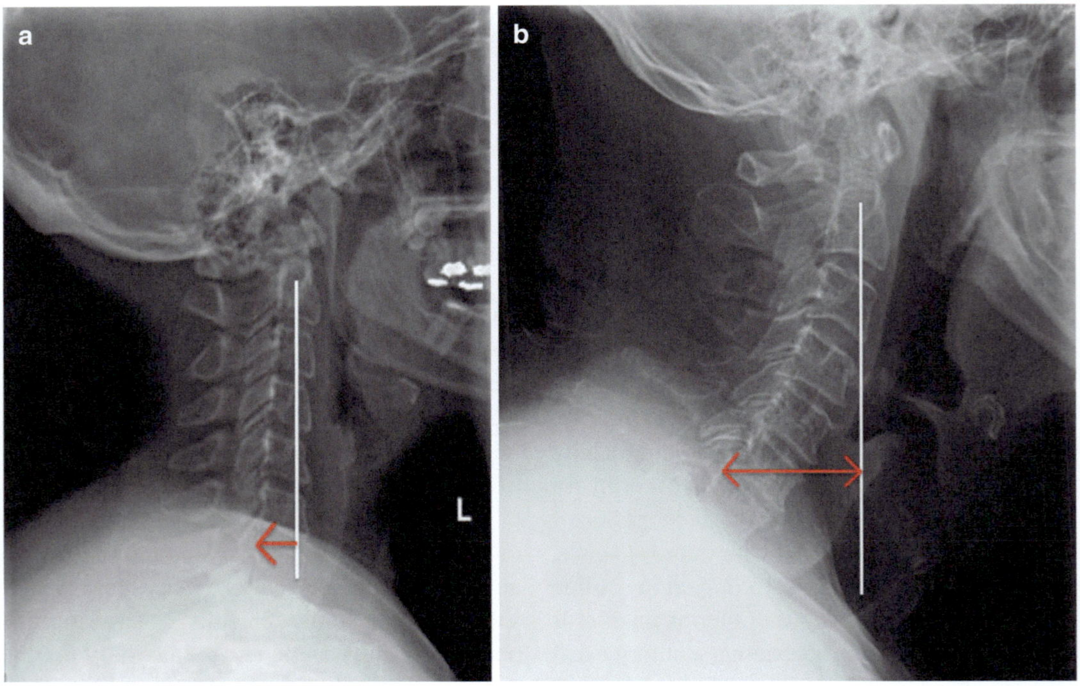

Fig. 3.3 (**a**) C2–C7 SVA (*red arrow*). (**b**) Positive C2–C7 SVA (*red arrow*)

Table 3.1 Important parameters of cervical sagital alignment

Cervical sagittal alignment	Measurements
Cobb angle	Line parallel to the inferior end plate of C2, a second line parallel to the inferior end plate of C7, and then perpendicular lines are drawn from each of the two
Harrison posterior tangent	Summation of parallel lines to the posterior surface of cervical vertebral bodies from C2 to C7
Jackson physiologic stress line	Parallel lines to posterior vertebral body of C2 and C7 and measuring the angle between them
CBV Chin-brow vertical angle (CBVA)A	Angle subtended by a vertical line intersecting a second line from the forehead to the chin
C2–C7 SVA	Plumb line from the centroid of C2 (or dens) and the posterosuperior aspect of C7
Neck tilt	Angle between 2 lines both originating from the upper end of the sternum with one being a vertical line and the other connecting to the center of the T1 end plate
Thoracic inlet angle	Angle between a line originating from the center of the T1 end plate and perpendicular to the T1 end plate and a line from the center of the T1 end plate and the upper end of the sternum
T1 slope	Angle between the horizontal plane and T1 end plate

Indeed, high preoperative SVA values are an independent predictor of high Neck Disability Index scores [27, 31]. Global alignment parameters (Table 3.1), particularly in instrumented patients, can also significantly impact quality of life. High postoperative SVA values, above 4 cm, have been shown to worsen HRQoL [29]. Similarly, Hyun et al. also showed a 5 cm cutoff for risk of poor quality of life [30].

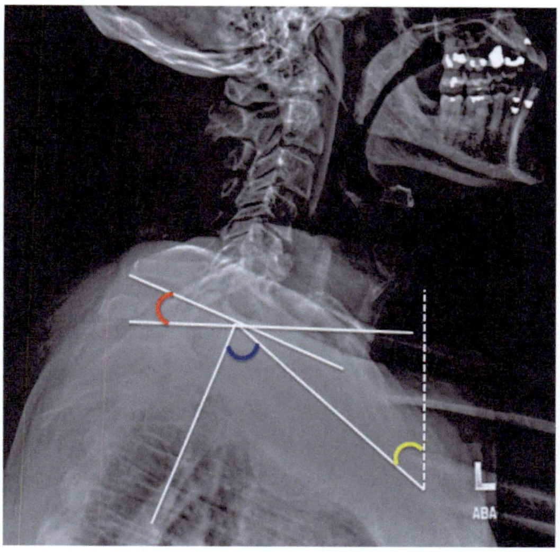

Fig. 3.4 Red: T1 slope. *Blue*: thoracic inlet angle. *Yellow*: neck tilt. Dashed line: vertical from manubrium

Thoracic Parameters

Similar to the how the pelvis controls the need for lumbar lordosis for the thoracolumbar spine, the upper thoracic spine determines the need for compensation for the cervical spine. Thoracic hyperkyphosis can result in chronic compensation of the cervical spine. As such thoracic parameters affecting cervical alignment have been identified [2]. The main parameters are T1 slope, neck tilt, and the thoracic inlet angle (Fig. 3.4). Neck tilt is defined as the angle between two lines both originating from the upper end of the sternum with one being a vertical line and the other connecting to the center of the T1 end plate. Thoracic inlet angle is the angle between a line originating from the center of the T1 end plate and perpendicular to the T1 end plate and a line from the center of the T1 end plate and the upper end of the sternum [2]. This measurement can be viewed as the cervical correlate to pelvic incidence. T1 slope is the angle between the horizontal plane and T1 end plate. T1 slope may be helpful in predicting physiologic alignment and guide deformity correction and is similar in concept to sacral slope. The sum of the T1 slope and the neck tilt results in the thoracic inlet angle.

The T1 slope, in conjunction with the SVA, can help determine the amount of subaxial cervical lordosis required to maintain CCOG in balance and maintain horizontal gaze. T1 slope can also be a useful predictor of post-laminoplasty kyphosis, as Kim et al. demonstrated [32]. Postoperative cervical laminoplasty patients with high T1 slope (>26.3°) were more likely to develop kyphotic changes (greater than 5° and 10°) at 2-year follow-up [32]. Despite its utility, only 11% of patients can have a full evaluation of T1 parameters on plain upright X-rays, limiting its application [33]. Upright kinematic MRIs can overcome this limitation; however such studies are not readily available at many institutions, and traditional MRIs and CT scans do not represent physiologic alignment as these images are obtained in the supine position.

To better assess cervical deformity after thoracolumbar surgery, T1 slope minus cervical lordosis (T1S-CL) can be employed. This has shown to be a useful tool to identify patients at risk of progression of cervical deformity following thoracolumbar deformity surgery [34]. It is also useful for determining the amount of cervical lordosis required to prevent increased SVA following cervical fusion. A postoperative mismatch greater than 20° corresponds with cervical SVA greater than 4 cm [35].

Thoracolumbar Deformity and Cervical Compensation

Global and local parameters of cervical deformity also are important considerations when evaluating patients for adult spinal deformity surgery. Interestingly 53% of this population also has cervical deformity [2, 36]. Patients can either have concomitant primary cervical deformity or physiologic compensatory changes in cervical alignment. As such, postoperatively, upper thoracic deformity correction can lead to new or worsened cervical deformity if such factors are not taken into account [35]. Lumbar posterior spinal osteotomies with adequate sagittal plane correction have been shown to result in spontaneous cervical deformity correction [37]. Other studies have not found such a link, and it may not always be apparent if cervical deformity patients have underlying thoracolumbar deformity [38]. To address this, Klineberg et al. demonstrated that a T1 slope greater than 32° correlates on chest X-ray with underlying thoracolumbar deformity and a T1 slope outside the range of 12–25° may warrant evaluation of global alignment [38, 39]. Protopsaltis et al. demonstrated that a mismatch between T1S-CL greater than 17° correlated with a primary cervical deformity [34]. These patients experienced progression of cervical deformity following thoracolumbar deformity correction instead of reciprocal improvement. Similarly, Ghobrial et al. showed that preoperative mismatch of greater than 15° was associated with an increased risk for postoperative deformity following corrective surgery [40].

Limitations and Areas for Future Investigation

Despite these numerous parameters established for evaluating cervical deformity, individually they fall short of providing a complete descriptor of a patient's clinical picture. Also, comparisons across studies can become difficult given the variety of parameters available for measuring alignment globally and even across segments. To this end, a cervical deformity classification system has been defined that incorporates the parameters described [41]. The system consists of five deformity descriptor groups that include three primary sagittal deformity groups at the cervical apex, cervicothoracic junction, and thoracic apex, primary cranio-vertebral junction deformity, and primary cervical coronal deformity. There are additional five modifiers that can be applied to those primary descriptors to account for SVA, horizontal gaze, T1S-CL, myelopathy, and the SRS-Schwab classification to address ASD, which is useful for standardizing descriptions. Similarly, a standardized system has also been developed to describe surgical deformity correction, with seven grades ranging from partial facetectomy to complete vertebral column resection [4, 5].

Discussion/Conclusion

In summary, cervical alignment has an extremely large physiologic range, and any surgical plan must address the individual patient's deformity, provide adequate correction at the pathologic site, and minimize perioperative risk. Kyphosis alone does not define symptomatic cervical deformity; however there is a relationship between cervical kyphosis and myelopathy that should be accounted for in a treatment plan. Cervical sagittal balance does correlate with quality of life metrics. A C2–C7 SVA of >4 cm corresponds with cervical deformity and is caused by a mismatch between thoracic slope and subaxial cervical lordosis (T1S-CL). This mismatch can be from a too high T1 slope (thoracolumbar deformity), not enough cervical lordosis (primary cervical deformity), or both. Assessment of global balance is key to defining the site of pathology that requires treatment. The goals of sagittal cervical deformity surgery are therefore to restore horizontal gaze, prevent dysphagia, alleviate neurologic compression, maintain or restore global balance, and promote fusion. Lastly, thoracolumbar deformity surgery, as well, should incorporate potential issues with cervical balance during operative planning to optimize cervical alignment.

References

1. Hann S, et al. An algorithmic strategy for selecting a surgical approach in cervical deformity correction. Neurosurg Focus. 2014;36(5):E5.
2. Scheer JK, et al. Cervical spine alignment, sagittal deformity, and clinical implications: a review. J Neurosurg Spine. 2013;19(2):141–59.
3. Kuntz CT, et al. Neutral upright sagittal spinal alignment from the occiput to the pelvis in asymptomatic adults: a review and resynthesis of the literature. J Neurosurg Spine. 2007;6(2):104–12.
4. Ames CP, et al. Cervical radiographical alignment: comprehensive assessment techniques and potential importance in cervical myelopathy. Spine (Phila Pa 1976). 2013;38(22 Suppl 1):S149–60.
5. Ames CP, et al. A standardized nomenclature for cervical spine soft-tissue release and osteotomy for deformity correction: clinical article. J Neurosurg Spine. 2013;19(3):269–78.
6. Hardacker JW, et al. Radiographic standing cervical segmental alignment in adult volunteers without neck symptoms. Spine (Phila Pa 1976). 1997;22(13):1472–1480; discussion 1480.
7. Grob D, et al. The association between cervical spine curvature and neck pain. Eur Spine J. 2007;16(5):669–78.
8. Le Huec JC, et al. Sagittal parameters of global cervical balance using EOS imaging: normative values from a prospective cohort of asymptomatic volunteers. Eur Spine J. 2015;24(1):63–71.
9. Shimizu K, et al. Spinal kyphosis causes demyelination and neuronal loss in the spinal cord: a new model of kyphotic deformity using juvenile Japanese small game fowls. Spine (Phila Pa 1976). 2005;30(21):2388–92.
10. Jarzem PF, et al. Spinal cord tissue pressure during spinal cord distraction in dogs. Spine (Phila Pa 1976). 1992;17(8 Suppl):S227–34.
11. Oshima Y, Seichi A, Takeshita K, Chikuda H, Ono T, Baba S, Morii J, Oka H, Kawaguchi H, Nakamura K, Tanaka S. Natural course and prognostic factors in patients with mild cervical spondylotic myelopathy with increased signal intensity on T2-weighted magnetic resonance imaging. Spine (Phila Pa 1976). 2012;37(22):1909–13.
12. Shamji MF, et al. The Association of Cervical Spine Alignment with neurologic recovery in a prospective cohort of patients with surgical myelopathy: analysis of a series of 124 cases. World Neurosurg. 2016;86:112–9.
13. Guerin P, et al. Sagittal alignment after single cervical disc arthroplasty. J Spinal Disord Tech. 2012;25(1):10–6.
14. Kim KT, et al. Surgical treatment of "chin-on-pubis" deformity in a patient with ankylosing spondylitis: a case report of consecutive cervical, thoracic, and lumbar corrective osteotomies. Spine (Phila Pa 1976). 2012;37(16):E1017–21.
15. Suk KS, et al. Significance of chin-brow vertical angle in correction of kyphotic deformity of ankylosing spondylitis patients. Spine (Phila Pa 1976). 2003;28(17):2001–5.
16. Lafage R, et al. Natural head posture in the setting of sagittal spinal deformity: validation of chin-brow vertical angle, slope of line of sight, and McGregor's slope with health-related quality of life. Neurosurgery. 2016;79(1):108–15.
17. Deviren V, Scheer JK, Ames CP. Technique of cervicothoracic junction pedicle subtraction osteotomy for cervical sagittal imbalance: report of 11 cases. J Neurosurg Spine. 2011;15(2):174–81.
18. Miyata M, et al. O-C2 angle as a predictor of dyspnea and/or dysphagia after occipitocervical fusion. Spine (Phila Pa 1976). 2009;34(2):184–8.
19. Morishima N, et al. The influences of halo-vest fixation and cervical hyperextension on swallowing in healthy volunteers. Spine (Phila Pa 1976). 2005;30(7):E179–82.
20. Yoshida M, et al. Upper-airway obstruction after short posterior occipitocervical fusion in a flexed position. Spine (Phila Pa 1976). 2007;32(8):E267–70.
21. Garfin SR, Botte MJ, Waters RL, Nickel VL. Complications in the use of the halo fixation device. J Bone Joint Surg Am. 1986;68(3):320–5.

22. Izeki M, et al. Reduction of atlantoaxial subluxation causes airway stenosis. Spine (Phila Pa 1976). 2013;38(9):E513–20.
23. Kaneyama S, et al. Dysphagia after Occipitothoracic fusion is caused by direct compression of oropharyngeal space due to anterior protrusion of mid-cervical spine. Clin Spine Surg. 2017;30(7):314–20.
24. Kaneyama S, et al. The prediction and prevention of dysphagia after Occipitospinal fusion by use of the S-line (swallowing line). Spine (Phila Pa 1976). 2017;42(10):718–25.
25. Bagley CA, et al. Assuring optimal physiologic craniocervical alignment and avoidance of swallowing-related complications after occipitocervical fusion by preoperative halo vest placement. J Spinal Disord Tech. 2009;22(3):170–6.
26. Matsuyama Y, et al. Long-term results of occipitothoracic fusion surgery in RA patients with destruction of the cervical spine. J Spinal Disord Tech. 2005;18(Suppl):S101–6.
27. Iyer S, et al. Impact of cervical sagittal alignment parameters on neck disability. Spine (Phila Pa 1976). 2016;41(5):371–7.
28. Smith JS, et al. Association of myelopathy scores with cervical sagittal balance and normalized spinal cord volume: analysis of 56 preoperative cases from the AOSpine North America myelopathy study. Spine (Phila Pa 1976). 2013;38(22 Suppl 1):S161–70.
29. Tang JA, et al. The impact of standing regional cervical sagittal alignment on outcomes in posterior cervical fusion surgery. Neurosurgery. 2012;71(3):662–669; discussion 669.
30. Hyun SJ, et al. Relationship between T1 slope and cervical alignment following multilevel posterior cervical fusion surgery: impact of T1 slope minus cervical lordosis. Spine (Phila Pa 1976). 2016;41(7):E396–402.
31. Lee JS, et al. Relationship between cervical sagittal alignment and quality of life in ankylosing spondylitis. Eur Spine J. 2015;24(6):1199–203.
32. Kim TH, et al. T1 slope as a predictor of kyphotic alignment change after laminoplasty in patients with cervical myelopathy. Spine (Phila Pa 1976). 2013;38(16):E992–7.
33. Weng C, et al. Influence of T1 slope on the cervical sagittal balance in degenerative cervical spine: an analysis using kinematic MRI. Spine (Phila Pa 1976). 2016;41(3):185–90.
34. Protopsaltis TS. et al. T1 slope minus cervical lordosis (TS-CL), the cervical analog of PI-LL defines cervical sagittal deformity in patients undergoing thoracolumbar osteotomy. Abstract presented at the 2013 Annual meeting of the Cervical Spine Research Society in Los Angeles; 2013.
35. Smith JS, et al. Prevalence and type of cervical deformity among 470 adults with thoracolumbar deformity. Spine (Phila Pa 1976). 2014;39(17):E1001–9.
36. Oh T, et al. Cervical compensatory alignment changes following correction of adult thoracic deformity: a multicenter experience in 57 patients with a 2-year follow-up. J Neurosurg Spine. 2015;22(6):658–65.
37. Smith JS, et al. Spontaneous improvement of cervical alignment after correction of global sagittal balance following pedicle subtraction osteotomy. J Neurosurg Spine. 2012;17(4):300–7.
38. Knott PT, et al. The use of the T1 sagittal angle in predicting overall sagittal balance of the spine. Spine J. 2010;10(11):994–8.
39. Klineberg EO, et al. Can measurements on cervical radiographs predict concurrent thoracolumbar deformity and provide a threshold for acquiring full-length spine radiographs? Spine J. 2015;15(10):S146.
40. Ghobrial GM, et al. Changes in cervical alignment after multilevel Schwab grade II thoracolumbar osteotomies for adult spinal deformity. Spine (Phila Pa 1976). 2018;43(2):E82–91.
41. Ames CP, et al. Reliability assessment of a novel cervical spine deformity classification system. J Neurosurg Spine. 2015;23(6):673–83.

Degenerative Cervical Myelopathy: A Spectrum of Degenerative Spondylopathies

4

Aria Nouri, Jean-Christophe Murray, and Michael G. Fehlings

Introduction

Degenerative cervical myelopathy (DCM) is an overarching term that describes the various age-related and progressive changes of intervertebral discs, ligaments, and vertebrae, which result in spinal cord impairment through static and dynamic injury mechanisms. At the present time, there remain a large number of ICD-10 codes that describe conditions that may fall under DCM (Table 4.1). The term DCM was recently introduced with the growing recognition that these patients present with a constellation of the aforementioned anatomical changes and that previous diagnostic delineation within this group had not been clear in the literature [54]. These factors have ultimately impeded knowledge dissemination and have resulted in under-recognition of the collective importance of this spectrum of disorders in the healthcare community. Following the introduction of the term, a guideline development for the management of patients with DCM, with sponsorship from the Cervical Spine Research Society and AOSpine, has been formulated. Previous guidelines by AANS/CNS focused on the surgical management of cervical spondylotic myelopathy and were published in 2009 [42]. However, these guidelines have been somewhat outdated given the recent introduction of the term DCM and publication of prospective and multicenter studies on the surgical management of DCM. The AANS/CNS spine section guidelines are slated to be updated in 2019.

Diagnostic entities that fall under DCM include degenerative disc disease, cervical osteoarthritis (spondylosis), spondylolisthesis or subluxation, and hypertrophy, calcification, or ossification of spinal ligaments (ligamentum flavum, posterior longitudinal ligament) (Fig. 4.1). These anatomical changes result in static compression of the cord due to spinal canal stenosis, cervical spine instability that can result in dynamic injury, and changes in the sagittal alignment that can result in altered cord tension and blood supply [3, 27, 54]. While the constellation of degenerative changes and underlying genetic predisposition uniquely affects individual patients, the unifying principle underlying the pathophysiology of DCM is spinal cord injury that is typically progressive in nature and a response to these changes.

In addition to neck pain and altered range of neck motion, DCM patients can present with great heterogeneity of clinical findings suggestive of

A. Nouri
Department of Neurosurgery, Yale University and University of Cincinnati, Cincinnati, OH, USA

J.-C. Murray · M. G. Fehlings (✉)
Division of Neurosurgery and Spine Program, Toronto Western Hospital, University of Toronto, Toronto, ON, Canada
e-mail: Michael.Fehlings@uhn.ca

M. G. Kaiser et al. (eds.), *Degenerative Cervical Myelopathy and Radiculopathy*,
https://doi.org/10.1007/978-3-319-97952-6_4

Table 4.1 International classification of diseases, tenth revision (ICD-10) list of condition that may be used to described cervical condition resulting in myelopathy

Classification group	Specific category
M25: Other joint disorders, not elsewhere classified	M25.3: Other instability of joint
	M25.7: Osteophyte
	M25.9: Joint disorder, unspecified
M43: Other deforming dorsopathies	M43.3: Recurrent atlantoaxial sub luxation with myelopathy
	M43.4: Other recurrent atlantoaxial subluxation
	M43.5: Other recurrent vertebral subluxation
M47: Spondylosis (including arthrosis or osteoarthritis, spine degeneration of facet joints)	M47.1: Other spondylosis with myelopathy
	M47.9: Spondylosis, unspecified
M48: Other spondylopathies	M43.0: Spinal stenosis
	M43.S: Other specified spondylopathies (including OPLL)
	M43.9: Spondylopathy, unspecified
M50: Cervical disc disorders (including cervical disc disorders with cervicalgia cervicothoracic disc disorders)	M50.0+: Cervical disc disorder with myelopathy
	M50.2: Other cervical disc displacement
	M50.3: Other cervical disc degeneration
	M50.8: Other cervical disc disorders
	M50.9: Cervical disc disorder unspecified

Nouri et al. [54]
OPLL indicates ossification of the posterior longitudinal ligament

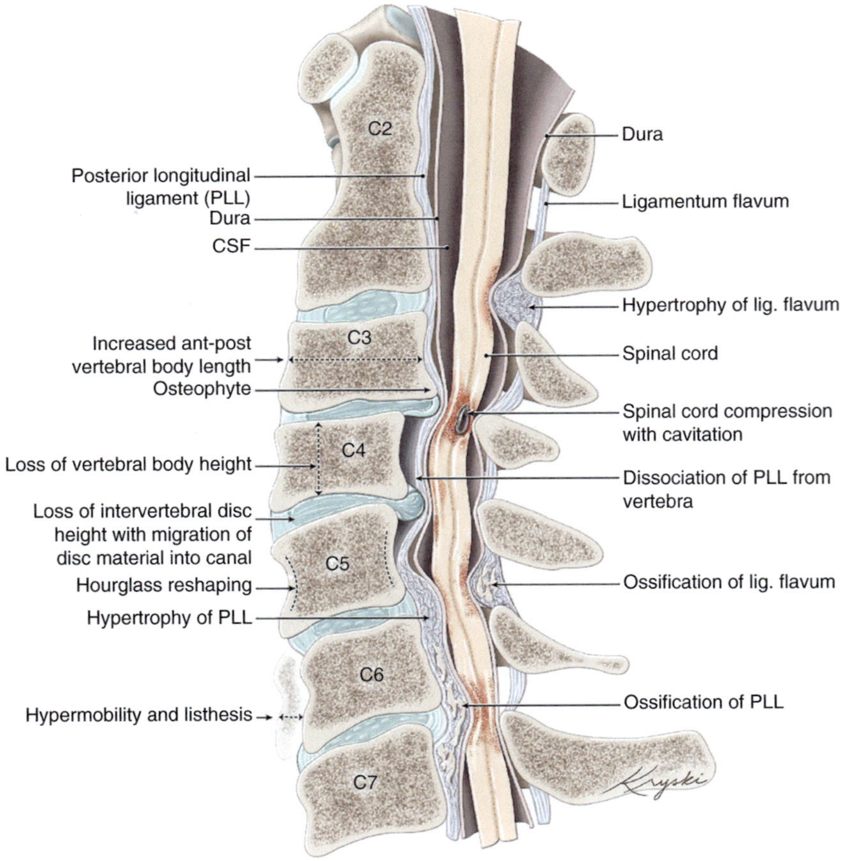

Fig. 4.1 An artistic depiction of the constellation of degenerative changes that may present in patients with DCM. (Conceptual design by Aria Nouri, edits by Michael Fehlings, and medical illustration by Diana Kryski (Kryski Biomedia))

myelopathy on physical examination. Symptoms include motor and sensory loss, usually most pronounced in the hands but also present in the lower limbs. In addition, patients typically present with loss of proprioception and impairment of gait, which is commonly broad-based in nature. These findings can be corroborated with the presence of clinical signs of myelopathy including hyperreflexia, Hoffman's sign, Babinski's response, a failed Romberg test, and ankle clonus [25, 65].

The present chapter will begin with a new perspective on the epidemiology of DCM. Subsequent sections of this chapter will describe the various pathophysiological processes of the aging spine and the impact of these changes on the spinal cord. Finally, genetic and anatomical risk factors that can predispose patients to DCM are briefly described.

Epidemiology

DCM is the most common cause of nontraumatic spinal cord injury in adults in developed nations [47, 54]. The average age at presentation has been estimated to be in the 50–60s [48, 54], but it is difficult to provide a precise estimate, as many patients who are mildly impaired or who do not seek treatment are not captured. This estimate is supported, however, by two recent AOSpine prospective and multicenter studies representing a global cohort of DCM patients undergoing surgical treatment, where the average age of patients was 56 years [14, 15]. It has also been widely reported that men present more commonly than women, with an estimated ratio of 3:2 and higher [48, 54]. It has been recently shown that despite comparable neurological impairment at presentation, men have worse MRI evidence of DCM than women (e.g., higher prevalence of T2 hyperintensity of the cord and more levels of spinal cord compression) [52].

Incidence and Prevalence of DCM

The incidence and prevalence of myelopathy due to degeneration of the spine are estimated at a minimum of 4.1 and 60.5 per 100,000 in North America, respectively [54], and the incidence of DCM-related hospitalization has been estimated at 4.04 per 100,000 person-years in Taiwan [75]. While some patients, particularly those with risk factors, can present at a younger age, the occurrence of DCM is largely dictated by age and accumulation of wear and tear. As a consequence, the aging population and increased recognition of potential DCM among elderly patients by primary care physicians are expected to result in an increased prevalence of the disorder. Indeed, research has indicated a rise in surgical treatments for DCM [35]. However, there remains only limited epidemiological data available at the present time to provide a clear picture of the increased impact of DCM in the coming years.

Spectrum of Degenerative Cervical Myelopathy Presentation

There has been little research describing the spectrum of pathologies present in patients with DCM. Recently, however, MRIs from the two AOSpine prospective and multicenter studies from a global cohort were analyzed to define the constellation of disorders presenting in patients with DCM. The authors described specific pathologies and criteria for their reporting (Table 4.2). Therein, it was reported that the vast majority of patients with DCM present with spondylosis (~90%) and accompanying ligamentum flavum hypertrophy (>50%). Single-disc pathology, spondylolisthesis, and OPLL were present in approximately 10% of patients in the global cohort, but Asians presented with a statistically greater prevalence of OPLL (Asia = 29% vs. others = 4.8%, $p = 0.3 \times 10^{-11}$), as has been previously reported [40, 54]. Interestingly, Asians also presented with a statistically lower rate of spondylolisthesis (Asia = 1.9% vs. others = 14.8%, $p = 0.002$). While not statistically significant, South Americans presented with an increased rate of ligamentum flavum hypertrophy (South America = 65.5% vs. others = 55.5%), and Europeans had a much lower rate of congenital stenosis (Europe = 2.3% vs. others = 9.4%).

The most common level of maximum spinal cord compression was C5–C6 region (39.5%), which reflects clinical experience and has also been reported by a smaller study [48]. The next

Table 4.2 Definition for the MRI diagnostic criteria

Diagnosis	Criteria
Isolated disc pathology	Single-level disc herniation/bulging disc, with no other disc pathology contributing to spinal cord compression at other levels
Multilevel disc pathology with or without bore changes (spondylosis)	Spinal cord compression at multiple levels due to multilevel cervical spine degeneration with two or more degenerated discs, with or without associated bony changes
Ossification of the posterior longitudinal ligament (OPLL)	OPLL appears hypointense on both T1 W1 and T2 W1. Effacement of the CSF anterior to the cord on T2 W1 as well as spinal cord compression that is contiguous across multiple levels, or in the absence of spondylotic changes, is highly suggestive of ligament pathology
Ligamentum flavum buckling, hypertrophy, calcification, or ossification	Any posterior enlargement of the ligamentum flavum contributing to stenosis of the cervical canal
Spondylo listhesis or subluxation	Anterior or posterior displacement of the vertebral body/bodies in relation to adjacent levels on sagittal imaging
Klippel-Feil syndrome	Vertebral levels without a complete disc and a wasp-waist sign. Absent discs due to degenerative autofusion were disregarded
Craniocervical junction abnormalities	Abnormal structural pathologies resulting in spinal cord or brain stem compression
Congenital stenosis	Patients with a spinal cord occupation ratio (SCOR) of ≥70% in the spinal canal at non-pathological sites

From Permission (Nouri et al. [52])

most common sites of maximum compression were in descending order of prevalence C4–C5, C3–C4, and C6–C7. In terms of cord signal changes on MRI, the prevalence of T2 hyperintensity across multiple studies has been reported within a range of 58–85% [51].

Pathophysiology of Degenerative Cervical Myelopathy

It is generally accepted that mechanical compression of the spinal cord is the primary pathophysiologic pathway leading to myelopathy. Several anatomic structures of the spine can be involved in spinal cord compression: a bulging or herniated intervertebral disc, posterior osteophytes protruding in the canal, an hypertrophied or ossified posterior longitudinal ligament, infolding or ossification of the flavum, and osteoarthritic uncovertebral and apophyseal joints (Fig. 4.2). In many cases, a combination of static compression coming from these structures, in addition to dynamic factors secondary to abnormal motion between unstable spine segments, can lead to myelopathy. Finally, altered cord tension, compromised vascular supply, and chronic repetitive microtrauma are likely to be contributory to the natural history of DCM.

In the following paragraphs, the discussion on the pathogenesis of DCM will be divided into (1) factors related to cervical osteoarthritis; (2) ossification, hypertrophy, and calcification of spinal ligaments (i.e., non-osteoarthritic causes); and (3) mechanisms and pathobiology of spinal cord compression as a result of the two previous factors.

Cervical Osteoarthritis

Degenerative osteoarthritis of the cervical spine, termed cervical spondylosis, is the result of multiple alterations in the normal anatomy of the vertebral body and intervertebral disc (Fig. 4.1). It is generally accepted that the disc degeneration is the initiating step in the development of a spondylotic spine [16, 26]. With progressive aging and wear of the cervical spine, the intervertebral disc and subsequently the uncovertebral joints degenerate and become flattened, altering the weight-bearing and load-transferring capacities of the vertebral segment. The facet joints become hypermobile and lax, causing abnormal cervical spine biomechanics, instability, and spondylolisthesis [51]. This puts greater stress on the cartilaginous end plates and promotes the formation of osteophytic spurs as a result of bone remodelling and in

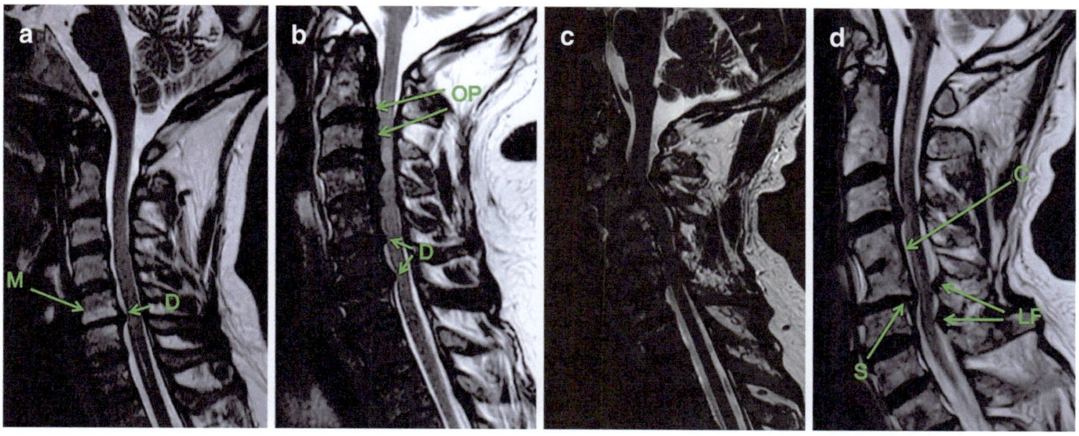

Fig. 4.2 Sagittal T2WI MRIs of patients with DCM. (**a**) A single-level disc degeneration resulting in spinal cord compression (D). Also shown here are hyperintensity changes of the end plate consistent with Type I or II Modic changes (M). (**b**) A patient with ossification of the posterior longitudinal ligament (OP) and disc degeneration (D). (**c**) A patient with severe multilevel bone and disc degeneration (spondylosis) and substantial kyphotic deformity. (**d**) A patient with congenital fusion of the C4 and C5 vertebrae (C) also referred to as Klippel-Feil syndrome. In addition, there is spondylolisthesis evident at the inferior end of the fused vertebrae (S) as well as enlargement of the ligamentum flavum (LF). (Nouri et al. [52])

an attempt to stabilize adjacent vertebrae [6, 16, 54]. In addition, there is loss of vertebral body height and an increase in the anterior-posterior diameter. This vertebral segment restructuring promotes canal size narrowing, which can be compounded by a preexisting congenitally narrow canal. In a study of 295 patients with neck pain with or without neurological symptoms, Morishita et al. [45] found that an anteroposterior cervical spinal canal diameter of less than 13 mm was associated with an increased risk of developing intervertebral disc degeneration and cervical spinal stenosis. In other words, a congenitally narrow canal lowers the threshold at which the various spondylotic changes in the cervical spine can ultimately encroach the spinal cord and cause myelopathy [8]. The final result of these degenerative changes is static and dynamic injury by repetitive microtrauma on the compressed cord during flexion and extension of the cervical spine [54].

Non-osteoarthritic Pathophysiology

In addition to degenerative changes affecting the intervertebral disc and segmental joints of the cervical spine, age-related changes to spinal ligaments (posterior longitudinal ligament (PLL) and ligamentum flavum (LF)) have been involved in the pathophysiology of DCM [54]. Both hypertrophy and ossification of these two ligaments, namely, ossification of the PLL (OPLL) and ossification of the ligamentum flavum (OLF), have been described. A multifactorial pathogenesis involving progressive age-related changes, local tissue characteristics, associated medical comorbidities, and genetic factors (described in details below) has been implicated in the final common pathway of hypertrophy and ossification of the spinal ligaments [4]. Hypertrophy of the PLL has been suggested to precede ossification [23] and can also result from a nucleus pulposus protrusion [43]. Stiffening and dynamic infolding of the LF have been linked to cervical joint spondylosis and loss of intervertebral disc height [6, 51]. OPLL is a well-studied form of spinal ligament ossification that is especially encountered in Asian populations with an incidence up to 3% [4, 52]. Radiographically, OPLL is classified based on its distribution into (1) localized, i.e., a solitary lesion involving one vertebral level; (2) segmental, i.e., multiple separate lesions; (3) continuous, i.e., a long, single lesion involving multiple levels; or (4) mixed, i.e., combining features of the previous three types [58, 68]. OPLL is typically a progressive disease that leads to increasingly severe cervical stenosis and myelopathy. In a cohort study of 207 patients followed during an average period of 10 years, myelopathy was diagnosed before or during the follow-up period in 70 patients (34%). The authors of this study highlighted the role of dynamic factors in the development of myelopathy in OPLL since patients with limited cervical motion tended to have less myelopathy progression [41]. OLF is another disease particularly common among Asians, where it has been radiographically found to some extent in >7% of volunteers greater than 45 years of age [18]. The occurrence of OLF is typically more common in the thoracic region; however, thoracic lesions are more likely to be asymptomatic than cervical [1]. In rare instances, OLF can occur concomitantly with OPLL, which has been referred to as "tandem ossification" [60]. Ultimately, OPLL and OLF result in anterior and posterior impingement on the spinal cord, respectively, and static cord compression.

Mechanisms and Pathobiology of Spinal Cord Compression

In addition to the aforementioned factors leading to anterior and/or posterior static cord compression, it has been shown that abnormal or excessive motion of the cervical spine by itself can be associated with progressive myelopathy [7, 20]. During daily range of motion, the cross-sectional diameter and space available for the spinal cord change as a result of dynamic compression [76] (Fig. 4.3). Flexion of the cervical spine may result in tensioning of the cord on an anterior disc bulge or osteochondral bar. In extension, LF infolding and hypertrophy can further increase cord compression [36]. This dynamic injury mechanism is exacerbated in patients with significant preexisting static compression. For example, in a prospective study on the natural history of patients with myelopathy from OPLL, Matsunaga et al. [39] found that patients with a space available for the cord (SAC) less than 6 mm all had myelopathy, whereas no myelopathy was present in patients with a SAC 14 mm or greater. Interestingly, when SAC was greater than 6 mm but less than 14 mm, myelopathy was preferentially found in those with increased range of motion of the cervical spine. Given these results, this study suggests that dynamic injury mechanism has a critical role in the development of myelopathy, especially in patients with a compromised canal diameter. In addition to excessive range of motion, dynamic injury may occur in the setting of cervical instability

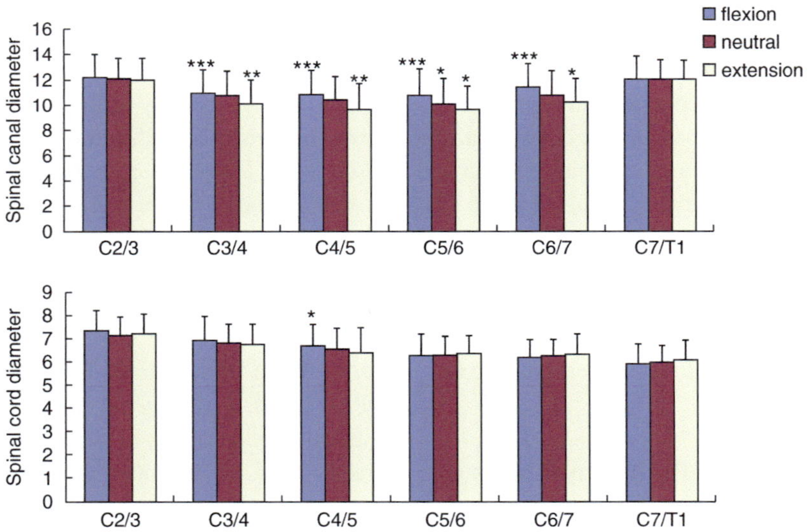

Fig. 4.3 The space available for the spinal cord. Comparing flexion with extension, neutral with flexion, and extension with neutral at each level. ASAC and PSAC were compared with each other at each level. *P < 0.05, **P < 0.01, ***P < 0.001. # represent the higher bar. #P < 0.05, ##P < 0.01, ###P < 0.001. ASAC indicates anterior space available for the cord; PSAC, posterior space available for the cord. (From Permission Xiong et al. [76])

(degenerative spondylolisthesis) and through minor repetitive trauma in the setting of preexisting DCM [54].

A number of pathobiological mechanisms have been studied in the setting of spinal cord compression, including hypoxic ischemic insult, chronic inflammatory response, demyelination, atrophy, and apoptosis of neural tissue [36]. These studies have investigated the role of vascular factors in the setting of cord compression, and it has been suggested that chronic cervical cord compression results in a reduction of the intraparenchymal spinal cord blood flow [27]. In addition it has been suggested that cord tension and kyphosis can result in flattening of blood vessels and reduction of blood flow as well [3]. In response to these changes, chronic ischemia generates a unique inflammatory response in the spinal cord parenchyma, characterized by persistent activation of microglia and macrophage recruitment and accumulation [26, 54]. It has been shown using rodent models of cervical myelopathy that chronic cervical spinal cord compression leads to compromise of the microvasculature, blood-spinal cord barrier disruption, inflammation, and activation of apoptotic signaling pathways, which inevitably potentiates the inflammatory response already initiated by immune cell accumulation and activation [29, 54, 78]. The final common pathway of this compression-mediated inflammatory reaction leads to white and gray matter degeneration, cystic cavitation, gliosis, and atrophy of the anterior horns associated with motoneuronal loss. These pathobiological changes are responsible for the clinical constellation of symptoms (fine motor dysfunction, spasticity, gait disturbances, etc.) seen in DCM [25]. The key pathophysiologic features seen in DCM are summarized in Fig. 4.4.

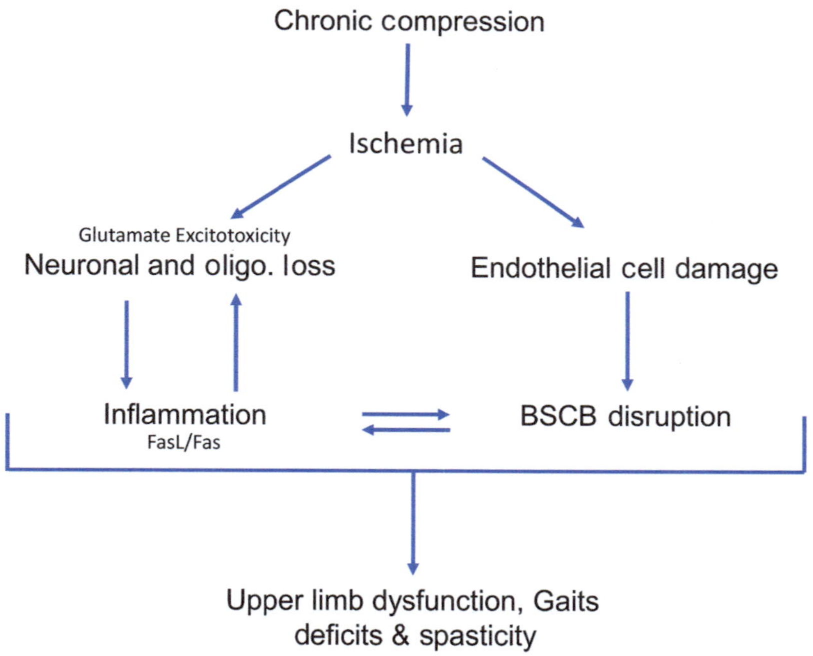

Fig. 4.4 Current knowledge about degenerative cervical myelopathy. Progressive compression of the cervical spinal cord causes a chronic hypoxic/ischemic insult that damages oligodendrocytes (oligo) and neurons, eliciting an inflammatory response. Furthermore, the compression-induced ischemic state leads to endothelial cell loss – disrupting the neurovascular unit (NVU) and leading to compromise of the blood-spinal cord barrier (BSCB). BSCB permeability and inflammation have been demonstrated in the chronic stages of DCM. Inflammation can potentiate the initial cellular loss and BSCB permeability. It is thought that the enhanced cross talk between the peripheral immune system and the spinal cord microenvironment, which occurs in DCM through the impaired BSCB, potentiates inflammation. Moreover, it has been suggested that inflammatory Fas ligand (FasL) signaling can lead to apoptosis of neurons and oligodendrocytes. Neuronal loss and axonal damage are responsible for the upper limb dysfunction, spasticity, and gait disturbances seen in humans with DCM. (Kalsi-Ryan et al. [25])

Greater understanding of these pathophysiological events has provided potential pharmacological targets for treatment of DCM. It has recently been shown, for instance, that apoptosis is mediated by Fas and that blocking the Fas ligand reduced neural inflammation mediated by macrophages, activated microglia, glial scar formation, and caspase-9 activation [78]. Furthermore, there is currently a Phase III investigation involving the perioperative administration of riluzole, which is a sodium glutamate channel blocker approved for the treatment of amyotrophic lateral sclerosis.[1] It is believed that decompression of the spinal cord during surgery can result in reperfusion injury via glutamate excitotoxicity, and it is believed that riluzole may be able to attenuate this phenomenon and improve surgical outcomes [28, 44].

Genetic and Congenital Factors

There is an increasing evidence that genetic and congenital factors play a role in the development of DCM [54, 61, 74]. Genetic factors can influence the natural degenerative process by predisposing disc degeneration and bone remodelling (spondylosis) or may promote the aberrant enlargement and ossification of intraspinal ligaments. Congenital factors that impact the typical anatomical architecture can promote the development of DCM by altering spine biomechanics, which may result in accelerated degeneration, or reduce the threshold of degenerative changes required to cause myelopathy (Table 4.2).

Genetic Factors

Genetic factors potentially involved in DCM development can be separated into two broad groups, those that impact disc degeneration and bone remodelling and those that influence the enlargement and ossification of spinal ligaments, including the posterior longitudinal ligament and ligamentum flavum. This segregation is largely based on the natural history of these conditions but also on genetic studies.

Disc Degeneration and Vertebral Remodelling (Spondylosis)

The first reports to investigate a potential genetic predisposition to spondylosis were studies that involved reviewing degenerative patterns on radiographs of identical twins [11, 59]. More recent studies have looked at specific allele polymorphism [66, 72, 73] and genealogical index of familiality [61]. Setzer et al. [66] investigated APOE, whose allele ε4 has shown to be associated with Alzheimer's disease, and assessed whether specific APOE alleles were related with DCM. The authors showed that APOE ε4 was significantly associated with cervical spondylotic myelopathy on multivariate analysis and concluded that it may be an independent predictor of cervical spondylotic myelopathy occurrence. Wang et al. [72] investigated specific polymorphism of the vitamin D receptor (VDR), given its role in bone metabolism and reports that certain VDR polymorphisms are associated with degenerative disc disease in the lumbar spine. The authors showed that the ApaI A and TaqI T alleles were associated with a significantly higher risk of DCM development with an odds ratio of 2.88 and 4.67, respectively. Another interesting genetic association was made between the collagen IX Trp2 allele and development of cervical spondylotic myelopathy [73]. Interestingly, these authors showed that this risk was directly related to smoking status, with greater consumption of cigarettes and presence of collagen IX Trp2 allele resulting in a significantly increased risk for cervical spondylotic myelopathy development [73]. Most recently, Patel et al. [61] assessed a genealogical database of over 2 million Utah residents and showed that there was a 5.21 relative risk ($p < 0.001$) for cervical spondylotic myelopathy development among first-degree relatives.

While a number of other genetic investigations have looked specifically at disc degeneration, these studies are likely to also indirectly associate with spondylosis, as the natural history of spondylosis begins with disc degeneration. These studies have implicated a wide array of

[1] https://clinicaltrials.gov/ct2/show/NCT01257828

Table 4.3 Genes associated with the development and progression of degenerative disc disease

Gene	Functions	
MMP-2	Degradation of collagen typo IV major structural component of basement membrane. Regulated in part by thrombospandins.	Inhibited by TIMP-2
MMP-3	Degradation of collagens II, III, IV, IX, and X; proteoglycans; fibronectin; laminin and elastin. Activator of MMP-1, -7, -9 and a facilitator of wound repair and initiation of tumorigenesis.	MMP-3 promoter stimulated by growth factors and cytokines as well as tumors and oncogenes. TIMP-1 inhibited
MMP-9	Key effector of ECV remodeling. Also known as a type IV collagenase (gelatinase-B). Increased activity in DDD.	
ADAMTS	ADAMTS-4 and -5 major players in degradation of cartilage in general and aggrecan in particular. ADAMTS4 in particular plays a major role in the progression of DDD.	
IL-1β	IL-1β is a critical cytokine involved with the regulation of the ECM and turnover of extracellular matrix.	
Vitamin D receptor	Polymorphisms associated with increased risk of DDD.	
Col9A2	Encodes part of the alpha chains of type IX collagen: a major collagen component of hyaline cartilage. Usually found in tissues containing type II collagen such as the MD NP.	
IL-1 receptor	11-1 RI gene expression and protein production reported to increase in degenerated compared with non-degenerated human discs. IL-1β is a predominant factor leading to accelerated ECM breakdown in progressive DDD.	

MMP matrix metalloproteinase, *TIMP* tissue inhibitors of matalloproteinases, *ECM* extracellular matrix, *DDD* degenerative disc disease, *ADAMTS* a disinterring and metalloproteinase with thombospondin motifs, *IL* interleukin, *IVD* intervertebral disc, *NP* nucleus pulposus

genes involving collagens, interleukins, the vitamin D receptor, ADAMTS, and matrix metalloproteinases (MMP) [13, 24]. A list of these implicated genetic products and their functions are described in Table 4.3.

Hypertrophy and Ossification of Intraspinal Canal Ligaments

Support for genetic predisposition to DCM development that is predominately related to intraspinal canal ligament aberrations, including OPLL and OLF, derives from the observation that such pathologies vary greatly in prevalence across geographic regions. Most notably, it has been shown that East Asian patients have a higher risk for OPLL development. Indeed, population prevalence rates have been reported to be as high as 4.3% in the Japanese [23, 54], and a survey on 1030 relatives from 347 Japanese families of patients with OPLL revealed that 26% of parents and 29% of siblings had radiographic evidence of OPLL [70]. Multiple genetic products have been studied and related to OPLL development, with the most significant and promising implicating single nucleotide polymorphisms in collagen 6 [COL6A1/Intron 32(−29)] and 11 [COL11A2/Intron 6(−4))] [33, 69, 74]. While others have shown associations with OPLL development with other genetic products including genes encoding retinoic X receptor β [56], BMP 2 [71] and 4 [64], and IL-15R [30], these have not been reproduced by other studies. Recently, it has also been proposed that genetic factors may differ depending on the morphology of OPLL (continuous vs. segmental) based on mRNA expression of Osterix production and alkaline phosphatase activity [34]. Overall, while these studies have provided some evidence to support a genetic association, the limited amount of literature and lack of validation studies require that further investigation be conducted to demonstrate a more definitive relationship [74].

As with OPLL, reports of higher prevalence rates of OLF among East Asians have suggested that there may be genetic factors involved. Animal studies have also supported a genetic role – a mouse model with a homozygous mutation in the NPPS gene (twy/twy) specifically develops OLF at C2–C3 [77]. Unfortunately, however, there is little evidence in terms of human studies to support a genetic predisposition. This may be partly due to its relatively low occurrence compared to OPLL. Furthermore, it is also challenging to ascribe specific genetic factors to OLF, as it has often been studied along with OPLL, making it challenging to determine whether there are genetic factors that are distinct from those implicated in OPLL. There is some evidence showing that haplotype 4 of the COL6A1 gene is related with OLF, whereas haplotype 1 was associated with OPLL [33]. However, the same authors found that that intron 33 (+20) and promoter (−572) SNPs of COL6A1 were associated with both OPLL and OLF [33]. It has also been shown that RUNX2 may be related with both OLF and OPLL [32, 38].

The observation that OLF and OPLL can occur in tandem suggests that genetic factors may be implicated in a general predisposition to ossification of spinal ligaments [32, 33, 38]. Indeed, this finding is not limited to only intraspinal ligaments. Diffuse idiopathic skeletal hyperostosis (DISH) is a condition where patients present with substantial ossification of the anterior longitudinal ligament, and it can manifest with diffuse ossification of the PLL and LF and result in myelopathy development [49]. Collectively, these findings indicate that there are likely to be distinct genetic factors that contribute to specific ligament ossification (such as OPLL) and others that are involved in a general increased propensity for cervical ligament ossification.

Congenital Factors

Congenital factors may accelerate degenerative changes in the cervical spine or reduce the threshold of degenerative changes necessary to cause DCM. These include congenital cervical fusions (Klippel-Feil syndrome), trisomy 21 (Down's syndrome), and congenital cervical spinal stenosis. Other conditions, particularly those which impact fibrous tissue, such as Ehlers-Danlos syndrome [19], may also predispose patients with DCM, but there is little research to support this relationship.

Klippel-Feil Syndrome (KFS)

A number of genetic conditions have been identified that impact vertebral segmentation during early gestation [17]. Many of these conditions tend to be quite severe however, while isolated cervical spine fusions are often discovered incidentally (Fig. 4.2d). Indeed, while most cases of KFS appear to occur sporadically, autosomal dominant, autosomal recessive, and X-linked genetic factors affecting PAXl, GDF6, and others have been reported [17].

It has been previously hypothesized that patients with KFS are predisposed to DCM due to increased wear and hypermobility at adjacent segments [50, 55, 63]. Biomechanically increased wear would be expected, as these fusions create a spontaneous lever arm, which places increased stress on the adjacent disc segment. Clinically, this mechanism is supported by the findings that patients receiving anterior surgical fusions for DCM are also predisposed to adjacent segment pathology [21, 22].

The prevalence of the KFS in the general population has been estimated at 0.71% [10], while the prevalence of the recent AOSpine global studies on DCM reported a prevalence of 2.4%. In this study it was estimated that the relative risk of DCM development in patients with KFS was 3.3 [50]. While baseline severity and surgical outcome did not appear to be different in patients with DCM with or without KFS, the degenerative pattern tended to be different. Adjacent segments tended to be more commonly affected, but more interestingly, pathology of adjacent segments preferentially occurred toward the mid-cervical regions.

Trisomy 21 (Down's Syndrome, DS)

Patients with DS have been reported to be at risk for DCM due to congenital abnormalities in the craniocervical junction including atlantoaxial instability, odontoid abnormalities, atlanto-occipital abnormalities, and hypoplasia of the posterior arch of C1 [9, 57]. It has been estimated that atlantoaxial instability occurs in 10–20% of patients with DS, of whom 1–2% present with symptomatic spinal cord compression [2]. While it is true that the average life expectancy of patients with DS is lower than the average, improvement in care has resulted in a significant increase in their life expectancy – it is therefore expected that the incidence of DCM among this population is likely to increase [54, 67].

Congenital Cervical Spinal Stenosis (CSS)

Cervical spinal stenosis (CSS) indirectly predisposes to the development of DCM due to two key factors: (1) it lowers the threshold of degenerative changes necessary to cause spinal cord compression and (2) due to a reduction in the amount of CSF surrounding the spinal cord, there is a reduced capacity to withstand dynamic forces directed at the spine [12, 53, 54]. This is supported by research showing that these CSS patients are predisposed to acute traumatic spinal cord injury and neurapraxia in athletes. Previous criteria for CSS include a Torg-Pavlov ratio of ≤0.82 [62] or an anteroposterior canal diameter of <12–13 mm [5, 37] (Fig. 4.5). Unfortunately, these parameters are applicable to patients without degenerative disease, largely derive from cadaveric studies, and do not take into account the size of the spinal cord within the canal. Recently, a new MRI diagnostic criterion called the spinal cord occupation ratio (SCOR) of ≥70% that measured the size of cord within the canal has been proposed to diagnose CSS to address these limitations [53] (Fig. 4.6). The technique measures the midsagittal spinal cord diameter and spinal canal diameter at the nearest normal adjacent segments above and below the site of compression in patients with DCM. As these patients typically present with compression in the mid-cervical levels, normal segments are typically measured at C3 and C7. SCOR is then calculated by dividing the mean cord diameter by the mean canal diameter and multiplying by 100. It has been demonstrated that patients with DCM and preexisting CSS presented 5.5 years younger on average and with worse neurological impairment; however, surgical outcome between patients with or without CSS did not differ [53].

The genetic basis for CSS is largely unknown, and it is likely simply a normal population

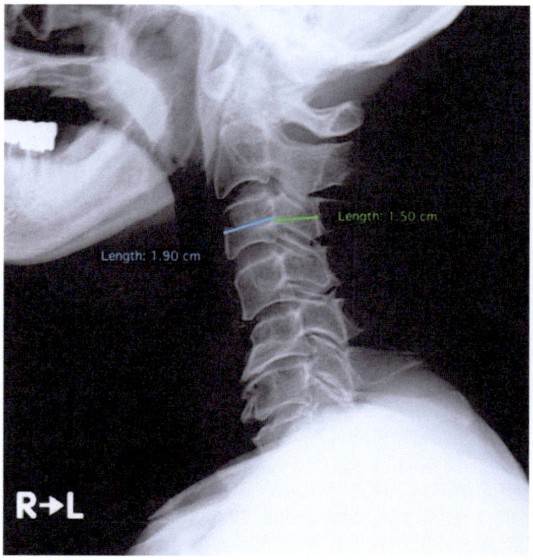

Fig. 4.5 A lateral radiograph of a patient with DCM with Torg-Pavlov measurements is presented. By dividing the spinal canal diameter (1.50 cm) and dividing it by the mid-vertebral anterior-posterior length (1.90 cm), a Torg-Pavlov ratio of 0.789 is computed at C3

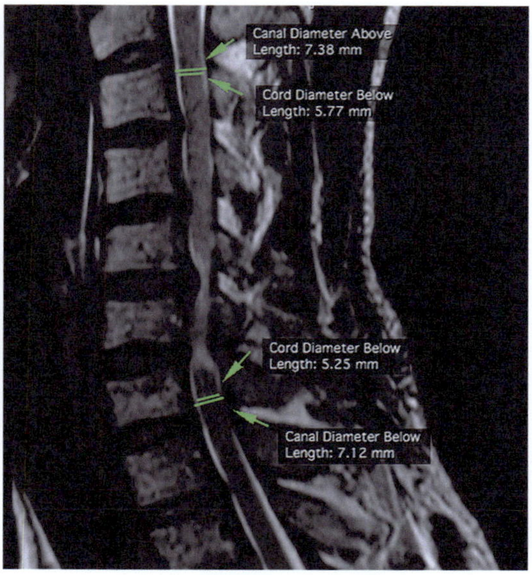

Fig. 4.6 A midsagittal T2WI MRI showing a patient with severe congenital cervical spinal stenosis. The spinal cord occupation rate (SCOR) in this patient was 76% [(5.77 + 5.25)/(7.38 + 7.12)] × 100. (Nouri et al. [52])

variation. However, some conditions have been reported to potentially present with CSS, including achondroplasia and KFS [31, 46].

Conclusion

A multitude of degenerative changes can present in patients with DCM, and patients with risk factors may have a greater predisposition to develop symptoms at an earlier age than otherwise expected. The unifying problem in patients with DCM remains spinal cord injury that is typically progressive in nature. However, this injury can manifest due to direct cord compression, dynamic forces directed at the cord, altered cord tension that can arise from tethering, and frequently a combination of these factors. Therefore, the disease process, natural history, and subsequent treatment strategies will remain unique to each patient.

It is clear that DCM is becoming increasingly prevalent worldwide, but there remain ongoing difficulties in identifying these patients at the primary care level due to the lack of awareness of the impact, prevalence, and importance of this condition by the public. Increasing awareness and understanding potential risk factors as well as the underlying pathologic process can help to identify patients before they become significantly neurologically impaired. Unfortunately, however, it remains unclear when and which asymptomatic patients with spinal cord compression will become myelopathic and require treatment. While guideline development will help to address this, longitudinal studies to evaluate the natural history of DCM are needed and would be a significant contribution to the field.

References

1. Al-Jarallah K, Al-Saeed O, Shehab D, Dashti K, Sheikh M. Ossification of ligamentum flavum in Middle East Arabs: a hospital-based study. Med Princ Pract. 2012;21:529–33.
2. Ali FE, Al-Bustan MA, Al-Busairi WA, Al-Mulla FA, Esbaita EY. Cervical spine abnormalities associated with down syndrome. Int Orthop. 2006;30:284–9.
3. Ames CP, Blondel B, Scheer JK, Schwab FJ, Le Huec JC, Massicotte EM, Patel AA, Traynelis VC, Kim HJ, Shaffrey CI, Smith JS, Lafage V. Cervical radiographical alignment: comprehensive assessment techniques and potential importance in cervical myelopathy. Spine (Phila Pa 1976). 2013;38:S149–60.
4. An HS, Al-Shihabi L, Kurd M. Surgical treatment for ossification of the posterior longitudinal ligament in the cervical spine. J Am Acad Orthop Surg. 2014;22:420–9.
5. Bajwa NS, Toy JO, Young EY, Ahn NU. Establishment of parameters for congenital stenosis of the cervical spine: an anatomic descriptive analysis of 1,066 cadaveric specimens. Eur Spine J. 2012;21:2467–74.
6. Baptiste DC, Fehlings MG. Pathophysiology of cervical myelopathy. Spine J. 2006;6:190S–7S.
7. Barnes MP, Saunders M. The effect of cervical mobility on the natural history of cervical spondylotic myelopathy. J Neurol Neurosurg Psychiatry. 1984;47:17–20.
8. Bernhardt M, Hynes RA, Blume HW, White AA 3rd. Cervical spondylotic myelopathy. J Bone Joint Surg Am. 1993;75:119–28.
9. Bosma GP, Van Buchem MA, Voormolen JH, Van Biezen FC, Brouwer OF. Cervical spondylarthrotic myelopathy with early onset in Down's syndrome: five cases and a review of the literature. J Intellect Disabil Res. 1999;43(Pt 4):283–8.
10. Brown MW, Templeton AW, Hodges FJ 3rd. The incidence of acquired and congenital fusions in the cervical spine. Am J Roentgenol Radium Therapy, Nucl Med. 1964;92:1255–9.
11. Bull J, El Gammal T, Popham M. A possible genetic factor in cervical spondylosis. Br J Radiol. 1969;42:9–16.
12. Countee RW, Vijayanathan T. Congenital stenosis of the cervical spine: diagnosis and management. J Natl Med Assoc. 1979;71:257–64.
13. Erwin WM, Fehlings MG. Intervertebral disc degeneration: genes hold the key. World Neurosurg. 2013;80:e131–3.
14. Fehlings MG, Ibrahim A, Tetreault L, Albanese V, Alvarado M, Arnold P, Barbagallo G, Bartels R, Bolger C, Defino H, Kale S, Massicotte E, Moraes O, Scerrati M, Tan G, Tanaka M, Toyone T, Yukawa Y, Zhou Q, Zileli M, Kopjar B. A global perspective on the outcomes of surgical decompression in patients with cervical spondylotic myelopathy: results from the prospective multicenter AOSpine international study on 479 patients. Spine (Phila Pa 1976). 2015;40:1322–8.
15. Fehlings MG, Wilson JR, Kopjar B, Yoon ST, Arnold PM, Massicotte EM, Vaccaro AR, Brodke DS, Shaffrey CI, Smith JS, Woodard EJ, Banco RJ, Chapman JR, Janssen ME, Bono CM, Sasso RC, Dekutoski MB, Gokaslan ZL. Efficacy and safety of surgical decompression in patients with cervical spondylotic myelopathy: results of the AOSpine North America prospective multi-center study. J Bone Joint Surg Am. 2013;95:1651–8.

16. Galbusera F, Van Rijsbergen M, Ito K, Huyghe JM, Brayda-Bruno M, Wilke HJ. Ageing and degenerative changes of the intervertebral disc and their impact on spinal flexibility. Eur Spine J. 2014;23(Suppl 3):S324–32.
17. Giampietro PF, Raggio CL, Blank RD, Mccarty C, Broeckel U, Pickart MA. Clinical, genetic and environmental factors associated with congenital vertebral malformations. Mol Syndromol. 2013;4:94–105.
18. Guo JJ, Luk KD, Karppinen J, Yang H, Cheung KM. Prevalence, distribution, and morphology of ossification of the ligamentum flavum: a population study of one thousand seven hundred thirty-six magnetic resonance imaging scans. Spine (Phila Pa 1976). 2010;35:51–6.
19. Halko GJ, Cobb R, Abeles M. Patients with type IV Ehlers-Danlos syndrome may be predisposed to atlantoaxial subluxation. J Rheumatol. 1995;22:2152–5.
20. Hayashi T, Wang JC, Suzuki A, Takahashi S, Scott TP, Phan K, Lord EL, Ruangchainikom M, Shiba K, Daubs MD. Risk factors for missed dynamic canal stenosis in the cervical spine. Spine (Phila Pa 1976). 2014;39:812–9.
21. Hilibrand AS, Carlson GD, Palumbo MA, Jones PK, Bohlman HH. Radiculopathy and myelopathy at segments adjacent to the site of a previous anterior cervical arthrodesis. J Bone Joint Surg Am. 1999;81:519–28.
22. Hilibrand AS, Robbins M. Adjacent segment degeneration and adjacent segment disease: the consequences of spinal fusion? Spine J. 2004;4:190S–4S.
23. Inamasu J, Guiot BH, Sachs DC. Ossification of the posterior longitudinal ligament: an update on its biology, epidemiology, and natural history. Neurosurgery. 2006;58:1027–39. discussion 1027-39
24. Kalb S, Martirosyan NL, Kalani MY, Broc GG, Theodore N. Genetics of the degenerated intervertebral disc. World Neurosurg. 2012;77:491–501.
25. Kalsi-Ryan S, Karadimas SK, Fehlings MG. Cervical spondylotic myelopathy: the clinical phenomenon and the current pathobiology of an increasingly prevalent and devastating disorder. Neuroscientist. 2013;19:409–21.
26. Karadimas SK, Erwin WM, Ely CG, Dettori JR, Fehlings MG. Pathophysiology and natural history of cervical spondylotic myelopathy. Spine (Phila Pa 1976). 2013;38:S21–36.
27. Karadimas SK, Gatzounis G, Fehlings MG. Pathobiology of cervical spondylotic myelopathy. Eur Spine J. 2015;24(Suppl 2):132–8.
28. Karadimas SK, Laliberte AM, Tetreault L, Chung YS, Arnold P, Foltz WD, Fehlings MG. Riluzole blocks perioperative ischemia-reperfusion injury and enhances postdecompression outcomes in cervical spondylotic myelopathy. Sci Transl Med. 2015;7:316ra194.
29. Karadimas SK, Moon ES, Yu WR, Satkunendrarajah K, Kallitsis JK, Gatzounis G, Fehlings MG. A novel experimental model of cervical spondylotic myelopathy (CSM) to facilitate translational research. Neurobiol Dis. 2013;54:43–58.
30. Kim DH, Jeong YS, Chon J, Yoo SD, Kim HS, Kang SW, Chung JH, Kim KT, Yun DH. Association between interleukin 15 receptor, alpha (IL15RA) polymorphism and Korean patients with ossification of the posterior longitudinal ligament. Cytokine. 2011;55:343–6.
31. King JA, Vachhrajani S, Drake JM, Rutka JT. Neurosurgical implications of achondroplasia. J Neurosurg Pediatr. 2009;4:297–306.
32. Kishiya M, Sawada T, Kanemaru K, Kudo H, Numasawa T, Yokoyama T, Tanaka S, Motomura S, Ueyama K, Harata S, Toh S, Furukawa K. A functional RNAi screen for Runx2-regulated genes associated with ectopic bone formation in human spinal ligaments. J Pharmacol Sci. 2008;106:404–14.
33. Kong Q, Ma X, Li F, Guo Z, Qi Q, Li W, Yuan H, Wang Z, Chen Z. COL6A1 polymorphisms associated with ossification of the ligamentum flavum and ossification of the posterior longitudinal ligament. Spine (Phila Pa 1976). 2007;32:2834–8.
34. Kudo H, Furukawa K, Yokoyama T, Ono A, Numasawa T, Wada K, Tanaka S, Asari T, Ueyama K, Motomura S, Toh S. Genetic differences in the osteogenic differentiation potency according to the classification of ossification of the posterior longitudinal ligament of the cervical spine. Spine (Phila Pa 1976). 2011;36:951–7.
35. Lad SP, Patil CG, Berta S, Santarelli JG, Ho C, Boakye M. National trends in spinal fusion for cervical spondylotic myelopathy. Surg Neurol. 2009;71:66–9. discussion 69
36. Lebl DR, Bono CM. Update on the diagnosis and management of cervical spondylotic myelopathy. J Am Acad Orthop Surg. 2015;23:648–60.
37. Lee MJ, Cassinelli EH, Riew KD. Prevalence of cervical spine stenosis. Anatomic study in cadavers. J Bone Joint Surg Am. 2007;89:376–80.
38. Liu Y, Zhao Y, Chen Y, Shi G, Yuan W. Runx2 polymorphisms associated with OPLL and OLF in the Han population. Clin Orthop Relat Res. 2010;468:3333–41.
39. Matsunaga S, Kukita M, Hayashi K, Shinkura R, Koriyama C, Sakou T, Komiya S. Pathogenesis of myelopathy in patients with ossification of the posterior longitudinal ligament. J Neurosurg. 2002;96:168–72.
40. Matsunaga S, Sakou T. Ossification of the posterior longitudinal ligament of the cervical spine: etiology and natural history. Spine (Phila Pa 1976). 2012;37:E309–14.
41. Matsunaga S, Sakou T, Taketomi E, Yamaguchi M, Okano T. The natural course of myelopathy caused by ossification of the posterior longitudinal ligament in the cervical spine. Clin Orthop Relat Res. 1994:168–77.
42. Matz PG, Anderson PA, Kaiser MG, Holly LT, Groff MW, Heary RF, Mummaneni PV, Ryken TC, Choudhri TF, Vresilovic EJ, Resnick DK. Introduction and methodology: guidelines for the surgical management of cervical degenerative disease. J Neurosurg Spine. 2009;11:101–3.

43. Mizuno J, Nakagawa H, Hashizume Y. Analysis of hypertrophy of the posterior longitudinal ligament of the cervical spine, on the basis of clinical and experimental studies. Neurosurgery. 2001;49:1091–7; discussion 1097-8.
44. Moon ES, Karadimas SK, Yu WR, Austin JW, Fehlings MG. Riluzole attenuates neuropathic pain and enhances functional recovery in a rodent model of cervical spondylotic myelopathy. Neurobiol Dis. 2014;62:394–406.
45. Morishita Y, Naito M, Hymanson H, Miyazaki M, Wu G, Wang JC. The relationship between the cervical spinal canal diameter and the pathological changes in the cervical spine. Eur Spine J. 2009;18:877–83.
46. Nagib MG, Maxwell RE, Chou SN. Identification and management of high-risk patients with Klippel-Feil syndrome. J Neurosurg. 1984;61:523–30.
47. New PW, Cripps RA, Bonne Lee B. Global maps of non-traumatic spinal cord injury epidemiology: towards a living data repository. Spinal Cord. 2014;52:97–109.
48. Northover JR, Wild JB, Braybrooke J, Blanco J. The epidemiology of cervical spondylotic myelopathy. Skelet Radiol. 2012;41:1543–6.
49. Nouri A, Fehlings MG. Diffuse idiopathic skeletal hyperostosis with cervical myelopathy. CMAJ. 2017;189:E410.
50. Nouri A, Martin AR, Lange SF, Kotter MRN, Mikulis DJ, Fehlings MG. Congenital cervical fusion as a risk factor for development of degenerative cervical myelopathy. World Neurosurg. 2017;100:531–9.
51. Nouri A, Martin AR, Mikulis D, Fehlings MG. Magnetic resonance imaging assessment of degenerative cervical myelopathy: a review of structural changes and measurement techniques. Neurosurg Focus. 2016;40:E5.
52. Nouri A, Martin AR, Tetreault L, Nater A, Kato S, Nakashima H, Nagoshi N, Reihani-Kermani H, Fehlings MG. MRI analysis of the combined prospectively collected AOSpine North America and international data: the prevalence and Spectrum of pathologies in a global cohort of patients with degenerative cervical myelopathy. Spine (Phila Pa 1976). 2016;42:1058.
53. Nouri A, Tetreault L, Nori S, Martin AR, Nater A, Fehlings MG. Congenital Cervical Spine Stenosis in a Multicenter Global Cohort of Patients With Degenerative Cervical Myelopathy: An Ambispective Report Based on a Magnetic Resonance Imaging Diagnostic Criterion. Neurosurgery. 2018;83(3): 521–8.
54. Nouri A, Tetreault L, Singh A, Karadimas S, Fehlings M. Degenerative cervical myelopathy: epidemiology, genetics and pathogenesis. Spine (Phila Pa 1976). 2015;40:E675–93.
55. Nouri A, Tetreault L, Zamorano JJ, Mohanty CB, Fehlings MG. Prevalence of Klippel-Feil syndrome in a surgical series of patients with cervical Spondylotic myelopathy: analysis of the prospective, multicenter AOSpine North America study. Global Spine J. 2015;5:294–9.
56. Numasawa T, Koga H, Ueyama K, Maeda S, Sakou T, Harata S, Leppert M, Inoue I. Human retinoic X receptor beta: complete genomic sequence and mutation search for ossification of posterior longitudinal ligament of the spine. J Bone Miner Res. 1999;14:500–8.
57. Olive PM, Whitecloud TS 3rd, Bennett JT. Lower cervical spondylosis and myelopathy in adults with Down's syndrome. Spine (Phila Pa 1976). 1988;13:781–4.
58. Ono K, Yonenobu K, Miyamoto S, Okada K. Pathology of ossification of the posterior longitudinal ligament and ligamentum flavum. Clin Orthop Relat Res. 1999;359:18–26.
59. Palmer PE, Stadalnick R, Arnon S. The genetic factor in cervical spondylosis. Skelet Radiol. 1984;11:178–82.
60. Park JY, Chin DK, Kim KS, Cho YE. Thoracic ligament ossification in patients with cervical ossification of the posterior longitudinal ligaments: tandem ossification in the cervical and thoracic spine. Spine (Phila Pa 1976). 2008;33:E407–10.
61. Patel AA, Spiker WR, Daubs M, Brodke DS, Cannon-Albright LA. Evidence of an inherited predisposition for cervical spondylotic myelopathy. Spine (Phila Pa 1976). 2012;37:26–9.
62. Pavlov H, Torg JS, Robie B, Jahre C. Cervical spinal stenosis: determination with vertebral body ratio method. Radiology. 1987;164:771–5.
63. Pizzutillo PD, Woods M, Nicholson L, Macewen GD. Risk factors in Klippel-Feil syndrome. Spine (Phila Pa 1976). 1994;19:2110–6.
64. Ren Y, Feng J, Liu ZZ, Wan H, Li JH, Lin X. A new haplotype in BMP4 implicated in ossification of the posterior longitudinal ligament (OPLL) in a Chinese population. J Orthop Res. 2012;30:748–56.
65. Rhee JM, Heflin JA, Hamasaki T, Freedman B. Prevalence of physical signs in cervical myelopathy: a prospective, controlled study. Spine (Phila Pa 1976). 2009;34:890–5.
66. Setzer M, Hermann E, Seifert V, Marquardt G. Apolipoprotein E gene polymorphism and the risk of cervical myelopathy in patients with chronic spinal cord compression. Spine (Phila Pa 1976). 2008;33:497–502.
67. Shin M, Besser LM, Kucik JE, Lu C, Siffel C, Correa A, Congenital Anomaly Multistate P, Survival C. Prevalence of down syndrome among children and adolescents in 10 regions of the United States. Pediatrics. 2009;124:1565–71.
68. Stapleton CJ, Pham MH, Attenello FJ, Hsieh PC. Ossification of the posterior longitudinal ligament: genetics and pathophysiology. Neurosurg Focus. 2011;30:E6.
69. Tanaka T, Ikari K, Furushima K, Okada A, Tanaka H, Furukawa K, Yoshida K, Ikeda T, Ikegawa S, Hunt SC, Takeda J, Toh S, Harata S, Nakajima T, Inoue I. Genomewide linkage and linkage disequilibrium

analyses identify COL6A1, on chromosome 21, as the locus for ossification of the posterior longitudinal ligament of the spine. Am J Hum Genet. 2003;73:812–22.

70. Terayama K. Genetic studies on ossification of the posterior longitudinal ligament of the spine. Spine (Phila Pa 1976). 1989;14:1184–91.
71. Wang H, Liu D, Yang Z, Tian B, Li J, Meng X, Wang Z, Yang H, Lin X. Association of bone morphogenetic protein-2 gene polymorphisms with susceptibility to ossification of the posterior longitudinal ligament of the spine and its severity in Chinese patients. Eur Spine J. 2008;17:956–64.
72. Wang ZC, Chen XS, Wang Da W, Shi JG, Jia LS, Xu GH, Huang JH, Fan L. The genetic association of vitamin D receptor polymorphisms and cervical spondylotic myelopathy in Chinese subjects. Clin Chim Acta. 2010;411:794–7.
73. Wang ZC, Shi JG, Chen XS, Xu GH, Li LJ, Jia LS. The role of smoking status and collagen IX polymorphisms in the susceptibility to cervical spondylotic myelopathy. Genet Mol Res. 2012;11:1238–44.
74. Wilson JR, Patel AA, Brodt ED, Dettori JR, Brodke DS, Fehlings MG. Genetics and heritability of cervical spondylotic myelopathy and ossification of the posterior longitudinal ligament: results of a systematic review. Spine (Phila Pa 1976). 2013;38:S123–46.
75. Wu JC, Ko CC, Yen YS, Huang WC, Chen YC, Liu L, Tu TH, Lo SS, Cheng H. Epidemiology of cervical spondylotic myelopathy and its risk of causing spinal cord injury: a national cohort study. Neurosurg Focus. 2013;35:E10.
76. Xiong C, Daubs MD, Scott TP, Phan KH, Suzuki A, Ruangchainikom M, Roe AK, Aghdasi B, Tan Y, Wang JC. Dynamic evaluation of the cervical spine and the spinal cord of symptomatic patients using a kinetic magnetic resonance imaging technique. Clin Spine Surg. 2016;30:8.
77. Yu WR, Baptiste DC, Liu T, Odrobina E, Stanisz GJ, Fehlings MG. Molecular mechanisms of spinal cord dysfunction and cell death in the spinal hyperostotic mouse: implications for the pathophysiology of human cervical spondylotic myelopathy. Neurobiol Dis. 2009;33:149–63.
78. Yu WR, Liu T, Kiehl TR, Fehlings MG. Human neuropathological and animal model evidence supporting a role for Fas-mediated apoptosis and inflammation in cervical spondylotic myelopathy. Brain. 2011;134:1277–92.

Pathobiology of Cervical Radiculopathy and Myelopathy

5

Cory J. Hartman and Daniel J. Hoh

Introduction

Symptomatic cervical spine disease commonly presents with signs and symptoms of radiculopathy and/or myelopathy. Understanding the pathobiologic mechanisms underlying radiculopathy and myelopathy is vital for appropriate and timely diagnosis and management. This chapter is an overview of current understanding of the pathophysiology of these two processes as it relates to their clinical presentation.

Cervical Radiculopathy

Cervical radiculopathy is the lower motor neuron and/or sensory manifestation of neurologic dysfunction in the distribution of a given cervical nerve root. While the true incidence of cervical radiculopathy is not known, a population-based study in Rochester, MN, from 1976 to 1990, showed an annual incidence of 107.3 per 100,000 men with a mean age of 47.6 and 63.5 per 100,000 females with a mean age of 48.2 [36]. Peak age-specific annual incidence was 202.9 per 100,000 people ages 50–54 [36]. More recently, Schoenfeld et al. found an incidence of cervical radiculopathy in the military population of 1.79 per 1000 person-years from 2000 to 2009 [39]. Risks factors in patients to develop cervical radiculopathy include axial load bearing, high-risk occupation (meat carriers, dentists, professional drivers), cigarette smoking, and prior lumbar radiculopathy [38]. Additional potentially implicated factors are prior cervical trauma, gender, race, and genetics [38]. Non-risk factors include repeated turning of the neck, sports, and sedentary occupations [38].

Cervical Radiculopathy Pathophysiology

The pathophysiology of degenerative cervical radiculopathy relates to age-related changes that occur within the intervertebral disc. Normally, the cervical intervertebral disc is characterized by a greater ventral disc height relative to dorsal, which is what contributes to the overall lordosis of this region. The annulus fibrosis of the ventral aspect contains multi-laminated, interweaving collagenous fibers of altering orientation; however the dorsal aspect is made of a thin layer of collagen [32]. With aging, however, the intervertebral disc diminishes the ability to retain water leading to decreased elasticity. This decrease in elasticity causes the disc to prolapse posteriorly, which can lead to compression of adjoining

C. J. Hartman · D. J. Hoh (✉)
Department of Neurosurgery, University of Florida, Gainesville, FL, USA
e-mail: Daniel.Hoh@neurosurgery.ufl.edu

M. G. Kaiser et al. (eds.), *Degenerative Cervical Myelopathy and Radiculopathy*,
https://doi.org/10.1007/978-3-319-97952-6_5

neural structures, radiculopathy and/or myelopathy, and concomitant loss of cervical lordosis.

Static Mechanical Compression-Induced Radiculopathy

A Rochester population-based study demonstrated that 21.9% of patients with cervical radiculopathy present with a cervical disc protrusion and 68.4% with degenerative cervical spondylosis, which may lead to static compression of the nerve root [36]. Less common presentations of compressive cervical radiculopathies include spinal neoplasm and infection [40]. The mechanism of symptomatic compressive radiculopathy is not fully understood; however, there are likely multiple contributing factors. One proposed etiology is direct mechanical compression of the nerve root including the dorsal root ganglia, which may be acute or chronic in nature. Acute compression is often secondary to herniated nucleus pulposus (Fig. 5.1), whereas chronic compression is commonly due to slowly progressive degenerative disc-osteophyte complex formation (Fig. 5.2) with superimposed facet and/or uncovertebral hypertrophy (Fig. 5.3). Compression of the nerve root proximal to the dorsal root ganglion (DRG) causes increased endoneurial fluid pressure and decreased blood flow to the DRG [52], leading to neuronal ischemic injury [52]. Patients with cervical radiculopathy have sensory axonal

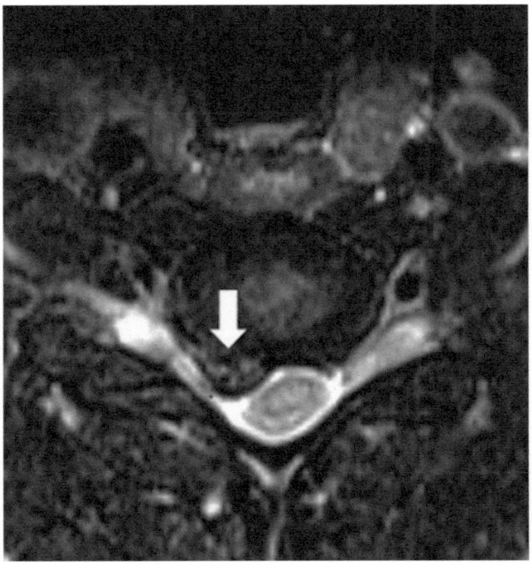

Fig. 5.1 MRI demonstrating an acute herniated nucleus pulposus (*arrow*) causing nerve root compression. The increased T2 signal within the paracentral disc herniation suggests an acute process

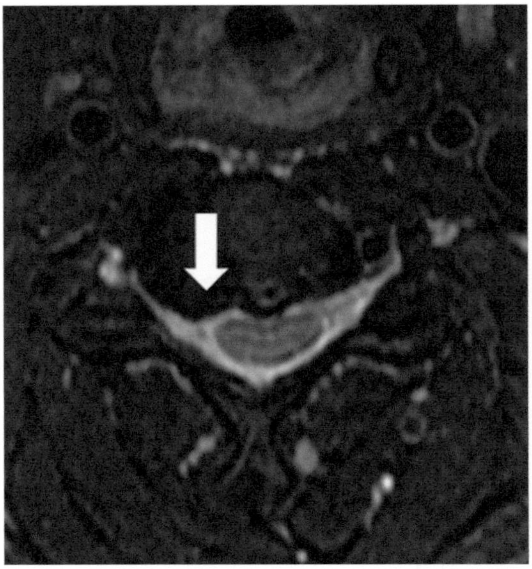

Fig. 5.2 MRI demonstrating a chronic disc-osteophyte complex (*arrow*) causing nerve root compression. The decreased T2 signal within the disc protrusion suggests a chronic process with likely possible osteophyte formation

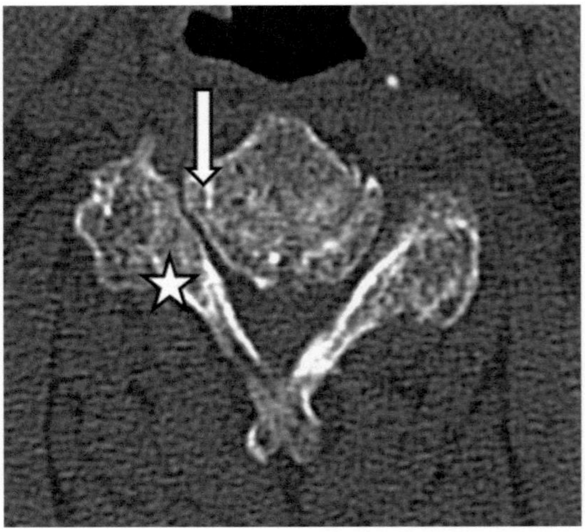

Fig. 5.3 CT demonstrating facet hypertrophy (star) and uncovertebral joint hypertrophy (*arrow*) causing neural foraminal stenosis and radiculopathy

dysfunction due to distal nerve axonal hyperpolarization thought to be due to Na+ -K+ ATPase over activation induced by proximal ischemia or remyelination of the axons [46]. Animal studies have revealed histologic, electrophysiologic, and functional changes in the nerve root as a result of chronic mechanical compression. Compressed nerve roots demonstrate thickened dura mater and arachnoid membrane with alterations in the blood-nerve barrier at 1 month, decreased number of large myelinated fibers at 3 months, and endoneurial fibrosis with Wallerian degeneration of nerve fibers at 6 months [53]. Jancalek and Dubovy showed a decreased number of myelinated axons in as little as 1 week of mechanical nerve compression [24]. Further, chronic compression of the dorsal root ganglia causes functional changes including enhanced excitability of sensory neurons, ectopic neuronal discharge, and hyperalgesia [44, 59].

Dynamic Compression-Induced Radiculopathy

Change in spinal alignment associated with cervical flexion, extension, and lateral bending may further cause dynamic compression or tension injury to cervical nerve roots. Rhee et al. report that the normal trajectory of nerve roots as they exit the cervical spine is at a 45° anterolateral angle toward the foramina, which may be subject to pathophysiologic stretch over ventral pathology with motion [37]. This repetitive dynamic compression may contribute to injury of the nerve root with associated radiculopathy over time.

Biochemical-Induced Radiculopathy

In addition to static and dynamic compression injury to the nerve, biochemical mediators released by the cervical disc also may have an important role in symptomatic radiculopathy. Burke et al. showed production of pro-inflammatory cytokines IL-6 and IL-8 from herniated nucleus pulposus in patients presenting with radiculopathy [8]. Release of TNF alpha causes upregulation of IL-1beta and nerve growth factor leading to hyperalgesia [50, 51]. Compared to normal disc material, herniated nucleus pulposus produces increased matrix metalloproteinases (MMP), nitric oxide, prostaglandin E2, and IL-6 [26, 60]. This pro-inflammatory chemical cascade is associated with increased pain and sensitization in the given nerve root distribution [50]. Compounding matters, it is thought that biochemical alterations of the nerve root may not only lead directly to symptoms but may also increase susceptibility to injury from static or dynamic forces.

Cervical Radiculopathy Clinical Presentation

Patients with cervical radiculopathy present with various neurologic sequelae, which may include pain, numbness, paresthesias (burning and/or tingling), weakness, or decreased upper extremity reflexes (Fig. 5.4a–c, Table 5.1). Radicular weakness typically follows a myotomal pattern, whereas sensory disturbance follows a distinct dermatome [37] (Table 5.2). A review of over 800 patients with cervical radiculopathy found arm pain in 99.4%, sensory deficits in 85.2%, scapular pain in 52.5%, anterior chest pain in 17.8%, headaches in 9.7%, anterior chest and arm pain in 5.9%, and left-sided chest pain and arm pain in 1.3% [20]. Another study found surgical pathology correlated with neurologic symptoms as follows: diminished reflexes (82%), motor weakness (77%), and diminished sensation (65%) [54].

C3 Nerve Root

Pure C3 radiculopathy is uncommon. The C3 nerve root exits the largest foramen at C2–C3 and is the smallest cervical nerve root [34]. There is no distinguishing motor function of the C3 nerve root, and symptoms of radicular pain may present as neck pain or occipital headaches.

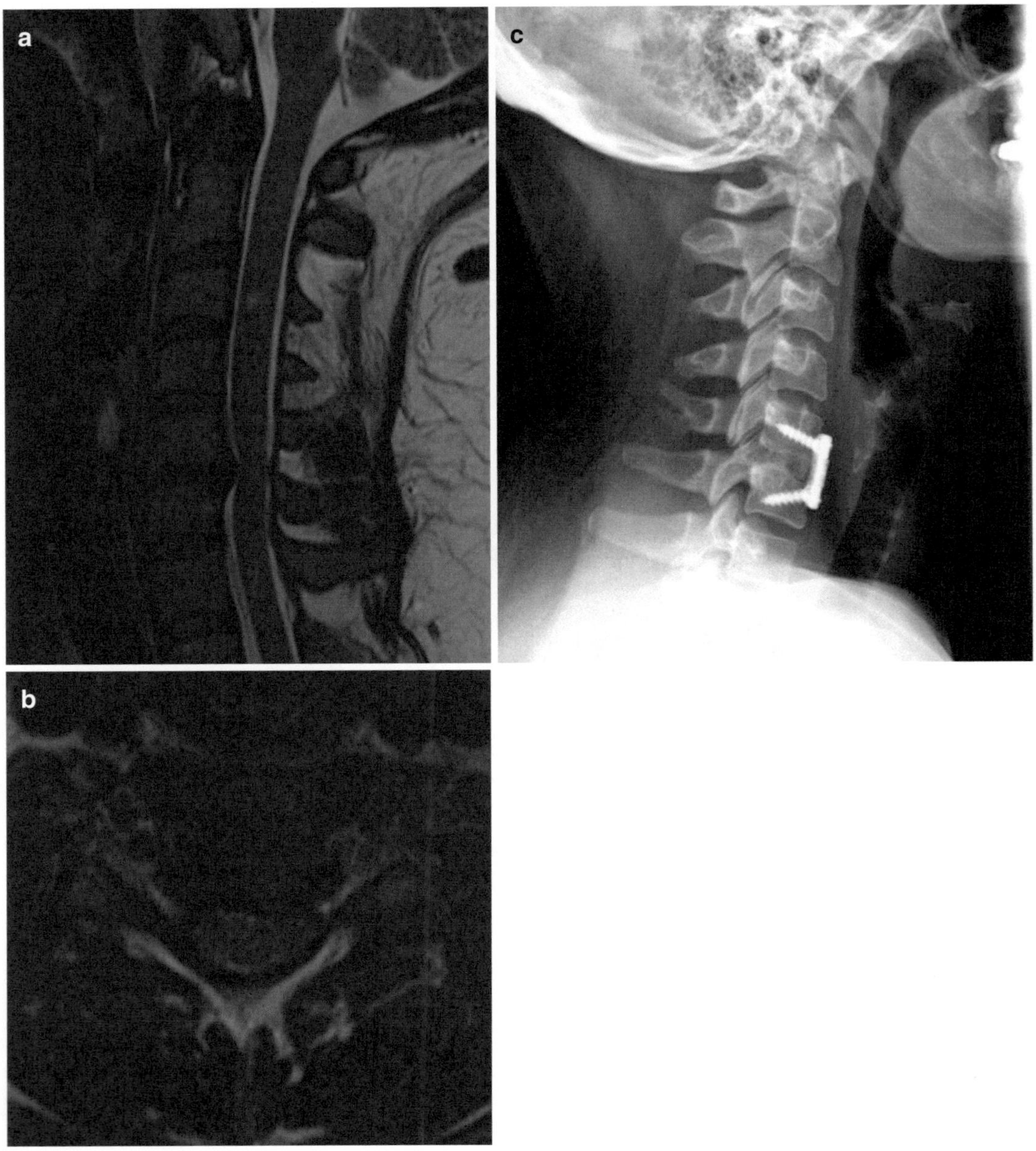

Fig. 5.4 (**a**-**c**) Case 1. A 37-year-old female presents with symptoms of mid-scapular pain and pain radiating down the left arm. On neurologic exam, the patient had subtle left wrist extension weakness and numbness to her left thumb. Reflexes were normal except for a slight diminished left brachioradialis reflex. Sagittal T2-weighted cervical MRI demonstrates a disc protrusion at the C5–C6 level (**a**). Axial T2-weighted cervical MRI at C5–C6 reveals left greater than right lateral recess and foraminal narrowing due to a broad-based disc protrusion. There is compression of the left C6 nerve root consistent with the patient's presenting radiculopathy (**b**). The patient eventually underwent surgical treatment with a C5–C6 anterior cervical discectomy and fusion (**c**)

Table 5.1 Cervical radiculopathy

Symptoms	Signs
Neck and/or radicular pain	Positive Spurling's test
Paresthesias	Hyporeflexia
Weakness	Shoulder abduction relief sign

C4 Nerve Root

Isolated C4 radiculopathy is also an uncommon presentation. C4 radiculopathy may present with pain radiating to the posterior neck, trapezius, and anterior chest.

Table 5.2 Cervical radiculopathy presentation

Disc Space	Nerve Root	Dermatome	Motor	Reflex
C1/C2	C2	Occiput		
C2/C3	C3	Upper 1/3 of neck	Diaphragm	
C3/C4	C4	Lower 2/3 of neck	Diaphragm	
C4/C5	C5	Lateral shoulder	Deltoid, biceps	Biceps
C5/C6	C6	Lateral forearm and thumb	Biceps, wrist extensors	Brachioradialis
C6/C7	C7	Posterior arm, digits 2 and 3	Triceps, wrist flexors	Triceps
C7/T1	C8	Ulnar palm, digits 4 and 5	Finger flexors	
T1/T2	T1	Medial arm	Interossei muscle	

C5 Nerve Root

C5 radiculopathy presents with pain and/or numbness over the lateral aspect of the shoulder and deltoid weakness. There may be minor weakness of the biceps, supraspinatus, and infraspinatus muscles. C5 radiculopathy may mimic shoulder pathology. Careful examination of the shoulder is crucial to make a correct diagnosis. The abductor relief sign, characterized by pain relief when placing one's hand over the head, is classic of cervical radiculopathy compared to pain with abduction seen with shoulder pathology. Of note, this sign is not limited to the C5 nerve root and may be seen with other lower cervical radiculopathies.

C6 Nerve Root

C6 radiculopathy is common and may lead to weakness of the biceps and particularly the extensor carpi radialis, which is only innervated by the C6 nerve root. C6 radicular weakness is characterized by impaired elbow flexion and wrist extension. Decreased biceps and/or brachioradialis reflexes may additionally be seen. C6 radicular sensation loss is over the thumb and lateral portion of the index finger. Radicular pain may start in the neck and radiate to the lateral arm and forearm into the thumb.

C7 Nerve Root

C7 radiculopathy is also a frequent presentation. The C7 nerve root innervates the triceps, and radiculopathy may lead to elbow extension or wrist flexion weakness and a diminished triceps reflex. Symptoms can include pain and sensory disturbance, including numbness and/or paresthesias radiating from the neck to the arm and digits 2–4. Horner's syndrome may also rarely be present [33].

C8 Nerve Root

The C8 nerve root innervates the hand intrinsic muscles and finger flexors. C8 radiculopathy may mimic ulnar neuropathy given their similar function. Weakness in the hand intrinsic muscles, wrist extensors, and wrist flexors may be present. Individuals may not be able to fully extend digits 4 and 5 (Benediction sign). Sensation over the medial forearm and digits 4 and 5 may be decreased, which can be distinguished from a pure ulnar neuropathy which results in splitting sensory loss of the ring finger. Pain typically radiates from the neck to the arm, medial forearm, and into digits 4 and 5. Horner's syndrome may also rarely be present in a C8 radiculopathy [33].

T1 Nerve Root

The T1 nerve root is a rare origin of radicular symptoms. Patients may present with hand intrinsic weakness without pain into the hand. Weakness of the first dorsal interosseous muscle (Froment's sign) may also be present. Similar to C7 or C8 radiculopathy, Horner's syndrome may also be a rare presentation [33].

Cervical Zygapophyseal and Discogenic Pain

It is important to note that cervical nerve roots are not the sole cause of neck, shoulder girdle, and upper extremity pain syndromes. Referred pain from small nociceptive neurons that innervate the zygapophyseal (facet) joints and disc space may mimic radicular pain symptoms [16, 43]. Unlike radicular symptoms, pain generated in the facet joints or disc space is not accompanied by sensory disturbance (i.e., numbness, paresthesias) or weakness. Radicular symptoms may be unilateral and/or bilateral, whereas pain associated with facet joints and/or the disc space is typically bilateral in nature. Table 5.2 summarizes the referred pain area from the facet joints and disc space [16, 43].

Cervical Myelopathy

Cervical myelopathy was first described in 1928 as neurologic signs or symptoms due to spinal cord dysfunction secondary to spinal canal narrowing or hypoperfusion of the spinal cord [34, 45] (Table 5.3). Cervical myelopathy is characterized by upper motor neuron and sensory impairment, often involving long ascending and descending spinal tracts. Cervical spondylosis and congenital spinal stenosis are the most common causes of cervical myelopathy [12], with cervical spondylotic myelopathy being the most common cause of spinal cord dysfunction in the elderly and the most common cause of nontraumatic spastic paresis. Other etiologies include ossification of the posterior longitudinal ligament, neoplasm, rheumatoid arthritis, infection, vascular disease, trauma, demyelinating disease, and metabolic disorders [55]. Cervical spondylotic myelopathy (CSM) is the most common worldwide cause of spinal cord dysfunction [27]. Early radiologic studies suggest 13% of men in the third decade and 100% of men over the age of 70, compared to 5% of women in the fourth decade and 96% of women over the age of 70, exhibit cervical degenerative changes that may lead to cervical myelopathy [23]. Multiple studies have assessed age as a risk factor for degenerative cervical myelopathy. Studies that have controlled for multiple cofounders show a positive association of age with myelopathy, whereas other conflicting studies fail to demonstrate correlation [10, 48, 58]. Gender has not been shown to be a risk factor for myelopathy [48, 58]. Radiologic studies and systematic reviews reveal that congenitally shortened canal and rheumatoid arthritis are factors associated with a high risk of developing cervical myelopathy [2, 30, 42].

Table 5.3 Cervical myelopathy

Symptoms	Signs
Paresthesias	Spastic gait
Gait disturbance	Positive Hoffman's reflex
Weakness	Positive Babinski's reflex
Problems with fine motor control	Hyperreflexia
Incontinence	Inverted radial reflex
Urinary retention	Weakness
Lhermitte's sign	Increased muscle tone

Cervical Myelopathy Pathophysiology

The pathophysiology of cervical spondylotic myelopathy is characterized by chronic progressive degenerative arthropathy. As described previously, age-related changes in the viscoelastic properties of the intervertebral disc lead to alterations in its biomechanical load-bearing capabilities. Ensuing redistribution of stress and strain across the cervical motion segment results in several pathologic changes. Initially, disc protrusion coincides with degenerative loss of disc height. Reactive endplate changes eventually progress to bridging osteophytic spur formation, in an attempt to minimize motion. The disc-osteophyte complex causes canal stenosis which may lead to cord compression and myelopathy (Fig. 5.5). Hypertrophy of the ligamentum flavum (Fig. 5.6) and progressive facet joint arthropathy develop to further off-load the

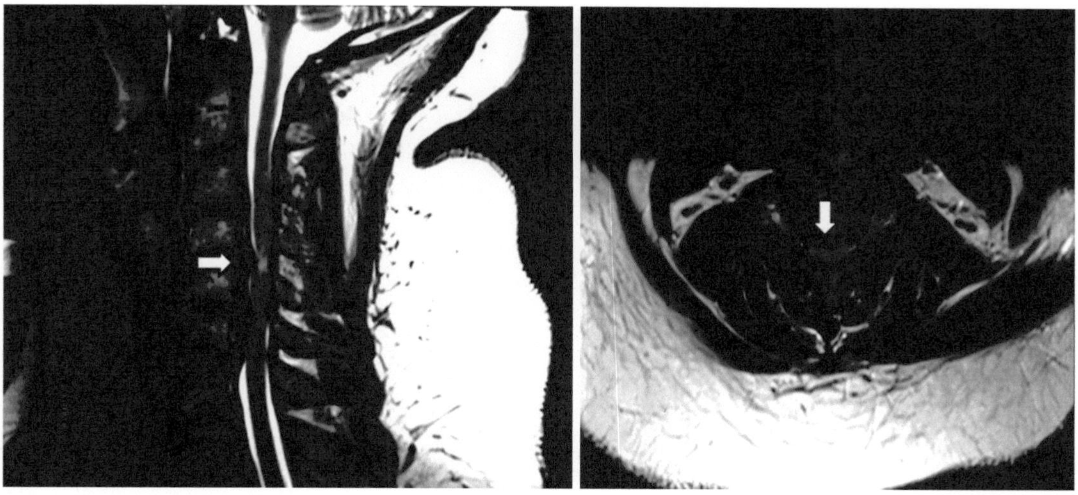

Fig. 5.5 MRI demonstrating multilevel disc-osteophyte complexes (*arrow*) causing canal stenosis and spinal cord compression. T2 signal change within the spinal cord suggests pathologic changes that correlate with myelopathy

degenerated disc. The combination of these factors (disc protrusion, osteophyte formation, ligamentum flavum hypertrophy, facet arthropathy) ultimately leads to narrowing of the spinal canal with potential compromise of the spinal cord. Congenital spinal stenosis and ossification of the posterior longitudinal ligament (Fig. 5.7) or ligamentum flavum are additional factors that may pathologically contribute to the development of cervical myelopathy.

Static Mechanical Compression-Induced Myelopathy

Static mechanical compression of the spinal cord leads to a cascade of pathophysiologic changes within the spinal cord ultimately resulting in spinal cord dysfunction and myelopathy. As discussed, common underlying etiologies of mechanical compression include spondylotic spinal stenosis, ossification of the posterior longitudinal ligament or ligamentum flavum, congenital stenosis, rheumatologic spinal disorders, and other acquired compressive pathologies (e.g., neoplasm or infection) [3]. Spinal cord histology in cervical myelopathy is characterized by cystic cavitation, gliosis, Wallerian degeneration of descending and ascending tracts, and loss of anterior horn cells [7, 47]. It deserves mention that mechanical compression injury from cervical spondylosis is distinct from that due to acute trauma. Unlike acute traumatic compression injury, in cervical spondylosis, there is no sudden mechanical insult, and consequently there is a noted absence of hemorrhagic necrosis within the spinal cord [27]. Further, the slow gradual

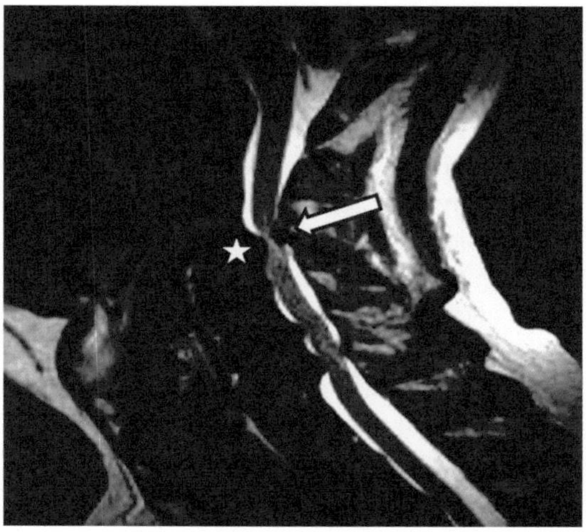

Fig. 5.6 MRI demonstrating ligament flavum hypertrophy (*arrow*) causing canal stenosis and spinal cord compression. A disc-osteophyte complex (star) with chronic degenerative anterolisthesis at the same level causing further stenosis and cord compression

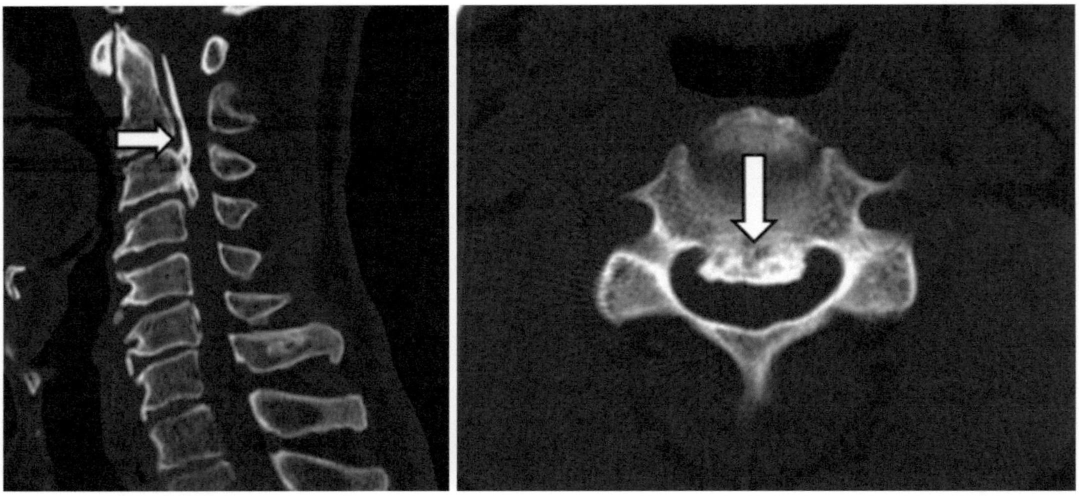

Fig. 5.7 CT demonstrating ossification of the posterior longitudinal ligament (*arrow*) causing canal stenosis and cord compression

development of spondylotic compression likely allows for coinciding compensatory neurologic and functional mechanisms to occur. This likely explains the chronic insidious symptoms, and often relatively minimal deficits in those with even severe radiologic spondylotic spinal cord compression, which is opposed to the immediate neurologic compromise seen in acute traumatic spinal cord injury (SCI) [27].

Static mechanical compression from cervical spondylosis is believed to cause myelopathy by direct injury to neurons via ischemic and apoptotic mechanisms. Gooding et al. first proposed the association of ischemic injury and myelopathy in a canine model of spinal cord compression [18]. They found hyalinization and hypertrophy in the walls of the anterior spinal artery after mechanical cord compression. Anterior and posterior compression of the spinal cord results in hypoperfusion through transverse arterioles originating from the anterior sulcal arteries and intramedullary branches to the central gray matter [15]. Foraminal stenosis compromises blood flow through the radiculo-medullary arteries leading to further decreased spinal cord perfusion [49]. Histologic evaluation of myelopathic spinal cords is characterized by areas of ischemic necrosis [14]. Corticospinal tracts are most affected by hypoperfusion and spinal cord ischemia [18], with the lower cervical spine being the most vulnerable to decreased perfusion [4]. Compression of spinal cord vasculature and hypoxia-induced cell injury of endothelial cells may additionally cause breakdown of the blood-spinal cord barrier (BSCB) leading to pathologic vasogenic edema [25]. A further distinction between pathologic changes in acute traumatic and spondylotic compression injury is that in traumatic SCI, there is repair to the BSCB, whereas in cervical spondylotic myelopathy, there is chronic disruption [29, 31]. While many studies suggest that alterations in spinal cord hemodynamics may play a role in myelopathy, other clinical and preclinical studies have countered with contradictory evidence of no or minimal spinal cord ischemia in the setting of myelopathy [1, 17, 21].

Apoptosis (programmed cell death) is the culmination of multiple biochemical processes resulting from primary and secondary injury to the spinal cord. In vivo models of cervical spondylotic myelopathy show that chronic extrinsic spinal cord compression results in Fas-mediated apoptosis of neurons and oligodendrocytes through action of caspase-8, caspase-9, and caspase-3 [56]. Animal models of spinal cord injury reveal apoptotic oligodendrocytes at the site of injury but more importantly distant demyelination of white matter tracts remote from the primary injury epicenter [13, 28]. Histologic analysis of human spinal cord injury demonstrates oligodendrocyte apoptosis occurs prior to axonal degeneration [6]. This demyelination process within the spinal cord secondary to compression may explain the long tract findings at clinical presentation in patients with cervical myelopathy.

Dynamic Compression-Induced Myelopathy

In addition to static compression, studies indicate that dynamic compression of the spinal cord may have a significant role in myelopathy development. Cadaveric research has shown alterations in the anteroposterior spinal canal diameter in response to tension-compression forces and flexion-extension changes [11]. From tension to compression, the canal diameter decreases 10.1% secondary to changes related to the disc and decreases 6.5% from the ligamentum flavum [11]. From flexion to extension, the canal diameter decreases 10.8% secondary to changes related to the disc and decreases 24.3% from the ligamentum flavum [11]. More recent clinical studies using dynamic magnetic resonance imaging demonstrate flexion-extension-induced spinal canal narrowing due to ligamentum flavum buckling and shingling of the lamina in hyperextension [9]. Narrowing of the spinal canal <11 mm during flexion-extension is correlated with cervical myelopathy [35]. Lhermitte's sign, electrical shock-like sensation, or pain radiating down the back with neck range of motion is a classic clinical manifestation of cervical extension-induced dorsal column compression.

Stretch and Shear Force-Induced Myelopathy

Dynamic movement of the cervical spine not only results in spinal canal narrowing but may further cause stretch and shear forces leading to axial strain-induced cord injury [19]. Yuan et al. showed an elongation of the spinal cord up to 10% of its length on the posterior surface and 6% on the anterior surface with full flexion from the neutral position [57]. Human cadaveric models show that the spinal cord is initially compliant to stretch but loses this compliance as axonal fibers straighten out and bear tensile load [5]. Histologic studies demonstrate that stretch and shear injury variably affects spinal cord gray and white matter, with gray matter being more rigid and thereby more susceptible to increased stretch of the spinal cord [22]. Stretch and shear injury leading to axonal dysfunction has been confirmed with in vitro electrophysiologic studies revealing stretch-induced disruption of compound action potentials [41].

Cervical Myelopathy Clinical Presentation

Patients with myelopathy may present with a variety of neurologic signs or symptoms that are often progressive in nature (Fig. 5.8a–c). Symptoms may include loss of fine motor coordination in the hands, numbness or paresthesias in upper or lower extremities, sensation of heaviness or weakness in the legs, gait imbalance, hyperreflexia, Lhermitte's sign, and, in late stages, bowel or bladder dysfunction [12]. Loss of fine motor control in the hands may present as dropping objects, difficulty writing, or trouble buttoning a shirt. Cervical myelopathy leads to characteristic signs noted on physical exam. Spastic gait and/or increased upper extremity tone are late-stage signs in cervical myelopathy secondary to loss of normal upper motor neuron tonic inhibition. Hoffman's and Babinski's signs are two common pathologic reflexes that may be seen in cervical myelopathy. Hoffman's sign is characterized by flexion and adduction of the thumb and concurrent flexion of the index finger with stimulation of the extensor tendon of the third digit. Babinski's sign (plantar reflex) is concurrent extension of the great toe with stimulation of the lateral aspect of the plantar surface of the foot. Another pathologic reflex

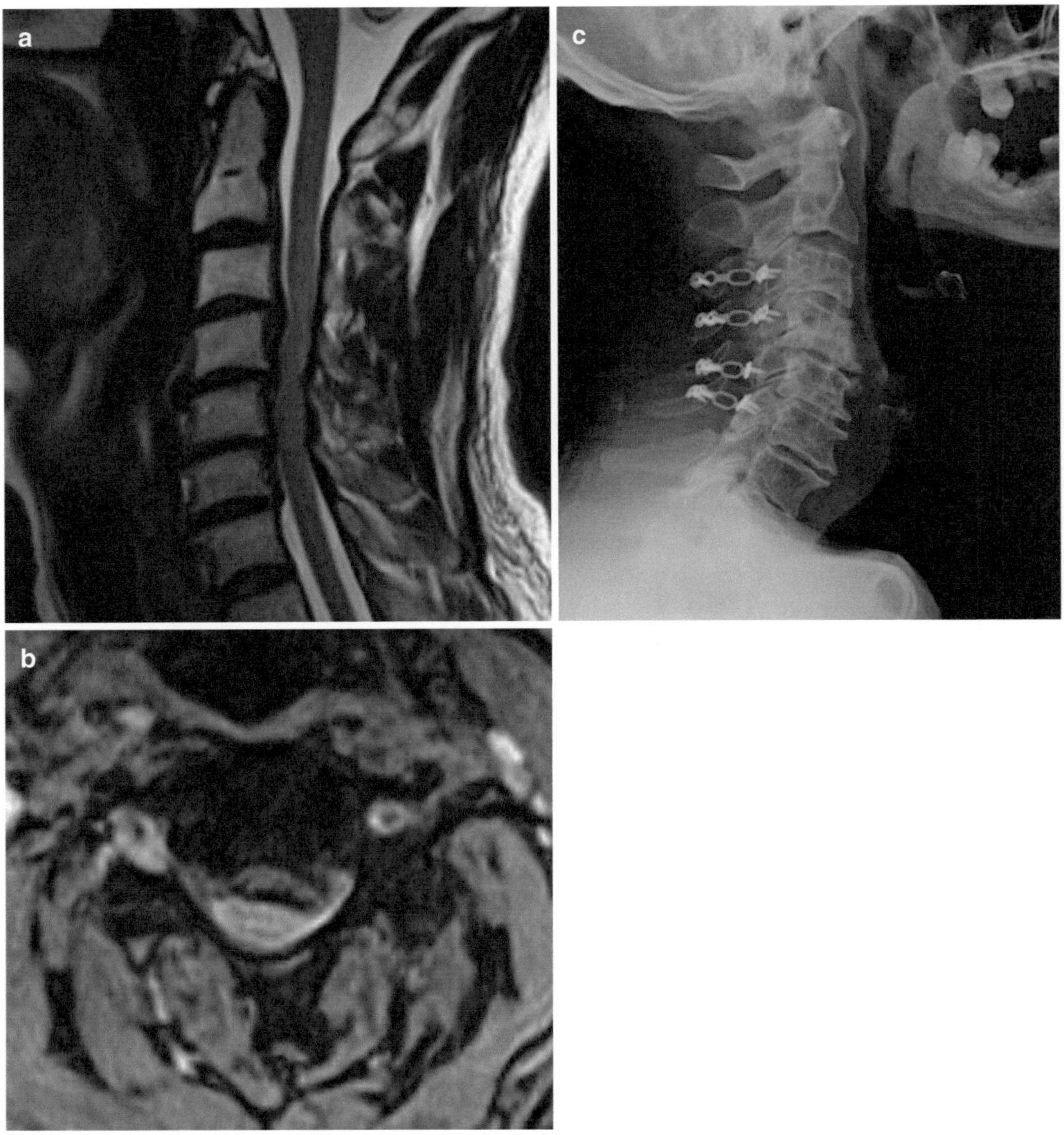

Fig. 5.8 (**a–c**) Case 2. A 55-year-old male presents with symptoms of progressive loss of hand coordination and gait instability. Neurologic examination was notable for impaired tandem gait, brisk patellar tendon reflexes, and positive Hoffman's sign. Sagittal T2-weighted cervical MRI demonstrates cervical spondylosis with spinal canal stenosis and cord compression from C3 to C6 (**a**). Axial T2-weighted cervical MRI demonstrates ventral spinal canal narrowing secondary to broad-based disc osteophyte formation with T2 signal abnormality within the spinal cord (**b**). The patient underwent surgical treatment via laminoplasty for posterior decompression (**c**)

that may be seen in cervical myelopathy is the inverted radial reflex; tapping the brachioradialis tendon causes wrist and finger flexion. Unlike cervical radiculopathy, significant neck or extremity pain is often notably absent in cervical myelopathy [12].

Conclusion

The pathobiology of cervical radiculopathy and myelopathy involves a combination of static and dynamic mechanical compressive factors, as well as biochemical processes that ultimately lead to nerve or spinal cord injury. In cervical radiculopathy, the pathophysiologic mechanisms result in motor and sensory loss in the distribution of select spinal nerve roots with clinical symptomatology along a myotome or dermatome. Cervical myelopathy is a more significant pathophysiologic process, which ultimately leads to disruption of long ascending and descending spinal cord pathways. As a result, the clinical manifestation of myelopathy is characterized by loss of combined motor and sensory function involving multiple spinal levels with the hallmark of upper motor neuron dysfunction. Improved understanding of the underlying pathobiology of radiculopathy and myelopathy may ultimately lead to improved management strategies.

References

1. al-Mefty O, Harkey HL, Marawi I, Haines DE, Peeler DF, Wilner HI, et al. Experimental chronic compressive cervical myelopathy. J Neurosurg. 1993;79(4):550–61. https://doi.org/10.3171/jns.1993.79.4.0550.
2. Arnold JG Jr. The clinical manifestations of spondylochondrosis (spondylosis) of the cervical spine. Ann Surg. 1955;141(6):872–89.
3. Baptiste DC, Fehlings MG. Pathophysiology of cervical myelopathy. Spine J. 2006;6(6 Suppl):190S–7S.
4. Baron EM, Young WF. Cervical spondylotic myelopathy: a brief review of its pathophysiology, clinical course, and diagnosis. Neurosurgery. 2007;60(1 Suppl 1):S35–41. https://doi.org/10.1227/01.NEU.0000215383.64386.82.
5. Bilston LE, Thibault LE. The mechanical properties of the human cervical spinal cord in vitro. Ann Biomed Eng. 1996;24(1):67–74.
6. Blight AR. Delayed demyelination and macrophage invasion: a candidate for secondary cell damage in spinal cord injury. Cent Nerv Syst Trauma. 1985;2(4):299–315. https://doi.org/10.1089/cns.1985.2.299.
7. Bohlman HH, Emery SE. The pathophysiology of cervical spondylosis and myelopathy. Spine. 1988;13(7):843–6.
8. Burke JG, Watson WG, McCormack D, Dowling FE, Walsh MG, Fitspatrick JM. Intervertebral discs which cause low back pain secrete high levels of proinflammatory mediators. J Bone Joint Surg. 2002;84-B(2):196–201.
9. Chen CJ, Hsu HL, Niu CC, Chen TY, Chen MC, Tseng YC, et al. Cervical degenerative disease at flexion-extension MR imaging: prediction criteria. Radiology. 2003;227(1):136–42. https://doi.org/10.1148/radiol.2271020116.
10. Chen IH, Liao KK, Shen WY. Measurement of cervical canal sagittal diameter in chinese males with cervical spondylotic myelopathy. Zhonghua Yi Xue Za Zhi (Taipei). 1994;54(2):105–10.
11. Chen IH, Vasavada A, Panjabi MM. Kinematics of the cervical spine canal: changes with sagittal plane loads. J Spinal Disord. 1994;7(2):93–101.
12. Coughlin TA, Klezl Z. Focus on cervical myelopathy. Br Ed Soc Bone Joint Surg. 2012:1–7.
13. Crowe MJ, Bresnahan JC, Shuman SL, Masters JN, Beattie MS. Apoptosis and delayed degeneration after spinal cord injury in rats and monkeys. Nat Med. 1997;3(1):73–6.
14. Dolan RT, Butler JS, O'Byrne JM, Poynton AR. Mechanical and cellular processes driving cervical myelopathy. World J Orthop. 2016;7(1):20–9. https://doi.org/10.5312/wjo.v7.i1.20.
15. Doppman JL. The mechanism of ischemia in anteroposterior compression of the spinal cord 1975. Invest Radiol. 1990;25(4):444–52.
16. Fukui S, Ohseto K, Shiotani M, Ohno K, Karasawa H, Nganuma Y, Yuda Y. Referred pain distribution of the cervical zygapophyseal joints and cervical dorsal rami. Pain. 1996;68:79–83.
17. Good DC, Couch JR, Wacaser L. "Numb, clumsy hands" and high cervical spondylosis. Surg Neurol. 1984;22(3):285–91.
18. Gooding MR, Wilson CB, Hoff JT. Experimental cervical myelopathy. Effects of ischemia and compression of the canine cervical spinal cord. J Neurosurg. 1975;43(1):9–17. https://doi.org/10.3171/jns.1975.43.1.0009.
19. Henderson FC, Geddes JF, Vaccaro AR, Woodard E, Berry KJ, Benzel EC. Stretch-associated injury in cervical spondylotic myelopathy: new concept and review. Neurosurgery. 2005;56(5):1101–13. discussion 1101-13.
20. Henderson CM, Hennessy RG, Shuey HM Jr, Shackelfor EG. Posterior-lateral foraminotomy as an exclusive operative technique for cervical radiculopathy: a review of 846 consecutively operated cases. Neurosurgery. 1983;12:504–12.
21. Hoff JT, Wilson CB. The pathophysiology of cervical spondylotic radiculopathy and myelopathy. Clin Neurosurg. 1977;24:474–87.
22. Ichihara K, Taguchi T, Sakuramoto I, Kawano S, Kawai S. Mechanism of the spinal cord injury and the cervical spondylotic myelopathy: new approach based on the mechanical features of the spinal cord white and gray matter. J Neurosurg. 2003;99(3 Suppl):278–85.
23. Irvine DH, Foster JB, Newell DJ, Klukvin BN. Prevalence of cervical spondylosis in a general practice. Lancet. 1965;1(7395):1089–92.
24. Jancalek R, Dubovy P. An experimental animal model of spinal root compression syndrome: an analysis of morphological changes of myelinated axons during compression radiculopathy and after decompression. Exp

Brain Res. 2007;179(1):111–9. https://doi.org/10.1007/s00221-006-0771-5.
25. Kalsi-Ryan S, Karadimas SK, Fehlings MG. Cervical spondylotic myelopathy: the clinical phenomenon and the current pathobiology of an increasingly prevalent and devastating disorder. Neuroscientist. 2013;19(4):409–21. https://doi.org/10.1177/1073858412467377.
26. Kang JD, Georgescu HI, McIntyre-Larkin L, Stefanovic-Racic M, Evans CH. Herniated cervical intervertebral discs spontaneously produce matrix metalloproteinases, nitric oxide, interleukin-6, and prostaglandin E2. Spine. 1995;20(22):2373–8.
27. Karadimas SK, Gatzounis G, Fehlings MG. Pathobiology of cervical spondylotic myelopathy. Eur Spine J. 2015;24(Suppl 2):132–8. https://doi.org/10.1007/s00586-014-3264-4.
28. Karadimas SK, Gialeli CH, Klironomos G, Tzanakakis GN, Panagiotopoulos E, Karamanos NK, et al. The role of oligodendrocytes in the molecular pathobiology and potential molecular treatment of cervical spondylotic myelopathy. Curr Med Chem. 2010;17(11):1048–58. BSP/CMC/E-Pub/065 [pii].
29. Karadimas SK, Moon ES, Yu WR, Satkunendrarajah K, Kallitsis JK, Gatzounis G, et al. A novel experimental model of cervical spondylotic myelopathy (CSM) to facilitate translational research. Neurobiol Dis. 2013;54:43–58. https://doi.org/10.1016/j.nbd.2013.02.013.
30. Kim HJ, Nemani VM, Riew KD, Brasington R. Cervical spine disease in rheumatoid arthritis: incidence, manifestations, and therapy. Curr Rheumatol Rep. 2015;17(2):9-014-0486-8. https://doi.org/10.1007/s11926-014-0486-8.
31. Loy DN, Crawford CH, Darnall JB, Burke DA, Onifer SM, Whittemore SR. Temporal progression of angiogenesis and basal lamina deposition after contusive spinal cord injury in the adult rat. J Comp Neurol. 2002;445(4):308–24. https://doi.org/10.1002/cne.10168. [pii]
32. Mercer S, Bogduk N. The ligaments and annulus fibrosus of human adult cervical intervertebral discs. Spine. 1999;24:619–28.
33. Murphy F, Simmons JC, Brunson B. Surgical treatment of laterally ruptured cervical discs: review of 648 cases—1939-1972. J Neurosurg. 1973;38:679–83.
34. Payne EE, Spillane JD. The cervical spine; an anatomico-pathological study of 70 specimens (using a special technique) with particular reference to the problem of cervical spondylosis. Brain. 1957;80(4):571–96.
35. Penning L. Some aspects of plain radiography of the cervical spine in chronic myelopathy. Neurology. 1962;12:513–9.
36. Radhakrishnan K, Litchy WJ, O'Fallon WM, Kurland LT. Epidemiology of cervical radiculopathy. A population-based study from rochester, minnesota, 1976 through 1990. Brain. 1994;117(Pt 2):325–35.
37. Rhee JM, Yoon T, Riew KD. Cervical radiculopathy. J Am Acad Orthop Surg. 2007;15(8):486–94. 15/8/486 [pii]
38. Roth D, Mukai A, Thomas P, Hudgins TH, Alleva JT. Cervical radiculopathy. Dis Mon. 2009;55(12):737–56. https://doi.org/10.1016/j.disamonth.2009.06.004.
39. Schoenfeld AJ, George AA, Bader JO, Caram PM Jr. Incidence and epidemiology of cervical radiculopathy in the United States military: 2000 to 2009. J Spinal Disord Tech. 2012;25(1):17–22. https://doi.org/10.1097/BSD.0b013e31820d77ea.
40. Shelerud RA, Paynter KS. Rarer causes of radiculopathy: spinal tumors, infections, and other unusual causes. Phys Med Rehabil Clin N Am. 2002;13(3):645–96.
41. Shi R, Pryor JD. Pathological changes of isolated spinal cord axons in response to mechanical stretch. Neuroscience. 2002;110(4):765–77. S0306452201005966 [pii].
42. Singh A, Tetreault L, Fehlings MG, Fischer DJ, Skelly AC. Risk factors for development of cervical spondylotic myelopathy: results of a systematic review. Evid Based Spine Care J. 2012;3(3):35–42. https://doi.org/10.1055/s-0032-1327808.
43. Slipman CW, Plastaras C, Patel R, Isaac Z, Chow D, Garvan C, Pauza K, Furman M. Provocative cervical discography symptom mapping. Spine J. 2005;5:381–8.
44. Song XJ, Hu SJ, Greenquist KW, Zhang JM, LaMotte RH. Mechanical and thermal hyperalgesia and ectopic neuronal discharge after chronic compression of dorsal root ganglia. J Neurophysiol. 1999;82(6):3347–58.
45. Stookey B. Compression of the spinal cord due to ventral extradural cervical chondromas. Arch Neurol Psychiatr. 1928;20:275–91.
46. Sung JY, Tani J, Hung KS, Lui TN, Lin CS. Sensory axonal dysfunction in cervical radiculopathy. J Neurol Neurosurg Psychiatry. 2015;86(6):640–5. https://doi.org/10.1136/jnnp-2014-308088.
47. Swagerty DL Jr. Cervical spondylotic myelopathy: a cause of gait disturbance and falls in the elderly. Kans Med. 1994;95(10):226–7. 229
48. Takamiya Y, Nagata K, Fukuda K, Shibata A, Ishitake T, Suenaga T. Cervical spine disorders in farm workers requiring neck extension actions. J Orthop Sci. 2006;11(3):235–40. https://doi.org/10.1007/s00776-006-1005-1.
49. Taylor AR. Mechanism and treatment of spinal-cord disorders associated with cervical spondylosis. Lancet. 1953;1(6763):717–20.
50. Van Boxem K, Huntoon M, Van Zundert J, Patijn J, van Kleef M, Joosten EA. Pulsed radiofrequency: a review of the basic science as applied to the pathophysiology of radicular pain: a call for clinical translation. Reg Anesth Pain Med. 2014;39(2):149–59. https://doi.org/10.1097/AAP.0000000000000063.
51. Woolf CJ, Allchorne A, Safieh-Garabedian B, Poole S. Cytokines, nerve growth factor and inflammatory

hyperalgesia: the contribution of tumour necrosis factor alpha. Br J Pharmacol. 1997;121(3):417–24. https://doi.org/10.1038/sj.bjp.0701148.
52. Yabuki S, Kikuchi S, Olmarker K, Myers RR. Acute effects of nucleus pulposus on blood flow and endoneurial fluid pressure in rat dorsal root ganglia. Spine. 1998;23(23):2517–23.
53. Yoshizawa H, Kobayashi S, Morita T. Chronic nerve root compression. Pathophysiologic mechanism of nerve root dysfunction. Spine. 1995;20(4):397–407.
54. Yoss RE, Kendall BC, MacCarthy CS, Love JG. Significance of symptoms and signs in localization of involved root in cervical disk protusion. Neurology. 1957;7:673–81.
55. Young WB. The clinical diagnosis of myelopathy. Semin Ultrasound CT MR. 1994;15(3):250–4.
56. Yu WR, Baptiste DC, Liu T, Odrobina E, Stanisz G, Fehlings M. Molecular mechanisms of spinal cord dysfunction and cell death in the spinal hyperostotic mouse: implications for the pathophysiology of human cervical spondylotic myelopathy. Neurobiol Dis. 2009;33:149–63.
57. Yuan Q, Dougherty L, Margulies SS. In vivo human cervical spinal cord deformation and displacement in flexion. Spine. 1998;23(15):1677–83.
58. Yue WM, Tan SB, Tan MH, Koh DC, Tan CT. The torg–pavlov ratio in cervical spondylotic myelopathy: a comparative study between patients with cervical spondylotic myelopathy and a nonspondylotic, nonmyelopathic population. Spine. 2001;26(16):1760–4.
59. Zhang JM, Song XJ, LaMotte RH. Enhanced excitability of sensory neurons in rats with cutaneous hyperalgesia produced by chronic compression of the dorsal root ganglion. J Neurophysiol. 1999;82(6):3359–66.
60. Zhuang HM, Xu GT, Wen SF, Guo YY, Huang Q. Altered expression of metalloproteinase-2 and tissue inhibitor of metalloproteinase-2 in cervical disc herniation patients. Genet Mol Res. 2016;15(2) https://doi.org/10.4238/gmr.15027594.

Natural History of Cervical Degenerative Disorders

6

John E. O'Toole and Joseph E. Molenda

Introduction

Cervical spondylosis is a naturally occurring, age-related phenomenon that can be seen radiologically in 95% of males and 70% of females over the age of 70 [13]. It is characterized by degenerative changes affecting the vertebrae, intervertebral discs, facets, and associated ligaments. Starting in the third decade of life, there is a progressive loss of water content of the intervertebral disc that continues with age. This is due to a loss of glycosaminoglycan proteins, which attract molecules of water due to their high molecular weight and overall negative charge, located in the nucleus pulposus. As water molecules leave the nucleus pulposus, this results in a less elastic and more compressible disc that bulges into the spinal canal [7]. At the same time, the vertebral bodies drift toward each other, and the ligamentum flavum and the facet joint capsule fold in dorsally [1]. The combination of these events ultimately decreases the dimensions of the neural foramen and spinal canal. The approximation of the vertebral bodies leads to a reactive process that produces osteophytes around the margins of the disc and at the uncovertebral and facet joints. Radiculopathy in cervical spondylosis is the result of compression either by a hypertrophied facet joint or uncovertebral joints, disc protrusion, spondylotic spurring of the vertebral body, or any combination of these processes [1]. Subacute radiculopathy occurs in patients with pre-existing cervical spondylosis, and these patients often develop symptoms which are polyradicular in nature.

A number of different factors have been implicated in increasing the risk for advanced pathological findings related to cervical spondylosis that include smoking, repetitive trauma (axial loading), Down syndrome, and genetics. Recently, an elevated relative risk of disease in both near and distant relatives of patients with cervical spondylosis has been demonstrated, confirming a genetic predisposition [27]. Additionally, smoking has been associated with disc degeneration and is thus a risk factor for cervical spondylosis [14]. This is particularly true for individuals with collagen IX Trp2 allele, where it is found that smoking amplifies this risk [31]. With disc degeneration, increased mechanical stresses occur at the end plates of the adjacent vertebral body, resulting in subperiosteal bone formation [21]. This bone formation has the potential to ventrally compress the spinal cord, which can result in cervical spondylotic myelopathy (CSM). CSM is the most common acquired cause of spinal cord dysfunction in patients older than 55 years [11]. However, the

J. E. O'Toole (✉) · J. E. Molenda
Department of Neurosurgery, Rush University Medical Center, Chicago, IL, USA
e-mail: JOHN_OTOOLE@rush.edu

M. G. Kaiser et al. (eds.), *Degenerative Cervical Myelopathy and Radiculopathy*,
https://doi.org/10.1007/978-3-319-97952-6_6

exact prevalence of CSM in the general population is not known [8]. Myelopathy is the end result of three important pathophysiological factors: static mechanical factors, dynamic mechanical factors, and spinal cord ischemia [2]. Unlike typical CSM, ossification of the posterior longitudinal ligament (OPLL) represents a distinct etiological entity with unique natural history [9] that is more commonly seen in certain Asian populations.

The natural history of CSM is very difficult to study due to heterogeneous patient populations, subjective questionnaires used to grade myelopathy and quality of life (QOL) outcomes, and the impossibility of verifying compliance with non-operative therapy. Although the use of the Japanese Orthopaedic Association (JOA) score is very popular among spine surgeons, the validity of the cutoff JOA score has not been formally tested, and cutoff JOA scores have been seldom used except in some studies. Other commonly used scales include the modified JOA (mJOA), as well as the Nurick scale, which primarily assesses function of the lower extremities. For the Nurick scale, a higher score indicates greater functional impairment (range 0–5). Alternatively, for the mJOA scale, a higher number is associated with normal function (range 1–18). QOL measures have become increasingly important, compared to relying solely on clinical signs/symptoms, in addressing subjective patient concerns when comparing outcomes.

The literature has historically been sparse on studies focusing on comparing outcome measures for patients with CSM. In a recent retrospective study of 119 patients undergoing surgery for CSM by Lubelski et al. [22], the authors compared measured QOL outcomes: health utility (EQ-5D), Patient Health Questionnaire-9 (PHQ-9), and Pain Disability Questionnaire (PDQ) of patients diagnosed with CSM for a 1-year period compared to the CSM-specific measures (mJOA, Nurick scale). The main goal of this study was to examine the convergent validity of QOL outcome measures for CSM, evaluate the responsiveness of each outcome measure, and assess the ability of each measure to predict positive or negative surgical outcomes via EQ-5D index scores [22]. They discovered that all measures demonstrated statistical significance with the EQ-5D and PDQ functional and total scores. The Nurick scale performed the worst in that it did not show significant correlation with either the PHQ-9 or the psychosocial component of the PDQ. Furthermore, the correlation of the Nurick scale was the lowest among those questionnaires with which it did achieve statistical significance. Among the myelopathy scores, the mJOA performed best. The substantially lower correlation between the mJOA and QOL outcomes suggests that these questionnaires are evaluating different aspects of the patient experience. The authors subsequently concluded that the mJOA is best used with the PDQ questionnaire to accurately evaluate the patient's experience following surgery for CSM.

Asymptomatic Cervical Spondylotic Stenosis

Much of our understanding of the natural history of patients with asymptomatic spondylotic cervical stenosis, and the risk for progression to symptomatic myelopathy, comes from prospective cohort studies performed by Bednarik et al. [3, 4, 5]. In the most recent study [3], the authors investigated 199 patients who received an MRI due to either moderate to severe cervical axial pain or clinical signs and symptoms of cervical radiculopathy. These patients were all admitted to the department of neurology between 1993 and 2005 and completed at least a 2-year follow-up. Inclusion criteria were MRI signs of spondylogenic or discogenic compression of the cervical spinal cord, axial pain and/or clinical signs and symptoms of radiculopathy, and the absence of clinical signs and symptoms that might be attributed to cervical cord involvement. The functional status of the patients was scored according to the modified Japanese Orthopaedic Association (mJOA) scale. 141 patients had a maximum entry score of 18, while 58 had a score of 16–17 resulting from motor and/or sensory signs of cervical radiculopathy. The primary end point was defined as the occurrence of clinical signs and symptoms of

CSM and a decrease in the mJOA scale of at least 1 point. Patients were examined at the beginning of the study, every 6 months for the first 2 years, and then annually.

During the follow-up period, 45 patients (22.6%) displayed clinical evidence of progression to symptomatic CSM with a decrease of at least 1 point in the mJOA scale. Sixteen of these patients (35.5%) progressed within 12 months of entry into the study. The 25th percentile time to clinical manifestation of myelopathy was 48.4 months.

Of the variables studied that might be associated with the development of symptomatic CSM, statistical significance was found for radiculopathy ($P < 0.001$), abnormal EMG ($P < 0.001$), abnormal MEP ($P < 0.001$), abnormal SSEP ($P < 0.001$), and MRI hyperintensity ($P = 0.049$). Male gender had an increased risk that did not reach significance ($P = 0.072$). Other risk factors investigated that were not associated with progression to myelopathy included age >50, type of compression (osteophytes and/or herniation), number of stenotic levels, Pavlov ratio <0.8, compression ratio <0.4, or cross-sectional spinal cord area <70 mm^2. Interestingly, risk of early progression (≤12 months) was predicted by the presence of clinically symptomatic radiculopathy, abnormal SEP, and abnormal MEP. Male gender and EMG abnormality were excluded from the set of independent risk factors and ultimately the multivariate regression model, due to highly significant positive correlation with radiculopathy ($P < 0.001$). Conversely, MRI hyperintensity predicted later (>12 months) development of CSM.

Findings such as these prompted the American Association of Neurological Surgeons/Congress of Neurological Surgeons (AANS/CNS) clinical practice guidelines workgroup to recommend that "in patients with cervical stenosis without myelopathy who have either abnormal EMG findings or clinical radiculopathy, decompression should be considered. The presence of EMG abnormalities or clinical radiculopathy is associated with development of symptomatic CSM (quality of evidence, Class I; strength of recommendation, B)" [25].

In an additional study by Bednarik et al. [6], the same 199 patients with asymptomatic spondylotic cervical stenosis as previously followed were analyzed for the risk of the development of symptomatic myelopathy after minor trauma. They concluded that there was no statistically significant association between traumatic events and the subsequent development of symptomatic myelopathy (OR 0.935; 95% CI, 0.247–3.535; $p = 0.921$).

Much of the data regarding the progression of asymptomatic patients with ossification of the posterior longitudinal ligament (OPLL) comes from two studies by Matsunaga et al. [23, 24]. These were both prospective cohort studies. In the first study, 323 patients did not have myelopathy on initial presentation and were treated conservatively. Of these patients, 55 (17%) developed myelopathic symptoms requiring surgery. Utilizing a Kaplan-Meier estimate of the remaining myelopathy-free patients, 71% remained that way at 30-year follow-up. All patients with OPLL-induced stenosis greater than 60% developed symptoms of myelopathy. Additionally, increased range of motion was found to be a significant risk factor for those patients with myelopathy and less than 60% stenosis. The authors measured the angle between C1 and the inferior margin of C7 on flexion and extension radiographs and found that the group of patients with myelopathy had a cervical ROM of 75.6° ± 18.3. Those patients without myelopathy had a cervical ROM of 36.5° ± 15.9 ($P < 0.05$). Therefore, the authors concluded that in patients with less than 60% stenosis, ROM appears to be an important variable in the development of myelopathy. In a later multicenter prospective cohort study [23], the same authors evaluated 156 patients from 16 institutions over an average 10.3-year period. They did not report on the time interval to the development of myelopathy. Similar to their previous work, all patients with greater than 60% OPLL-induced stenosis had symptoms of myelopathy. 57 (49%) of the remaining 117 with <60% stenosis were myelopathic. Once again, an increased ROM was associated with the development of myelopathy. Additionally, a lateral-deviated-type OPLL opposed to central OPLL was more commonly seen in patients who developed myelopathy.

With regard to OPLL in asymptomatic patients and their risk for progression after minor trauma, 1 study found that 13/19 (68%) of patients developed myelopathy [19]. This would suggest that asymptomatic patients with underlying OPLL may be at increased risk for the development of myelopathy after minor trauma, as opposed to those patients with CSM *not* caused by OPLL.

Mild CSM

The evidence for how best to manage a patient with mild CSM is weak to moderate at best. This is due to a heterogeneous patient population, inconsistent follow-up, and variation in nonoperative treatments. Additionally, the majority of studies rely on the JOA (Japanese Orthopedic Association), mJOA, motor function JOA, or Nurick scale for use as an objective measure of myelopathy.

Kadanka et al. [15, 16, 17] in a prospective study attempted to look at patients with mild or moderate clinical myelopathy (mJOA score ≥12) by randomizing them into two groups: those treated surgically and those treated conservatively. In their first study of 68 patients, 33 were treated surgically and 35 nonoperatively. Nonoperative treatment consisted of intermittent cervical immobilization with a soft collar, anti-inflammatory medications, intermittent bed rest for patients with pain, and active discouragement of high-risk activities. Inclusion criteria consisted of clinical signs and symptoms of myelopathy, MRI evidence of cord compression caused by spondylosis (with or without congenital narrowing of the spinal canal), age <75, mJOA score ≥12, and consent to surgery. Outcomes evaluated were a patient self-evaluation, mJOA, 10-meter timed walk, and daily activities (evaluated by two independent physicians blinded to the treatment). The results of this study did not show any difference in outcomes between those patients treated nonoperatively and those treated surgically. However, they acknowledged the goal with surgery is not for improvement but to stop progression and/or sudden deterioration. The same study population was assessed again at the 10-year mark [15], and at that time point, no significant difference between the groups was observed. The authors further acknowledged that according to the power analysis, these results could not definitively answer the question as to whether surgical versus nonsurgical treatment was appropriate in this patient population due to the low number of patients available for final evaluation.

Sumi et al. [30] added to the work of Kadanka with a prospective study of nonoperatively treated patients with mild CSM (JOA ≥13). Sixty patients with mild CSM (42 males and 18 females, average age 57.2 years) were initially treated conservatively. Patients with OPLL were excluded from the study. Follow-up records were available for 55. The mean overall follow-up period was 78.9 ± 39.0 months (range 5–147 months), with those that did not deteriorate being followed for more than 5 years. Surgery was offered with deterioration of myelopathy, defined as a decline in JOA score to less than 13 with a decrease of at least 2 points. Deterioration occurred in 14 of 55 (25.5%) cases between 5 and 96 months after the initial visit. There was not a significant difference seen in mean JOA score between the initial visit (14.5 ± 1.3) and the end point (14.1 ± 2.2; $p = 0.227$). Those patients that deteriorated had a decrease in JOA from 14.3 ± 1.0 to 10.9 ± 1.0 at the end point ($p = 0.001$). No statistical difference was seen between sex, age, or JOA score at the initial visit between the groups that deteriorated and those that remained clinically stable. 74.5% of mild CSM cases maintained the same level of symptoms without deterioration over more than 5 years, with a tolerance rate of 70%. The major prognostic factor in this study that predicted deterioration was the presence of angular-edged deformity, opposed to an ovoid deformity on T1-weighted axial MR imaging. Of those patients with ovoid deformity, only 1/19 (5.3%) deteriorated. This is in stark contrast to those with angular-edged deformity, of which 13/14 (92.9%) deteriorated and 23/41 (56.1%) remained stable during the follow-up period ($p = 0.006$).

Oshima et al. [26] performed a retrospective review of patients with mild myelopathy, as defined by a motor JOA score of 3 or more in both upper and lower extremities, in addition to cervical spinal cord compression with ISI (increased signal intensity) on T2-weighted MRI. They did not include patients with OPLL or disc herniation. The mean follow-up period was 78 months (range, 24–208 mo), and the end point was conversion to surgery. Of the 45 patients at the beginning of the study, 16 deteriorated and underwent surgery, while 27 remained neurologically stable. Two of the patients worsened after minor trauma and consequently received surgery. Kaplan-Meier survival analysis indicated that 82% of the patients continued to be followed without surgery at 5 years and 56% at 10 years. Prognostic factors of the 16 patients that gradually deteriorated were compared to the 27 patients who were followed without surgery, and significance was found for local slip, as well as the segmental lordotic angle at the maximum compression segment. Cox proportional hazard analysis revealed that total ROM between C2 and C7 larger than 50°, segmental kyphosis in the maximum compression segment, and existence of a local slip were all risk factors for surgery. The authors concluded that even in the presence of ISI on MRI, mild CSM is well tolerated in most patients. However, patients should be counseled on the possibility of acute spinal cord injury after minor trauma.

Similarly, Shimomura et al. [29] prospectively analyzed prognostic factors for deterioration in patients with mild CSM. The prognostic factors analyzed included age, gender, follow-up period, developmental or dynamic canal factors of the cervical spine on lateral radiographs, presence or absence of ISI, and the extent of cord compression at the maximum compression segment. The extent of cord compression was further divided into that of partial and circumferential. The mean follow-up period was 35.6 ± 25.2 months. Seventy patients with mild CSM were included in the analysis. Fifty-six of these 70 were observed for the duration of the study, of which 11 deteriorated (moderate or severe forms of myelopathy). The only factor that had a significant effect was circumferential spinal cord compression on axial MRI. Indeed, 10/11 patients with this finding deteriorated. Nonsurgical treatment is generally well tolerated as the first choice of treatment in mild CSM; however, the authors concluded that surgery can be considered for those patients with circumferential compression on axial MRI.

One of the most informative studies in the patient population with mild CSM (JOA ≥13) was performed by Kong et al. [20]. In this study, 78 patients were followed prospectively, and initial management was conservative (traction for 8 h/day for 2 weeks). After discharge, these patients were followed every 3 months and instructed to present earlier should myelopathic symptoms progress. Surgery was subsequently performed when JOA became <13 or a decrease of ≥2 points was observed. All surgeries were performed within 1 month of deterioration, and all surgically treated patients were followed for ≥1 year postoperatively. Twenty-one patients were ultimately treated surgically with a mean reduction in JOA score of 2.9 points (range 2–5) at the time of treatment. The remaining 57 patients had an average JOA score at presentation of 14.2 ± 1.0, compared to 14.0 ± 1.1 in the surgically treated group with a nonsignificant *p*-value of 0.62. The mean JOA score of the surgically treated group decreased to 11.1 ± 0.8 at the time of surgical treatment but improved to 13.4 ± 2.5 following timely surgical intervention. This work and the recent systematic review by Karadimas et al. [18] suggest that patients with mild CSM can be safely managed conservatively with close follow-up and surgical intervention performed acutely once progression of myelopathy is observed, since these patients can generally be expected to return to a level of neurological function similar to those patients who did not experience a decline in JOA scores.

Ultimately, treatment decision-making in mild CSM requires a balancing in understanding the above evidence base, clinician expertise, and patient choice. This is largely why the AANS/CNS spine section clinical practice guidelines recommend that "patients with mild CSM (aged younger than 75 years with a mJOA scale score

>12) be offered both operative and nonoperative management options (quality of evidence: Class I; strength of recommendation, B) [25]. Furthermore, evidence suggests that clinical gains after nonoperative treatment in this patient population are maintained over 3 years in 70% of cases (quality of evidence, Class III; strength of recommendation, D)" [25].

Spinal Cord Injury and CSM

Estimating the risk of acute spinal cord injury (SCI) or central cord syndrome from even minor trauma in patients with cervical stenosis is impossible due to the unknown prevalence of asymptomatic stenosis in the population. Some attempts at estimating this risk through administrative database reviews have been performed. In cases of mild CSM, Wu et al. [33] found a worst-case incidence of SCI of 13.9/1000 person-years for nonoperative care vs 9.4/1000 person-years for operative care. However, this study suffers from the typical problems associated with administrative database studies including lack of clinical granularity and likely incorrect coding issues. In patients with OPLL, however, some data suggests that the risk of SCI is higher than in typical CSM [10, 32], and so clinicians may have a lower threshold for surgical intervention in cases of mild myelopathy with OPLL.

Although patients with asymptomatic or minimally symptomatic CSM should be counseled regarding the possible risk of SCI in the absence of operative treatment, they should also be aware that this risk is very small [9]. Similarly, when contrasting the risks and benefits of treatment for asymptomatic/mild CSM, the clinician need also acknowledge the risks of operative intervention. Total complication rates (early and late) for CSM surgery in one prospective multicenter study [12] have been calculated to be 20%. Though a true "number needed to treat" when considering surgery to prevent a SCI cannot be accurately calculated, perhaps a true "number needed to harm" can be when analyzing surgical complications. Regardless, as mentioned earlier, the decision for or against surgery for asymptomatic or mild CSM should derive from a nuanced discussion between patient and surgeon that is driven by the limited evidence available, rational consideration of the risks, surgeon judgment, and patient preferences.

Moderate to Severe CSM

There is a consensus that patients with moderate to severe CSM should undergo surgical decompression [28]. These patients have a low likelihood of improvement with nonoperative measures [25].

Conclusions, Key Recommendations, and Guidelines

- For asymptomatic patients with evidence of cervical cord compression (without evidence of radiculopathy), prophylactic surgery should not be offered. These patients should be closely followed clinically and understand the relevant signs and symptoms for which to watch. For patients with clinical evidence of a radiculopathy or abnormal findings on EMG, SEP, or MEP, a surgical discussion is appropriate once the patient has failed conservative measures. Class I evidence shows that electromyographic abnormalities (as well as presence of radiculopathy) are predictive of the development of myelopathy in minimally symptomatic patients with cervical stenosis and spinal cord compression [11]. Class II evidence suggests that somatosensory evoked potentials have prognostic value in patients with CSM [11].
- For patients with mild CSM, 20–60% will progress over time without surgical intervention [18]. A supervised trial of nonoperative management may be appropriate in this group. Class II evidence suggests that in patients with mild to moderate CSM (mJOA ≥12), the clinical condition remains stable when observed over a 3-year period in patients younger than 75 [11]. If, however, they fail to improve or demonstrate subsequent neuro-

logical deterioration, prompt operative intervention is warranted.

- The presence of low signal on T1-weighted images and high signal on T2-weighted images and the presence of cord atrophy on preoperative MRI in CSM are indicators of poorer outcome as well as lack of improvement after surgical intervention [11].
- Class III evidence suggests that the duration of symptoms and possibly advancing age negatively affect outcome in patients with CSM [11].
- All patients with moderate and severe CSM should undergo surgical intervention [25].

References

1. Abbed KM, Coumans JV. Cervical radiculopathy: pathophysiology, presentation, and clinical evaluation. Neurosurgery. 2007;60:S28–34.
2. Baron EM, Young WF. Cervical spondylotic myelopathy: a brief review of its pathophysiology, clinical course, and diagnosis. Neurosurgery. 2007;60:S35–41.
3. Bednarik J, Kadanka Z, Dusek L, et al. Presymptomatic spondylotic cervical myelopathy: an updated predictive model. Eur Spine J. 2008;17:421–31.
4. Bednarik J, Kadanka Z, Dusek L, et al. Presymptomatic spondylotic cervical cord compression. Spine (Phila Pa 1976). 2004;29:2260–9.
5. Bednarík J, Kadanka Z, Vohánka S, et al. The value of somatosensory and motor evoked potentials in preclinical spondylotic cervical cord compression. Eur Spine J. 1998;7:493–500.
6. Bednarik J, Sladkova D, Kadanka Z, et al. Are subjects with spondylotic cervical cord encroachment at increased risk of cervical spinal cord injury after minor trauma? J Neurol Neurosurg Psychiatry. 2011;82:779–81.
7. Blumenkrantz N, Sylvest J, Asboe-Hansen G. Local low-collagen content may allow herniation of intervertebral disc: biochemical studies. Biochem Med. 1977;18:283–90.
8. Boogaarts HD, Bartels RH. Prevalence of cervical spondylotic myelopathy. Eur Spine J. 2015;24(Suppl 2):139–41.
9. Chang H, Song KJ, Kim HY, et al. Factors related to the development of myelopathy in patients with cervical ossification of the posterior longitudinal ligament. J Bone Joint Surg Br. 2012;94:946–9.
10. Chikuda H, Seichi A, Takeshita K, et al. Acute cervical spinal cord injury complicated by preexisting ossification of the posterior longitudinal ligament: a multicenter study. Spine (Phila Pa 1976). 2011;36:1453–8.
11. Fehlings MG, Arvin B. Surgical management of cervical degenerative disease: the evidence related to indications, impact, and outcome. J Neurosurg Spine. 2009;11:97–100.
12. Fehlings MG, Smith JS, Kopjar B, et al. Perioperative and delayed complications associated with the surgical treatment of cervical spondylotic myelopathy based on 302 patients from the AOSpine North America cervical Spondylotic myelopathy study. J Neurosurg Spine. 2012;16:425–32.
13. Gore DR, Sepic SB, Gardner GM. Roentgenographic findings of the cervical spine in asymptomatic people. Spine (Phila Pa 1976). 1986;11:521–4.
14. Hadley MN, Reddy SV. Smoking and the human vertebral column: a review of the impact of cigarette use on vertebral bone metabolism and spinal fusion. Neurosurgery. 1997;41:116–24.
15. Kadaňka Z, Bednařík J, Novotný O, et al. Cervical spondylotic myelopathy: conservative versus surgical treatment after 10 years. Eur Spine J. 2011;20:1533–8.
16. Kadanka Z, Mares M, Bednaník J, et al. Approaches to spondylotic cervical myelopathy: conservative versus surgical results in a 3-year follow-up study. Spine (Phila Pa 1976). 2002;27:2205–10. discussion 10-1
17. Kadanka Z, Mares M, Bednarík J, et al. Predictive factors for spondylotic cervical myelopathy treated conservatively or surgically. *Eur J Neurol*. 2005;12:55–63.
18. Karadimas SK, Erwin WM, Ely CG, et al. Pathophysiology and natural history of cervical spondylotic myelopathy. Spine (Phila Pa 1976). 2013;38:S21–36.
19. Katoh S, Ikata T, Hirai N, et al. Influence of minor trauma to the neck on the neurological outcome in patients with ossification of the posterior longitudinal ligament (OPLL) of the cervical spine. Paraplegia. 1995;33:330–3.
20. Kong LD, Meng LC, Wang LF, et al. Evaluation of conservative treatment and timing of surgical intervention for mild forms of cervical spondylotic myelopathy. Exp Ther Med. 2013;6:852–6.
21. Kumaresan S, Yoganandan N, Pintar FA, et al. Contribution of disc degeneration to osteophyte formation in the cervical spine: a biomechanical investigation. J Orthop Res. 2001;19:977–84.
22. Lubelski D, Alvin MD, Nesterenko S, et al. Correlation of quality of life and functional outcome measures for cervical spondylotic myelopathy. J Neurosurg Spine. 2016;24:483–9.
23. Matsunaga S, Nakamura K, Seichi A, et al. Radiographic predictors for the development of myelopathy in patients with ossification of the posterior longitudinal ligament: a multicenter cohort study. Spine (Phila Pa 1976). 2008;33:2648–50.
24. Matsunaga S, Sakou T, Taketomi E, et al. Clinical course of patients with ossification of the posterior longitudinal ligament: a minimum 10-year cohort study. J Neurosurg. 2004;100:245–8.

25. Matz PG, Anderson PA, Holly LT, et al. The natural history of cervical spondylotic myelopathy. J Neurosurg Spine. 2009;11:104–11.
26. Oshima Y, Seichi A, Takeshita K, et al. Natural course and prognostic factors in patients with mild cervical spondylotic myelopathy with increased signal intensity on T2-weighted magnetic resonance imaging. Spine (Phila Pa 1976). 2012;37:1909–13.
27. Patel AA, Spiker WR, Daubs M, et al. Evidence of an inherited predisposition for cervical spondylotic myelopathy. Spine (Phila Pa 1976). 2012;37:26–9.
28. Rhee JM, Shamji MF, Erwin WM, et al. Nonoperative management of cervical myelopathy: a systematic review. Spine (Phila Pa 1976). 2013;38:S55–67.
29. Shimomura T, Sumi M, Nishida K, et al. Prognostic factors for deterioration of patients with cervical spondylotic myelopathy after nonsurgical treatment. Spine (Phila Pa 1976). 2007;32:2474–9.
30. Sumi M, Miyamoto H, Suzuki T, et al. Prospective cohort study of mild cervical spondylotic myelopathy without surgical treatment. J Neurosurg Spine. 2012;16:8–14.
31. Wang ZC, Shi JG, Chen XS, et al. The role of smoking status and collagen IX polymorphisms in the susceptibility to cervical spondylotic myelopathy. Genet Mol Res. 2012;11:1238–44.
32. Wu JC, Chen YC, Liu L, et al. Conservatively treated ossification of the posterior longitudinal ligament increases the risk of spinal cord injury: a nationwide cohort study. J Neurotrauma. 2012;29:462–8.
33. Wu JC, Ko CC, Yen YS, et al. Epidemiology of cervical spondylotic myelopathy and its risk of causing spinal cord injury: a national cohort study. Neurosurg Focus. 2013;35:E10.

Part II

Evaluation and Diagnosis of Cervical Spondylotic Disorders

Fundamentals of Cervical Neurological Exam

7

Meena Thatikunta and Maxwell Boakye

Pearls and Pitfalls

- The neurological exam provides the foundation for clinical decision-making; clinicians should be adept at distinguishing normal from abnormal findings on exam.
- Physical examination should be thorough and relevant to suspected pathology.
- Cervical radiculopathy and cervical myelopathy are common clinical scenarios; however there are a host of other disease entities with similar presentations. Distinguishing these non-neurosurgical entities is imperative to appropriate patient management.

Introduction

History and physical examination are critical in the evaluation of cervical myelopathy and radiculopathy. Physical examination guides the decision to pursue surgery, the potential benefit of surgery, as well as surgical approach. Operative decisions should be questioned when physical examination findings are incongruent with diagnosis and/or radiological findings.

Neurological testing should be thorough and include relevant examinations of cervical alignment, skin, muscle bulk, range of motion, tone, motor, sensory modalities, reflexes, and gait [1].

In this chapter, we review the signs, symptoms, and physical findings consistent with axial neck pain, radiculopathy, and myelopathy or myeloradiculopathy. Importantly, radiculopathy and myelopathy must be distinguished from imitators of cervical degenerative myelopathy and radiculopathy. At the end of the chapter is a brief overview of neurosurgical and non-neurosurgical entities that must be distinguished from radiculopathy and/or myelopathy through pointed history and physical examination.

Components of the Neurological Examination

Examiners should have an organized framework which addresses cervical alignment, skin, muscle bulk, range of motion, tone, motor strength, sensory modalities, reflexes, and special maneuvers [1]. As examiners progress in their training, the exam may become more focused and relevant to certain pathologies. Patients may also present

M. Thatikunta · M. Boakye (✉)
Department of Neurosurgery, University of Louisville, Louisville, KY, USA
e-mail: max.boakye@louisville.edu

M. G. Kaiser et al. (eds.), *Degenerative Cervical Myelopathy and Radiculopathy*,
https://doi.org/10.1007/978-3-319-97952-6_7

with non-neurological diagnosis, necessitating physical examination of other organ systems, i.e., left arm paresthesias in a patient with acute myocardial infarction. Examiners should also recognize when physical exam findings do not follow an anatomical pattern, e.g., ipsilateral facial and body numbness, indicating that there may not be an organic cause.

Cervical Alignment

Cervical alignment refers to the curvature of the cervical bodies in the sagittal and coronal planes. Normal sagittal alignment is lordotic. Abnormal cervical alignment may include kyphosis, scoliosis, and/or torticollis [1]. Alignment is best assessed on imaging, rather than on physical examination. See Fig. 7.1 for examples of kyphotic and lordotic alignment.

Muscle Bulk and Tone

The source of muscle bulk changes can localize to any portion of the neuromuscular system including the central nervous system, peripheral nervous system, neuromuscular junction, and primary muscle. Upper motor neuron disorders will exhibit weakness, decreased muscle bulk over time, and increased tone. Lower motor neuron pathology will exhibit weakness, muscle atrophy, and flaccidity [7]. Examiners should inspect muscle bulk for any wasting in the extremities. If wasting is identified, then note differences between right and left, proximal and distal, and upper extremity and lower extremity [1]. While there is no formal grading system for muscle bulk, examiners can assess for atrophy, hypertrophy, or pseudohypertrophy through visual inspection [19]. Generally, muscle wasting is indicative of a long-standing pathology.

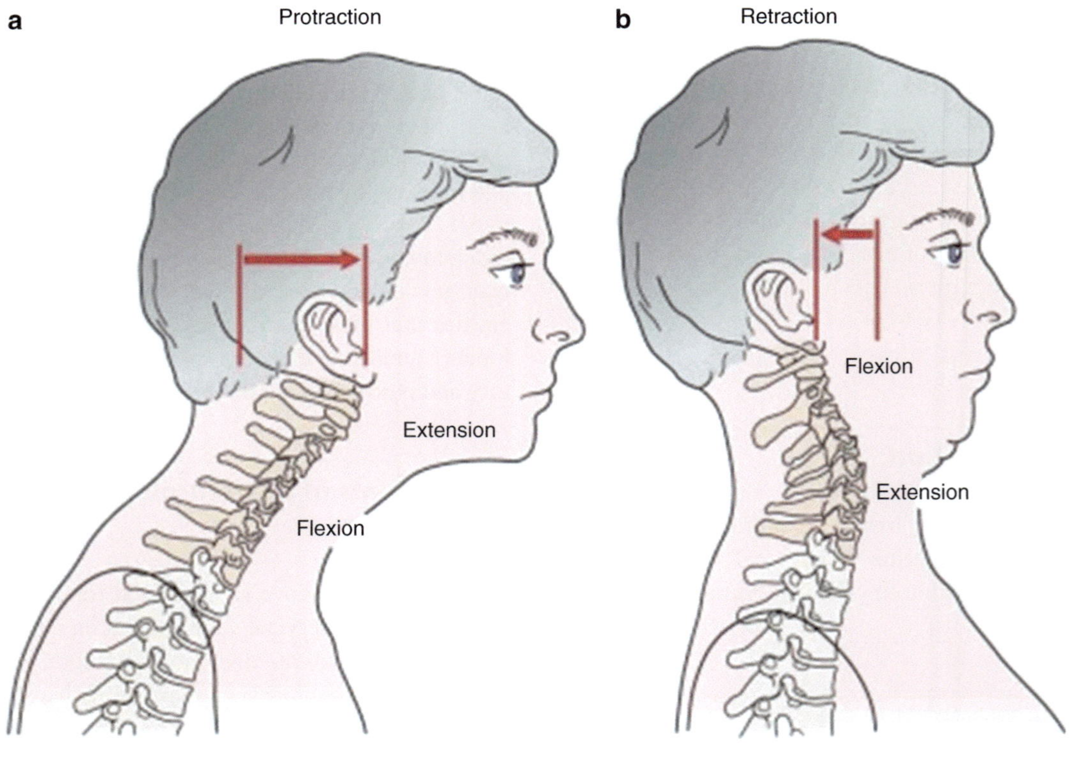

Fig. 7.1 Panel A demonstrating a kyphotic cervical alignment and panel B demonstrating a lordotic alignment. (Magee [10])

Table 7.1 Modified Ashworth scale

Grade	Tone
0	No increase in muscle tone
1	Slight increase in muscle tone, catch, or resistance at the end of range of motion
1+	Catch proceeded by slight increase in muscle tone through less than half range of motion
2	Increase muscle tone throughout range of motion but extremities still easily moved
3	Marked increase in tone, resistance to passive movement
4	Rigid flexion or extension

Tone should be assessed for multiple reasons: (1) preoperative to postoperative comparison, (2) elucidation of other neurological pathologies, and (3) understanding of upper motor neuron damage in the spinal cord or brain. Muscle tone is subjectively defined as hypotonia or hypertonia. The Ashworth scale objectifies findings of hypertonia and is commonly used in patients with spasticity. Please see Table 7.1 for description of the scale. In cervical myelopathy, spasticity is common [1, 12].

Range of Motion

Range of motion can be limited by a combination of factors, including pain, muscular strain, degenerative bony changes, and/or cervical fusion. Range of motion is tested simply through flexion, extension, and lateral bending. Degrees of deficit can be detected through passive and active motion, as well as against resistance [1].

Motor

Motor testing should be completed in all extremities with special attention to areas of expected deficit. Motor testing can be graded according to the schema provided in Table 7.2. Of note, extremities may exhibit different velocities and contraction forces based on the muscle length. Maximal contraction of the muscle fiber is reached when shortening occurs but then decreases with extreme shortening and lengthening of the muscle fiber, in parabolic fashion. This is termed the "length-strength" principle (Fig. 7.2). For optimal examination, one should place large muscles at somewhat of a mechanical disadvantage (when muscle not optimally shortened) and small muscles at an advantage (optimally shortened) to exploit the "length-strength" principle.

Table 7.2 Motor grading

Grading	Strength
0	No muscle twitch
1	Muscle twitch present but no movement
2	Able to move with elimination of gravity
3	Moves antigravity but not against resistance
4	Moves against some resistance
5	Moves against full resistance

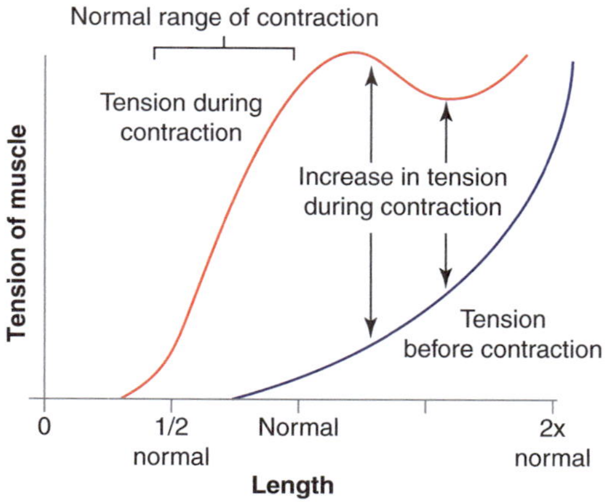

Fig. 7.2 Tension versus length of muscle in the muscle. (Hall [9])

Examiners should note whether motor deficits follow a nerve root versus peripheral nerve distribution. Specific nerve roots can be tested through isolated muscle group assessment, for example, the triceps muscle corresponds well to the C7 nerve root. In comparison, the C6 nerve root cannot be isolated and supplies multiple muscle groups. See Fig. 7.3 for dedicated enumeration of cervical myotomes and dermatomes.

Sensory

Light Touch, Pain, Temperature, and Vibration

While multiple modalities are available for sensory testing, generally light touch with the examiner's fingers or a tissue is adequate for the

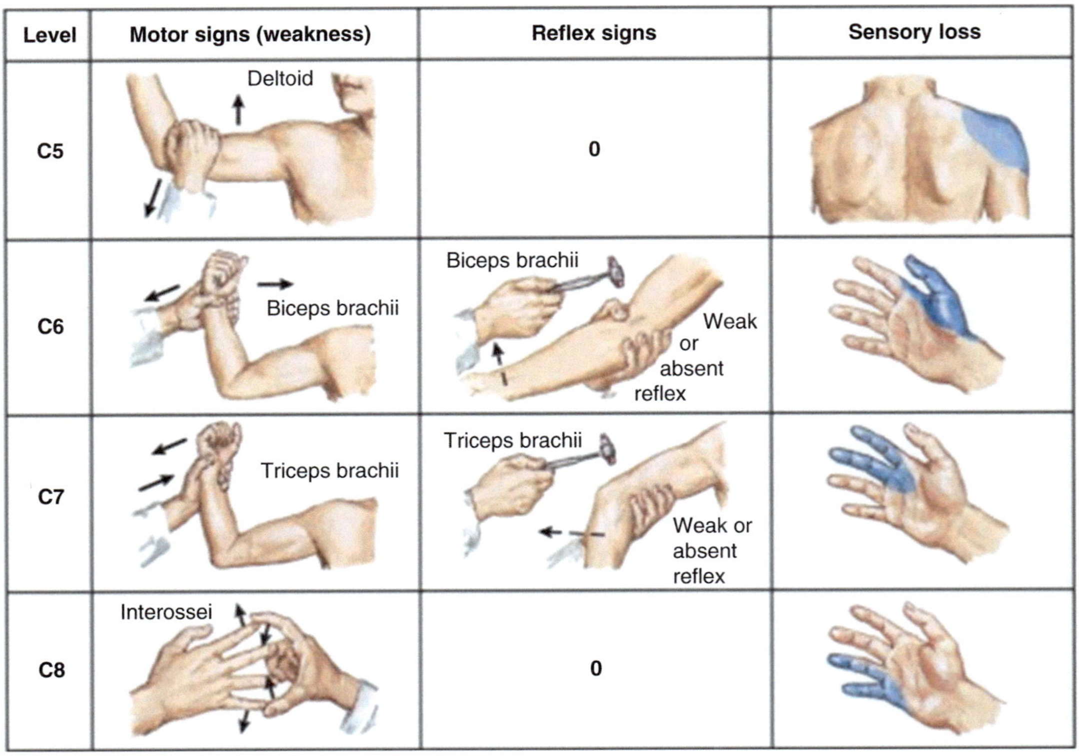

Fig. 7.3 Cervical dermatomes and myotomes. (Royden et al. [16])

determination of sensory loss. If there is suspicion for a Brown-Sequard pattern, then pain and temperature testing should also be performed. Figure 7.3 enumerates cervical dermatomes [1].

Pain should be tested with a pin tip. Begin the examination by testing an area known to be normal to establish a baseline for the patient. Then proceed to the necessary dermatomes. Examiners should be careful to induce pain but not pressure with the pin tip. Pain is carried primarily in the anterolateral system which crosses immediately at that level but may be carried in other ascending spinal pathways [1].

Temperature can be tested with hot or cold. Similar to pain, begin the exam by testing an area known to be normal to establish a baseline. Then proceed to relevant dermatomes [1]. Temperature is solely carried in the anterolateral system and is more specific than pain.

Vibration can be tested with the use of a tuning fork, preferably 256 Hz which activates the Pacinian corpuscles [1].

Position Sense

The patient should close their eyes before position sense testing. The examiner may then elevate or depress a phalange and then ask the patient which direction their phalange has been displaced [1]. The examiner should be careful to place their own fingers in a neutral position, such as on either side of the patient's finger so as not to bias the patient's perception. Placing the examiner's fingers on the ventral and dorsal aspects of the patient's phalanges places directional pressure which the patient can sense and is a confounder of position sense pathways.

Position sense is an important discriminator in certain pathologies, i.e., position sense is spared in anterior spinal syndrome, and position sense is lost in tabes dorsalis or vitamin B12 deficiency which affects the posterior columns [12]. Position sense should not be altered in radiculopathy.

Table 7.3 Reflex grading

Grading	Reflex response
0	No reflex response
1+	Hyporeflexic
2+	Normal reflex response
3+	Hyperreflexic
4+	Hyperreflexic with clonus

Table 7.4 Reflex levels

Reflex	Level
Biceps	C5
Brachioradialis	C6
Triceps	C7
Patellar	L2–L4
Ankle	L5–S1

Reflexes

Reflexes are tested by placing the thumb over the tendon of interest and then striking the thumb with a reflex hammer. Reflexes have a standard grading system from 0 to 4. These are outlined in Table 7.3. Abnormal reflexes should be correlated with their cervical level. These are outlined in Table 7.4 [1]. Crossed radial reflex may occur when the reflex arc extends to the next joint; as in, the biceps reflex is tested, the patient displays a normal biceps response, and in addition the wrist extends. This is a sign of spinal cord compression, myelopathy, or spasticity. Inverted radial reflex is flexion of the fingers and diminished wrist extension in response to tapping the distal brachioradialis tendon. Inverted radial reflex is thought to localize to C5 to C6 [6].

Babinski

Babinski sign indicates an upper motor neuron lesion. Babinski is tested by dragging the tip of a hard object from the heel, upward along the lateral edge of the foot and then medially across dorsum of the foot. An abnormal response is extension of the first toe. A normal response is plantar flexion of the first toe [1].

Hoffman's

Hoffman's test indicates an upper motor neuron lesion and is routinely tested in the cervical neurological exam. The patient's hand should remain relaxed. The examiner flicks the middle fingernail, and if Hoffman's sign is present, then the patient will reflexively flex the fingers [1].

Clonus

Clonus is performed by forcefully dorsiflexing the patient's ankle. A positive response is seen with "beating back" of the foot. Clonus is graded on the number of beats. Severe clonus displays sustained beating of the foot [1]. There is no consensus on the number of beats considered abnormal, but in general, four or more beats should raise suspicion of an upper motor neuron lesion.

Maneuvers

Maneuvers should be used as adjuncts to the cervical neurological examinations. These are described in the following section. Sensitivities and specificities of each maneuver are listed in Table 7.5.

Spurling's

Spurling's tests assess for foraminal compression in the cervical spine. In the upright position, the patient's head should be slightly extended, rotated, and laterally flexed to one side. Once in position, the examiner applies downward axial force on top of the patient's head. If this worsens the patient's radiculopathy, then this indicates compression of the nerve root at the foramen [1, 4].

L'Hermitte's Sign

L'Hermitte's sign indicates upper motor neuron disease and is classically seen in multiple sclerosis; however, it can be seen in other neurologic conditions such as cervical degenerative myelopathy. L'Hermitte's sign is tested by placing the head in flexion and applying downward force on the head. The patient should subjectively feel an electric shock sensation through the spine [1].

Table 7.5 Specificity and sensitivity of cervical maneuvers

Maneuver	Specificity	Sensitivity
Spurling's sign	95%	92%
	93%	30%
L'Hermitte's sign	97%	28%
Distraction test	100%	40–43%
Hoffman's	78%	28–94%
Clonus	96–100%	7–13%
Babinski	92–100%	7–53%
Adson's test	Not reported	Not reported
Broad or spastic gait	94%	19%
Hand withdrawal reflex	63%	41%
Finger escape sign	100%	50%

Cook et al. [6], Malanga et al. [11], Rhee et al. [13], Shah and Rajshekar [14], Tong et al. [17]

Distraction Test

Distraction testing mimics the effects of traction on the spine by widening the neural foramina. The distraction test is performed by placing one hand behind the head and the other under the chin, placing the head in slight extension or flexion, and then pulling gently upward. If the patient experiences relief of their radiculopathy, this indicates a foraminal etiology which may be alleviated by surgical intervention such as foraminotomy or laminectomy [1].

Adson's Test

Adson's test can demonstrate subclavian artery compression which can be from subclavian artery stenosis, the presence of cervical rib, or tightened scalenus and medius muscles. The test is performed by placing the arm in an abducted, externally rotated position above the level of the clavicle. Ask the patient to breathe in and hold their breath and turn their head toward the raised arm. Meanwhile, the examiner is palpating the radial pulse. If there is subclavian artery compression, then the pulse will be reduced or lost [1].

Hand Withdrawal Reflex

While holding the patient's hand so the fingers hang limply in the air, the dorsum of the hand is tapped with a reflex hammer. An abnormal response is finger flexion. Hand withdrawal reflex is seen in cervical myelopathy [6].

Finger Escape Sign

Finger escape sign can be elicited in myelopathic patients by instructing the patient to hold fingers extended and adducted. A positive finger escape sign is seen when the last digit spontaneously abducts and flexes due to intrinsic weakness in the hand [6].

Grip and Release Test

The patient is asked to make a tight grip and then release their grip 20 times in 10 seconds. This repetitive action is slowed in myelopathic patients [6].

Cervical Pathology: Axial Neck Pain, Radiculopathy, and Myelopathy

Axial Neck Pain

Axial neck pain is a challenging pathology, particularly for neurosurgeons. The etiology of neck pain is vast and may not be due to cervical pathology; degenerative changes are common and may not be the source of neck pain; and lastly, operating on cervical pathology may not alleviate the patient's neck pain. Alternatively, degenerative disc disease and facet disease can present with axial neck pain, headache, or scapular pain. Complaints of solely pain can complicate operative decisions. As a principle, surgeons should attempt to correlate levels of disease with distribution of pain, i.e., C7–T1 degenerative disease can present as interscapular pain. See Fig. 7.4 for further depiction of pain distributions related to degenerative cervical pathology. Palpation is useful in ruling out myofascial pain, weakness, or overuse [1].

Radiculopathy by Group

C2 to C4 Radiculopathy

Upper cervical radiculopathies should be considered in patients presenting with headache and pure neck pain. Due to the distribution, there may be no associated sensory or motor deficits; how-

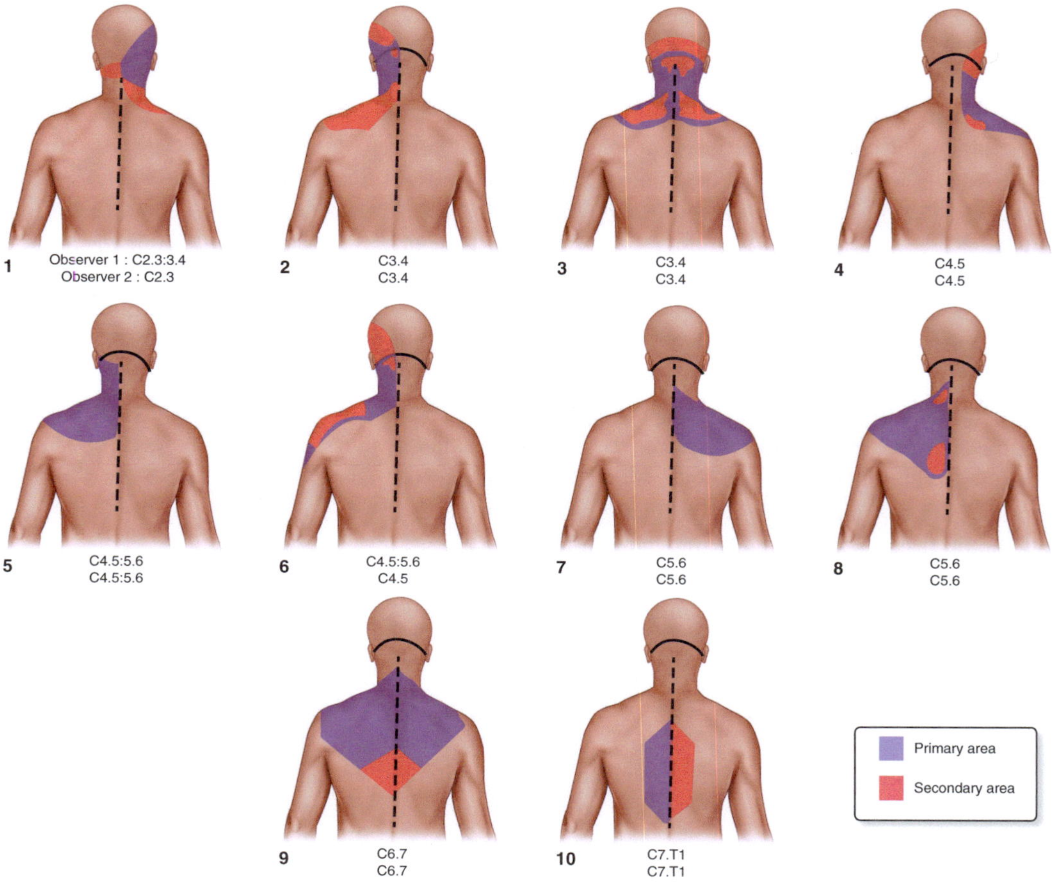

Fig. 7.4 Distributions of pain related to cervical degenerative disease. (Aprill et al. [2])

ever, CN XI deficits may be noted due to their cervical origin in the lateral aspect of the anterior horn cell. The C2 to C4 dermatome covers the posterior skull, neck, and upper chest and scapular areas [1, 15].

C5 to C6 Radiculopathy

C5 to C6 radiculopathy presentation overlaps significantly with shoulder pathology and brachial plexus pathology engendering the physical examination critical in the differentiation process. Shoulder abduction supplied by the deltoid (C5), elbow flexion supplied by biceps (C5, C6), supination supplied by multiple muscle groups (C5), internal and external rotation of the shoulder supplied by multiple muscle groups (C5, C6), and wrist extension supplied by multiple muscle groups (C6) may be weak. Sensory loss is seen in the C5 (axillary nerve) and C6 (lateral antebrachial cutaneous nerve) distribution over the lateral aspect of the arm. The biceps reflex supplied by C5 or the brachioradialis supplied by C6 may be abnormal [1, 7, 15].

C7 Radiculopathy

Weakness of elbow extension supplied by the triceps (C7) and wrist flexion (C7, C8) may be evident in C7 radiculopathy. C7 nerve root provides sensation to the middle digit. The triceps reflex is supplied by C7 [1, 15].

C8 Radiculopathy

The C8 nerve root contributes to finger flexion and thumb adduction. C8 dermatome covers the medial portion of the forearm, fourth and fifth digits [1, 15].

T1 Radiculopathy

Finger abduction and adduction are controlled by the interossei (C8, T1). Medial brachial cutaneous nerve (T1) provides sensation to the medial arm [1, 15].

Myelopathy

Myelopathy is a common neurosurgical entity in spine practice. Presenting symptoms may be subtle, including incoordination and gait abnormalities. Patients may complain of difficulty with fine motor tasks, such as buttoning buttons or using zippers. Severe myelopathy is characterized by neck pain, extremity weakness, distal extremity numbness, spasticity, and gait abnormalities.

Physical examination generally reveals signs of upper motor neuron injury:

- Motor examination may reveal weakness in the extremities, more likely the distal upper extremities and proximal lower extremities.
- Sensory examination may show numbness, classically in the distal extremities.
- Reflex testing may show hyperreflexia and perhaps inverted or crossed radial signs.
- Hoffman's sign and sustained clonus are signs of more severe myelopathy.
- Tone may be increased, characteristic of spasticity.
- Gait may display slowness, stiffness, broad-based steppage, and hesitancy.
- In the case of acute injury in chronic myelopathy, such as hyperextension injuries in pre-existing spinal stenosis and myelopathy, urinary changes should be assessed, and rectal tone should be noted. Patients with urinary retention, incontinence, and/or poor rectal tone should be considered for emergent surgical decompression.

Myelopathy presents on a spectrum and may overlap with radiculopathy resulting in myeloradiculopathy. Radiculopathy is present in approximately half of myelopathy patients. Myelopathy and radiculopathy may be difficult to separate in these patients. Common myelopathy signs may be present including hand weakness, hyperreflexia, and abnormal gait. Superimposed radiculopathy will present as pain or paresthesias following a radicular distribution. Weakness and paresthesias of the hand are generally attributable to compression of the anterior horn cells rather than nerve root compression. Spurling's sign and shoulder abduction relief test are specific for radiculopathy. Most commonly, the C5–C6 level is affected, and 59% of cases show multilevel pathology [5]. Myelopathy may be induced by metabolic abnormalities or radiation; these entities are non-operative [12, 15].

Imitators of Cervical Pathology

Shoulder Pathology

Cervical pathology may closely resemble shoulder pathology, including rotator cuff tear, frozen shoulder, impingement syndrome, osteoarthritis, and shoulder dislocation. History may relay pain over the shoulder joint or difficulty with shoulder abduction which should be distinguished from C5/C6 radiculopathy. Physical examination is particularly helpful in identifying presence and/or concomitance of shoulder pathology. Palpation of the clavicle, acromioclavicular joint, humeral head, and glenohumeral joint can elicit tenderness which localizes well to the pathologic area. The strength of subscapularis muscle can be tested with internal rotation and lift-off test. Lift-off testing is performed by the patient placing the dorsal surface of their hand on his/her back (internal rotation at the shoulder) and pressing the said hand into the examiner's hand against resistance. Weakness against resistance is positive indicator. Lift-off testing reveals subscapularis weakness in patients with shoulder pathology. Infraspinatus and teres minor can be tested with external rotation. Supraspinatus is commonly affected by impingement syndrome and can be tested through several maneuvers. Hawkin's maneuver is tested by placing the arm in front of the body at shoulder level with the elbow flexed at 90°. The examiner then places upward pressure at the elbow and downward pressure at the wrist. Neer's test is performed by stabilizing the scapula and raising the patient's arm while in full internal rotation. Both maneuvers will exacerbate shoulder pain in a patient with true shoulder pathology. Importantly, this sign may also relieve pain in the patient with cervical radiculopathy and is alternately termed the shoulder abduction relief sign [12].

Brachial Plexitis

Brachial plexitis (Parsonage-Turner syndrome) is a predominantly painful pathology affecting a single limb. Classically, the patient experiences extreme pain followed by profound weakness. Brachial plexitis is a self-limiting condition with the expectation of (near) complete recovery over the course of months. Motor weakness may not follow a single nerve root or trunk distribution [7, 12]. The absence of axial neck pain and self-limitation distinguishes from cervical pathology. Confirmation of diagnosis can be made by (a) an MRI of the brachial plexus which will show enlargement and increased intensity on T2 and STIR sequences on the affected nerves and (b) electromyographic (EMG) studies which will show denervational changes. EMG result will be abnormal within 3 weeks and will show evidence of reinnervation at 3 months [3]. Because of the presumed autoimmune etiology, steroids may be used as treatment [7, 12].

Neuropathy

Peripheral neuropathy classically follows a "stocking-glove" distribution and is often symmetrical. Patients may complain of sensory loss and clumsiness which may mimic cervical myelopathy. Sensory loss may be subtle and may necessitate the use of two-point discrimination. Reflexes will be hyporeflexic in contrast with myelopathy. Patients may exhibit stigmata of the offending disease, such as Charcot joints in diabetes [12]. Common causes of peripheral neuropathy include diabetic neuropathy, renal failure, alcoholic neuropathy, and immune-mediated neuropathies (Guillain-Barre syndrome) [20]. Peripheral neuropathy is distinguished from cervical pathology by the "stocking-glove" and often symmetric presentation.

Compressive neuropathies include carpal tunnel syndrome, cubital tunnel syndrome, or ulnar nerve compression at the elbow. Carpal tunnel syndrome (compression of the median nerve) is classically described by the patient as paresthesias in the first three digits and worsened by activities which flex the wrist, including sleeping. Pertinent physical examination findings include Tinel's sign which is performed by tapping of the median nerve at the wrist. Tinel's sign indicates carpal tunnel pathology when tapping reproduces symptoms. Phalen's sign is performed by forcible flexion of the wrist. Traditionally, the patient places the dorsal surfaces on their hands together. Phalen's sign is positive if flexion reproduces their paresthesias. Muscle wasting of the thenar eminence may be seen in long-standing disease. Carpal tunnel is distinguished from cervical pathology by its classic distribution in the first three digits and absence of symptoms proximal to the wrist. While bilateral carpal tunnel is possible, this should raise suspicion for a cervical origin. Pronator syndrome, referring to forearm compression of the median nerve, is similar in presentation to carpal tunnel but is marked by the absence of nocturnal symptoms. The palm is numb in pronator syndrome due to the involvement of the palmar cutaneous branch. Cubital tunnel syndrome leads to ulnar distribution numbness and tingling in the hand and results from compression of the ulnar nerve at the medial epicondyle or the arcade of Struthers. Tinel's sign may be elicited at the medial epicondyle [4, 8].

Amyotrophic Lateral Sclerosis

The hallmark of amyotrophic lateral sclerosis (ALS) is concomitant upper and lower motor neuron signs including weakness, muscle wasting, and fasciculations (lower motor neuron) with spasticity or hyperreflexia (upper motor neuron). The monomelic variant of ALS which occurs in a single limb and may follow a radicular distribution may mimic radiculopathy. Sensory loss is not present in ALS; thus the presence of sensory disturbances should heighten suspicion for another pathology [7, 12]. Lower motor neuron findings generally should not be present in cervical degenerative pathology. However, there is at times overlap between these two conditions: ALS may not have characteristic bulbar symptoms and radiographic degenerative changes may be present on cervical MRI. Cervical myelopathy may show signs of lower motor neuron damage (muscle wasting and fasciculations) secondary to degeneration of anterior horn cells. Helpful adjuncts in distinguishing these two entities include the El Escorial diagnostic criteria for ALS which classify symptomatology into definite, probable, possible, and suspected probability of ALS based on history, physical examination, EMGs, and radiographic evidence [18].

Brachial Plexus Pathology

A thorough review of brachial plexus pathology and presentation is outside the scope of this chapter; a thorough understanding of brachial plexus innervation is required to diagnose these lesions. However, some general principles can be noted. The presence of upper motor neuron signs generally rules out the presence of peripheral pathology. Historical clues of trauma or radiation (usually breast carcinoma) to the area can indicate possible brachial plexus pathology. Traumatic brachial plexus pathology usually affects the upper trunk. Chronic usage of a crutch and Pancoast's tumor can cause lower trunk injuries [12].

Syringomyelia

Syringomyelia is an easily missed diagnosis if not suspected or tested for properly. The patient will relate a history of pain, numbness, and loss of pain and temperature sensation. The patient may present with unintentional injuries (classically burn injuries) due to an inability to sense pain and temperature. On physical examination, patients will have progressive wasting and weakness of the intrinsic muscles of the arm and hand. Sensory modalities should be thoroughly tested with emphasis on pain and temperature sensation, as these are the only expected areas of deficit. Importantly, syringomyelia is often found with Arnold-Chiari malformations and scoliosis [7, 12].

Multiple Sclerosis

Multiple sclerosis has been called the great imitator. Multiple sclerosis can cause transient neurological findings including weakness and paresthesias which may mimic cervical radiculopathy or spasticity which may mimic cervical myelopathy. L'Hermitte's sign is non-specific but may be seen in multiple sclerosis [12]. Multiple sclerosis can be distinguished from cervical pathology by a history of remitting-relapsing neurologic deficits that arise from any area of the central nervous system.

Thoracic Outlet Syndrome

Thoracic outlet syndrome can produce weakness and paresthesias, generally in a C8 to T1 distribution, which may mimic a cervical radiculopathy. Vascular compression symptoms including pallor or cyanosis may be present. Adson's test provokes vascular compression in thoracic outlet syndrome. Similarly, applying pressure in the supraclavicular fossa may reproduce paresthesias [1, 12]. Cervical pathology should not produce any vascular phenomena.

Summary

Cervical radiculopathy, myelopathy, and myeloradiculopathy comprise a significant portion of a spinal neurosurgical practice. Effective treatment of patients with cervical degenerative pathology requires mastery of the neurological examination. Furthermore, the examiner should be able to distinguish these operable conditions from imitators outlined in this chapter. This requires a thorough history and directed neurological examination on the part of the clinician.

Key Recommendations

- Physical examination should be performed in a thorough manner and address relevant areas of expected deficit.
- Special maneuvers should be used to increase or decrease suspicion for certain pathologies.
- Examiners should distinguish between mimics of cervical radiculopathy and myelopathy through the history and physical examination.

References

1. Albert T, Vaccaro A. Physical examination of the spine. New York: Thieme; 2005.
2. Aprill C, Dwyer A, Bogduk N. Cervical zygapophyseal joint pain patterns II: A clinical evaluation. Spine. 1990;15:458–61.
3. Aydin S, Abuzayed B, Bozkus H, Keles Boyaciyan A, Cetin Sarioglu A. Posttraumatic brachial plexitis. J Trauma. 2011;71:E136.
4. Benzel B, editor. Spine surgery: techniques, complication avoidance and management. Philadelphia: Elsevier/Saunders; 2012.
5. Choi B, Kim S, Lee DH, Kim J. Cervical radiculopathy combined with cervical myelopathy: prevalence and characteristics. Eur J Orthop Surg Traumatol. 2017. (epub).
6. Cook C, Wilhelm M, Cook A, Petrosino C, Isaacs C. Clinical tests for screening and diagnosis of cervical spine myelopathy: a systematic review. J Manip Physiol Ther. 2011;34:539–46.
7. Daroff R, Jankovic J, Mazziota J, Pomeroy S, editors. Bradley's neurology in clinical practice. London: Elsevier; 2015.
8. Goldman L, Schafer A. Goldman-Cecil medicine. 25th ed. Philadelphia: Saunders; 2016.
9. Hall. Textbook of medical physiology. Philadelphia: Saunders; 2016.
10. Magee D. Orthopedic physical assessment: St. Louis: Saunders; 2014.
11. Malanga G, Landes P, Nadler S. Provocative tests in cervical spine examination: historical basis and scientific analysis. Pain Physician. 2003;6:199–205.
12. Patten J. Neurological differential diagnosis. London: Springer; 1996.
13. Rhee J, Heflin J, Hamasaki T, et al. Prevalence of physical signs in cervical myelopathy: a prospective, controlled study. Spine. 2009;34:890–5.
14. Shah K, Rajshekar V. In soft lateral disc prolapse reliability of diagnosis of soft cervical disc prolapse using Spurling's test. Br J Neurosurg. 2004;18:480–3.
15. Shen F, Samartzis D, Fessler R, editors. Textbook of the cervical spine: Maryland Heights; Saunders; 2015.
16. Royden J, Srinivasan J, Allam G, Baker R. Netter's Neurology. Philadelphia: Saunders; 2012.
17. Tong H, Haig A, Yamakawa K. The Spurling test and cervical radiculopathy. Spine. 2002;27:156–9.
18. Truffert A, Rosler K, Magistris M. Amyotrophic lateral sclerosis versus cervical spondylotic myelopathy. Clin Neurophysiol. 2000;111:1031–8.
19. Walker H, Hall W, Hurst J. Clinical methods: the history, physical, and laboratory examinations. 3rd ed. Boston: Butterworth-Heinemann; 1990.
20. Winn H. Youmans and Winn neurological surgery. 7th ed. Philadelphia: Elsevier; 2017.

8 Clinical Assessment Tools

Jian Guan and Zoher Ghogawala

Introduction

The prevalence of degenerative cervical myelopathy (DCM) in the population [1] results in an outsized impact on global health. DCM is the most common cause of spinal cord dysfunction in the world. It is associated with a significant decline in patient-reported quality of life. Evaluation of patients with DCM is complex, frequently involving a combination of physical examination, electrophysiological testing, and advanced imaging. An increasingly important component of the outcome of treatment involves the use of clinical assessment tools, sometimes referred to as "patient-reported outcomes."

Clinical assessment tools allow for the quantification of health status from the patient's perspective, and their use makes it possible for multiple stakeholders to assess the benefits of therapy. On an individual patient level, observing changes in reported scores of these outcome instruments makes it possible to objectively monitor a patient's response to any type of intervention for DCM. Increasingly, these measures are also being used to track the performance of individual providers and hospitals, inexorably becoming tied to reimbursement and accreditation [2]. Objective, validated, and widely understood clinical assessment tools are also necessary for the successful design and interpretation of high-quality clinical trials [3]. Studies for DCM are no exception, with many recent studies reporting a number of clinical assessment tool measures as outcomes [1, 3].

From a healthcare systems perspective, objective, standardized outcome assessments allow for the study of management effectiveness, allowing for optimization of healthcare value [4]. One example of this is the use of quality-adjusted life year (QALY) measurements to compare the cost-effectiveness of interventions. In studies utilizing QALYs, one QALY is representative of a year of perceived "perfect" health, with various disease states reducing this value, with a score of zero representing death. By utilizing QALY, researchers can assess the burden of a disease or the benefit of a treatment as it pertains to both quality and quantity of life. Whitmore et al. performed such an analysis on DCM patients, using QALY measures to calculate the incremental cost-effectiveness ratio (difference in costs of two

J. Guan
Department of Neurosurgery, University of Utah, Salt Lake City, UT, USA

Alan L. and Jacqueline Stuart Spine Center, Department of Neurosurgery, Lahey Hospital and Medical Center, Burlington, MA, USA

Z. Ghogawala (✉)
Department of Neurosurgery, Lahey Hospital and Medical Center, Burlington, MA, USA

Department of Neurosurgery, Tufts University School of Medicine, Boston, MA, USA
e-mail: Zoher.Ghogawala@lahey.org

M. G. Kaiser et al. (eds.), *Degenerative Cervical Myelopathy and Radiculopathy*,
https://doi.org/10.1007/978-3-319-97952-6_8

interventions divided by the difference in QALY gains) of ventral versus dorsal surgery, suggesting an advantage for ventral operations [5]. Such analyses also suggest that not only are such comparisons increasingly vital but that the methodology for making such comparisons must be carefully considered.

A vast array of clinical assessment tools exist – a recent review identified over 50 unique instruments [6]. In this chapter, we will discuss these tools, both their basic overarching characteristics, and some of the details of more commonly used assessments.

General Characteristics of Clinical Assessment Tools

The vast majority of clinical assessment tools are presented in questionnaire form and can be administered by a clinician/researcher or filled out by the patient without supervision from a healthcare provider. Two broad categories of clinical assessment tools exist. The first are those that measure what is referred to as "health-related quality of life" (HRQOL) global health domains not related to a particular pathology but which may be impacted by a range of disease states [7]. The results of HRQOL testing can be reported as either an instrument specific score or as a utility score which may be converted into a more universally applicable "quality-adjusted life year" (QALY) measure. The second category of outcome tool includes all of the disease specific measures, instruments that measure limitations specific for the disease process in question. For DCM pathology, these tools assess variables such as upper extremity motor function, ability to perform common tasks of daily living, and localized neck pain.

An important part of any clinical assessment tool is the identification of the minimal clinically important difference (MCID), the point at which a change in score is associated with significant clinical improvement or deterioration for any patient [8]. This value can be determined via a number of methods, though the two most commonly used are the so-called "anchor" method, where scores are classified based on an external value that can divide patients into those who have improved or not, and the "distribution-based" method, where scores are classified based on the statistical distribution of responses. With any grading schema, it is important to note that MCID is not universal and may vary based on demographic and other variables [9]. One example is the MCID for the Neck Disability Index – described in greater detail later on in this chapter – which has been found to have an MCID as low as 2.41 points (on a 50-point scale) for patients undergoing surgery for degenerative spine disorders [10], to 9.5 points in nonoperative patients receiving physical therapy alone [11]. Such differences are not uncommon within the same grading scale across various pathologies, treatment strategies, and study methodologies, and careful knowledge of all these factors is necessary for a well-balanced interpretation of results.

Clinical assessment tools are not without limitations, and researchers must be aware of these in order to properly assess their results. The interpretation of assessment results can be influenced by a variety of cultural factors that must be taken into account. These can be as basic as differences in wording across questionnaire translations [12] to deep-seated cultural differences in interpretation/reporting of pain and societal norms [13]. The utility of a clinical assessment tool in practice is also limited by the time available to the subject to complete the questionnaire. Longer surveys, while able to provide more data points and ask more in-depth questions, can result in reduced rates of completion and poorer data quality [14]. Longer surveys are also more difficult to integrate into frequently busy clinic schedules and may lead to significant issues in accrual of patients for studies using these instruments if enrollment becomes prohibitively disruptive to patient care [15].

Assessment of Clinical Assessment Tools

Three major criteria are important in the evaluation of a clinical assessment tool – reliability, validity, and responsiveness [16]. Reliability is a measure of the reproducibility of a tool's results. This includes reproducibility between observers (interobserver reliability), with multiple instances of testing by the same observer (intraobserver reliability for a static subject, test-retest reliability for a subject between time points), and for different subsections of the test compared to the overall test's results (internal consistency) [17]. Validity refers to a test's ability to properly act as a measurement for the variable being tested. Testing for validity can either be done by measuring test-specific values such as floor and ceiling effects – the percentage of subjects that have the maximum or minimum result, with a value of ≥15% suggesting an instrument with poor validity – or by comparing the test in question to existing, previously validated measures [18]. The responsiveness of a tool is a measure of whether an instrument can detect changes in the outcome being measured. A variety of statistical analyses can be used for the assessment of reliability, validity, and responsiveness for any given instrument – Cronbach α for reliability, Pearson correlation coefficient for validity, and area under the curve of a receiver-operating characteristic curve for responsiveness [19].

Individual Clinical Assessment Tools

As previously stated, a wide array of clinical assessment tools currently exist in the literature, with the majority being used only in the context of their initial publication [6]. For this section, we will focus on five of the most frequently used, validated instruments for DCM patients. Two of these, the EuroQOL-5D (EQ-5D) and the Short Form-36 (SF-36), are HRQOL measures (Table 8.1). The remaining three, the modified Japanese Orthopedic Association score (mJOA), the Neck Disability Index (NDI), and Nurick grade, are specifically for cervical pathology (Table 8.2).

Table 8.1 Health-related quality of life (HRQOL) clinical assessment tools

Name	Brief description	Advantages	Disadvantages
EQ-5D	Short questionnaire assessing five areas of life quality with either three or five options within each domain. Includes patient assessment of overall health status with a score from 0 to 100	Brief Simple Increasingly widespread usage	Possible oversimplification of health status Variable reported MCID values
SF-36	Thirty-six-item questionnaire assessing eight domains including both physical and mental functioning	Most widely used HRQOL tool Comprehensive	Time-consuming to administer

Table 8.2 Cervical pathology specific clinical assessment tools

Name	Brief description	Advantages	Disadvantages
mJOA	Four questions assessing upper extremity motor function, upper extremity sensory function, lower extremity motor/sensory function, and bladder function. Grading is on a scale of 0–17, with lower scores corresponding to worsening pathology	Simple, concise Widely used in the cervical spine literature	Some questions involve a subjective component
NDI	Ten questions assessing disability in ten realms of functioning related to cervical pathology. Grading is from 0 to 50, with higher values corresponding to worsening pathology	Simple, concise Encompasses a variety of functional domains influenced by cervical pathology Widely used in the cervical spine literature	May ignore a number of clinically important signs and symptoms related to cervical myelopathy
Nurick grade	Grading scale of patient difficulty with ambulation. Scored from 0 to 5, with higher values corresponding to worsening disability	Simple, measure of single variable	May fail to capture significant signs of cervical myelopathy unrelated to ambulation

EQ-5D

Originally developed in 1990 by the EuroQol Group [20], the EQ-5D is a HRQOL measure based on questions regarding the realms of mobility, self-care, usual activities, pain/discomfort, and anxiety/depression. Two versions of the EQ-5D exist, one with three options in each realm (EQ-5D 3L) and one with five options in each realm (EQ-5D 5L). Both versions also ask for a grade for overall health state from 0 to 100. Choices in the EQ-5D are converted into a utility score where 0 represents death and 1 represents ideal health, though negative results are possible in this scale, signifying a health status worse than death. Scores are calibrated based on population-based studies in a variety of countries, ranging from the United States and Europe to Japan and Zimbabwe.

The simplicity of the EQ-5D is a major advantage of the scale, allowing for ease of explanation and completion by patients [6]. As a result, the EQ-5D has been used in a variety of DCM studies to date [3, 21] and has been adopted by national agencies such as the UK Department of Health [22]. Criticisms of the EQ-5D include concerns that it may represent an oversimplification of health status and that it may be subject to a significant ceiling effect [4]. The MCID of the EQ-5D is also unclear, with a wide range of values reported in differing publications from as low as 0.074 to as high as 0.54 [23, 24].

SF-36

The SF-36 is a 36-item questionnaire and is itself a simplification of an earlier 116-question survey produced by the RAND corporation [25]. The results are divided into eight "domains" – social role limitations due to physical or emotional problems, role limitations due to physical problems, role limitations due to emotional problems, physical activity limitations because of health problems, bodily pain, mental health, vitality, and general health perceptions. These domains can be more broadly synthesized into the physical component summary (PCS) and emotional component summary (MCS). Scoring for each subsection ranges from 0 to 100, normalized with a mean score of 50 and a standard deviation of 10 [26]. Utility scores can also be generated from these results.

The benefits of the SF-36 are its widespread use – it is the most commonly used HRQOL measure among recently published articles on degenerative cervical disease [6] – and its more comprehensive question set compared to instruments such as the EQ-5D. The length of the questionnaire, however, inevitably increases the amount of effort required to complete testing. Abbreviated versions of the SF-36, specifically a 12-question tool known as the SF-12, have been developed in response to this issue. Studies have also called into account the validity of the SF-36 for cervical spine surgery, especially when using the summary measures alone [27]. One recent study found MCID values for the SF-36 PCS of 5.56 and for MCS of 5.73 [28].

mJOA

The mJOA is one of the most commonly used cervical myelopathy specific clinical assessment tools [6]. Initially formulated in the 1980s by a group of Japanese investigators, the scale was modified by Benzel et al. in 1991 to produce the mJOA [29]. The instrument consists of questions related to upper extremity motor function, upper extremity sensory function, lower extremity motor/sensory function, and bladder function. The scale is scored out of a total of 17 points, with lower values indicating more severe disease.

The mJOA is short and straightforward to administer, and its widespread use allows for comparison to previously published studies. Recent psychometric testing by Kopjar et al. also suggests the mJOA has appropriate reliability, validity, and responsiveness [30]. One disadvantage is that the scale does have some subjective components ("slight difficulty" versus "great difficulty" in relation to motor tasks, "mild" versus "severe" sensory loss). The MCID of the mJOA appears to vary depending on the severity of myelopathy, with a value of 1 for mild (score of 15–17), 2 for moderate (score of 12–14), and 3 for severe (score <12) [31].

NDI

The NDI is the cervical modification of the Oswestry Disability Index for lower back pathology [32]. The questionnaire is comprised of ten questions in the categories of pain intensity, personal care, lifting, reading, headaches, concentration, work, driving, sleeping, and recreation. Each question has five choices and is scored from 0 (no disability) to 5 (total disability). The focus of each category in the NDI is primarily on the pain associated with each domain, versus the mJOA that has questions on both pain and other domains of neurological functioning. The total score may be out of the raw value of 50 or presented as a percentage.

Advantages of the NDI are its simplicity and its incorporation of a variety of realms important to acts of daily living that may be influenced by cervical myelopathy. The scale is also widely used within the cervical myelopathy literature. One significant disadvantage of the NDI is the limited ability of the scale to discern several classic findings of DCM including arm weakness and bowel/bladder dysfunction. The MCID of the NDI also varies fairly significantly from study to study from 5 points on the raw score up to as high as 19 points [33].

Nurick Grade

The Nurick grade was initially proposed by Nurick in 1972 and is a simple classification of a patient's difficulty with ambulation [34]. Scored from 0 (signs/symptoms attributable to root dysfunction but without spinal cord-related signs/symptoms) to 5 (wheelchair bound or bedridden), the instrument is less a patient-reported outcome and more a healthcare professional-administered clinical assessment tool.

The primary advantage of the Nurick grade is its simplicity and ease of use. Similar to the NDI, however, the Nurick grade may miss common symptoms of DCM such as upper extremity dysfunction and bowel/bladder dysfunction. The fact that some of the Nurick grades require assessment by someone familiar with cervical pathology (differentiating root-related signs/symptoms from cord-related signs/symptoms) means the Nurick grade is a significantly less useful indicator of patient health status and is, as a result, less commonly used [6].

Conclusion

Clinical assessment tools form an important component of the armamentarium in the treatment of DCM. Apart from their obvious benefits as a means to track individual patient response to treatment, they also enable a set of accepted indices to promote discussion and research between clinicians, policy makers, and patients (along with patient advocates). A wide variety of clinical assessment tools exist for DCM. In 2009, the Joint Spine Section of the American Association of Neurological Surgeons and Congress of Neurological Surgeons released guidelines on the use of clinical assessment tools for cervical degenerative disease, recommending their routine utilization and highlighting a variety of tools described above such as the mJOA and SF-36 as well validated instruments in cervical pathology [35]. Then, as now, there remains a need for further investigations into which tools are most appropriate for specific contexts. More work is needed to develop tools that maximize validity, reliability, and responsiveness without sacrificing ease of use.

References

1. Fehlings MG, Wilson JR, Kopjar B, Yoon ST, Arnold PM, Massicotte EM, Vaccaro AR, Brodke DS, Shaffrey CI, Smith JS, Woodard EJ, Banco RJ, Chapman JR, Janssen ME, Bono CM, Sasso RC, Dekutoski MB, Gokaslan ZL. Efficacy and safety of surgical decompression in patients with cervical spondylotic myelopathy: results of the AOSpine North America prospective multi-center study. J Bone Joint Surg Am. 2013;95(18):1651–8.
2. Godil SS, Parker SL, Zuckerman SL, Mendenhall SK, McGirt MJ. Accurately measuring the quality and effectiveness of cervical spine surgery in registry efforts: determining the most valid and responsive instruments. Spine J. 2015;15(6):1203–9.
3. Ghogawala Z, Benzel EC, Heary RF, Riew KD, Albert TJ, Butler WE, Barker FG 2nd, Heller

JG, McCormick PC, Whitmore RG, Freund KM, Schwartz JS. Cervical spondylotic myelopathy surgical trial: randomized, controlled trial design and rationale. Neurosurgery. 2014;75(4):334–46.
4. Nayak NR, Coats JM, Abdullah KG, Stein SC, Malhotra NR. Tracking patient-reported outcomes in spinal disorders. Surg Neurol Int. 2015;6(Suppl 19):S490–9.
5. Whitmore RG, Schwartz JS, Simmons S, Stein SC, Ghogawala Z. Performing a cost analysis in spine outcomes research: comparing ventral and dorsal approaches for cervical spondylotic myelopathy. Neurosurgery. 2012;70(4):860–7.
6. Ueda H, Cutler HS, Guzman JZ, Cho SK. Current trends in the use of patient-reported outcome instruments in degenerative cervical spine surgery. Global Spine J. 2016;6(3):242–7.
7. Whitmore RG, Ghogawala Z, Petrov D, Schwartz JS, Stein SC. Function outcome instruments used for cervical spondylotic myelopathy: interscale correlation and prediction of preference-based quality of life. Spine J. 2013;13(8):902–7.
8. Copay AG, Subach BR, Glassman SD, Polly DW Jr, Schuler TC. Understanding the minimum clinically important difference: a review of concepts and methods. Spine J. 2007;7:541–6.
9. Revicki D, Hays RD, Cella D, Sloan J. Recommended methods for determining responsiveness and minimally important differences for patient-reported outcomes. J Clin Epidemiol. 2008;61(2):102–9.
10. Auffinger B, Lam S, Shen J, Thaci B, Roitberg BZ. Usefulness of minimum clinically important difference for assessing patients with subaxial degenerative cervical spine disease: statistical versus substantial clinical benefit. Acta Neurochir. 2013;155(12):2345–54.
11. Cleland JA, Childs JD, Whitman JM. Psychometric properties of the neck disability index and numeric pain rating scale in patients with mechanical neck pain. Arch Phys Med Rehabil. 2008;89(1):69–74.
12. Hahn EA, Bode RK, Du H, Cella D. Evaluating linguistic equivalence of patient-reported outcomes in a cancer clinical trial. Clin Trials. 2006;3(3):280–90.
13. Watanabe K, Lenke LG, Bridwell KH, Hasegawa K, Hirano T, Endo N, Cheh G, Kim YJ, Hensley M, Stobbs G, Koester L. Cross-cultural comparison of the Scoliosis Research Society Outcomes Instrument between American and Japanese idiopathic scoliosis patients: are there differences? Spine (Phila Pa 1976). 2007;32(24):2711–4.
14. Diehr P, Chen L, Patrick D, Feng Z, Yasui Y. Reliability, effect size, and responsiveness of health status measures in the design of randomized and cluster-randomized trials. Contemp Clin Trials. 2005;26(1):45–58.
15. Mark TL, Johnson G, Fortner B, Ryan K. The benefits and challenges of using computer-assisted symptom assessments in oncology clinics: results of a qualitative assessment. Technol Cancer Res Treat. 2008;7(5):401–6.
16. Ghogawala Z, Resnick DK, Watters WC 3rd, Mummaneni PV, Dailey AT, Choudhri TF, Eck JC, Sharan A, Groff MW, Wang JC, Dhall SS, Kaiser MG. Guideline update for the performance of fusion procedures for degenerative disease of the lumbar spine. Part 2: assessment of functional outcome following lumbar fusion. J Neurosurg Spine. 2014;21(1):7–13.
17. Karanicolas PJ, Bhandari M, Kreder H, Moroni A, Richardson M, Walter SD, Norman GR, Guyatt GH, Collaboration for Outcome Assessment in Surgical Trials (COAST) Musculoskeletal Group. Evaluating agreement: conducting a reliability study. J Bone Joint Surg Am. 2009;91(Suppl 3):99–106.
18. McHorney CA, Tarlov AR. Individual-patient monitoring in clinical practice: are available health status surveys adequate? Qual Life Res. 1995;4:293–307.
19. Terwee CB, Bot SD, de Boer MR, van der Windt DA, Knol DL, Dekker J, Bouter LM, de Vet HC. Quality criteria were proposed for measurement properties of health status questionnaires. J Clin Epidemiol. 2007;60(1):34–42.
20. EuroQol Group. EuroQol – a new facility for the measurement of health-related quality of life. Health Policy. 1990;16:199–208.
21. Ravindra VM, Guan J, Holland CM, Dailey AT, Schmidt MH, Godzik J, Hood RS, Ray WZ, Bisson EF. Vitamin D status in cervical spondylotic myelopathy: comparison of fusion rates and patient outcome measures: a preliminary experience. J Neurosurg Sci. 2016.; Epub ahead of print.
22. Devlin NJ, Parkin D, Browne J. Patient-reported outcome measures in the NHS: new methods for analyzing and reporting EQ-5D data. Health Econ. 2010;19(8):886–905.
23. Parker SL, Godil SS, Shau DN, Mendenhall SK, McGirt MJ. Assessment of the minimum clinically important difference in pain, disability, and quality of life after cervical discectomy and fusion: clinical article. J Neurosurg Spine. 2013;18:154–60.
24. Xiao R, Miller JA, Lubelski D, Alberts JL, Mroz TE, Benzel EC, Krishaney AA, Machado AG. Quality of life outcomes following cervical decompression for coexisting Parkinson's disease and cervical spondylotic myelopathy. Spine J. 2016;16(11):1358–66.
25. Ware JE Jr, Shelbourne CD. The MOS 36-item short-form health survey (SF-36). I. Conceptual framework and item selection. Med Care. 1992;30:473–83.
26. Ware JE, Kosinski M. Interpreting SF-36 summary health measures: a response. Qual Life Res. 2001;10(5):405–13.
27. Baron R, Elashaal A, Germon T, Hobart J. Measuring outcomes in cervical spine surgery: think twice before using the SF-36. Spine (Phila Pa 1976). 2006;31(22):2575–84.
28. Auffinger BM, Lall RR, Dahdaleh NS, Wong AP, Lam SK, Koski T, Fessler RG, Smith ZA. Measuring surgical outcomes in cervical spondylotic myelopathy patients undergoing anterior cervical discectomy and

fusion: assessment of minimum clinically important difference. PLoS One. 2013;8(6):e67408.
29. Benzel EC, Lancon J, Kesterson L, Hadden T. Cervical laminectomy and dentate ligament section for cervical spondylotic myelopathy. J Spinal Disord. 1991;4(3):286–95.
30. Kopjar B, Tetreault L, Kalsi-Ryan S, Fehlings M. Psychometric properties of the modified Japanese Orthopaedic Association scale in patients with cervical spondylotic myelopathy. Spine (Phila Pa 1976). 2015;49(1):E23–8.
31. Tetreault L, Nouri A, Kopjar B, Côté P, Fehlings MG. The minimum clinically important difference of the modified Japanese Orthopaedic association scale in patients with degenerative cervical myelopathy. Spine (Phila Pa 1976). 2015;40(21):1653–9.
32. Vernon H, Mior S. The neck disability index: a study of reliability and validity. J Manip Physiol Ther. 1991;14:409–15.
33. MacDermid JC, Walton DM, Avery S, Blanchard A, Etruw E, McAlpine C, Goldsmith CH. Measurement properties of the neck disability index: a systematic review. J Orthop Sports Phys Ther. 2009;39(5):400–17.
34. Nurick S. The pathogenesis of the spinal cord disorder associated with cervical spondylosis. Brain. 1972;95:87–100.
35. Holly LT, Matz PG, Anderson PA, Groff MW, Heary RF, Kaiser MG, Mummaneni PV, Ryken TC, Choudhri TF, Vresilovic EJ, Resnick DK, Joint Section on Disorders of the Spine and Peripheral Nerves of the American Association of Neurological Surgeons and Congress of Neurological Surgeons. Functional outcomes assessment for cervical degenerative disease. J Neuosurg Spine. 2009;11(2):238–44.

Radiographic Modalities

9

Ha Son Nguyen and Shekar N. Kurpad

Pitfalls/Pearls Outline

1. Degenerative cervical myelopathy (DCM) and radiculopathy refer to a host of age-related disorders that can inflict ongoing spinal cord and/or nerve root injury in the cervical spine, causing substantial disability. Consequently, accurate and timely assessment of these disorders is paramount, which may require advanced radiographic modalities for diagnostic and therapeutic purposes.
2. Conventional magnetic resonance imaging (MRI) has been the radiographic modality of choice for the diagnosis and treatment of DCM and radiculopathy.
3. Unfortunately, conventional MRI findings do not convey reliable data regarding the health status of the spinal cord parenchyma. As such, these findings are not predictive of neurological status or treatment outcomes.
4. Advanced MRI techniques—namely, diffusion tensor imaging (DTI), magnetization transfer (MT), myelin water fraction (MWF), magnetic resonance spectroscopy (MRS), and functional MRI (fMRI)—may help elucidate details regarding the microscopic structure and functional composition of the spinal cord parenchyma.

Introduction

Degenerative cervical myelopathy (DCM) and radiculopathy refer to a host of age-related disorders that can inflict ongoing spinal cord and/or nerve root injury in the cervical spine, causing substantial disability [1, 2]. This term incorporates spondylosis, disc herniation, facet arthropathy, spondylolisthesis, and ligamentous degeneration (hypertrophy, calcification, or ossification) [1–3]. In due course, these age-related degenerative changes constrict the spinal canal and/or foramen, compressing spinal cord parenchyma and/or nerve roots. Persistent compression of the spinal cord and nerve roots leads to anatomic distortion (flattening and/or widening), vascular compromise, and pathophysiological consequences (viz., endothelial cell loss, disruption of vascularization, compromise of the blood-spinal

H. S. Nguyen · S. N. Kurpad (✉)
Department of Neurological Surgery, Medical College of Wisconsin, Milwaukee, WI, USA
e-mail: skurpad@mcw.edu

M. G. Kaiser et al. (eds.), *Degenerative Cervical Myelopathy and Radiculopathy*,
https://doi.org/10.1007/978-3-319-97952-6_9

cord barrier, neuroinflammation, and apoptosis) [4] that result in lasting features of spinal cord damage (cystic cavitation, gliosis, central gray and white matter degeneration, Wallerian degeneration of posterior columns and posterolateral tracts, and anterior horn cell loss) [5].

To diagnose DCM and radiculopathy, the clinician must rely on the clinical exam as well as advanced radiographic modalities that demonstrate compromise of the neural elements [6]. Conventional MRI has been the imaging modality of choice to confirm the diagnosis of DCM and radiculopathy. However, several studies have noted that signal intensity changes observed via conventional MRI do not convey structural changes within the spinal cord parenchyma [7]. Moreover, findings may not convincingly correspond with disease severity or surgical outcomes in DCM [7, 8]. As such, new advanced MRI techniques have been studied to improve the understanding, diagnosis, and treatment of DCM [3].

Imaging Modalities

X-Rays

Plain radiographs are generally the initial imaging modality for assessment of DCM and radiculopathy. To obtain an image, a generator directs a beam of X-rays toward an object, which absorbs a variable quantity of X-rays based on its density and composition. X-rays that pass through the object are captured by a detector, which provides an image. Though limited when compared to sophisticated techniques, such as CT and MRI, plain lateral radiographs are typically obtained with the patient in the upright position and provide valuable information regarding sagittal alignment, distinguishing normal lordosis from a pathologic kyphosis, and define the extent of disc disease [1].

Accumulating evidence imply that sagittal alignment might be a contributor to disease severity in patients with DCM; indeed, close to 12% DCM patients can possess spondylolisthesis/subluxation [3], where dynamic motion can cause sporadic spinal cord compromise. Moreover, extent of cervical kyphosis or lordosis can alter the decision between an anterior versus posterior surgical approach. In addition, if movement-dependent instability is suspected, dynamic flexion and extension radiographs can be obtained.

Dynamic lateral X-rays (such as flexion and extension films) may also be used to detect cervical instability. From cervical trauma studies [9, 10], concerns for cervical instability include (1) a translational displacement $\geq$ 3.5 mm and (2) angulation between adjacent vertebra $\geq$ 11 degrees. On the other hand, limited studies exist regarding instability associated with degenerative spondylosis; White et al. [11] evaluated this condition, where concerns for instability were a translational displacement $\geq$ 2 mm; overall, the authors concluded that ~1% exhibited spondylolisthesis only on dynamic films and 3% exhibited change in spondylolisthesis. Dynamic films may have limited information if patient's mobility is compromised by neck pain.

CT

A computed tomography (CT) scan incorporates numerous X-ray images obtained from various angles to yield cross-sectional depictions of a scanned object. Moreover, modern scanners offer multiplanar reconstruction, such as orthogonal planes (coronal and sagittal), that can enhance visualization of the spinal column. This permits better assessment of the intervertebral disc spaces, which can be difficult to visualize on axial images, and of the relative relationship of the vertebral bodies, since multiple spinal levels can be studied simultaneously.

CT imaging can visualize bony anatomy effectively. This is particularly significant for assessment of calcified pathology, such as OPLL. CT has been regarded as the noninvasive modality of choice to assess calcified pathology, since a strong relationship exists between tissue density and extent of calcification/ossification. The correlation is not exact, as tissue density can be influenced by other compositions (i.e., hemosiderin content in hemorrhages). Ideally, the gold standard for diagnosis of OPLL is histological confirmation. However, no studies have formally addressed the accuracy of CT for the diagnosis of OPLL, correlating radiographic findings to histological confirmation.

For other calcified pathology, such as hemorrhagic brain tumors [12], gallstones [13, 14], and atherosclerotic plaques [15], CT may not be sensitive for certain patterns.

Nevertheless, the modality remains the preferred method to assess ossification (i.e., OPLL). Compared to CT, MRI has much lower sensitivity for cervical OPLL; large studies have shown that only 33–44% of ossified pathology could be recognized on sagittal T1 sequences and 44–57% on sagittal T2 sequences; axial T1 and T2 sequences were more sensitive (up to 91%) [16–18]. Moreover, a recent study involving 41 patients yielded an overall MR sensitivity of 49% [18].

CT Myelography

With CT myelography (CTM), a CT scan is obtained once radiographic contrast has been introduced into the CSF space. The contrast helps to visualize the spinal cord and nerve roots. This imaging modality is an alternative option if MRI is contraindicated (i.e., due to body habitus, metallic foreign bodies, stimulators/batteries/pacemakers, or severe claustrophobia) [19] or compromised due to the previous insertion of spinal instrumentation. The procedure however is associated with more risk, including spinal headaches associated with a dural puncture, and greater radiation exposure. Moreover, given a theoretical danger of seizures, patients are asked to hold certain medications pre- and post-myelogram, (such as phenothiazines, MAO inhibitors, antidepressants, and antipsychotics).

For most parameters (characterization of facet joint disease, lateral recess disease, spinal canal stenosis, cord size, and neural foraminal stenosis), the agreement between the interpretation of CTM compared to MRI remains modest at best [20]. CTM tends to stress more severe findings with respect to spinal canal stenosis and neural foraminal stenosis [21]. CTM can help outline bony anatomy and the nature of the pathology (i.e., OPLL). Unfortunately, depiction of soft issue pathology (including disc herniation and spinal cord edema) can be lacking; CTM fails to depict intrinsic spinal cord pathology, and if the pathology completely obliterates the CSF space, visualization distal to the block may be hampered.

MRI

With an MR scanner, a strong magnet applies an external magnetic field that orients hydrogen atoms either in a "north" or "south" direction. Pulses of radio waves can provide enough energy where the atoms "spin" the other way; once the pulse is removed, these atoms will return to their original position, releasing energy that is captured and converted into an image. By adjusting the parameters of the pulse sequence, different types of tissues can be discerned based on the relaxation properties of the hydrogen atoms. Consequently, MRI can depict impressive images of the spinal cord, nerve roots, intervertebral disc, ligament, and cerebrospinal fluid. Compared to CTM, MRI is noninvasive; moreover, the modality can visualize intrinsic spinal cord pathologies and can reveal findings distal to a complete myelographic obstruction. However, MRI can be hampered by a larger section thickness and ongoing artifacts from CSF dynamics [21].

For conventional MRI, the scan is performed with the patient supine and enclosed in a long, narrow tube (close configuration). Contraindications include large body habitus, implanted metal (foreign bodies, stimulators/batteries/pacemakers), or severe claustrophobia. An open-configuration scanner reduces claustrophobia and permits the imaging of obese patients; however, imaging quality may be diminished due to a theoretically greater inhomogeneity of the magnetic field [22].

Upright/Dynamic MRI

Supine imaging can be misleading. Approximately 20–30% of individuals who have disc protrusions or disc ruptures discovered through MRI are completely asymptomatic [23]. Moreover, symptoms may be alleviated in the supine position but exacerbate in an upright/flexion/extension position. Via cadaveric studies, nerve root compression has been associated with decreased foramen width and area [24]; moreover, flexion increases foramen width while extension decreases foramen width [25].

Upright/dynamic MRI in the cervical spine has sparsely been reported in the literature [23, 26–31]. The technique permits imaging of patients with relative contraindications (obesity, claustrophobia, severe spinal kyphosis, severe congestive heart failure, or severe chronic obstructive pulmonary disease) [23]. The technique provides reasonable resolution without artifact [32]. On the other hand, the scan time is lengthened, which increases the risk for image degradation with patient movements [23, 33].

With upright/dynamic MRI, there is a potential to diagnose occult stenosis, disc protrusion, or instability [23]. Patients can be scanned in a position that elicits symptoms [23]. Employing MRI in asymptomatic patients, Muhle et al. [34] noted that flexion significantly increased the foramen height, width, and cross-sectional area (CSA), while extension significantly decreased these parameters. In a group of symptomatic patients, Muhle et al. [35] concluded that exacerbated pain was related to a decrease in foramen size and to nerve root motion, often associated with extension and axial rotation to the side of the pain. Through a qualitative assessment of symptomatic patients, Ferreiro et al. [36] found that 4 of 31 diagnosed posterior disc herniations were only discovered in the upright-sitting position. However, focal posterior disc herniations were seen to comparatively enlarge in size for 21 patients but reduce in size for 5 patients.

MRI: Imaging Modality of Choice for DCM Patients

The introduction of MRI in the mid-1980s offered clinicians high-resolution anatomic images to facilitate clinical decision-making [8]. Conventional T1 and T2 sequences (along axial and sagittal planes) are typically employed for detailed visualization of the cervical spine anatomy. The normal cervical spinal cord travels through the lordotic spinal column, bounded anteriorly by vertebral bodies (VBs) and posterior longitudinal ligament (PLL), posteriorly by ligamentum flavum (LF) and lamina, and laterally by pedicles (Fig. 9.1). Kato et al. [37] described the normal morphology, age-related changes, and abnormal findings on MRI in 1211 asymptomatic patients to establish mean values for the cervical spinal canal, dural tube, and spinal cord. Spinal canal size is dependent on many factors, including spinal level, age (decreasing size with increasing age) [6, 37], gender [38], and underlying pathology (congenital stenosis or degenerative changes) [37].

With conventional MRI, degenerative changes can be visualized along the spinal column, neural foramen, and spinal cord. Spondylosis, defined as multilevel disc and bone changes, can be seen in up to 89.7% in a recent large prospective cohort study regarding DCM [3]. On both T1 and T2

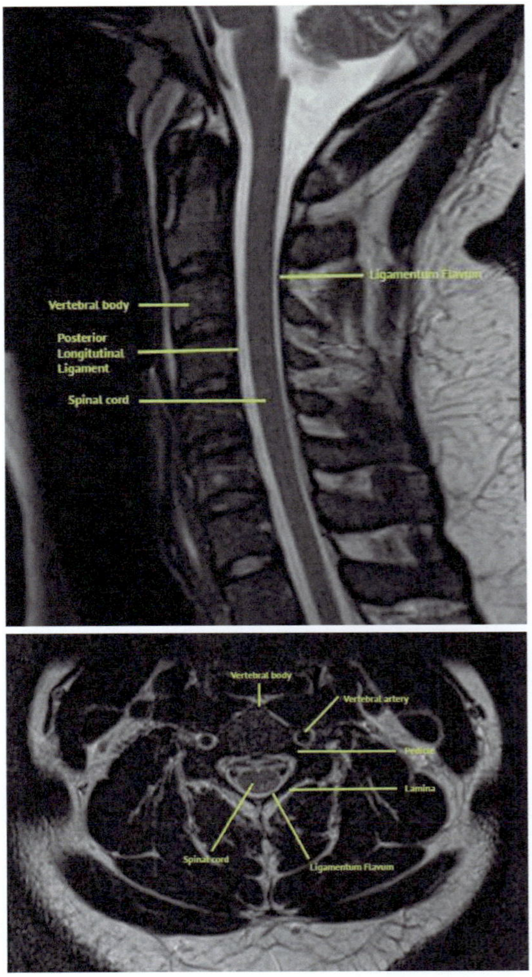

Fig. 9.1 Sagittal (*left*) and axial T2 images of a normal C spine with various labels

sequences, the nucleus pulposus tends to be hyperintense relative to the surrounding annulus [6]. With age, the nucleus pulposus can exhibit (1) loss of T2 hyperintensity, whereby the boundaries between the nucleus pulposus and annulus become obscured; (2) loss of height, associated with the collapse of the intervertebral disc space and potential auto-fusion of adjacent VBs; and (3) herniation, which can be associated with a compromised annulus, with extrusion of disc material into the spinal canal [6, 39].

With perpetual static and dynamic stresses, VBs can exhibit morphologic alterations (such as increased anteroposterior dimensions and formation of osteophytes that border degenerated discs) [1]. Disc herniation into VB (Schmorl's nodes) can also be seen in the cervical spine. As described by Modic et al. [40], signal intensity variation within the VBs and their end plates on MRI imply bone marrow changes associated with degenerative disc disease. Modic changes (MCs) have been classified into three types: (1) low intensity on T1W and high intensity on T2W (reflects disruption of end plates and inflammation), (2) high intensity on both T1W and T2W (reflects yellow marrow replacement), and (3) low intensity in both T1W and T2W (reflects sclerotic changes). The cervical segments with MCs were significantly more likely to have disc degeneration and spinal canal stenosis [41, 42]. The C5/C6 and C6/C7 levels are most affected [41]. Some studies have suggested that MCs denote cervical instability at the same level [43], while others found that such levels exhibit less angular motion, implying loss of mobility [42].

Finally, ligamentous pathology may be evident on MRI. Anterior compression of the cord can occur through hypertrophy (HPLL) or ossification (OPLL) of the posterior longitudinal ligament. Unfortunately, conventional MRI does not convey a clear delineation between the PLL and disc material, as both appear hypointense on T1 and T2 sequences [6]. Some sources have observed that HPLL appears isointense or mildly hyperintense to paravertebral muscles on T1, while OPLL and osteophytes look hypointense to paravertebral muscles [6, 44]. With the absence of significant spondylosis and/or with the presence of multilevel anterior compression, OPLL is suggested [6]. The pathology can be observed in up to 10.5% DCM patients [3]. CT remains the modality of choice for diagnosis of OPLL [18]. The presence of OPLL can alter surgical approach [1]. Similarly, posterior compression of the spinal cord can occur through either hypertrophy or ossification of the LF, which can be evident in up to 56.8% [3].

Diagnosis of DCM requires evidence of spinal cord compression with associated clinical signs of myelopathy [6]. Degenerative changes eventually constrict the spinal canal and compress the spinal cord parenchyma. Spinal cord compression has been quantified through various definitions. The compression ratio (CR) [45, 46], the ratio between the anteroposterior diameter and the transverse diameter, and the method of maximum spinal cord compression (MSCC) [47] have been utilized frequently. Both have limitations, as both do not account for lateral compression, while MSCC neglects variation of spinal cord size along the spinal column [6]. The C5/C6 level is the most common site of MSCC, followed by C4/C5 and C3/C4 [3]. Overall, spinal cord compression is a sensitive feature of myelopathy, but it can also present in approximately 5.3–13.3% of asymptomatic patients [37, 39, 48]. Moreover, spinal cord re-expansion (or lack thereof) may be associated with surgical outcomes [49, 50].

As the extent of spinal cord damage increases, the water content increases; this affects changes to tissue relaxation, which equates to changes on T1 and T2 sequences. With more water content, tissue exhibits hypointensity on T1 and hyperintensity on T2. Overall, as T2 is more sensitive to variation in water content than T1, changes on T2 are frequently observed prior to changes on T1. DCM patients frequently demonstrate T2 hyperintensity and, less commonly, T1 hypointensity, at the level of compression [6]. Both features are helpful diagnostic findings [6]. In particular, T2 hyperintensity can be present in up to 85% of patients with DCM [6]. Moreover, the extent of T2 hyperintensity (including size of signal change, relative intensity of signal change, and pattern of signal change) has been linked to clinical impairment in DCM patients [51]. On the other hand, T1 hypointensity, which can indicate cavitation and disruption of fiber tracts, may be a specific feature for poorer baseline neurological function and worse surgical results [52–54]. Snake-eye appearance, where symmetric hyperintensity of the spinal cord is observed on axial T2 sequences, is a rare finding. Through autopsy studies, this imaging feature has been associated with cystic necrosis due to mechanical compression and venous infarction, corresponding to damage of gray matter and neuronal loss in the anterior horn [55]. Not surprisingly, snake-eye appearance has been considered a poor prognostic factor for surgical outcome [55].

Limitations of Conventional MRI

Despite the utility of MRI in the assessment of DCM patients, findings can be nonspecific and do not reveal data pertaining to pathophysiology at the microscopic level. Degenerative changes on MRI can be seen in asymptomatic patients. In particular, evidence of disc degeneration (annular tears and/or disc bulge/protrusions/herniations) can be observed in up to 36.7 to 89% of patients [37, 39, 48]. Cervical OPLL can also be observed in asymptomatic patients. Several demographic factors have been associated with the pathology. National background has a profound role, as up to 3.6% patients exhibit radiographic evidence of OPLL in the Japanese population; this remains markedly higher than other Asian countries and non-Asian countries [18]. Less demonstrated, older age and male gender appear to be risk factors for disease development as well [1]. Overall, spinal cord compression can occur in up to 5.3% to 13.3% of asymptomatic patients [37, 48]; furthermore, up to 2.3% and 3.1% display T2 signal change and cord deformity, respectively [37, 39]. Per a recent systematic review by Wilson et al. [56], for patients without clinical myelopathy, but evident canal stenosis and cord compromise due to degenerative changes, 8% will exhibit clinical myelopathy at 12-month follow-up, and 23% will do so at 44-month follow-up; surprisingly, the lack of T2 hyperintensity was associated with early progression to myelopathy, while the presence of T2 hyperintensity was associated with late progressive myelopathy [56]. Risk of early progression to symptomatic myelopathy (≤12 months) was predicted by the presence of clinically symptomatic radiculopathy and abnormal SEP and MEP [57].

On the other hand, MRI findings noted in DCM patients can exhibit inadequate correlates with clinical status. Studies have observed that T2 signal changes can be delayed manifestations and may forecast worse prognosis despite surgical intervention [58]. To complicate matters, not all T2 signal changes are the equivalent; there are two broad characterizations based on the level of signal intensity and pattern of signal change [3, 51]. In addition, although T1 hypointensity is considered a specific finding of poorer baseline neurological function and worse postoperative recovery, the imaging feature is less common compared to T2 hyperintensity and can be tougher to observe as consistently as T2 hyperintensity [52–54, 59]. A recent systematic review [8] assessed the role of MRI characteristics to direct treatment (surgery versus conservative management) and to predict postsurgical outcomes. There are three MRI features that may be considered negative predictors of postsurgical outcomes (number of high-signal intensity segments, combined T1/T2 signal change, and signal intensity ratio) [8].

Overall, the current literature offers weak recommendations based on low strength of evidence: (1) MRI can help with the diagnosis of DCM, but physicians should depend on clinical history and examination to assess progression and severity of DCM; (2) T2 signal may be a helpful prognostic factor but should be used in combination with other features (such as signal intensity on T1 or compression ratios) [8]. These conclusions underlie the variable tolerance of spinal cord compression in different patients, where minimal degenerative changes/"mild" stenosis can be observed on conventional MRI despite prominent clinical cervical myelopathy and vice versa.

In addition, the diagnosis of DCM depends on the assessment of spinal canal stenosis in the setting of degenerative changes. Definitive guidelines for the assessment of this feature remain deficient. Spinal canal stenosis can occur through acquired degenerative disease or congenital stenosis. Unfortunately, no clear quantitative criteria have been established to differentiate these two etiologies [6]. Recently, authors have defined an "occupation rate" of the spinal cord within the dural tube (the ratio between the sagittal diameter of the spinal cord parenchyma to the sagittal diameter of the neural tube on T2 sequences), where ≥70% threshold was used to establish a working diagnosis of congenital stenosis [3]. With this demarcation, roughly 8.4% DCM patients can exhibit congenital stenosis [3]. Unfortunately, this definition requires further studies for validation [3].

Advanced MRI Techniques

Over the last decade, MRI has continued to evolve. These novel imaging protocols have significantly improved our ability to gather information pertaining to the microstructure and intrinsic functional properties of the spinal cord. This information may prove very useful in predicting operative outcome, overcoming limitations observed with conventional MRI. The following is a brief description of some of these novel modalities.

Diffusion Tensor Imaging (DTI)

DTI aims to analyze the presence, strength, and directionality of water particles—properties that can be distorted in DCM [60]. In particular, findings can implicate degeneration of white matter tracts [61–65]. Various metrics have been introduced, including fractional anisotropy (FA), apparent diffusion coefficient, mean diffusivity, tractography, and fiber tractography ratio [60]. FA, which ranges from 0 for isotropic diffusion [same in all directions] to 1 for anisotropic [all in 1 direction], has gained the most traction [6]. A recent systematic review delineated nine studies, where Level 3 evidence suggests that DTI is associated with preoperative severity and postsurgical outcomes in DCM patients and may be a good adjunct to assess those that may benefit from surgery [60].

Magnetization Transfer (MT)

MT offers a measure of myelin quantity [3, 66]; values can implicate the extent of demyelination [67]. The protocol employs a pre-pulse that evaluates the relative chemical and magnetization exchange between protons bound to lipid macromolecules and those neighboring water protons [3]. The feature is expressed as a ratio between scans with and without the pre-pulse or between the spinal cord and cerebrospinal fluid [3]. The method has been predominantly evaluated in multiple sclerosis [3, 67]. Nevertheless, recent preliminary data suggest that DCM patients have reduced MT ratio compared to healthy patients; moreover, MT ratio may correlate with mJOA scores [65].

Myelin Water Fraction (MWF)

MWF, also a modality to assess demyelination, is designed to measure myelin by taking advantage of T2 relaxation of water compartmentalized within different tissue (white matter, gray matter, and CSF) [3, 6]. The method has been studied in multiple sclerosis, but limited studies have focused on DCM [3, 66, 68].

MR Spectroscopy (MRS)

MRS offers a measure of different molecules within a single voxel, namely, N-acetyl aspartate, myoinositol, choline, creatine, and lactate [66]. Two studies [69, 70] discovered that the N-acetyl aspartate/creatine ratio was significantly reduced in DCM patients compared to healthy subjects; however, when Holly et al. [69] included mJOA scores, there was no significant correlation with N-acetyl aspartate/creatine ratio. On the other hand, Salamon et al. [71] showed that choline/N--acetyl aspartate ratio was increased in DCM patients compared to healthy subjects and that the ratio significantly correlated mJOA scores.

Functional MRI (fMRI)

fMRI attempts to correlate changes in neurological function (via motor tasks or sensory stimuli) with either neurovascular coupling (where fluctuations in function parallel fluctuations in local blood flow) or signal enhancement by extravascular protons (where fluctuation in intracellular and extracellular volumes may correspond with neural activity) [3]. The method has been studied in multiple sclerosis and chronic spinal cord injury but has not been pursued in DCM [3]. For multiple sclerosis, cervical cord demonstrated increased number of active voxels, increased mean signal intensity change in active voxels, and increased distribution of activation outside expected ipsilateral dorsal horns [66]. For chronic spinal cord injury, fMRI demonstrated increased bilateral activation compared to healthy controls [66].

Case Presentations

A. Significant stenosis/T2 signal with no myelopathy: 71-year-old male who presented with bilateral hand numbness in the first to third digits, where workup included MRI C spine and electromyography. The former demonstrated severe stenosis at C3/C4; the latter was consistent with bilateral carpal tunnel syndrome. He underwent carpal tunnel releases, with improvement of symptoms (Fig. 9.2).
B. Significant stenosis/T2 signal and clinical myelopathy: 72-year-old male who presented with progressive weakness in the hands/arms/legs, now requiring wheelchair for mobilization. MRI C spine demonstrated multilevel cervical stenosis (Fig. 9.3).
C. Minimal stenosis/T2 signal and clinical myelopathy: 44-year-old female who presented with frequent falls, hand dexterity issues, and bilateral Hoffman's signs. MRI C spine demonstrated C5/C6 canal stenosis. Though there was slight CSF signal posterior to the spinal cord, there was a concern for dynamic spinal cord damage with the pronounced herniated disc and the loss of cervical lordosis. After an ACDF C5/C6, she noted improvement with balance and with fine motor skills (Fig. 9.4).

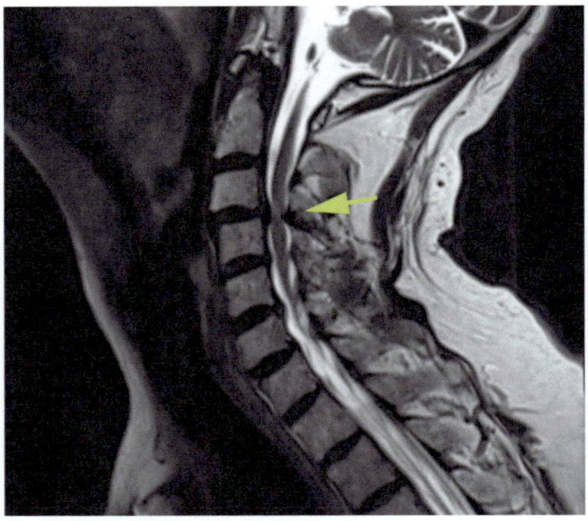

Fig. 9.2 71-year-old male who presented with bilateral hand numbness in the first to third digits, where workup included MRI C spine and electromyography. The former demonstrated severe stenosis at C3/C4 (*arrow*); the latter was consistent with bilateral carpal tunnel syndrome. He underwent carpal tunnel releases, with improvement of symptoms

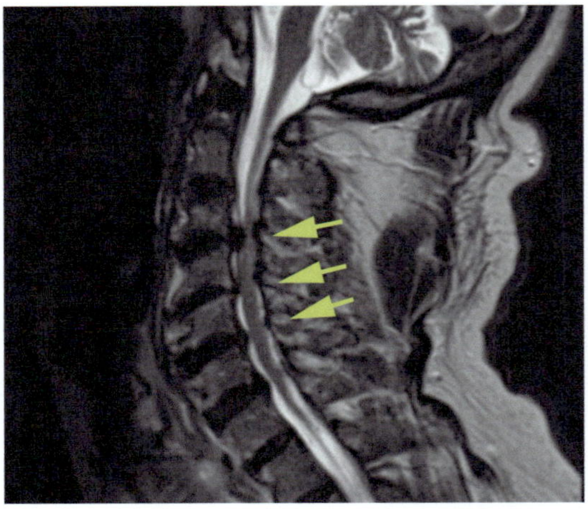

Fig. 9.3 72-year-old male who presented with progressive weakness in the hands/arms/legs, now requiring wheelchair for mobilization. MRI C spine demonstrated multilevel cervical stenosis (*arrows*)

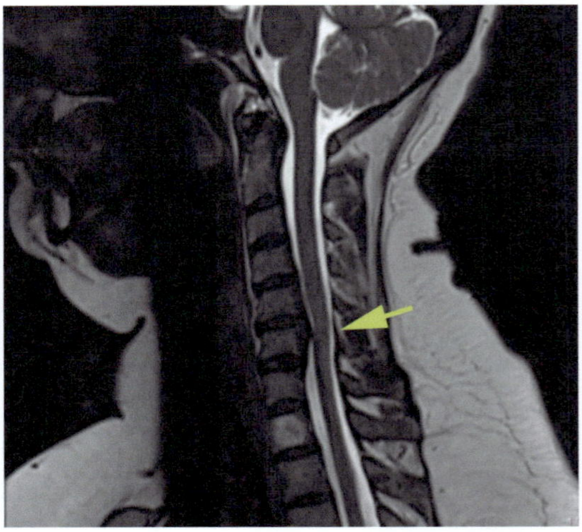

Fig. 9.4 44-year-old female who presented with frequent falls, hand dexterity issues, and bilateral Hoffman's signs. MRI C spine demonstrated C5/C6 canal stenosis (*arrow*). Though there was slight CSF signal posterior to the spinal cord, there was a concern for dynamic spinal cord damage with the pronounced herniated disc and the loss of cervical lordosis. After an ACDF C5/C6, she noted improvement with balance and with fine motor skills

Conclusions

Degenerative cervical myelopathy and radiculopathy comprise a host of age-related disorders which can cause significant damage to the spinal cord and/or nerve root. For the past 30 years, conventional magnetic resonance imaging has been the primary imaging protocol for the assessment of DCM. Unfortunately, imaging findings can be nonspecific and do not convey data regarding the health status of the spinal cord parenchyma. Advanced MRI techniques may help elucidate details regarding the microscopic structure and functional composition of the spinal cord parenchyma.

Key Recommendations

1. Conventional MRI is a useful imaging tool for diagnosis of DCM, but it has significant limitations.
2. Radiographs and CT imaging continue to have supplementary roles in the management of DCM.
3. Clinical judgment remains a key component to assess disease severity and surgical prognosis.
4. Emerging advanced MRI techniques, specifically DTI, can potentially offer more details regarding the health status of the spinal cord with respect to DCM.
5. Extensive prospective studies that correlate advanced MRI data to clinical examination and outcome need to be completed before the techniques can become clinically relevant.
6. Advanced MRI techniques will likely be a valuable adjunct to surgical decision-making and prognosis in the future for patients with DCM.

References

1. Tetreault L, Goldstein CL, Arnold P, et al. Degenerative cervical myelopathy: a spectrum of related disorders affecting the aging spine. Neurosurgery. 2015;77(Suppl 4):S51–67.
2. Nouri A, Tetreault L, Singh A, Karadimas SK, Fehlings MG. Degenerative cervical myelopathy: epidemiology, genetics, and pathogenesis. Spine. 2015;40:E675–93.
3. Nouri A, Martin A, Tetreault L, et al. MRI analysis of the combined prospectively collected AOSpine North America and International Data: the prevalence and spectrum of pathologies in a global cohort of patients with degenerative cervical myelopathy. Spine. 2017;42:1058–67.
4. Karadimas SK, Erwin WM, Ely CG, Dettori JR, Fehlings MG. Pathophysiology and natural history of cervical spondylotic myelopathy. Spine. 2013;38:S21–36.
5. Kalsi-Ryan S, Karadimas SK, Fehlings MG. Cervical spondylotic myelopathy. Neuroscientist. 2012;19:409–21.
6. Nouri A, Martin AR, Mikulis D, Fehlings MG. Magnetic resonance imaging assessment of degenerative cervical myelopathy: a review of structural changes and measurement techniques. Neurosurg Focus. 2016;40:E5.
7. Wada E, Ohmura M, Yonenobu K. Intramedullary changes of the spinal cord in cervical spondylotic myelopathy. Spine. 1995;20:2226–32.
8. Tetreault LA, Dettori JR, Wilson JR, et al. Systematic review of magnetic resonance imaging characteristics that affect treatment decision making and predict clinical outcome in patients with cervical spondylotic myelopathy. Spine. 2013;38:S89–110.
9. Nasir S, Mahmud R, Hussain M, Min D, Shuang-ming S. Flexion/extension cervical spine views in blunt cervical trauma. Chin J Traumatol. 2012;15:166–9.
10. Khan SN, Erickson G, Sena MJ, Gupta MC. Use of flexion and extension radiographs of the cervical spine to rule out acute instability in patients with negative computed tomography scans. J Orthop Trauma. 2011;25:51–6.
11. White AP, Biswas D, Smart LR, Haims A, Grauer JN. Utility of flexion-extension radiographs in evaluating the degenerative cervical spine. Spine. 2007;32:975–9.
12. Berberat J, Grobholz R, Boxheimer L, Rogers S, Remonda L, Roelcke U. Differentiation between calcification and hemorrhage in brain tumors using susceptibility-weighted imaging: a pilot study. AJR Am J Roentgenol. 2014;202:847–50.
13. Sarva RP, Farivar S, Fromm H, Poller W. Study of the sensitivity and specificity of computerized tomography in the detection of calcified gallstones which appears radiolucent by conventional roentgenography. Gastrointest Radiol. 1981;6:165–7.
14. Middleton WD, Thorsen MK, Lawson TL, Foley WD. False-positive CT diagnosis of gallstones due to thickening of the gallbladder wall. AJR Am J Roentgenol. 1987;149:941–4.
15. Pham PH, Rao DS, Vasunilashorn F, Fishbein MC, Goldin JG. Computed tomography calcium quantification as a measure of atherosclerotic plaque morphology and stability. Investig Radiol. 2006;41:674–80.
16. Otake S, Matsuo M, Nishizawa S, Sano A, Kuroda Y. Ossification of the posterior longitudinal ligament: MR evaluation. AJNR Am J Neuroradiol. 1992;13:1059–67; discussion 1068–1070.

17. Yamashita Y, Takahashi M, Matsuno Y, et al. Spinal cord compression due to ossification of ligaments: MR imaging. Radiology. 1990;175:843–8.
18. Wong J, Leung O, Yuen M. Questionable adequacy of magnetic resonance for the detection of ossification of the posterior longitudinal ligament of the cervical spine. Hong Kong J Radiol. 2011;14:78–83.
19. Houser OW, Onofrio BM, Miller GM, Folger WN, Smith PL. Cervical spondylotic stenosis and myelopathy: evaluation with computed tomographic myelography. Mayo Clin Proc. 1994;69:557–63.
20. Shafaie FF, Wippold FJ 2nd, Gado M, Pilgram TK, Riew KD. Comparison of computed tomography myelography and magnetic resonance imaging in the evaluation of cervical spondylotic myelopathy and radiculopathy. Spine. 1999;24:1781–5.
21. Song KJ, Choi BW, Kim GH, Kim JR. Clinical usefulness of CT-myelogram comparing with the MRI in degenerative cervical spinal disorders: is CTM still useful for primary diagnostic tool? J Spinal Disord Tech. 2009;22:353–7.
22. Enders J, Rief M, Zimmermann E, et al. High-field open versus short-bore magnetic resonance imaging of the spine: a randomized controlled comparison of image quality. PLoS One. 2014;8:e83427.
23. Gilbert JW, Wheeler GR, Lingreen RA, Johnson RR. Open stand-up MRI: a new instrument for positional neuroimaging. J Spinal Disord Tech. 2006;19:151–4.
24. Sohn HM, You JW, Lee JY. The relationship between disc degeneration and morphologic changes in the intervertebral foramen of the cervical spine: a cadaveric MRI and CT study. J Korean Med Sci. 2004;19:101–6.
25. Yoo JU, Zou D, Edwards WT, Bayley J, Yuan HA. Effect of cervical spine motion on the neuroforaminal dimensions of human cervical spine. Spine. 1992;17:1131–6.
26. Hughes TB Jr, Richman JD, Rothfus WE. Diagnosis of Os odontoideum using kinematic magnetic resonance imaging. A case report. Spine. 1999;24:715–8.
27. Muhle C, Weinert D, Falliner A, et al. Dynamic changes of the spinal canal in patients with cervical spondylosis at flexion and extension using magnetic resonance imaging. Investig Radiol. 1998;33:444–9.
28. Muhle C, Wiskirchen J, Weinert D, et al. Biomechanical aspects of the subarachnoid space and cervical cord in healthy individuals examined with kinematic magnetic resonance imaging. Spine. 1998;23:556–67.
29. Vives MJ, Harris C, Reiter MF, Drzala M. Use of stand-up magnetic resonance imaging for evaluation of a cervicothoracic injury in a patient with ankylosing spondylitis. Spine J. 2008;8:678–82.
30. Suzuki F, Fukami T, Tsuji A, Takagi K, Matsuda M. Discrepancies of MRI findings between recumbent and upright positions in atlantoaxial lesion. Report of two cases. Eur Spine J. 2008;17(Suppl 2):S304–7.
31. Gilbert JW, Wheeler GR, Lingreen RA, et al. Imaging in the position that causes pain. Surg Neurol. 2008;69:463–5; discussion 465.
32. Jinkins JR, Dworkin JS, Damadian RV. Upright, weight-bearing, dynamic-kinetic MRI of the spine: initial results. Eur Radiol. 2005;15:1815–25.
33. Janssen M, Nabih A, Moussa W, Kawchuk GN, Carey JP. Evaluation of diagnosis techniques used for spinal injury related back pain. Pain Res Treat. 2011;2011:478798.
34. Muhle C, Resnick D, Ahn JM, Sudmeyer M, Heller M. In vivo changes in the neuroforaminal size at flexion-extension and axial rotation of the cervical spine in healthy persons examined using kinematic magnetic resonance imaging. Spine. 2001;26:E287–93.
35. Muhle C, Bischoff L, Weinert D, et al. Exacerbated pain in cervical radiculopathy at axial rotation, flexion, extension, and coupled motions of the cervical spine: evaluation by kinematic magnetic resonance imaging. Investig Radiol. 1998;33:279–88.
36. Ferreiro Perez A, Garcia Isidro M, Ayerbe E, Castedo J, Jinkins JR. Evaluation of intervertebral disc herniation and hypermobile intersegmental instability in symptomatic adult patients undergoing recumbent and upright MRI of the cervical or lumbosacral spines. Eur J Radiol. 2007;62:444–8.
37. Kato F, Yukawa Y, Suda K, Yamagata M, Ueta T. Normal morphology, age-related changes and abnormal findings of the cervical spine. Part II: magnetic resonance imaging of over 1,200 asymptomatic subjects. Eur Spine J. 2012;21:1499–507.
38. Ulbrich EJ, Schraner C, Boesch C, et al. Normative MR cervical spinal canal dimensions. Radiology. 2013;271:172–82.
39. Matsumoto M, Fujimura Y, Suzuki N, et al. MRI of cervical intervertebral discs in asymptomatic subjects. J Bone Joint Surg. 1998;80:19–24.
40. Modic MT, Steinberg PM, Ross JS, Masaryk TJ, Carter JR. Degenerative disk disease: assessment of changes in vertebral body marrow with MR imaging. Radiology. 1988;166:193–9.
41. Mann E, Peterson CK, Hodler J. Degenerative marrow (modic) changes on cervical spine magnetic resonance imaging scans: prevalence, inter- and intra-examiner reliability and link to disc herniation. Spine. 2011;36:1081–5.
42. Hayashi T, Daubs MD, Suzuki A, Phan K, Shiba K, Wang JC. Effect of Modic changes on spinal canal stenosis and segmental motion in cervical spine. Eur Spine J. 2014;23:1737–42.
43. Tong T, Gao XD, Li J, et al. Do modic changes affect cervical sagittal alignment and motion in symptomatic patients? Eur Spine J. 2017;26:1945–52.
44. Inamasu J, Guiot BH, Sachs DC. Ossification of the posterior longitudinal ligament: an update on its biology, epidemiology, and natural history. Neurosurgery. 2006;58:1027–39; discussion 1027–1039.
45. Fujiwara K, Yonenobu K, Hiroshima K, Ebara S, Yamashita K, Ono K. Morphometry of the cervical spinal cord and its relation to pathology in cases with compression myelopathy. Spine. 1988;13:1212–6.
46. Okada Y, Ikata T, Yamada H, Sakamoto R, Katoh S. Magnetic resonance imaging study on the results of

surgery for cervical compression myelopathy. Spine. 1993;18:2024–9.
47. Fehlings MG, Rao SC, Tator CH, et al. The optimal radiologic method for assessing spinal canal compromise and cord compression in patients with cervical spinal cord injury. Part II: results of a multicenter study. Spine. 1999;24:605–13.
48. Ernst CW, Stadnik TW, Peeters E, Breucq C, Osteaux MJ. Prevalence of annular tears and disc herniations on MR images of the cervical spine in symptom free volunteers. Eur J Radiol. 2005;55:409–14.
49. Mastronardi L, Elsawaf A, Roperto R, et al. Prognostic relevance of the postoperative evolution of intramedullary spinal cord changes in signal intensity on magnetic resonance imaging after anterior decompression for cervical spondylotic myelopathy. J Neurosurg Spine. 2007;7:615–22.
50. Arvin B, Kalsi-Ryan S, Karpova A, et al. Postoperative magnetic resonance imaging can predict neurological recovery after surgery for cervical spondylotic myelopathy: a prospective study with blinded assessments. Neurosurgery. 2011;69:362–8.
51. Vedantam A, Rajshekhar V. Does the type of T2-weighted hyperintensity influence surgical outcome in patients with cervical spondylotic myelopathy? A review. Eur spine J. 2013;22:96–106.
52. Alafifi T, Kern R, Fehlings M. Clinical and MRI predictors of outcome after surgical intervention for cervical spondylotic myelopathy. J Neuroimaging. 2007;17:315–22.
53. Arvin B, Kalsi-Ryan S, Mercier D, Furlan JC, Massicotte EM, Fehlings MG. Preoperative magnetic resonance imaging is associated with baseline neurological status and can predict postoperative recovery in patients with cervical spondylotic myelopathy. Spine. 2013;38:1170–6.
54. Morio Y, Teshima R, Nagashima H, Nawata K, Yamasaki D, Nanjo Y. Correlation between operative outcomes of cervical compression myelopathy and mri of the spinal cord. Spine. 2001;26:1238–45.
55. Mizuno J, Nakagawa H, Inoue T, Hashizume Y. Clinicopathological study of "snake-eye appearance" in compressive myelopathy of the cervical spinal cord. J Neurosurg Spine. 2003;99:162–8.
56. Wilson JR, Barry S, Fischer DJ, et al. Frequency, timing, and predictors of neurological dysfunction in the nonmyelopathic patient with cervical spinal cord compression, canal stenosis, and/or ossification of the posterior longitudinal ligament. Spine. 2013;38:S37–54.
57. Bednarik J, Kadanka Z, Dusek L, et al. Presymptomatic spondylotic cervical myelopathy: an updated predictive model. Eur Spine J. 2008;17:421–31.
58. Suri A, Chabbra RPS, Mehta VS, Gaikwad S, Pandey RM. Effect of intramedullary signal changes on the surgical outcome of patients with cervical spondylotic myelopathy. Spine J. 2003;3:33–45.
59. Nouri A, Tetreault L, Zamorano JJ, et al. Role of magnetic resonance imaging in predicting surgical outcome in patients with cervical spondylotic myelopathy. Spine. 2015;40:171–8.
60. Rindler RS, Chokshi FH, Malcolm JG, et al. Spinal diffusion tensor imaging in evaluation of preoperative and postoperative severity of cervical spondylotic myelopathy: systematic review of literature. World Neurosurg. 2017;99:150–8.
61. Koskinen E, Brander A, Hakulinen U, et al. Assessing the state of chronic spinal cord injury using diffusion tensor imaging. J Neurotrauma. 2013;30:1587–95.
62. Li X, Cui JL, Mak KC, Luk KD, Hu Y. Potential use of diffusion tensor imaging in level diagnosis of multilevel cervical spondylotic myelopathy. Spine. 2014;39:E615–22.
63. Cui JL, Li X, Chan TY, Mak KC, Luk KD, Hu Y. Quantitative assessment of column-specific degeneration in cervical spondylotic myelopathy based on diffusion tensor tractography. Eur Spine J. 2015;24:41–7.
64. Maki S, Koda M, Ota M, et al. Reduced field-of-view diffusion tensor imaging of the spinal cord shows motor dysfunction of the lower extremities in patients with cervical compression myelopathy. Spine. 2018;43(2):89–96.
65. Martin AR, De Leener B, Cohen-Adad J, et al. 163 microstructural MRI quantifies tract-specific injury and correlates with global disability and focal neurological deficits in degenerative cervical myelopathy. Neurosurgery. 2016;63(Suppl 1):165.
66. Martin AR, Aleksanderek I, Cohen-Adad J, et al. Translating state-of-the-art spinal cord MRI techniques to clinical use: a systematic review of clinical studies utilizing DTI, MT, MWF, MRS, and fMRI. NeuroImage Clin. 2016;10:192–238.
67. Lema A, Bishop C, Malik O, et al. A comparison of magnetization transfer methods to assess brain and cervical cord microstructure in multiple sclerosis. J Neuroimaging. 2017;27:221–6.
68. Liu H, MacMillian EL, Jutzeler CR, et al. Assessing structure and function of myelin in cervical spondylotic myelopathy: evidence of demyelination. Neurology. 2017;89:602–10.
69. Holly LT, Freitas B, McArthur DL, Salamon N. Proton magnetic resonance spectroscopy to evaluate spinal cord axonal injury in cervical spondylotic myelopathy. J Neurosurg Spine. 2009;10:194–200.
70. Taha Ali TF, Badawy AE. Feasibility of 1H-MR spectroscopy in evaluation of cervical spondylotic myelopathy. Egypt J Radiol Nucl Med. 2013;44:93–9.
71. Salamon N, Ellingson BM, Nagarajan R, Gebara N, Thomas A, Holly LT. Proton magnetic resonance spectroscopy of human cervical spondylosis at 3T. Spinal Cord. 2013;51:558–63.

10 Alternative Diagnostic Tools

Kurt M. Eichholz

Pearls and Pitfalls

- EMG/NCV should not be used as a replacement for a detailed history and physical examination, and should be used sparingly and only when necessary, as these tests increase cost and discomfort to the patient.
- EMG/NCV should be performed by an appropriate and well-trained physician. In some states, these tests may legally be performed by physical therapists or chiropractors. The study should be performed with the interpreting neurologist or physiatrist on site and not performed by a technician and interpreted at a later time.
- Electrophysiologic studies should be reviewed in the appropriate clinical context. For example, a study that determines that a radiculopathy is present based solely on paraspinal muscle denervation, in a patient that has already had one or more spine surgeries, should be viewed with suspicion.
- EMG/NCV studies should be obtained when a patient has clinical signs and symptoms that cannot be correlated to one specific finding on imaging or when imaging shows compression at several different levels that may be similar in nature. In this setting, EMG may be useful in delineating which are of compression is the causative agent.
- EMG/NCV may also be useful in helping determine if a patient has a specific cervical radiculopathy versus a distal entrapment neuropathy, such as median or ulnar neuropathy.
- While cervical transforaminal selective nerve root blocks may be performed as a diagnostic tool in order to determine if a specific neural foramen is the location of neural compression, this injection is not without significant risk of vertebral artery injury, which should be taken into account prior to obtaining or ordering such a test.

Introduction

Cervical radiculopathy and myelopathy are among the more common causes of patients presenting to a spinal specialist. Radiculopathy typically presents with a combination of neck pain, paresthesias, numbness, and/or weakness in a

K. M. Eichholz
St. Lcuis Minimally Invasive Spine Center,
St. Lcuis, MO, USA
e-mail: kurt@stlmisc.com

M. G. Kaiser et al. (eds.), *Degenerative Cervical Myelopathy and Radiculopathy*,
https://doi.org/10.1007/978-3-319-97952-6_10

specific cervical nerve root distribution in one or both arms. There may be absence of reflexes in the affected distribution as well. Cervical myelopathy may present with neck pain as well as upper motor neuron signs, which include hyperreflexia, including a positive Hoffman's sign, and symptoms related to increased spasticity, such as difficulty with fine motor skills, balance, Lhermitte's sign, paresthesias in the arms and legs, and increased muscle tone.

The annual age-adjusted incidence of cervical radiculopathy is 83.2 per 100,000 person-years [1]. There is age adjusted incidence, and then there is age specific incidence for the age group 50–54 years old, where it reaches a peak of 202.9 per 100,000 person-years. The incidence and prevalence of cervical myelopathy have been estimated to be 41 and 605 per million in North America, respectively, while the incidence of cervical spondylotic myelopathy-related hospitalizations has been estimated at 4.04 per 100,000 person-years [2].

The basis of surgical decision-making for patients with cervical radiculopathy or myelopathy is a detailed history and physical examination, with correlation of radiographic studies. For patients who have distinct and well-delineated symptoms, with appropriate findings on physical examination, and corresponding radiographic findings, the causative agent in most cases need not be confirmed with additional testing.

However, in cases in which the differential diagnosis continues to encompass more than one possible etiology for the patient's presentation, other diagnostic tools may be required to determine the most effective treatment paradigm. In most cases, these adjuvant tests have a lower sensitivity and/or specificity than imaging studies. But in situations where the diagnosis is not definitive based on history, physical/neurological examination, and imaging, supplementing with these additional studies may be necessary in order to confirm the diagnosis and determine treatment.

This chapter will focus on diagnostic studies apart from imaging studies such as magnetic resonance imaging, which are used in the evaluation of patients with cervical radiculopathy or myelopathy. The most commonly used adjuvant diagnostic test is electromyography and nerve conduction testing. Some are used relatively often, while others are used rarely. These studies may be a useful adjuvant when used in combination with imaging and a detailed history and physical/neurological examination.

Electromyography and Nerve Conduction Study

Electromyography and nerve conduction studies are some of the most commonly used adjuvant diagnostic tools used in patients with potential cervical radiculopathy. Laws regarding what type of practitioner is qualified to perform an EMG/NCV vary state to state and can include neurologists, physiatrists, chiropractors, or physical therapists. The American Association of Neuromuscular & Electrodiagnostic Medicine issued a position statement recommending that this testing only be performed by physicians who specialize in neurology or physical medicine and rehabilitation in order to ensure high-quality testing [3]. Because this testing is directed at electrophysiologic testing of a specific nerve root, it is of limited value in a patient with cervical myelopathy. In fact, a patient may have an obvious cervical myelopathy and have a normal electromyography and nerve conduction study. Electromyography (EMG) is a separate test from nerve conduction studies (NCS), but both are commonly performed together.

EMG utilizes an electromyograph to determine the electric potential or difference in voltage which is generated by muscle tissue when stimulated. EMG uses either surface electrodes or intramuscular leads to measure this difference; however, intramuscular needle EMG testing is typically more accurate [3]. Most commonly, a monopolar EMG needle is inserted in the muscle with a surface electrode used as reference.

The intramuscular needle inserted for EMG will measure insertional activity and resting activity in the muscle. Insertional activity is the short burst activation that occurs with insertion of the needle into the muscle. This short activation is typically less than 100 milliseconds. Insertion of the needle or subsequent movement of the needle will cause a short burst of depolarization from muscle fibers, which should cease once the movement is stopped. Prolonged insertional activity may be pathologic in patients who have myopathy, or in patients with early neuropathy, prior to more advanced neuropathy in which fibrillation potentials are present. Increased insertional activity may occur in partially denervated muscles, which become progressively more irritable as denervation progresses. Increased insertional activity is not a specific finding, but an indication of irritability and early denervation. Decreased insertional activity can be seen in patients with advanced muscle loss or necrosis. Once inserted into the muscle, resting activity is measured, and pathology may be seen if the resting muscle displays fasciculations or fibrillations.

Further EMG study measures the electrical potential during active muscle contraction. The resultant size, frequency, and shape of electrical activity during muscle contraction are used to determine the functional capability of the muscle being analyzed. See Fig. 10.1 for an example of a normal EMG waveform. Additional parameters measured by EMG include the maximal voluntary contraction, which measures the peak force generated by the muscles being measured. In addition, muscle fatigue can be measured during the test by monitoring the degradation of the signal amplitude and duration through the course of the test. EMG may also delineate pathology at the neuromuscular junction, by measuring decreased recruitment of muscle activity in a motor unit action potential.

EMG is typically performed with a concurrent nerve conduction study test. While EMG measures electrical potential, or difference in electrical voltage, neve conduction studies measure the time it takes for an electrical stimulus to travel from the site of stimulation to the site of recording. There are four parts to a complete nerve conduction study test. These include motor NCS, sensory NCS, F-wave study, and H-reflex study. See Fig. 10.2 for a normal NCS waveform. While the study is often called nerve conduction velocity, or NCV, this is a misnomer, as the velocity is just one component of the entire study.

Motor NCS measures the time interval for an electrical stimulus to reach the muscle supplied by the nerve stimulated, which is called latency, and is measured in milliseconds. Once the stimulus reaches the muscle, the amplitude of the response is measured in millivolts. Measurements done on two or more locations along the same nerve allow the nerve conduction velocity to be measured by determining the difference in latencies against the difference between the distances of the stimulating electrodes.

Sensory nerve conduction studies are recorded from a sensory area of the nerve stimulated. In most cases, this is a distal area, such as a finger. Again, latency and amplitude are measured, but sensory amplitudes are smaller than motor amplitudes and are measured in microvolts rather than millivolts. The sensory nerve conduction velocity

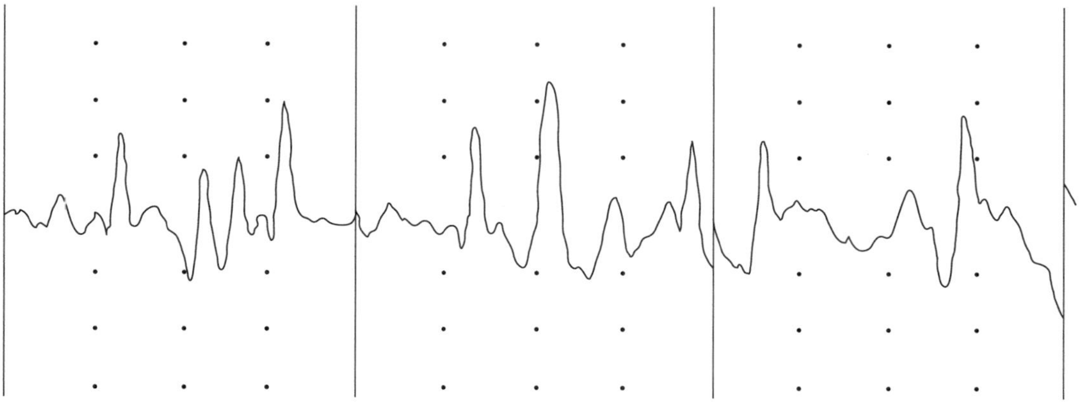

Fig. 10.1 Normal EMG waveform

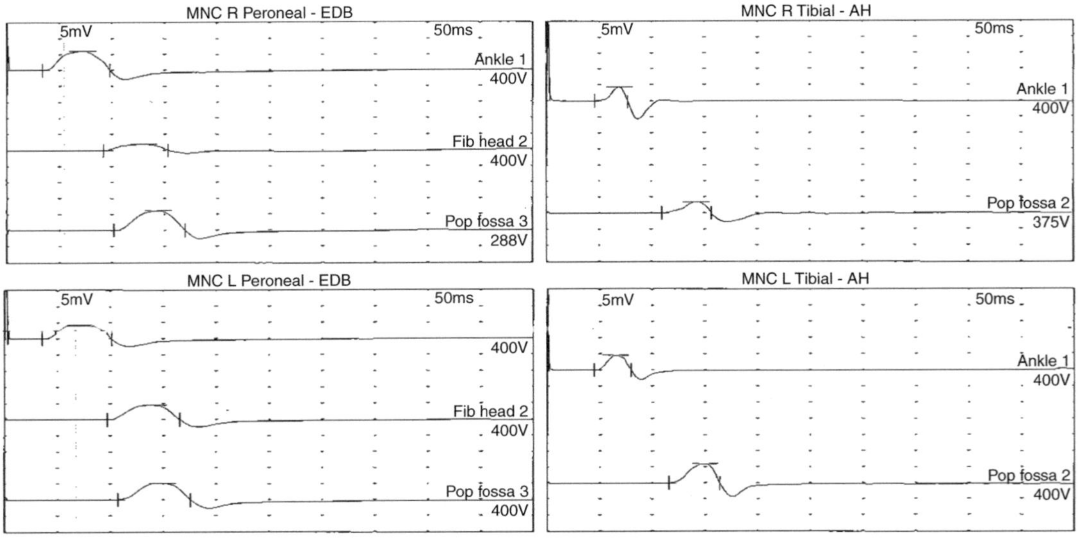

Fig. 10.2 Normal NCS waveform

is again calculated using the latency and the distance between electrodes.

One key component in interpretation of nerve conduction studies is that the neural cell bodies for the sensory nerves are located in the dorsal ganglion. Therefore, in cervical radiculopathy, the lesion will be proximal to the cell bodies, and the sensory NCS will be normal, while electromyography will be positive. In the setting of a positive NCS, lesions distal to the dorsal root ganglion must be considered, such as brachial plexitis or median or ulnar neuropathy [4].

F-wave is a measurement of action potentials from a muscle during supramaximal stimulation. Stimulation occurs in the limb, and travels to the ventral horn of the spinal cord, and then returns to the limb in the same nerve. The stimulation creates both antidromic (distal to proximal, i.e., toward the spinal cord) and orthodromic (proximal to distal) impulses. Once the antidromic response reaches the motor neuron cell bodies, a reflex compound muscle action potential (CMAP) response called the F-wave travels back distally down the nerve. The time difference measured between when the orthodromic response reaches the distal recording electrode, and when the F-wave reaches the recording electrode is the latency. The latency is then used to determine the conduction velocity between the spine and the distal nerve.

The H-reflex is a measurement of both the afferent and efferent reflex aspects of the peripheral nerves. In this case, the sensory nerve is stimulated (the afferent impulse), and the reflex motor response (the efferent impulse) is measured.

EMG/NCS Utilization in Practice

While cervical radiculopathy is often due to nerve root compression in the cervical spine from either a disc herniation or other spondylotic compression, there are several other entities that could present with a similar clinical constellation of symptoms. A detailed physical examination by a well-trained clinician should achieve a high level of certainty as to the clinical diagnosis when attempting to differentiate between cervical radiculopathy and median or ulnar entrapment neuropathy. However, the first-line diagnostic test of choice may be more of a function of the specialty of the physician to whom the patient presents. Those presenting to a neurologist may be sent first for electrophysiologic testing, while those presenting to a primary care physician or spinal specialist may obtain MRI or imaging studies as the first-line test.

Other pathologies that should be in the differential diagnosis include entrapment neuropathies of the upper limb, such as median neuropathy at the wrist or ulnar neuropathy at the elbow, idiopathic brachial neuritis or plexitis, radiation plexopathy, intramedullary spinal cord lesion or neoplasm, multifocal motor neuropathy, diabetes mellitus, thoracic outlet syndrome, leptomeningeal carcinomatosis, or other inflammatory polyneuropathies. While these are less common, the clinician must keep other potential causes of such symptoms in the differential diagnosis until it is reasonable to rule them out.

One of the most common indications for EMG/NCS in the clinical setting is the differentiation between cervical radiculopathy and entrapment neuropathies, such as carpal tunnel syndrome and ulnar neuropathy, or as a confirmation tool for evaluation of peripheral neuropathy.

In the case of median neuropathy at the wrist, or carpal tunnel syndrome, the presentation may be similar to that of a distinct C6 radiculopathy. While there is a similar sensory deficit in both cases, primarily involving the thumb, index, and middle fingers, there is a specific difference between the motor involvement of the two different entities. Median neuropathy will cause a motor deficit of the abductor pollicis brevis, innervated by the recurrent branch of the median nerve. The recurrent branch of the median nerve splits off distal to the carpal tunnel. However, a C6 nerve root compression will also affect the postaxial muscles of the forearm, specifically the brachioradialis. On clinical examination, a Tinel's sign at the wrist, as well as Phalen's sign, exacerbates the signs and symptoms of median neuropathy, but will not do so for a patient with cervical radiculopathy. In addition, a Spurling's maneuver may be positive in the patient with cervical radiculopathy, but not in the patient with median neuropathy at the wrist.

Distinguishing between ulnar neuropathy at the elbow and C8 radiculopathy is another common indication for EMG/NCS testing. In general, the sensory difference between the two entities is that ulnar neuropathy will cause sensory loss in the fifth digit and the medial aspect of the fourth digit, while a C8 radiculopathy will affect the entire fourth digit. This is a relatively small difference in sensation, and in some cases, the variability in the overlapping dermatomes may account for such a difference. However, isolated ulnar neuropathy should not have a component of axial neck pain, which one would expect with a cervical radiculopathy.

Interpretation of Results

In general, the literature supports the utilization of needle EMG for evaluation of cervical radiculopathy and NCS in the evaluation of entrapment neuropathy. The American Association of Electrodiagnostic Medicine performed a literature review and made practice guidelines for electrophysiologic testing in 1999 [5]. These guidelines state that for a properly performed EMG, examination should be performed of at least one muscle innervated by the C5, C6, C7, C8, and T1 spinal roots in a symptomatic limb, and cervical paraspinal muscles in at least one or more levels as appropriate to the clinical presentation. If there is suspicion for a radiculopathy of a specific root, it is recommended that one of two additional muscles innervated by the suspected root be examined or demonstration of normal muscles above and below the involved root. These guidelines also recommend that at least one motor and one sensory NCS should be performed in order to determine if concomitant polyneuropathy or nerve entrapment exists.

The effectiveness of EMG/NCS is highly dependent upon having a specially trained physician perform the test, as well as a clinician who is able to apply the results of the test to the patient's clinical scenario. It is imperative that the entire report be read by the clinician, to ensure that the results are based on conduction differences in distal muscles affected by a specific nerve root, rather than just on denervation of paraspinal muscles. If an EMG report states that a specific cervical radiculopathy is present, and that result is based purely on paraspinal muscle denervation, that result should be viewed with suspicion. Paraspinal musculature has overlapping innervation throughout the spine. To be able to delineate an isolated cervical radiculopathy based purely on paraspinal denervation is highly suspect, as EMG testing is not performed with any concurrent radiographic imaging which would corroborate which nerve would innervate a specific portion of the paraspinal musculature. One study [6] showed that positive sharp waves were present in 92% of patients older than 40 years, and fibrillations were present in 8% of those patients. These findings were not found in patients under 40 years old. Date et al. [7] showed positive sharp waves in 12% of the paraspinal muscles of asymptomatic patients. These findings exemplify how EMG changes in the paraspinal musculature may be erroneous and should not be the sole criteria for a positive EMG test. However, positive findings in the paraspinal muscles when combined with findings in the extremities increase the sensitivity for cervical radiculopathy [8]. In addition, in the setting of a patient who has undergone a prior surgical procedure through a posterior cervical approach, the cervical paraspinal musculature will be partially denervated from the prior surgical procedure. Therefore, in patients who have undergone a prior posterior cervical surgical procedure, the utilization of EMG changes in the paraspinal musculature of limited value in determining a specific cervical radiculopathy.

Specific EMG and NCV changes will be seen in various pathologies. As mentioned above, entrapment neuropathy at the wrist or elbow will cause decreased motor latency as well as decreased conduction velocity distal to the area of entrapment. Radiation plexopathy will display myokymia, or spontaneous discharges accompanied by wavelike muscle quivering. Multifocal motor neuropathy will cause reduction in CMAP at proximal sites compared to distal sites, with multifocal conduction block, decreased velocities, prolonged terminal latencies, and delayed or absent F-waves. Sensory NCS will be normal across the same segments. Diabetes mellitus causes abnormal spontaneous potentials, positive sharp waves, decreased CMPA amplitude, and fibrillation potentials on EMG while also causing slowing of the nerve conduction velocities due to demyelination.

Sensitivity and Specificity

In the abovementioned literature review, 22 articles provided data which addressed the diagnostic value of needle EMG confirmation [5]. These studies showed that needle EMG examination provided confirmation of cervical root pathology in patients with signs and symptoms of cervical radiculopathy in 30–72% of cases. In studies based on patients with clear neurological or radiological signs, sensitivity was estimated between 50% and 71%. It was shown that needle EMG abnormalities highly correlated with motor weakness. In patients with motor weakness, EMG findings correlated with imaging studies in 65–85% of cases. This shows that needled EMG testing confirms the diagnosis of cervical radiculopathy with a moderate degree of sensitivity and a high degree of specificity. For the well-trained clinician, the more severe of a radiculopathy that is present, the less likely a confirmatory electrophysiologic test will be required.

However, in a study by Askhan et al. [9] comparing the sensitivity for MRI and neurophysiological studies in diagnosing cervical radiculopathy, it found that MRI was predictive 93% of the time, compared to 42% for EMG. The positive predictive values were similar between MRI and EMG (91% vs. 85%); however, the negative predictive value was higher in MRI (25% vs. 7%). Alwari et al. [10] performed a small prospective study to attempt to determine whether EMG could accurately predict outcome in patients undergoing anterior cervical fusion. In 20 patients who were described as having borderline surgical findings on preoperative CT myelogram, those who underwent a preoperative EMG that confirmed radiculopathy had a better postoperative Prolo score than those that did not ($p = 0.001$). However, this study should be viewed with trepidation, as the Prolo scale is a non-validated outcome measure, and in this study, reviewers were unblinded for outcome measure and patient selection. Therefore, based on this information, EMG/NCS should be used as a supplemental diagnostic test and not as a replacement for a detailed physical examination or imaging.

In the clinical setting, the surgeon must determine if EMG/NCS testing will change his or her clinical decision-making. If the clinician has an imaging study that shows a specific neural compressive lesion which would correlate with the patient's presenting signs and symptoms, he or she must determine if there is enough uncertainty in the cause of the symptoms to warrant the additional electrophysiologic testing. Considerations that should be made prior to ordering the test include the delay in care due to the time taken to order, schedule, and obtain the results of the test, the additional cost of obtaining the EMG, as well as the discomfort caused to the patient during the test.

Evoked Potential Studies

Somatosensory evoked potentials and motor evoked potential recordings may further delineate the extent of pathology in patients with cervical spondylotic disease. SEPs are recorded after the electrical stimulation of a nerve in either the upper or lower extremity. In the lower extremities, the posterior tibial nerve, sural nerve, or common peroneal nerve are used, while in the upper limb, the median, radial, and ulnar nerves are used. In patients with cervical myelopathy, diminished SEPs from the posterior tibialis are used for diagnosis. In patients with radiculopathy, several nerves supplied by different spinal segments must be used to ascertain the appropriate level [11].

Motor evoked potentials, first described by Baker in 1985 [12], involve transcranial stimulation of the cerebral cortex with short magnetic pulses that stimulate the peripheral nerves and then record muscle action potentials from muscles in the upper and lower extremities. Muscles typically tested during MEPs are abductor pollicis, adductor minimi, quadriceps, tibialis anterior, gastrocnemius, extensor halluces, and abductor hallucis. Again, segmental innervation of the muscles determines the level affected. In general terms, MEPs measure efferent signals, while SEPs measure afferent signals.

SEPs and MEPs are most often used intraoperatively to monitor electrophysiologic changes during surgical intervention. While these studies may be obtained in the preoperative setting, the availability of MEPs and SEPs in the preoperative setting may be limited when compared to the availability of EMGs. As mentioned previously, the surgeon must take into account whether the diagnosis and appropriate surgical treatment will be altered by ordering such studies.

Some studies have utilized transcranial MEPs as a screening tool or confirmatory test in the evaluation of patients with cervical myelopathy. Lo et al. [13] evaluated the sensitivity and the specificity of MEPs in relation to the severity of pathology present on MRI. The purpose was to show that MEPs could be used as a rapid, inexpensive, and noninvasive screening tool prior to obtaining imaging with MRI. This study grouped 231 patients into 4 cohorts based on the severity of cord compression on MRI. Group 1 had spondylosis with or without contact with the cord, but no cord deformity. Group 2 showed mild indentation or flattening of the cord, with AP cord diameter not less than two-thirds of the original size. Group 3 showed significant cord indentation with AP cord diameter less than two-thirds of the original size, with absence of hyperintense T2 cord signal. Group 4 had indentation of the cord, with AP cord diameter less than two-thirds of original, with hyperintense T2 cord signal present. Transcranial MEPs were obtained in these patients and compared to the results of 45 control patients. As expected, patients who had more severe pathology (groups 3 and 4) had significant findings on physical examination and correlated over 90% of the time. However, for less severe pathology (group 2), correlation was 70%. EMG correlation was approximately the same as physical examination, which is not unexpected, as EMG is utilized for radiculopathy rather than myelopathy. When MEPs were positive in all four parameters used, there was high sensitivity in patients in group 2, as well as groups 3 and 4.

The basis for these findings may be that myelopathy, especially from anterior compression syndromes, will produce abnormalities in the corticospinal tract which are seen on MEPs, rather than from compression of the dorsal columns.

SSEPs and MEPs have also been studied as a predictor of progression of cervical spondylotic myelopathy or as a predictor of conservative vs. surgical outcomes. Bedarnik et al. [14] showed that cord dysfunction detected by SSEPs or MEPs was associated with early development of myelopathy (less than 12 months), while the presence of T2 hyperintense cord signal abnormality predicted later progression (more than 12 months) to symptomatic myelopathy. This indicates that MEP and SSEP changes, i.e., electrophysiologic changes, occur early in the pathogenesis of myelopathy, while T2 cord signal abnormality may be a sign of prolonged cord compression. In terms of prediction of outcome, Kadanka et al. [15] performed a 3-year prospective randomized study that evaluated outcome in conservatively and surgically treated patients with myelopathy in relation to clinical, electrophysiological, and imaging parameters. Those that had a good outcome when treated conservatively were those of older age and normal MEPs and those with a larger transverse area of the spinal cord (over 70 mm^2). Those that had a good outcome when treated surgically had a worse modified JOA score and slower walk and thus more severe myelopathy. This would indicate that the more severe that cord compression is at presentation, the more likely it is that surgery will be necessary as treatment.

Mazur et al. [16] looked at MEPs as an objective measure of improvement of cervical myelopathy after surgery, which may be more appropriate than as a diagnostic or predictive tool. While only 17 patients were evaluated in this study, patients underwent MEP evaluation before surgery and at 1, 3, 6, and 12 months after surgery. Other objective tests were performed as well, including the 10-m walk test, the 9-hole peg task, and grip and release test. It was found that the MEPs correlated with these objective tests both before and after surgery and suggested that MEPs could be used to monitor disease severity and recovery of neurological function before and after surgical intervention. It was also shown that prolonged baseline MEPs were associated with worse surgical outcome, most likely due to worse myelopathy prior to surgery.

However, MEPs do not provide an anatomic picture that can be used for surgical planning. Therefore, the surgeon will need to take the entire clinical picture into account to determine if MEPs would change the course of clinical action if a patient is suspected of having cervical compression.

Cervical Transforaminal Selective Nerve Root Blocks

Cervical epidural steroid injections are a frequent treatment modality in patients with cervical radiculopathy. It is most commonly used in patients who have mild to moderate nerve root compression with signs and symptoms consistent with radiculopathy, rather than in those with large disc herniations or severe nerve root compression, in whom surgery would be a more appropriate and definitive treatment option.

The two approaches for epidural steroid injections are translaminar and transforaminal. In the cervical spine, the translaminar approach can be performed safely and in most cases in the office setting. This approach is effective, and in addition, the injected medication can cover more than one level of the cervical spine, as it spreads through the epidural space.

The transforaminal approach allows the physician to place the tip of the needle in the foraminal space, thus applying steroid medication to just one exiting nerve root, rather than multiple. In this way, this injection can be both therapeutic and diagnostic. If there is question as to which specific nerve root is causing the patient's radicular symptoms, a transforaminal selective nerve root block may be performed. If the patient experiences relief with a transforaminal selective nerve root block, even temporary, then that block may confirm the presence of the causative radiculopathic agent at the site of the transforaminal injection. However, if the patient received no benefit from such an injection, then consideration should be given to other potential causes of the symptoms.

However, the transforaminal approach for selective nerve root blocks has increased the risk of complication than the translaminar approach.

Due to the location of the vertebral artery in such close proximity to the foramen, there is a higher risk of inadvertent injection or damage to the vertebral artery. Therefore, some practitioners will utilize CT guidance during these injections in order to reduce the risk of vertebral artery injection. Fitzgerald et al. [17] reviewed the position of the vertebral artery relative to the typical injection point for a transforaminal injection at 70 cervical levels in 68 patients. It was found that the more advanced the foraminal degenerative narrowing present in a patient, the higher the risk of the vertebral artery compromising the course of the injection. The needle trajectory intersected with the vertebral artery in 46% of injections. Using oblique fluoroscopic technique, the trajectory intersected with the vertebral artery in 39%. In patients with severely narrowed foramen, 65% of patients had complete or near-complete covering of the foramen.

Diagnostic transforaminal selective nerve root blocks are done with far more frequency in the lumbar spine due to the lower risk of complications, and some pain management physicians will therefore not perform transforaminal injections in the cervical spine. When considering obtaining a cervical transforaminal selective nerve root block, the surgeon must take into account how useful this injection will be in determining the treatment in relation to the risk of such an injection, as well as the availability of a practitioner willing and capable of performing such an injection.

Other Diagnostic Tests

While there are other tests that may be of use in the diagnosis of cervical radiculopathy or entrapment neuropathy, they are of limited value at this point in time. Recently, advanced imaging studies of the peripheral nervous system have been utilized, including high field strength MRI and ultrasound. Recent advances in MRI and ultrasound now have been shown to have the ability to demarcate nerve compression and inflammatory conditions within the extremity. In the case of MRI, signal changes on T2-weighted sequences of the peripheral nerve can show demyelinating segments or inflammatory changes that were not previously seen with lower strength magnets [18]. Newer, high strength ultrasound can also see localized edema in larger peripheral nerves in patients with localized nerve inflammation. However, the clinician must make the determination of whether this testing will alter the clinical course prior to obtaining such a study.

Finally, provocative cervical discography is a controversial diagnostic test utilized to determine if the degeneration of the disc itself is a causative agent for axial neck pain. Typically, when this test is being performed, it is for a patient with axial neck pain without radicular or myelopathic signs or symptoms, in order to justify a surgical procedure. While there are some studies that have shown that a positive discogram can lead to good results for patients undergoing a cervical fusion [19], there are many confounding factors that can lead to a high false-positive rate, both in the cervical and lumbar spine [20]. While the degeneration of cervical discs may cause spondylotic changes such as disc osteophyte complexes which result in nerve root or spinal cord compression, these anatomical entities which cause radiculopathy or myelopathy should be the indication for surgical intervention, rather than studies such as a discogram.

Conclusion

The indication for surgical intervention for the patient should be based upon the patient's presenting symptoms and physical signs, as determined by a detailed history and physical examination and by their correlation with appropriate imaging studies such as MRI and CT myelogram. In cases where there is a diagnostic quandary in terms of either which cervical nerve root is responsible for the clinical syndrome or whether there is another causative agent that cannot be definitively eliminated from the differential diagnosis by physical examination or imaging (i.e., entrapment neuropathy or peripheral neuropathy), then electrophysiologic testing such as electromyography and nerve conduction studies may be a useful adjuvant to ensure that the appropriate surgical intervention is being performed. When considering a diagnostic cervical selective nerve root block, the surgeon must take into consideration the additional risk of vertebral artery injury using a transforaminal approach, as well as the availability of a pain management physician willing and able to perform such an injection. These tests should be used as a supplement to the physician's history, examination, and clinical judgment and not as a replacement or substitution for a detailed physical examination.

Case Review: GM 3-28-68

Patient GM is a 49-year-old male construction worker who presented primarily with neck pain and radicular pain down both arms. He has had a chronic history of numbness in both of his hands, but that has been getting worse. He now wakes up in the middle of the night and shakes out his hands. The pain in his neck started approximately 2 months prior to presentation. There was no traumatic inciting event. He has been taking tramadol and Celebrex for the past 6 weeks and has not done any therapy, injections, or chiropractic manipulation. He is otherwise healthy but does smoke 1 pack per day for 35 years. The patient had already obtained both an EMG and an MRI prior to presenting to his surgeon.

On examination, the patient has no focal motor deficits. He has non-dermatomal sensory loss that involves all of his fingers except for his fifth digit. His reflexes are 1+ and symmetric, and he has no Hoffman's sign. He has a positive Tinel's sign bilaterally and a positive Phalen's test.

The patient presented with an EMG which showed bilateral median neuropathy at the wrist, but no acute cervical radiculopathy. There was

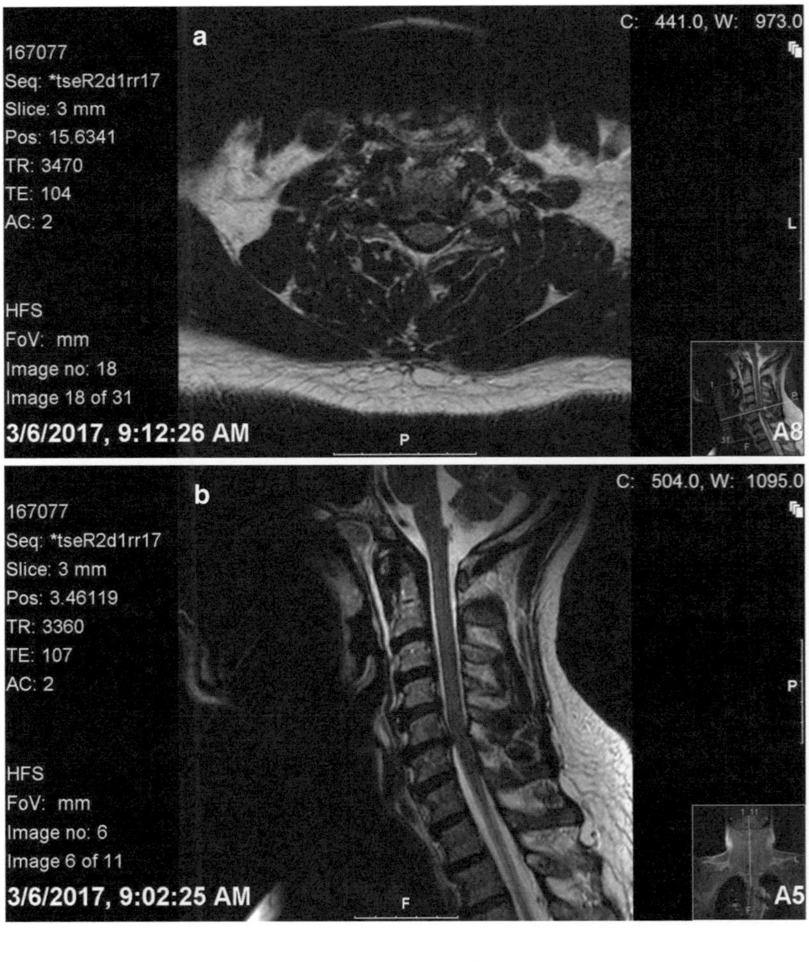

Fig. 10.3 (**a**) Axial T2 MRI image of patient described in case study showing disc-osteophyte complex at the C5-6 intervertebral level. (**b**) Sagittal T2 MRI image of patient described in case study, showing disc-osteophyte complex at the C5-6 intervertebral level

no spontaneous insertional activity in any of the tested muscles. On the right side, the nerve conduction velocity across the wrist was 35.1 M/s, compared to 62.1 M/s proximal to the wrist. On the left side, the nerve conduction velocity was 34.7 M/s across the wrist, compared to 64.2 M/s proximal to the wrist.

His MRI is shown below in Fig. 10.3. He has a C5–C6 disc osteophyte complex which causes significant central canal stenosis and bilateral neural foraminal stenosis.

As the patient was clearly symptomatic from both his C5–C6 disc osteophyte complex and his longstanding bilateral median neuropathy at the wrist, he ultimately underwent both an anterior cervical discectomy and fusion at C5–C6 and also bilateral carpal tunnel release. Due to the patient's smoking history and the increased risk of pseudoarthrosis, the patient first underwent a right carpal tunnel release while he underwent smoking cessation. Three weeks later, he underwent a C5–C6 anterior cervical fusion and then, 2 weeks after that, a left carpal tunnel release. Now 3 months out from his first surgery, the patient has minimal neck pain, has had complete resolution of his radicular arm pain as well as the longstanding numbness in his hands, and has returned to work.

References

1. Radhakrishnan K, Litchy W, O'Fallon W, et al. Epidemiology of cervical radiculopathy. A population-based study from Rochester, Minnesota, 1976 through 1990. Brain J Neurol. 1994;117(Pt 2):325–35.
2. Nouri A, Teteault L, Sing A, Karadimas S, Fehlings M. Degenerative cervical myelopathy: epidemiology, genetics, and pathogenesis. Spine. 2015;40(12):E675–93.
3. American Association of Neuromuscular & Electrodiagnostic Medicine. Position statement: who is qualified to practice electrodiagnostic medicine? Muscle Nerve.1999;(Suppl. 8):S263–265.
4. Hakimi K, Spanier D. Electrodiagnosis of cervical radiculopathy. Phys Med Rehabil Clin N Am. 2013;24:1–12.
5. American Association of Electrodiagnostic Medicine, American Academy of Physical Medicine and Rehabilitation. The electrodiagnostic evaluation of patients with suspected cervical radiculopathy: literature review on the usefulness of needle electromyography. Muscle Nerve. 1999;22(Supplement 8):S213–221.
6. Gilad R, Dabby M, Boaz M, et al. Cervical paraspinal electromyography: normal values in 100 control subjects. J Clin Neurophysiol. 2006;23:573–6.
7. Date ES, Kim B, Yoon JS, et al. Cervical paraspinal spontaneous activity in asymptomatic subjects. Muscle Nerve. 2006;34:361–4.
8. Dillingham TR, Lauder TD, Andary M, et al. Identification of cervical radiculopathies: optimizing the electromyographer screen. Am J Phys Med Rehabil. 2001;80:84–91.
9. Ashkan K, Johnston P, Moore AJ. A comparison of magnetic resonance imaging and neurophysiological studies in the assessment of cervical radiculopathy. Br J Neurosurg. 2002;16(2):146–8.
10. Alrawi MF, Khalil NM, Mitchell P, Hughes SP. The value of neurophysiological and imaging studies in predicting outcome in the surgical treatment of cervical radiculopathy. Eur Spine J. 2007;16(49):5–500.
11. Dvorak J, Sutter M, Herdmann J. Cervical myelopathy: clinic and neurophysiological evaluation. Eur Spine J. 2003;12(Suppl 2):S181–7.
12. Barker AT, Jalinous R, Freeston IL. Non-invasive magnetic stimulation of human motor cortex. Lancet. 1985;1(8437):1106–7.
13. Lo YL, Chan LL, Lim W, Tan SB, Tan CT, Chen JLT, Fook-Chong S, Patnagopal P. Transcranial magnetic stimulation screening for cord compression in cervical spondylosis. J Neurol Sci. 2006;224:17–21.
14. Bedarnik J, Kadanka Z, Dusek L, Kerkovsky M, Vohanka S, Novotny O, Urbanek I, Kratochvilova D. Presymtomatic spondylotic cervical myelopathy: an updated predictive model. Eur Spine J. 2008;17:421–31.
15. Kadanka Z, Mares M, Bedarnik J, Smrcka V, Krbec M, Chaloupka R, Dusek L. Predictive factors for mild forms of spondylotic cervical myelopathy treated conservatively or surgically. Eur J Neurol. 2005;12:16–24.
16. Mazur MD, White A, McEvoy S, Bisson EF. Transcranial magnetic stimulation of the motor cortex correlated with objective clinical measures in patients with cervical spondylotic myelopathy. Spine. 2014;39(14):1113–20.
17. Fitzgerald RT, Bartynski WS, Collins HR. Vertebral artery position in the setting of cervical degenerative disease: implications for selective cervical transforaminal epidural injections. Interv Neuroradiol. 2013;19(4):425–31.
18. Stoll G, Wilder-Smith E, Bendszus M. Imaging of the peripheral nervous system. Handb Clin Neurol. 2013;115:137–53.
19. Motimaya A, Arici M, George D, Ramsby G. Diagnostic value of cervical discography in the management of cervical discogenic pain. Conn Med. 2000;64(7):395–8.
20. Carragee EJ, Tammer CM, Khurana S, Hayward C, Welsh J, Date E, Truong T, Rossi M, Hagle C. The rates of false-positive lumbar discography in select patients without low back symptoms. Spine (Phila Pa 1976). 2000;25(11):1373–80; discussion 1381.

Part III

Surgical Decision-Making

11 Failure of Nonoperative Management

Hamadi Murphy, Scott C. Wagner, Alex Vaccaro, and Stephen Silva

Cervical myelopathy and radiculopathy can be debilitating conditions that result in significant functional impairments. As one of the more common reasons that patients seek evaluation from spinal specialists, these degenerative disorders of the cervical spine place a substantial functional, psychosocial, and economic burden upon patients. The treating physician's goal should be the rapid diagnosis and treatment of this condition in order to help patients return to their normal state of health. The majority of initial treatment strategies utilize conservative modalities and primarily focus on rehabilitation. Conservative, nonoperative treatments should be initiated on all patients with new-onset radiculopathy, unless there are signs of significant motor deficit or myelopathy [1]. The objectives of these treatment strategies are pain relief, improvements in function, and prevention of recurrence.

This chapter will primarily focus on the nonoperative modalities for the treatment of cervical myelopathy and radiculopathy. In addition, it will also describe the endpoints used to define the failure of those treatment strategies before advancing to surgical intervention. Many of the conservative measures employed to manage degenerative cervical disorders are supported primarily by anecdotal evidence, making it difficult to standardize an ideal treatment regimen. In 2010, the North American Spine Society (NASS) published the evidence-based guidelines, "Diagnosis and Treatment of Cervical Radiculopathy from Degenerative Disorders," the first known multidisciplinary collaborative statement on this subject [2]. The nonoperative treatment strategies for cervical myelopathy and radiculopathy have not been compared in large-scale, randomized controlled trials. Despite the high incidence of symptomatic cervical degeneration and the widespread use of nonoperative management, the number of comparative trials in the literature is small and usually of poor quality. Any current recommendations are based on recent evidence, comparatively smaller case series, and anecdotal experience.

Nonsurgical treatment is typically the most appropriate course of initial management for cervical radiculopathy, with surgical intervention being utilized in mild, moderate, or severe myelopathy or in cases with continuous and progressive symptoms that have failed nonoperative treatments [3]. In addition, systematic reviews of the literature have demonstrated that up to 90% of patients with radiculopathy will have resolution of symptoms with nonoperative care alone, often observing a time to recovery ranging from 24 to 36 months [1, 4, 5]. Various conservative modalities include pharmacological strategies,

H. Murphy · S. C. Wagner · A. Vaccaro (✉) · S. Silva
Department of Orthopaedics, Rothman Institute at Thomas Jefferson University Hospital, Philadelphia, PA, USA
e-mail: Alex.Vaccaro@Rothmaninstitute.com

M. G. Kaiser et al. (eds.), *Degenerative Cervical Myelopathy and Radiculopathy*,
https://doi.org/10.1007/978-3-319-97952-6_11

cervical steroid injections, physical therapy, manipulation techniques, alternative medicine, and other ancillary treatments. While there is a lack of high-quality evidence comparing these strategies to surgical approaches, the following is a compilation of the most recent evidence-based guidelines and peer-reviewed resources addressing the utility of these measures.

Several pharmacological treatments have been used in the treatment of cervical myelopathy and radiculopathy. Common first-line medications include oral analgesics such as nonsteroidal anti-inflammatories, opioids, or oral steroids [2, 4, 6, 7]. Nonsteroidal anti-inflammatory medications (NSAIDs) are one of the mainstay treatment options in the acute relief of symptoms due to their analgesic and anti-inflammatory properties which target the inflammatory response pathway [8]. A short trial of NSAIDs can be effective at relieving symptoms or allowing the patient to tolerate and participate in other treatment modalities [6]. Despite the widespread use of NSAIDs, there lacks high-quality evidence to support their use in the treatment of degenerative cervical disorders. Oral corticosteroids can also be used to acutely manage pain symptoms by inhibiting the inflammatory cascade. Similar to NSAIDs, corticosteroids also lack substantial evidence to support their use in cervical disorders and can lead to riskier adverse effects such as increased susceptibility to infection, osteonecrosis, and hyperglycemia [1, 6].

Opioid narcotics are another pharmacologic strategy for pain control. When possible, the clinician should avoid the use of opioid medications as they can lead to physiologic dependence and result in secondary effects that can make postoperative pain management more difficult [8]. However, if the patient presents with poorly controlled pain, a short and closely monitored course of oral opioids can be beneficial. Other pharmacological options that are often used to address the symptoms of degenerative cervical disorders include antidepressants, antiepileptics, neuropathic medications, and muscle relaxants [9]. While there have been case reports of patients achieving relief of symptoms, the 2010 NASS systematic review demonstrated that no literature adequately examined the role of these pharmacologic treatments and therefore could not provide a statement on their utility in the management of cervical radiculopathy [2]. When suggesting pharmacologic treatments for patients, it is important to design an individualized strategy that incorporates appropriate considerations such as age of the patient, potential drug interactions, and other comorbidities.

Cervical steroid injections may also be considered in the nonsurgical management of cervical radiculopathy and myelopathy. The epidural steroid injections performed under fluoroscopic or CT guidance function by decreasing inflammation at the site of the irritated cervical nerve roots with the hopes of providing symptomatic relief to the patient. Often these injections are utilized as a method of subsiding any pain in order for the patient to tolerate other methods of nonoperative care. The injections may consist of transforaminal or interlaminar epidurals, as well as selective nerve blocks. Certain studies have shown that patients respond well to cervical steroid injections if they had previously confirmed pathology by advanced imaging, such as CT or MRI, and had experienced improvements while taking oral corticosteroids [6]. In addition, a systematic review of the literature has shown some support for epidural steroid injections in the treatment of cervical radiculopathy, with up to 60% of patients experiencing symptomatic relief in the long term with transforaminal epidural steroid injections [2, 4]. In addition, approximately 25% of patients were shown to obtain short-term pain relief thereby negating the need for surgery despite prior clear surgical indications. Due to limited high-quality evidence, it is still unclear whether the benefits seen with cervical epidurals are demonstrating a true treatment response to the injections or whether it is a reflection of the natural progression of the disease course. Likewise, all of the reviewed studies had used transforaminal epidural injections, making it impossible to derive any conclusions or recommendations regarding the safety or efficacy of interlaminar injections as a treatment modality for cervical radiculopathy.

While cervical epidural injections are considered safe and well tolerated, the provider and patient must be aware that these procedures are not without significant risks and potential complications. In particular, cervical transforaminal and interlaminar steroid injections can result in neurological deficits, epidural hematomas, vascular infarcts, or death [4]. As of 2014, the Federal Drug Administration felt that these risks were significant enough to result in the addition of a black box warning for the use of corticosteroids in the epidural space [1, 10]. While evidence suggests that corticosteroid injections may lead to short-term, symptomatic improvement in radicular symptoms, there is no current method of predicting which patients will experience improvements from these injections [4, 6]. Transforaminal epidural steroid injections under imaging guidance may be considered as a nonoperative strategy when designing a treatment plan for patients suffering from cervical degenerative disorders. However, it is important for the physician to be cautious in recommending cervical epidural injections, and consideration should be given to the potential complications. In the setting of overt moderate or severe myelopathy with image-documented cord compression, many clinicians recommend against the use of epidural injections in order to avoid further potential epidural compression.

Physical therapy is another nonoperative modality that is often utilized as a stand-alone treatment strategy or in conjunction with other treatment methods for cervical degenerative disorders. The aim of physical therapy is to restore range of motion and strengthen the neck and chest musculature with the goal of decreasing symptoms and preventing recurrence. A carefully tailored physical therapy regimen should progress through stages, as the patient's pain improves [8]. Early on in the treatment regimen, the patient should begin with gentle range of motion exercises and stretching techniques. As the pain subsides, stretching techniques, isometric strengthening, and active range of motion and resistance exercises may be incorporated as tolerated [5]. In addition, most programs will also include components of postural and ergonomic training with the hopes of preventing recurrence of radicular symptoms.

The difficulty in comparing the overall effectiveness of physical therapy as a treatment modality is that exercise regimens vary widely in their frequency, duration, and intensity [8]. On average, these regimens consist of 15–20 sessions lasting 30–45 min in duration over a 3-month period [3]. Several trials and systematic reviews have evaluated the utility of physical therapy for the treatment of cervical radiculopathy and myelopathy. Those studies demonstrated a moderate benefit in providing relief of neck pain and improvements in muscle strength. However, these benefits were shown to be short term and dissipate after 6 months to a year. The overall review of the literature highlights a lack of trials that adequately assess the utility of physical therapy as a treatment modality in the management of cervical myelopathy and radiculopathy.

Similar to physical therapy, manipulative therapy involves numerous techniques often focused on the cervical spine in order to provide relief and prevent the recurrence of symptoms. Manual therapy includes options such as immobilization, muscle energy techniques, traction, or soft-tissue and neural mobilization [11]. Some studies have promoted the benefits of immobilization and cervical traction at decreasing the symptoms associated with cervical radiculopathy [4]. The concept behind these techniques is that short-term immobilization would allow for a decrease in inflammation, while cervical traction would increase the dimensions of the neural foramen. Both methods result in a decompression of the nerve root with the goal of improving symptoms [7].

Cervical traction can play a major contribution toward rehabilitation in cervical radiculopathy, especially if incorporated with other conservative modalities, though high-quality literature examining the topic remains lacking. A recently published case report described successful management of cervical radiculopathy utilizing traction: A 52-year-old woman with a 2-month history of cervicobrachial pain and a presentation consistent with cervical radiculopathy underwent a simultaneous combination of cervical traction and slider neural mobilization [12]. Neural mobilization techniques have also been advocated in the management of cervical radiculopathy as a method of relieving nerve adherence and facilitating nerve gliding. These concepts are thought to normalize the cervical nerve root's structure and function, thereby decreasing any symptoms. While both techniques have been used and studied independently in treatment plans, there is a lack of sufficient data regarding the efficacy of combining both strategies. After undergoing the combination treatment, the patient noted improvements in all outcomes measured after a period of 4 weeks. The patient noted that her pain had almost disappeared and she was able to perform her activities of daily living without any limitations or difficulty. A recent prospective randomized clinical trial discovered similar findings by demonstrating that the addition of mechanical traction to a strengthening regimen in patients suffering from cervical radiculopathy resulted in better 6-month and 1-year outcomes when compared to strengthening exercises alone [13]. The findings of these reports support the concept of combining cervical traction with other treatment modalities in order to provide significant improvements in the treatment of cervical radiculopathy.

These manipulative techniques are often utilized in various methods, frequencies, intensities, or durations making it difficult to standardize their efficacy and determine their optimal therapeutic benefit [11]. Although there has been no established cause and effect relationship between these manipulative techniques and an improvement in radicular symptoms, the results for short-term benefits have been generally promising. However, there is a lack of high-quality evidence in the literature to support the use of cervical traction in the long-term management of cervical radiculopathy [5]. A recent Cochrane Review stated that current research cannot adequately support or refute the efficacy of cervical traction in the management of cervical radiculopathy as compared to other conservative treatment modalities [14].

In addition, manipulative therapy is not without risk, with complications such as worsening radiculopathy, myelopathy, or spinal cord injury [5]. A systematic review also identified several case reports describing serious vascular and non-vascular complications associated with manipulation including vertebral artery compression and disc herniation, with most serious complications requiring emergent surgical treatment [14]. As the efficacy of manipulation in the treatment of cervical radiculopathy is not completely understood, careful consideration should be given prior to incorporating these techniques within a treatment strategy as there is evidence suggesting that manipulation may lead to worsened symptoms or significant complications [11]. Well-conducted randomized controlled trials are needed to clarify the safety and efficacy of traction and establish clear and effective treatment protocols for patients with cervical degenerative disorders.

Finally, examples of other ancillary treatments often utilized by patients include transcutaneous electrical nerve stimulation, acupuncture, or ozone injections [2, 15, 16]. These methods have recently started gaining attraction due to their associations with improvements in pain in uncontrolled case series. However, the research has yet to distill whether the observed improvements were truly from the treatment modalities or a natural progression of the disease course. Further ongoing research will be required in order to be able to determine the efficacy of incorporating these other nonoperative modalities in treatment regimens.

Nonoperative treatment is a labor-intensive, collaborative effort requiring the physician to carefully select treatment strategies specific to each patient's needs and to routinely monitor their progression. Despite the high incidence of symptomatic cervical degeneration and the widespread use of nonoperative management, there is currently no high-quality evidence comparing nonoperative and operative treatment modalities. However, a typical conservative approach would have patients attempt to control their symptoms using primarily a combination of physical therapy, manipulation techniques, and pharmacotherapy. More invasive conservative treatment options, such as cervical epidural injections, may benefit those patients that have not responded to simpler nonoperative alternatives. If patients fail to improve with nonoperative treatments or exhibit progressively worsening symptoms, surgical intervention should be considered.

References

1. Woods BI, Hilibrand AS. Cervical radiculopathy: epidemiology, etiology, diagnosis, and treatment. J Spinal Diord Tech. 2015;28:251–9.
2. Bono CM, Ghiselli G, Gilbert TJ, North American Spine Society, et al. An evidence-based clinical guideline for the diagnosis and treatment of cervical radiculopathy from degenerative disorders. Spine J. 2011;11(1):64–72.
3. Hirpara KM, Butler JS, Dolan RT, O'Byrne JM, Poynton AR. Nonoperative modalities to treat symptomatic cervical spondylosis. Adv Orthop. 2012;2012:294857.
4. Wong JJ, Cote P, Quesnele JJ, et al. The course and prognostic factors of symptomatic cervical disc herniation with radiculopathy: a systematic review of the literature. Spine J. 2014;14:1781–9.
5. Caridi JM, Pumberger M, Hughes AP. Cervical radiculopathy: a review. HSS J. 2011;7:265–72.
6. Corey DL, Comeau D. Cervical radiculopathy. Med Clin N Am. 2014;4:791–9.
7. Eubanks J. Cervical radiculopathy: nonoperative management of neck pain and radicular symptoms. Am Fam Physician. 2010;81(1):33–40.
8. Iyer S, Kim HJ. Cervical radiculopathy. Curr Rev Musculoskelet Med. 2016;9:272–80.
9. Onks CA, Billy G. Evaluation and treatment of cervical radiculopathy. Prim Care Clin Office Pract. 2013;40:837–48.
10. Food Drug Administration Center for Drugs Evaluation Research. FDA drug safety communication: FDA requires label changes to warn of rare but serious neurologic problems after epidural corticosteroid injections for pain (FDA Maryland). 2014.
11. Boyles R, Toy P, Mellon J Jr, Hayes M, Bradley H. Effectiveness of manual physical therapy in the treatment of cervical radiculopathy: a systematic review. J Man Manip Ther. 2011;19(3):135–42.
12. Savva C, Giakas G. The effect of cervical traction combined with neural mobilization on pain and disability in cervical radiculopathy. A case report. Man Ther. 2013;18:443–6.
13. Jellad A, Salah ZB, Boudokhane S, Migaou H, Bahri I, Rejeb N. The value of intermittent cervical traction in recent cervical radiculopathy. Ann Phys Rehabil Med. 2009;52:638–52.
14. Graham N, Gross A, Goldsmith CH, et al. Mechanical traction for neck pain with or without radiculopathy. Cochrane Database Syst Rev. 2008;(3):CD006408.
15. Bocci V, Borrelli E, Zanardi I, Travagli V. The usefulness of ozone treatment in spinal pain. Drug Des Devel Ther. 2015;9:2677–85.
16. Walsh D, Howe T, Johnson M, et al. Transcutaneous electrical nerve stimulation for acute pain. Cochrane Database Syst Rev. 2009;(2):CD006142.

12 Timing of Operative Intervention

Alexander M. Tucker, Tianyi Niu,
Daniel T. Nagasawa, and Langston T. Holly

Pitfalls/Pearls

- Asymptomatic and mild cervical spondylotic myelopathy patients can be treated with nonoperative therapy.
- Surgical decompression should be offered in cases of progressive, moderate, or severe cervical spondylotic myelopathy or in those who have failed nonoperative treatment.
- Surgical decision-making requires careful consideration in elderly, chronically ill, or mildly symptomatic patients.

Introduction

Cervical spondylotic myelopathy (CSM) is the result of progressive degenerative narrowing of the spinal canal causing spinal cord compression. The pathophysiology of CSM involves both primary mechanical and secondary biological injury to the spinal cord. Primary mechanical spinal cord injury is frequently caused by a combination of disc degeneration, facet hypertrophy, and ligamentum flavum thickening. This results in compressive, distracting, or shear forces on the spinal cord. Secondary biological injury is multifactorial and involves elements of glutamate-related toxicity, cell injury from free radicals, apoptosis, or spinal cord ischemia [5]. While surgery is able to relieve primary mechanical compression of the spinal cord, it does not directly treat secondary biological injury. As the inherent recuperative capacity of the spinal cord is unpredictable, neurological recovery should never be guaranteed to patients considering surgery – although this is commonly the case.

The prevalence of CSM is estimated at 604 per million in North America, with 16 per million requiring surgery [3, 17]. Although over half of all middle-age people have radiographic evidence of cervical spondylosis, only 10% have myelopathic or radicular symptoms [13]. Furthermore, for patients with cervical spondylotic myelopathy, approximately 20% to 60% will deteriorate neurologically overtime without surgery [12]. In order to prevent this deterioration and irreversible neurological injury, some surgeons offer decompression surgery to all patients with radiographic evidence of cervical spinal cord compression, regardless of symptom severity. However, a small but significant risk of neurological injury or other complications exists with any surgical intervention.

A. M. Tucker · T. Niu · D. T. Nagasawa ·
L. T. Holly (✉)
Department of Neurosurgery, University of California-Los Angeles, Los Angeles, CA, USA
e-mail: lholly@mednet.ucla.edu

M. G. Kaiser et al. (eds.), *Degenerative Cervical Myelopathy and Radiculopathy*,
https://doi.org/10.1007/978-3-319-97952-6_12

Based on data [2] from the National Inpatient Sample of CSM patients undergoing surgery from 1993 to 2002, the postoperative complication rate was 13.4%. A single postoperative complication led to a 4-day increase in mean length of hospital stay, increased the mortality rate twofold, and added more than $10,000 to hospital charges. Patients aged 65–84 years had 8- and 14-fold increases in complications and mortality, respectively, compared to patients less than 64 years of age.

Despite a high prevalence of this disease and different surgical treatment options, there remains a lack of universally accepted guidelines regarding the timing of operative intervention for patients with CSM. This chapter aims to provide evidence-based recommendations to determine the need and timing for surgical decompression in patients with cervical spondylotic myelopathy (Table 12.1).

Assessment and Treatment

Evaluation

History and Physical Examination

Each patient with suspected cervical spondylotic myelopathy should have a detailed history and physical exam. Signs and symptoms of myelopathy may be subtle, including changes in axial balance, dysfunctional bladder control, decreased dexterity, distorted proprioception, or abnormal gait. The interviewer should explore risk factors that may accelerate the degenerative processes of cervical spondylosis, including occupational or lifestyle hazards (carrying objects on the head or contact sports), as well as associated comorbidities, such as Down syndrome, rheumatoid arthritis, or Klippel-Feil syndrome. Additionally, patient lifestyle may have an impact on whether patients considered "on the bubble" for surgery

Table 12.1 CSM clinical presentation, radiographic findings, and treatment plan

	Presentation	Imaging	Clinical grades	Initial treatment	Follow-up or treatment
Asymptomatic spondylosis	No symptoms of myelopathy, may have radiculopathy Neck pain common	Spinal canal narrowing with spinal cord effacement or compression	Nurick grade 0 mJOA score 18	Observation Physical therapy	3–6 months
Mild spondylotic myelopathy	Mild symptoms, frequently upper extremity predominant	Spinal cord effacement or compression; commonly no MRI signal abnormality in cord	Nurick grade 0–1 mJOA score 15–17	Physical therapy, dangerous behavior avoidance, external bracing	3 months
Moderate spondylotic myelopathy	Moderate symptoms, often diminished fine motor skills, may have mild to moderate gait abnormality	Spinal cord compression; frequently high T2, but not as often low T1 signal change in cord	Nurick grade 2–3 mJOA score 12–14	Surgical decompression	1–2 months
Severe spondylotic myelopathy	Severe symptoms, often progressive, significant dexterity and gait dysfunction	Severe cord compression; high T2, low T1 signal change in cord	Nurick grade 4–5 mJOA score 0–11	Surgical decompression	2 weeks

(*summary of diagnostic and treatment recommendations*). The typical clinical presentation, radiographic findings, and clinical grades are described for patients with asymptomatic spondylosis, mild spondylotic myelopathy, moderate spondylotic myelopathy, and severe spondylotic myelopathy. Recommendations for initial treatment and time to follow-up are also listed for each group of patients based on rather modest symptomatology would be more optimally treated with surgical intervention. This could include individuals who engage in recreational or occupational high-impact activities, (e.g., surfing) or those with a history of frequent falls.

A comprehensive physical examination is critically important and should focus on strength testing, evaluation of reflexes, and sensation. Objective clinical findings of myelopathy include increased deep tendon reflexes, positive pathological reflexes, and sensory disturbances. Finally, consideration should be given to other etiologies of myelopathy, such as syringomyelia, trauma, amyotrophic lateral sclerosis, multiple sclerosis, progressive polyarthritis, congenital pathologies, or vitamin B12 deficiency.

The presence and severity of cervical myelopathy can be assessed with multiple quantitative scales, including Nurick grade, Japanese Orthopaedic Association score, modified Japanese Orthopaedic Association (mJOA) score, the short form-36, walking test, and grip and release test. We typically use the mJOA score, one of the most frequently used measurements, which utilizes a functional assessment scale in patients with CSM [14]. It cannot be stressed enough, however, that although quantitative scores may be used to evaluate patients and improve documentation, they should be considered adjunctive, and not the primary tool used in surgical decision-making.

Radiographical Imaging

All patients with presumed cervical stenosis should have AP/lateral X-rays with dynamic flexion and extension views, as well as MRI of the cervical spine. X-ray imaging is important to visualize bony anatomy, evaluate cervical stability, assess cervical alignment, and accurately localize spinal levels. CT scans are helpful in diagnosing lesions that are poorly evaluated with MRI such as ossification of the posterior longitudinal ligament or calcified intervertebral discs. However, MRI is the most useful imaging modality overall, as it provides a detailed visualization of soft tissue anatomy and high-resolution imaging of the spinal cord macrostructure. It is believed that an anteroposterior compression ratio (anterior-posterior cord diameter divided by the transverse cord diameter) of less than 40%, a reduction in the size of the spinal cord by 30%, or a transverse area less than 60 sq mm are likely to result in myelopathic symptoms [8, 18]. Many surgeons also use an AP diameter cutoff of 7 mm to assess for potential cervical cord compression. In 2009, the Joint Section on Disorders of the Spine and Peripheral Nerves of the American Association of Neurological Surgeons published Guidelines for the Surgical Management of Cervical Degenerative Disease, which concluded that multilevel T2 hyperintensity, T1 focal hypointensity combined with T2 focal hyperintensity, and spinal cord atrophy were all associated with poor prognosis after surgery [16]. Some believe that areas of increased T2-weighted signal change represent edema, gliosis, ischemia, and potentially reversible change, whereas corresponding areas of T1 hypointensity have been correlated histopathologically with late stages of myelomalacia or cystic necrosis and, thus, represent irreversible spinal cord injury [19].

Electrophysiological Testing

Some surgeons report that electrophysiological testing before and after surgery can aid in preoperative diagnosis, assist with disease monitoring, and provide accurate prognostic information [9]. However, we do not advocate routine electrophysiological testing. Yet in cases when distinguishing myelopathy from radiculopathy is challenging (or when myelopathy and radiculopathy coexist), then electrophysiological testing should be considered. Of note, this type of testing is distinct from intraoperative electrophysiological monitoring that alerts the surgeon to intraoperative neurophysiological changes, although it's overall intraoperative utility remains controversial.

At present, no radiographic, serologic, or electrophysiological sign is regularly used clinically for predicting functional impairment due to CSM. Recent research has pointed to advanced imaging techniques, such as diffusion tensor imaging, as potentially showing promising results which may be useful in the future [6]. Until a reliable and reproducible biomarker is discovered, determination of when to offer surgery to patients with CSM requires integrating physical exam findings, imaging results, and careful analysis of the patient's history. Patients should then be stratified into asymptomatic, mild, moderate, and severe categories, which will be reviewed here.

Non-myelopathic Spondylosis

Non-myelopathic spondylosis refers to patients without symptoms of myelopathy but with imaging evidence of cord compression (Fig. 12.1). The diagnosis of cervical spondylosis in this patient population is often made incidentally after imaging has been obtained for other reasons such as neck pain or trauma.

Cervical spondylosis is an expected consequence of aging, with an incidence of 10% at age 25 and 95% by the age of 65 [22]. Senior citizens are the fastest-growing age group in the United States, and by the middle of this century, it is predicted that they will represent 23% of the population [23]. Thus, asymptomatic cervical spondylosis is likely to be encountered with increasing frequency in the coming years.

Non-myelopathic spondylosis patients can be subdivided into those with and without radiculopathy. The rationale for this distinction is that the presence of symptomatic radiculopathy, either clinical or electrophysiological, has been reported as a significant predictor of myelopathy development. Utilizing multivariate analysis, in a recent systematic review, Wilson et al. determined that clinically symptomatic radiculopathy ($p = 0.007$; moderate level evidence) and prolonged somatosensory (SEP) ($p = 0.007$; moderate level evidence) and motor evoked potentials (MEP) ($p = 0.033$; moderate level evidence) were

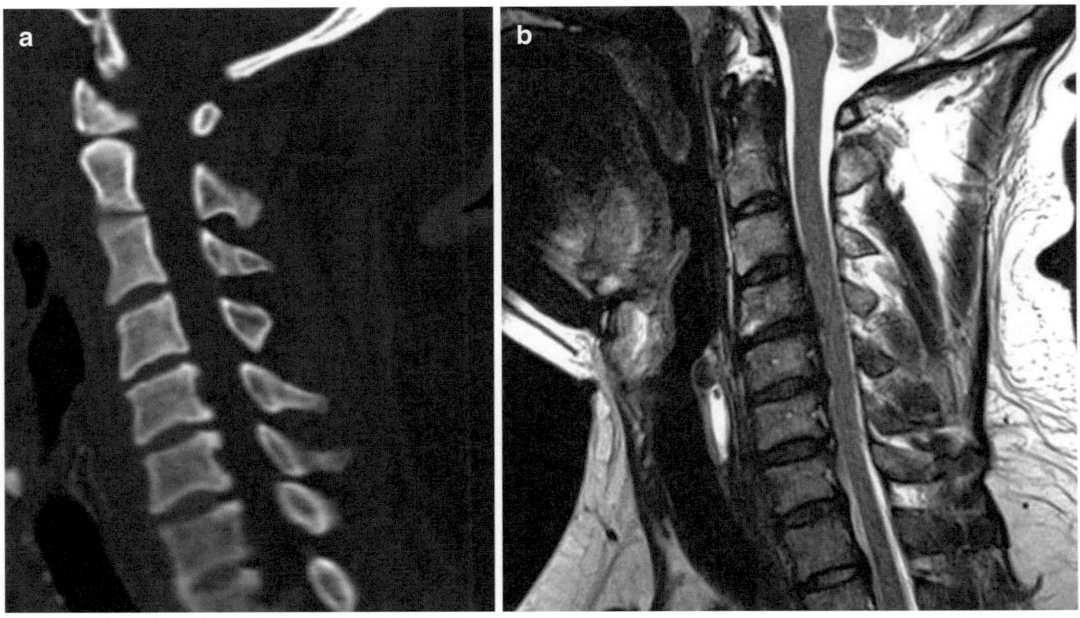

Fig. 12.1 Asymptomatic spondylosis. A 38-year-old male with neck pain, found to have hyperreflexia but no weakness, sensory change, or gait abnormality (mJOA 18). He was treated with physical therapy and has not required surgical intervention (mJOA 18). (**a**) CT cervical spine showing areas of osteophyte formation. (**b**) MRI cervical spine with mild spondylosis and ventral cord effacement without spinal cord signal change

significantly associated with early (≤1 year) myelopathic development [25]. Additionally, a diagnosis of radiculopathy was encountered in 63% of patients that developed myelopathy within 1 year compared to only 23% that did not develop myelopathy. Expectedly, abnormal SEP and MEP were present in a much larger percentage of patients that developed myelopathy than those that did not. One of the most cited clinical studies in this patient population was performed by Bednarik et al., who longitudinally evaluated the clinical examination, EMG, and SEP in a group of 66 non-myelopathic patients with spinal cord compression [1]. Development of myelopathy was defined by neurological examination and a decrease in mJOA score of 1 point or greater. Approximately 20% of the cohort developed CSM, and radiculopathy was encountered in 92% of those that developed CSM and 24% of those that did not ($p < 0.0001$). EMG abnormalities were observed in 61% of those that developed CSM and 11% of those that did not ($p < 0.01$).

However, there is no evidenced-based consensus to support prophylactic surgical decompression in asymptomatic patients with spinal cord compression. These patients should be informed about the signs and symptoms of myelopathy, the risks of progression, and observed clinically. In contrast, the treatment of non-myelopathic patients with spinal cord compression and radiculopathy is more controversial. While there have been no published studies comparing operative to nonoperative treatment in this patient population, there is mounting evidence that the presence of radiculopathy is associated with the development of myelopathy [1]. Moreover, some of these patients will require surgery for significant radiculopathy that is refractory to nonoperative therapy. As such, surgery can be considered in this patient population, and consideration should be made to treat both the radiculopathy and the spinal cord compression. These entities may be located at different spinal levels, and a multilevel procedure may be required, even if the radiculopathy originates from a single level. Nonoperative intervention consisting of close longitudinal follow-up or a supervised trial of structured rehabilitation can also be offered and, in fact, may be the most appropriate initial option for the majority of these patients. However, if myelopathy develops during the course of nonoperative treatment, surgical management should be entertained.

Mild Spondylotic Myelopathy

Mild spondylotic myelopathy refers to patients with subtle or relatively minor myelopathic symptoms that may not be disabling in any one category but with objective radiographic or physical exam findings of spinal cord narrowing. These patients typically have a mJOA score of 15–17. As with non-myelopathic patients with spinal cord compression and radiculopathy, controversy remains regarding optimal treatment of patients with mild CSM due to a relative lack of high-level published data directly comparing operative to nonoperative treatment for this patient population. Kadanka et al. [10] performed a prospective study that included both mild and moderate CSM patients ($n = 68$) that were randomized to either surgical ($n = 33$) or nonoperative treatment ($n = 35$). The patients were evaluated using the mJOA scale, a timed 10-meter walk, video assessment of daily activity performance, and self-reported evaluation at standardized time points over a 3-year period. There was no significant deterioration in the mJOA score in the two groups over the 3-year follow-up period. However, there was a significant difference in the time walk that favored the nonoperative group. Nonetheless, the mJOA score demonstrated no difference between groups. The authors concluded that there was no significant difference between surgery and nonoperative therapy in the treatment of patients with mild to moderate CSM. This initial cohort was subsequently followed for a total of 10 years, and the results were reported in a separate publication [11]. Once again the authors did not find a significant difference between nonoperative and surgical intervention at the latter time point. However, it must be noted that the lack of improvement following surgical intervention in these two studies is contrary to the results from a number of other investigations [20].

Although nonoperative management has been demonstrated to stabilize disease progression in some mildly affected CSM patients, the ability of this modality to effect neurological improvement is another matter. Based on the available literature, it appears as though neurological improvement that reaches the minimal clinically important difference (MCID) may be possible in a cohort of nonoperatively treated patients with soft disc herniation and/or dynamic myelopathy [15]. Intuitively this makes sense as a soft disc herniation may resorb with immobilization, and cessation of movement is a well-known treatment of dynamic myelopathy. However, nonoperative treatment is less likely to induce neurological recovery that reaches the MCID in patients with severe static compression from spondylotic bars or ossified spinal elements. In contrast, surgery may result in neurological improvement in patients with a wide variety of pathophysiology and radiographic findings compared to immobilization alone. Results from the AOSpine North America prospective multicenter study have suggested that mildly affected CSM patients can achieve statistically significant improvements in both the mJOA and Nurick scores despite the ceiling effect associated with these functional assessment tools [7].

Based on the aforementioned data, it is therefore reasonable to offer surgical intervention or a supervised trial of structured rehabilitation for patients with mild CSM. In patients treated nonoperatively, surgery should be recommended if there is neurological deterioration during the observation period. Although there are no published guidelines regarding the duration of observation, many surgeons offer surgery if symptoms persist after 3 or more months of nonoperative therapy. There is no convincing available data that mild or asymptomatic patients should undergo prophylactic decompression surgery to prevent the occurrence of paralysis following a traumatic event, such as a fall or motor vehicle accident. A recent study by Chang et al. [4] prospectively followed 55 asymptomatic or mildly affected patients with cervical stenosis that were treated nonoperatively. Thirty-one patients (56%) were previously recommended surgery by a previous physician. Twenty-six patients (47%) were told that they would be paralyzed after a motor vehicle accident or fall unless surgery was performed. The patients were followed for a mean of 2.3 years. Ten patients (18%) experienced a traumatic event during the follow-up, with none sustaining an SCI. The authors concluded that occurrence of SCI in this patient population after minor trauma is likely smaller than many physicians surmise, yet a prospective study with a large cohort of patients is necessary to fully elucidate their true risk stratification.

Moderate Spondylotic Myelopathy

Moderate spondylotic myelopathy refers to patients with clear signs and symptoms of myelopathy and that typically have a mJOA score of 12–14 (Fig. 12.2). They may present with mild to moderate hand coordination and gait difficulty or relatively profound isolated impairment in one of these functions. Although nonoperative treatment may be attempted in patients at the cusp of mild to moderate myelopathy, current literature suggests that patients with moderate CSM should undergo surgical intervention. In fact, patients are 1.22 times more likely to achieve a postoperative mJOA score of >16 for every 1-point increase in preoperative mJOA [24]. Conversely, in a study of patients with a mJOA score of 11–14 who were treated nonoperatively, the change in mJOA score was minimal (0–2.3), and up to 54% of patients eventually required surgery [25]. As such, nonoperative treatments are typically considered stopgap measures prior to surgery. Part of the rationale with this recommendation is that spinal cord compression severe enough to result in moderate spinal cord dysfunction can be associated with progressive permanent microstructural changes that cannot be reversed through decompression surgery. Therefore, pursing nonoperative treatment in this patient population confers the risk of neurological functional decline. As part of a large multicenter study, Fehlings et al. prospectively followed 110 moderately affected CSM patients that under-

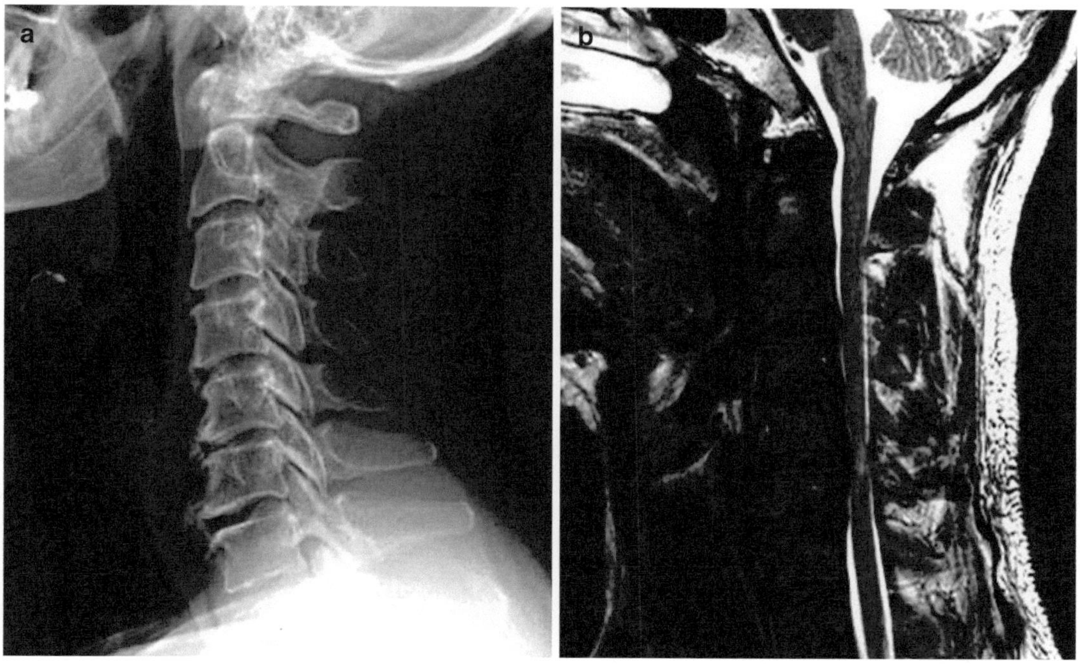

Fig. 12.2 Moderate CSM. A 40-year-old male with bilateral hand weakness, paresthesias, and positive Hoffman's sign (mJOA 14). Per patient wishes, conservative therapy was trialed for 3 months with persistent symptoms, and thus, the patient underwent C3–6 laminoplasty. Postoperatively the patient's hand strength and sensation improved significantly (mJOA 16). (**a**) X-ray cervical spine showing cervical straightening and moderate osteophyte formation. (**b**) MRI cervical spine with diffuse spondylosis and focal stenosis at C5–6, with corresponding spinal cord T2-weighted signal hyperintensity

went surgical decompression [7]. The mean improvement in the mJOA score was 2.58, the Nurick grade 1.51, and the NDI 9.79. All of these were statically significant improvements compared to the preoperative baseline and surpassed the MCID measurements for moderate CSM.

This sentiment was also found in a study by Sampath et al. who prospectively compared the results of operative versus nonoperative treatment for moderate to severe CSM [21]. Surgical patients had improved functional status and overall pain but with nonsignificant improvement in preoperative neurological symptoms. In contrast, nonoperative patients had significant worsening of their functional status and nonsignificant worsening of their baseline neurological symptoms. The fact that the operative cohort noted functional improvement while the nonoperative group declined infers a benefit to operative management in this patient population.

Nonoperative treatment may be appropriate in this patient population under certain circumstances, including severe medical comorbidities that significantly increase surgical risk, personal aversion to surgery, or improving symptomatology. However, if a nonoperative strategy is pursued, patients in this moderate category must be closely monitored for progressive symptoms or red flags, such as bowel/bladder symptoms, sexual dysfunction, or new-onset paresis.

Severe Spondylotic Myelopathy

Severe spondylotic myelopathy refers to patients with significant signs and symptoms of myelopathy or those with rapidly progressive disease (Fig. 12.3). These patients typically have a mJOA score of 0–11 and may be wheelchair bound or completely dependent on a walking assist device. MRI characteristics frequently include an AP

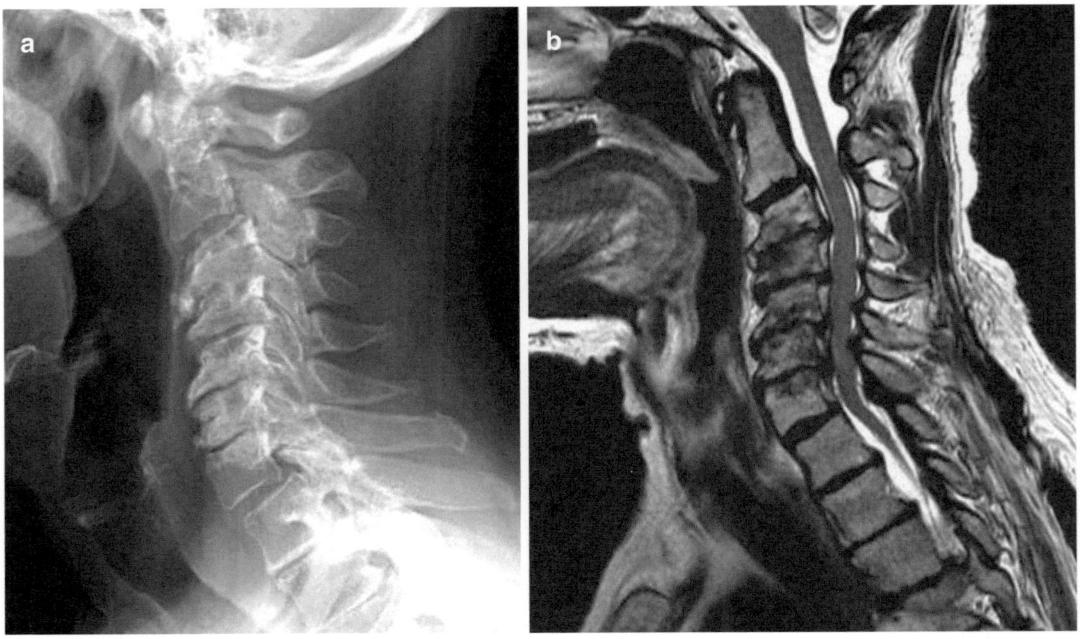

Fig. 12.3 Severe spondylosis. An 82-year-old male with hand weakness, progressive gait abnormality, and hyperreflexia (mJOA 7). The patient underwent C3–7 laminectomy and fusion 1 week after consultation. Postoperatively, the patient's dexterity and ability to ambulate improved, although some gait dysfunction persisted (mJOA 11). (**a**) X-ray cervical spine demonstrating severe degenerative changes, kyphosis, osteophyte formation, and auto-fusion. (**b**) MRI cervical spine with multilevel stenosis and T2 signal change at C6–7

diameter of 7 mm or less, suggesting severe spinal canal narrowing with cord compression, and may demonstrate evidence of spinal cord injury. This includes high T2-weighted intramedullary signal intensity, corresponding low T1-weighted intramedullary signal intensity or spinal cord atrophy.

A recent study of patients with severe spondylotic myelopathy found that with surgery, the average mJOA score improved by 4.91 and Nurick score improved by 1.74 [7]. Although the nearly 5-point increase in mJOA appears impressive, these patients with severe CSM still have a relatively low postoperative mJOA score, suggesting only a minimal change in true functional capacity. Therefore, surgery should ideally be performed before the symptoms become severe. Nonetheless, Yoshimatsu et al. [26] performed a retrospective study in which CSM patients chose to either undergo operative intervention or nonoperative treatment. Patients that underwent surgery had more severe CSM, with a mean JOA of 9.1, compared to those in the nonoperative group. In the immediate surgery group, 78% improved their JOA score at last follow-up, whereas only 23% of patients in the nonoperative group improved from their baseline scores. Accordingly, results of this study advocate for urgent surgical decompression in this patient population, typically within a few weeks. Nonoperative treatments are of limited utility and could delay surgical intervention, resulting in further neurological injury.

Specific Time Frame of Surgery

There are no published studies that support a specific time frame for surgery, and the majority of previous investigations and guidelines have assessed this important question by stratifying timing based on severity of disease, as presented in this chapter. However, we have provided some time frames based on our experience and interpretation of the available medical literature in Table 12.1. The overall concept of erring toward earlier instead of later surgical intervention appears to be supported in a large prospective multicenter study of CSM patients undergoing surgical intervention [24]. They found that the odds of a successful outcome decreased by 22% when the duration of symptoms increased from ≤ to 3 months to at least 3 but less than 6 months.

Conclusions

Surgical decision-making for cervical spondylotic myelopathy requires careful integration of patients' subjective symptoms, objective physical exam findings, radiographic evidence, patient lifestyle, and overall health. Based upon this analysis, patients may be stratified into asymptomatic, mild, moderate, and severe disease categories. Patients with non-myelopathic disease do not require treatment, per se, but should be followed closely, particularly if there is evidence of concurrent radiculopathy. Patients with mild disease may improve or stabilize with nonoperative treatment, but surgical management has been also demonstrated to provide benefit. Patients with moderate disease usually require surgery, which should be considered first-line treatment. Conservative measures may be offered to patients who refuse surgery or who have elevated operative risk. However, these patients require vigilant monitoring for signs of disease progression, including gait dysfunction or loss of dexterity. Finally, patients with severe spondylotic myelopathy should be managed with surgical decompression, as delays in utilizing nonoperative management may result in further irreversible neurologic decline.

References

1. Bednarik J, Kadanka Z, Dusek L, Novotny O, Surelova D, Urbanek I, et al. Presymptomatic spondylotic cervical cord compression. Spine. 2004;29:2260–9.
2. Boakye M, et al. Cervical spondylotic myelopathy: complications and outcomes after spinal fusion. Neurosurgery. 2008;62:455–61; discussion 461–452.
3. Boogaarts HD, Ronald HM. Prevalence of cervical Spondylotic myelopathy. Eur Spine J. 2013;24(S2):139–41.
4. Chang V, Ellingson BM, Salamon N, Holly LT. The risk of acute spinal cord injury after minor trauma in patients with preexisting cervical stenosis. Neurosurgery. 2015;77(4):561–5; discussion 565.
5. Dolan RT, Butler JS, O'Byrne JM, Poynton AR. Mechanical and cellular processes driving cervical myelopathy. World J Orthop. 2016;7(1):20–9.
6. Ellingson BM, Salamon N, Grinstead JW, Holly LT. Diffusion tensor imaging predicts functional impairment in mild-to-moderate cervical spondylotic myelopathy. Spine J. 2014;14(11):2589–97.
7. Fehlings MG, Wilson JR, Kopjar B, Yoon ST, Arnold PM, Massicotte EM, Vaccaro AR, et al. Efficacy and safety of surgical decompression in patients with cervical spondylotic myelopathy: results of the AOSpine North America Prospective Multi-Center Study. J Bone Joint Surg Am. 2013;95(18):1651–8.
8. Fujiwara K, Yonenobu K, Ebara S, Yamashita K, Ono K. The prognosis of surgery for cervical compression myelopathy. An analysis of the factors involved. J Bone Joint Surg. 1989;71(3):393–8.
9. Hu Y, Ding Y, Ruan D, Wong YW, Cheung KMC, Luk KDK. Prognostic value of somatosensory-evoked potentials in the surgical management of cervical spondylotic myelopathy. Spine. 2008;33(10):E305–10.
10. Kadanka Z, Mares M, Bednanik J, Smrcka V, Krbec M, Stejskal L, et al. Approaches to spondylotic cervical myelopathy: conservative versus surgical results in a 3-year follow-up study. Spine. 2002;27:2205–10; discussion 2210–2201.
11. Kadanka Z, Bednarik J, Novotny O, et al. Cervical spondylotic myelopathy: conservative versus surgical treatment after 10 years. Eur Spine J. 2011;20:1533–8.
12. Karadimas SK, Mark Erwin W, Ely CG, Dettori JR, Fehlings MG. Pathophysiology and natural history of cervical spondylotic myelopathy. Spine. 2013;38(22 Suppl 1):S21–36.
13. Klineberg E. Cervical spondylotic myelopathy: a review of the evidence. Orthop Clin North Am. 2010;41(2):193–202.
14. Kopjar B, Tetreault L, Kalsi-Ryan S, Fehlings M. Psychometric properties of the modified Japanese Orthopaedic Association scale in patients with cervical spondylotic myelopathy. Spine. 2015;40(1):E23–8.
15. Matsumoto M, Chiba K, Ishikawa M, Maruiwa H, Fujimura Y, Toyama Y. Relationships between outcomes of conservative treatment and magnetic resonance imaging findings in patients with mild cervical myelopathy caused by soft disc herniations. Spine. 2001;26(14):1592–8.
16. Matz PG, Anderson PA, Kaiser MG, Holly LT, Groff MW, Heary RF, Mummaneni PV, et al. Introduction and methodology: guidelines for the surgical management of cervical degenerative disease. J Neurosurg Spine. 2009;11(2):101–3.
17. Nouri A, Tetreault L, Singh A, Karadimas SK, Fehlings MG. Degenerative cervical myelopathy: epidemiology, genetics, and pathogenesis. Spine. 2015;40(12):E675–93.

18. Ono K, Ota H, Tada K, Yamamoto T. Cervical myelopathy secondary to multiple Spondylotic protrusions. Spine. 1977;2(2):109–25.
19. Ramanauskas WL, Wilner HI, Metes JJ, Lazo A, Kelly JK. MR imaging of compressive myelomalacia. J Comput Assist Tomogr. 1989;13(3):399–404.
20. Rhee JM, Shamji MF, Erwin WM, et al. Nonoperative management of cervical myelopathy: a systematic review. Spine (Phila Pa 1976). 2013;38:S55–67.
21. Sampath P, Bendebba M, Davis JD, et al. Outcome of patients treated for cervical myelopathy. A prospective, multicenter study with independent clinical review. Spine (Phila Pa 1976). 2000;25:670–6.
22. Steinmetz MP, Benzel EC. Benzel's spine surgery: techniques, complication avoidance, and management. 2017.
23. Stevens JA, Olson S. Reducing falls and resulting hip fractures among older women. MMWR Recomm Rep. 2000;49:3–12.
24. Tetreault LA, Kopjar B, Vaccaro A, Yoon ST, Arnold PM, Massicotte EM, Fehlings MG. A clinical prediction model to determine outcomes in patients with cervical spondylotic myelopathy undergoing surgical treatment: data from the prospective, Multi-Center AOSpine North America Study. J Bone Joint Surg Am. 2013;95(18):1659–66.
25. Wilson JR, Barry S, Fischer DJ, Skelly AC, Arnold PM, Daniel Riew K, Shaffrey CI, Traynelis VC, Fehlings MG. Frequency, timing, and predictors of neurological dysfunction in the nonmyelopathic patient with cervical spinal cord compression, canal stenosis, and/or ossification of the posterior longitudinal ligament. Spine. 2013;38:S37–54.
26. Yoshimatsu H, Nagata K, Goto H, et al. Conservative treatment for cervical spondylotic myelopathy. Prediction of treatment effects by multivariate analysis. Spine J. 2001;1:269–73.

Surgical Approach Decision-Making

13

Mena G. Kerolus and Vincent C. Traynelis

Pearls/Pitfalls

- Plain neutral, flexion, and extension films are essential for a full radiographic evaluation of degenerative cervical myelopathy and radiculopathy. Evaluation of this imaging provides valuable information regarding cervical alignment, stability, and preoperative planning.
- In order to provide successful surgical management of cervical spondylosis in the patient with radiculopathy and/or myelopathy, evaluating the need for decompression, maintenance, or improvement of cervical alignment and long-term stabilization is necessary.
- Most patients with multilevel myelopathy suffer from cord compression at the interspace as opposed to directly posterior to the vertebral body and thus are excellent candidates for anterior segmental decompression and fusion.
- Posterior cervical approaches are reserved for lateral soft disc herniations and myelopathy due to multilevel congenital stenosis or ossification of the posterior longitudinal ligament which cannot be safely or adequately addressed with an anterior approach.
- In patients where larger foraminal decompression is desired after posterior cervical instrumentation, interfacet spacers have shown to increase foraminal area and provide high fusion rates while maintaining lordosis.

Introduction

Cervicalspondylotic myelopathy is the most common cause of spinal cord dysfunction in the elderly [1]. The surgical approach must address the patient's neurologic symptoms, provide adequate decompression of the neural elements, and maintain or improve alignment and stability. Ideally the surgical approach should be cost-effective and have a low complication rate [2, 3]. The patient's clinical symptoms, location of compressive pathology, number of levels

M. G. Kerolus · V. C. Traynelis (✉)
Department of Neurosurgery, Rush University Medical Center, Chicago, IL, USA
e-mail: vincent_traynelis@rush.edu

M. G. Kaiser et al. (eds.), *Degenerative Cervical Myelopathy and Radiculopathy*,
https://doi.org/10.1007/978-3-319-97952-6_13

involved, and overall cervical spine alignment are critical when considering the surgical approach. Other factors to be noted include the body habitus, prior cervical procedures, and comorbidities especially smoking and steroid usage that may affect fusion potential. These components contribute to the decision process for a particular surgical approach to the cervical spine.

Technological advancements in instrumentation along with a better understanding of cervical spine biomechanics and alignment parameters have improved surgical outcomes, but the optimal approach is still defined by the specific details of each particular case [4]. Systematic-based reviews comparing the superiority or efficacy of different cervical spine approaches have been published; however given the heterogeneity of patient population and the variety of surgical techniques, drawing blanket conclusions can be difficult. There is evidence that provides direction in choosing a particular surgical approach, but in some instances, there is equipoise between anterior and posterior surgical strategies. This chapter presents a systematic approach to the surgical management of degenerative cervical radiculopathy and myelopathy.

General Considerations

Radiographic Evaluation

Determining the appropriate surgical approach requires a comprehensive evaluation of all pertinent radiographic data. Asymptomatic patients with imaging findings of degenerative changes do not require surgical intervention [5, 6]. The radiographic evaluation of symptomatic patients should include plain films in neutral, as well as flexion and extension, views. Sophisticated imaging to evaluate the neural structures is critical, and this may be accomplished with magnetic resonance imaging (MRI) or a postmyelogram computed tomography (CT). Patients with suspected ossification of the posterior longitudinal ligament, significant facet arthropathy, or bony foraminal stenosis should be evaluated with both MRI and CT. In these cases, myelography is frequently unnecessary if there is an adequate MRI. Radionuclide bone scans are occasionally helpful to verify whether a facet joint is the potential pain generator but are not required in all patients.

Neutral, flexion, and extension radiographs are used for the evaluation of overall cervical alignment, instability, extent of spondylosis, disc height, facet changes, endplate sclerosis, and osteophytes. Baseline films are also useful to assess numerous alignment parameters after surgical intervention which are important to correlate clinical outcomes with radiographic data during follow-up [7]. Flexion and extension films are the most efficient means of accurately evaluating instability which is key to planning a successful surgery. Reversal of cervical lordosis and the presence of kyphosis on neutral radiographs are key drivers for performing an anterior surgery.

The imaging modality of choice for evaluation of the effect of cervical degenerative disease on the neural elements is MRI as it clearly outlines the subarachnoid space, central canal, and neural foramina. It also may demonstrate T1- and T2-weighted signal changes in the spinal cord which may be of prognostic significance. MRI can demonstrate a herniated disc and synovial cysts among other neural compressive entities [8].

CT is invaluable as a means to evaluate osseous anatomy, osteophyte formation, endplate sclerosis, facet degeneration, and bony foraminal stenosis. It is critical to obtain a CT in patients in whom ossification of the posterior longitudinal ligament (OPLL) is suspected on the MRI [6]. CT can direct the management in many ways. For example, patients with significant endplate changes or facet arthropathy as determined by CT are not optimal candidates for cervical arthroplasty [9].

If MRI or CT fails to provide clear visualization of the necessary structures, CT myelogram should be obtained. This is commonly the case in patients who have had prior instrumented fusions or where the pathology is at the cervical thoracic junction. CT myelography is the imaging modality of choice in patients who cannot undergo an MRI.

Cervical Spine Deformity

Our understanding of sagittal alignment has evolved especially in the last decade. Cervical lordosis and overall sagittal alignment have been correlated to the severity of myelopathy and general health scores. Cervical alignment also appears to be related to thoracolumbar spinal pelvic alignment [10]. Thoracolumbar deformity can influence cervical alignment and vice versa. Patients in whom a thoracolumbar deformity is suspected should also be evaluated with full-standing anteroposterior and lateral scoliosis radiographs. Patients symptomatic due to a cervical deformity in the absence of myelopathy or radiculopathy will benefit from correction of cervical deformity. The correction of symptomatic cervical deformities requires complex planning and frequently employs multiple sequential operative techniques, the review of which is outside the parameters of this chapter [11].

Surgical Decision-Making

The treatment of cervical spondylosis varies, and surgical decision-making is essential for an optimal outcome. Cervical radiculopathy often resolves with nonoperative therapy and the passage of time, but the same is not true of myelopathy. All of the literature supports the concept that cervical myelopathy is a progressive disease which only responds to surgical intervention [12–14].

Successful surgical management of cervical spondylosis in the patient with radiculopathy and/or myelopathy must address the following three elements: decompression of the neural elements, maintenance or improvement of alignment, and long-term stabilization. A secondary goal would be the preservation of motion, but this is only important if the first two issues are dealt with in a positive manner. The critical factors which help dictate the approach include the location of pathology in relationship to the spinal cord and/or nerve root(s), number of involved levels, presence of instability, and segmental and overall sagittal alignment. The treatment of malalignment in the myelopathic patient also is directed by whether the deformity is fixed or reducible.

Anterior Cervical Approach

Anterior cervical approaches include anterior cervical foraminotomy, anterior cervical discectomy(ies) and fusion or arthroplasty, and cervical corpectomy(ies). Anterior approaches directly address pathology that involves the disc space and the vertebral body and are a key means of correcting or maintaining proper sagittal/alignment. It is important to assess vocal cord function in all patients with previous anterior neck surgery. Patients with significant swallowing dysfunction or those who have had extensive cervical radiation may not be candidates for an anterior approach.

Anterior Cervical Foraminotomy

Patients with purely cervical radiculopathy may benefit from an anterior cervical foraminotomy. Since this chapter is focused on myeloradiculopathy, the anterior foraminotomy is not a treatment choice. Anterior microforaminotomy was first performed in 1968 and most recently described by Choi et al. [15]. This surgical approach is associated with an increased risk of Horner's syndrome and a high recurrence rate of symptoms. It should be reserved for very specialized indications [16].

Anterior Cervical Discectomy and Fusion

Anterior cervical discectomy and fusion (ACDF) is used in patients with cervical instability, kyphosis or paracentral or central disc herniation, radiculopathy, or myelopathy. An anterior cervical approach provides direct decompression of the neural foramina and central canal and stabilization of the disc space and is often an excellent means of restoring or at least maintaining proper sagittal alignment. ACDF is not ideal in cases where the primary vector of spinal cord compression is posterior, such as may occur with ligamentum hypertrophy and multilevel congenital stenosis. Dural involvement in cases of OPLL is a relative contraindication to an ACDF. In patients with multilevel cervical disease with minimal involvement posterior to the vertebral body, ACDF is superior to corpectomy because of its increased ability to correct cervical alignment and superior immediate stabilization due to segmental grafting and fixation [17]. Most patients with multilevel myelopathy suffer from cord compression at the interspace as opposed to directly posterior to the vertebral body and thus are excellent candidates for anterior segmental decompression and fusion. ACDF allows for bilateral foraminal decompression at each treated level which is useful in many patients. In patients with radiculopathy alone, ACDF and posterior foraminotomy have comparable results [18]. The decision to treat posterior in these patients is predicated on the location of the neural compression of the exiting nerve root. If it is due to a lateral disc herniation or proximal neural foraminal narrowing, the outcomes are similar [19]. If not, the results may be disparate. Fusion rates at 12 months in one- and two-level ACDF have been reported to be 97% and 94% although the actual number may be lower given the fact that patients with myelopathy are more likely to have comorbidities which adversely affect fusion [20]. Although it has been reported that anterior and posterior approaches for the treatment of cervical spondylotic myelopathy are equal in terms of efficacy and safety, there is a growing body of literature which supports the anterior approach as being associated with better neurological improvement, better alignment, increased cost utility, and greater patient satisfaction [2, 17, 21–25].

Anterior Cervical Corpectomy and Fusion

Anterior cervical corpectomy and fusion is utilized in cases of anterior spinal cord compression that cannot be addressed with discectomy and fusion alone. In some patients, the pathology extends beyond the disc space and is behind the vertebral body and cannot be adequately addressed with an ACDF alone. These are rather rare occurrences but they do present from time to time. There is a conception that to perform a corpectomy to decompress multiple levels is more efficient in terms of operative time but that has not been our experience. The same meticulous decompression of the foramina at each interspace is required in both instances, and this requires time. Additionally, it is more efficient in terms of time to place interbody devices as opposed to the cages or grafts to needed to reconstruct a vertebral body resection. Multilevel corpectomies require posterior instrumentation which further decreases the value of this technique [26, 27]. Patients with extensive cervical disease involving the retrovertebral space are probably best managed using a hybrid approach combining corpectomy(ies) and anterior cervical discectomy as opposed to corpectomies alone [28].

Cervical Arthroplasty

Motion-preserving options in the treatment of cervical degenerative disc disease can be accomplished with cervical arthroplasty [29]. The Food and Drug Administration (FDA) has approved the clinical effectiveness of cervical arthroplasty in one- and two-level applications with non-inferiority and superiority when compared to ACDF [30]. As the inherent goal of arthroplasty is motion preservation, patients with baseline limited neck movement are unlikely to achieve any additional benefit with cervical arthroplasty as opposed to decompression and fusion. Additionally, patients with osteoporosis or endplate damage are not good candidates for arthroplasty. There are 7-year data available to show superiority of arthroplasty over ACDF in appropriately selected cases [31].

Posterior Cervical Approach

Posterior cervical approaches include posterior cervical foraminotomy(ies), laminectomy, laminoplasty, and fusion. These procedures are generally reserved for lateral soft disc herniations, foraminal stenosis, and myelopathy due to multilevel congenital stenosis or OPLL which cannot be safely or adequately addressed with an anterior approach. Posterior cervical approaches are sometimes advocated because of physician comfort and avoidance of perceived difficult anterior cervical anatomy; however, in a retrospective nationwide database study of 8548 patients, the incidence of mortality and inpatient complications was higher in those patients undergoing posterior fusion [32]. A single institution study in patients with cervical spondylotic myelopathy alone showed overall complication rates were similar [22].

Posterior Cervical Foraminotomy

Patients with purely cervical radiculopathy without myelopathy may benefit from posterior cervical foraminotomy. It is used when clinical symptoms correlate to the involved nerve root on imaging. Compression can be from osteophyte formation, foraminal stenosis (frequently secondary to facet arthropathy), or a herniated disc. In rare cases, a synovial cyst may cause neural foraminal compression. A foraminotomy is not the best treatment strategy in patients with compression medial to the foramen, with myelopathy, instability, or kyphosis.

Cervical Laminectomy

Cervical laminectomy allows for multilevel decompression but can increase the risk of developing a deformity. While this technique may be useful in older individuals with very stiff spines, over 20% of patients who undergo laminectomy for cervical spondylotic myelopathy will develop kyphosis [33]. Because of the risk of kyphosis, the authors do not recommend laminectomy. Those with perceived "stiff" spines will not suffer from adding a fusion to the laminectomy procedure, and this is a safer and more complete treatment than laminectomy alone.

Cervical Laminoplasty

Cervical laminoplasty is utilized in relatively young patients with myelopathy due to congenital stenosis and good cervical spinal mobility [34]. It is critical that patients who have at least some lordosis are not kyphotic [35]. Primary anterior compression is a negative prognostic factor for neurologic recovery after laminoplasty [36]. We fully evaluate the C45 neural foramina with CT preoperatively and consider significant foraminal stenosis at this level as a contraindication to laminoplasty since it may increase the risk of developing a postoperative C5 palsy.

Cervical Laminectomy and Fusion

Patients with multilevel cervical stenotic myelopathy without irreducible kyphosis may benefit from laminectomy and fusion. As in other posterior approaches, the neurologic compression should be posterior to the cervical cord. If it is primarily anterior and there is relatively preserved lordosis, then a posterior decompression will usually allow for adequate indirect decompression. Posterior cervical instrumentation with lateral mass fixation is advocated as the method of choice for fixation given low complication rate. Posterior cervical instrumentation and fusion has been shown to improve neck pain significantly after surgery compared to those undergoing laminoplasty; however, there is a higher reoperation rate and increased cost associated with posterior cervical lateral mass fixation [37, 38]. In patients where larger foraminal decompression is desired after posterior cervical instrumentation, interfacet spacers have shown to increase foraminal area and provide high fusion rates while maintaining lordosis [39, 40]. Laminectomy and fusion does not appear to be a favorable means of improving sagittal alignment, and it is associated with a decrease in lordosis in most series [37, 41–43]. It is our practice to try and reposition the patient intraoperatively after decompression to optimize lordosis.

Combined Anterior and Posterior Approach

Combined cervical approaches are primarily used in cases of anterior and posterior compression of the spinal cord. Additionally, patients with multilevel anterior pathology requiring corpectomy involving three or more levels require supplemental posterior instrumentation, and patients with kyphosis undergoing posterior decompression for dorsal pathology will also need anterior decompression and fusion to address ventral draping of the spinal cord. Finally, patients with poor bone quality secondary to metabolic disease such as osteoporosis and severe renal disease or patients who are smokers may require supplemental fixation [44]. These are also used for the management of complex patients and require a level of decision-making which is outside the context of this chapter.

Case Presentations

Several case examples are illustrated to highlight key thought process in pursuing surgical approach decision-making.

Anterior Cervical Discectomy and Fusion

A 65-year-old male with history of right arm discomfort. On motor examination, there was slight weakness of his right triceps and tingling dysesthesias to light cutaneous stimulation in the C6 and C7 dermatomes on right. There were no long tract signs. Plain cervical radiographs reveal C2–C7 SVA of 35.1 mm, C2–C7 lordosis of 20.5 degrees, and no instability on flexion/extension views (Fig. 13.1a). MRI revealed degenerative changes at C5–C6 and C6–C7 with disc collapse, disc bulging with osteophyte formation, and bilateral neural foraminal narrowing, right greater than left (Fig. 13.1b, c). Given he has failed conservative management, and imaging findings of severe nerve compression, he was an excellent candidate for a two-level ACDF at C5/C6 and C6/C7 (Fig. 13.1d).

Discussion In this case, given the disc collapse and bilateral neural foraminal narrowing, an ACDF was an appropriate option.

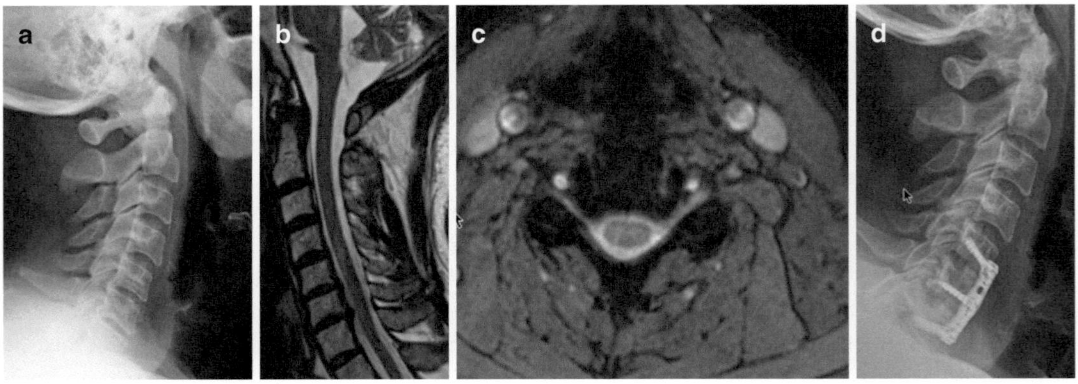

Fig. 13.1 (**a**) Plain neutral cervical radiograph demonstrating a C2–C7 SVA of 35.1 mm and C2–C7 lordosis of 20.5 degrees. (**b**) Sagittal and (**c**) axial T2-weighted magnetic resonance imaging (MRI) demonstrates degenerative changes at C5–C6 and C6–C7 with disc collapse, disc bulging with osteophyte formation, and bilateral neural foraminal narrowing, right greater than left. (**d**) Plain cervical postoperative radiographs demonstrated C5/C6 and C6/C7 anterior cervical discectomy and fusion (ACDF)

Posterior Cervical Foraminotomy

A 35-year-old male with 1-year history of left neck, scapular, and arm pain who failed conservative management. The pain was worse when extending his neck or tilting it to the left. He also experienced numbness and tingling in the third–fifth digits and weakness in his left hand. On motor examination, he had a positive Spurling's maneuver, tenderness in his neck to palpation, focal weakness in his handgrip and hand intrinsics, and tingling dysesthesias to light cutaneous stimulation in the left C7 and C8 dermatomes. On neutral, flexion, and extension radiographs, there were degenerative changes from C3 to C7 and loss of disc height at multiple levels (Fig. 13.2a). On MRI, he has congenital stenosis with two large disc herniations at C6/C7 and C7/T1 eccentric to the left causing significant compromise of the foramina and nerve root compression (Fig. 13.2b–d). He underwent C6/C7 and C7/T1 foraminotomies which produced an excellent result.

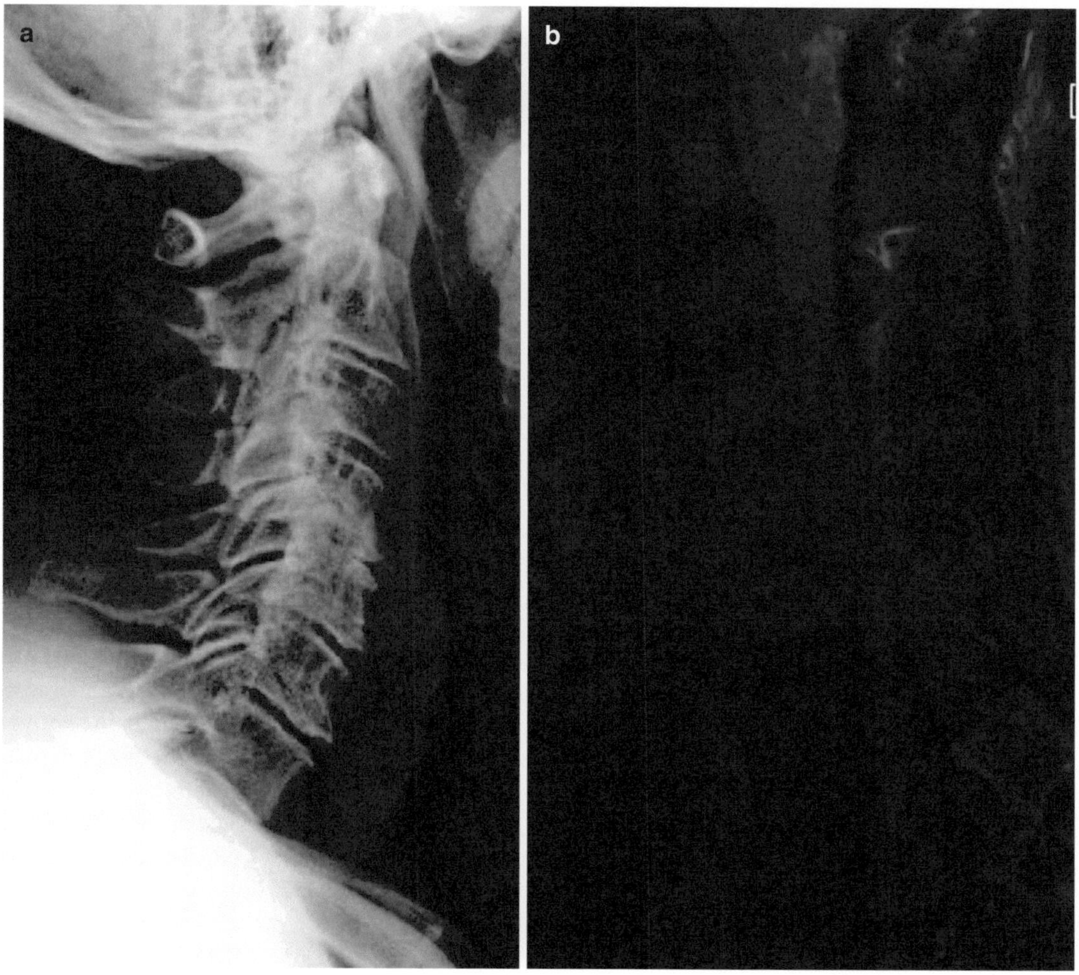

Fig. 13.2 (**a**) Plain neutral cervical radiograph demonstrates degenerative changes from C3 to C7 and loss of disc height at multiple levels. (**b**) Sagittal T2-weighted MRI demonstrates congenital stenosis with two large disc herniations. Axial T2-weighted MRI demonstrates (**c**) C6/C7 and (**d**) C7/T1 disc herniations eccentric to the left causing significant compromise of the foramina and nerve root compression

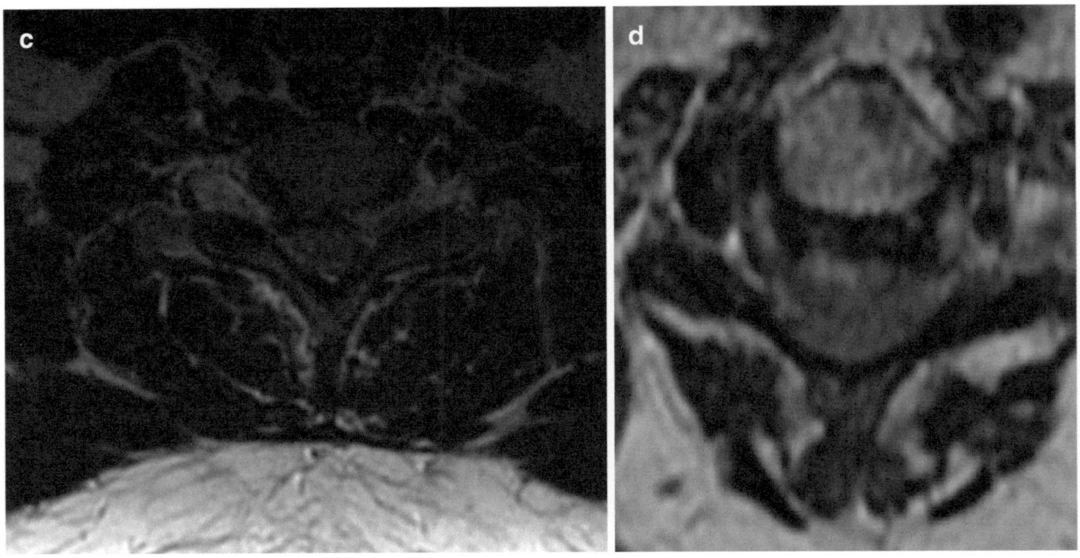

Fig. 13.2 (continued)

Discussion The patient did not want to proceed with ACDF because he wanted to spare motion. Posterior foraminotomy was an adequate treatment option given the lateral location of the disc herniation.

Posterior Cervical Laminectomy and Fusion

A 72-year-old male with recent history of recurrent falls, right constant lateral neck pain, and progressive weakness in his hands and his legs. On examination, he had difficulty with rapid movements of his hands, hyperactive reflexes, and positive Hoffman's and Babinski signs. Plain radiographs revealed good lordosis (Fig. 13.3a). MRI of the cervical spine revealed marked stenosis from C3 to C6 and cord signal change at the cord at C3 (Fig. 13.3b, c). The patient underwent C3–C5 laminectomies and C3–C6 posterior fusion.

Discussion This patient has progressive cervical myelopathy due to stenosis. Options discussed with the patient included laminoplasty or a laminectomy and fusion. Given his age and radicular symptoms which are likely due to C4 radiculopathy, laminectomy and fusion was a better option.

Anterior Cervical Arthroplasty

A 49-year-old female presented with right and shoulder pain, posterior neck pain eccentric to the right, and paresthesias radiating down in her arm. She did not have any gait abnormalities. On examination, she did not have neck tenderness. On motor testing, she has 4/5 strength in her right triceps and hypesthesia in the right C7 dermatome. She did not have any long tract signs. On neutral radiographs, there is disc collapse at C5/C6 and some collapse at C6/C7. The C2–C7 SVA is 30.2 mm; C2–C7 lordosis is 3.4 degrees (Fig. 13.4a). Flexion and extensions with minimal movement at C5/6. MRI revealed degenerative changes at C5/C6 and C6/C7. At C6/C7 there is disc herniation which is central and eccentric

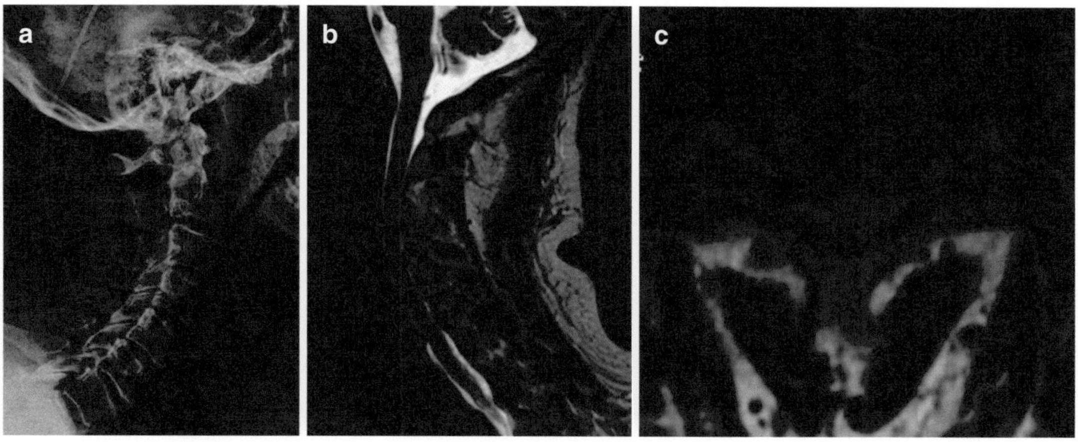

Fig. 13.3 (**a**) Plain neutral cervical radiograph demonstrates appropriate cervical lordosis. (**b**) Sagittal and (**c**) axial T2-weighted MRI demonstrates marked stenosis from C3 to C6 and cord signal change at the cord at C3

to the right causing significant neural foraminal stenosis of the exiting nerve root (Fig. 13.4b, c). She underwent a C6/C7 arthroplasty without complication (Fig. 13.4d).

Discussion Although the patient does have a narrow canal, there is no hypertrophy of the posterior ligamentous structures. Given her radiculopathy symptoms, age, and baseline neck mobility, arthroplasty was the chosen surgical option.

Posterior Cervical Laminoplasty

A 46-year-old male with several months of numbness and tingling in his hands as well as difficulty using his hands and trouble walking. On examination, he had difficulty with rapid movements of his hands. MRI of the cervical spine reveals marked spinal cord compression. Radiographs reveal good lordosis and no motion on flexion or extension films (Fig. 13.5a). MRI of the cervical spine reveals marked spinal cord compression (Fig. 13.5b, c). The patient underwent a C3 laminectomy and C4–C7 laminoplasty which resulted in the resolution of his symptoms (Fig. 13.5d).

Discussion Although a two-level decompression and arthrodesis would decompress the stenosis, there is significant posterior compression secondary to the congenital stenosis. There are also degenerative changes in the lower cervical spine which if he does become symptomatic would 1 day almost certainly require fusion.

Anterior-Posterior 360° Cervical Reconstruction

A 70-year-old man with a history of myelopathy was treated with a C3–C6 laminectomy. His myelopathy did not improve, and he developed significant neck pain which was most likely due to the postlaminectomy kyphosis (Fig. 13.6a). He was successfully treated with a multilevel anterior decompression and fusion followed with placement of posterior instrumentation (Fig. 13.6b). His neck pain resolved, and he improved in terms of his myelopathy.

Discussion Sagittal alignment is needed to be restored. A multilevel ACDF was able to restore alignment, while a posterior construct provided stability.

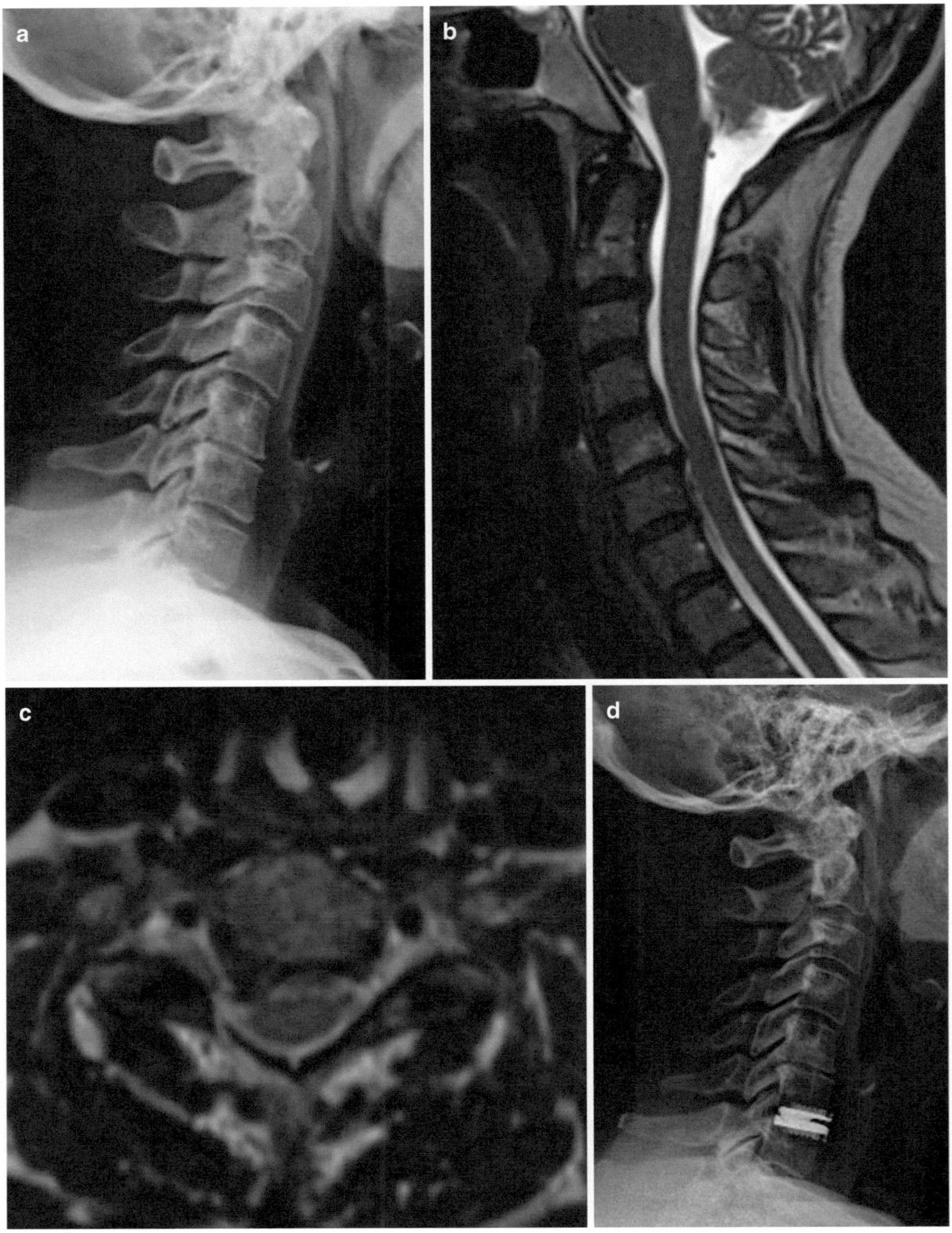

Fig. 13.4 (**a**) Plain neutral cervical radiograph demonstrates disc collapse at C5/C6 and some collapse at C6/C7. The C2–C7 SVA is 30.2 mm; C2–C7 lordosis is 3.4 degrees. Flexion and extension radiographs revealed minimal movement at C5/C6 (not pictured). (**b**) Sagittal T2-weighted MRI revealed degenerative changes at C5/C6 and C6/C7. An (**c**) axial T2-weighted MRI at C6/C7 demonstrated a disc herniation primarily central and eccentric to the right causing significant neural foraminal stenosis of the exiting nerve root. (**d**) Postoperative plain neutral cervical radiographs revealing a C6/C7 arthroplasty

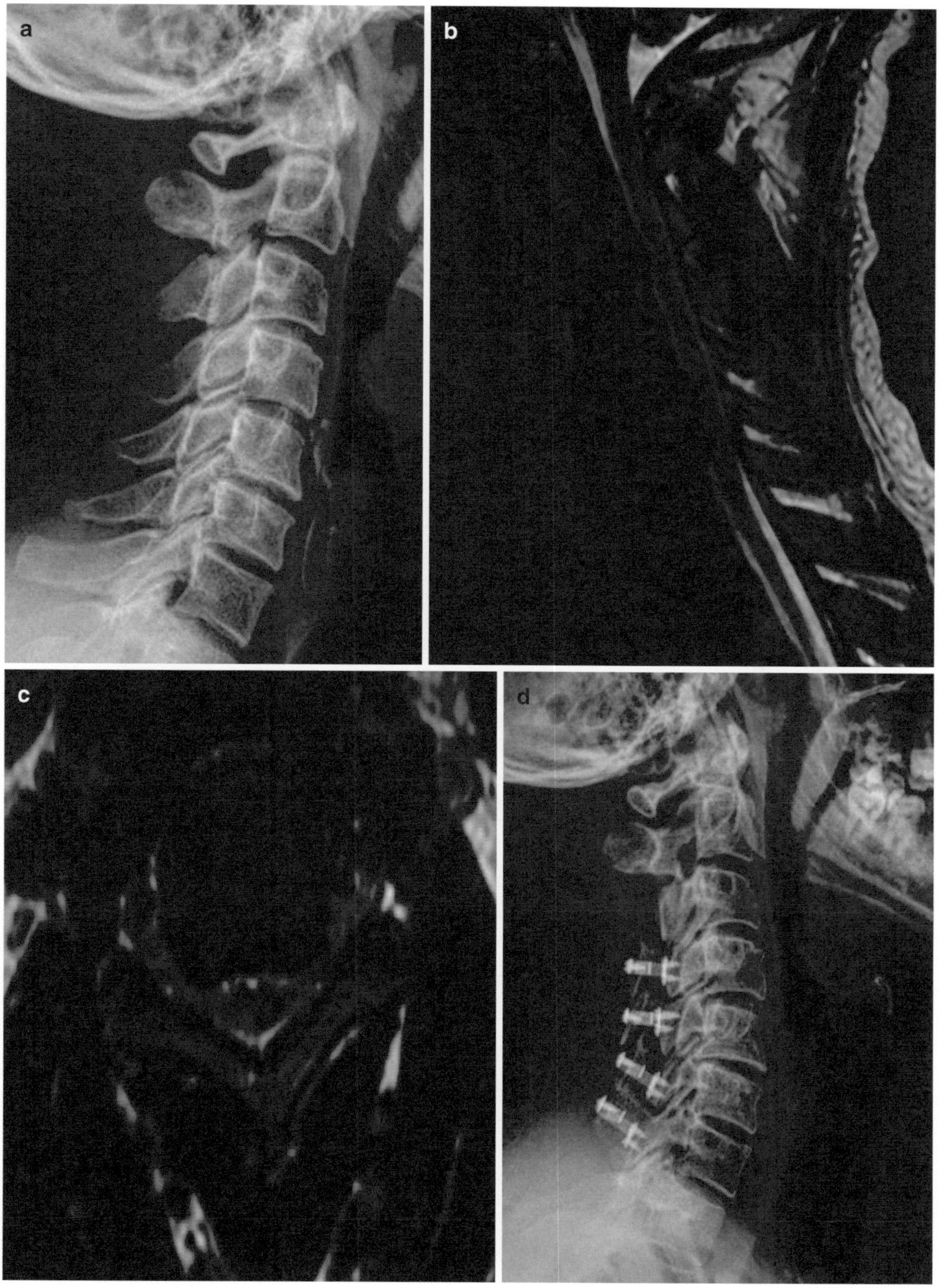

Fig. 13.5 (**a**) Plain neutral cervical radiographs reveal appropriate cervical lordosis and no motion on flexion or extension films (not pictured). (**b**) Sagittal and (**c**) axial T2-weighted MRI of the cervical spine reveals marked spinal cord compression. (**d**) Postoperative plain neutral radiographs demonstrating a C3 laminectomy and C4–C7 laminoplasty

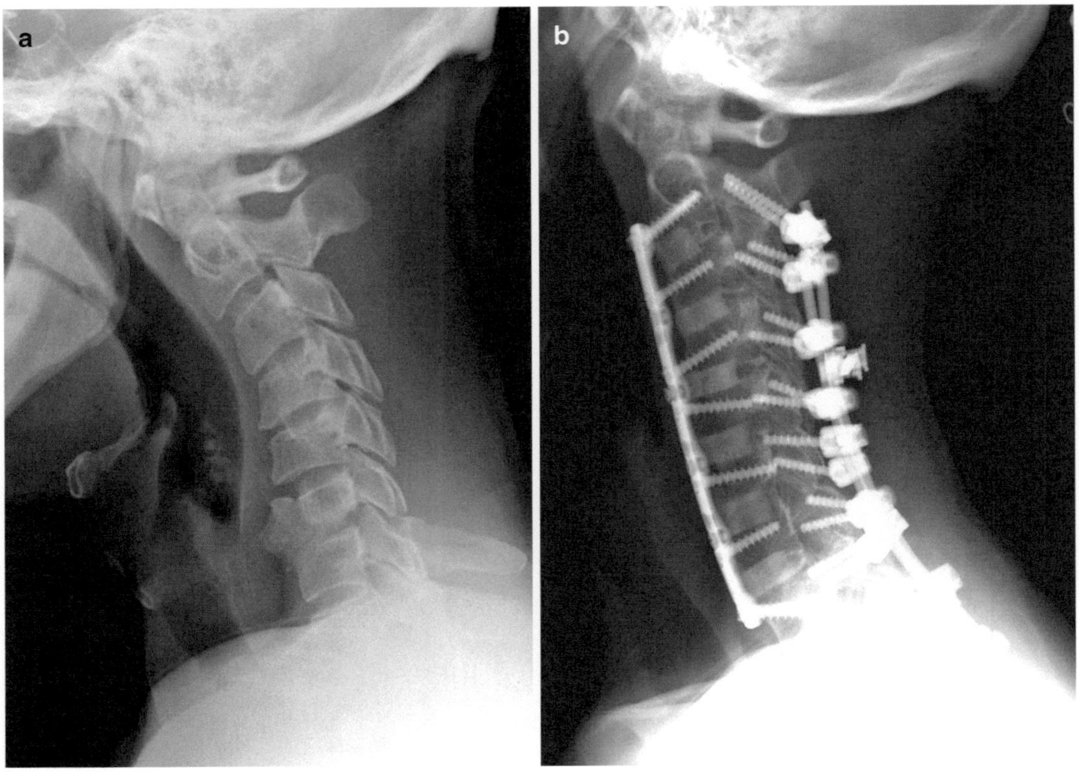

Fig. 13.6 (**a**) Plain neutral cervical radiograph revealing postlaminectomy kyphosis after a C3–C6 laminectomy. (**b**) Postoperative neutral cervical radiograph demonstrating a multilevel ACDF with posterior instrumentation from C2 to T3 with correction of cervical lordosis

Conclusion

Due to the heterogeneity of presentation, no stringent recommendations for one surgical approach over another for the treatment of cervical spondylotic myelopathy can be advocated. Rather it is an individualized decision-making process. It is clear that surgery is beneficial for patients with cervical spondylotic myelopathy. Systematic-based reviews have suggested surgical approaches with varying radiographic and clinical findings that are likely to be of benefit when addressing cervical degenerative disease.

References

1. Klineberg E. Cervical spondylotic myelopathy: a review of the evidence. Orthop Clin North Am. 2010;41:193–202. https://doi.org/10.1016/j.ocl.2009.12.010.
2. Fehlings MG, Jha NK, Hewson SM, Massicotte EM, Kopjar B, Kalsi-Ryan S. Is surgery for cervical spondylotic myelopathy cost-effective? A cost-utility analysis based on data from the AOSpine North America prospective CSM study. J Neurosurg Spine. 2012;17:89–93. https://doi.org/10.3171/2012.6.AOSPINE111069.
3. Witiw CD, Tetreault LA, Smieliauskas F, Kopjar B, Massicotte EM, Fehlings MG. Surgery for degenerative cervical myelopathy: a patient-centered quality of life and health economic evaluation. Spine J. 2017;17:15–25. https://doi.org/10.1016/j.spinee.2016.10.015.
4. Hukuda S, Mochizuki T, Ogata M, Shichikawa K, Shimomura Y. Operations for cervical spondylotic myelopathy. A comparison of the results of anterior and posterior procedures. J Bone Joint Surg Br. 1985;67:609–15.
5. Boden SD, McCowin PR, Davis DO, Dina TS, Mark AS, Wiesel S. Abnormal magnetic-resonance scans of the cervical spine in asymptomatic subjects. A prospective investigation. J Bone Joint Surg Am. 1990;72:1178–84.
6. Kalsi-Ryan S, Karadimas SK, Fehlings MG. Cervical spondylotic myelopathy the clinical phenomenon and

the current pathobiology of an increasingly prevalent and devastating disorder. Neuroscientist. 2013;19:409–21. https://doi.org/10.1177/1073858412467377.
7. Gillis CC, Kaszuba MC, Traynelis VC. Cervical radiographic parameters in 1- and 2-level anterior cervical discectomy and fusion. J Neurosurg Spine. 2016;25:421–9. https://doi.org/10.3171/2016.2.SPINE151056.
8. Carette S, Fehlings MG. Clinical practice. Cervical radiculopathy. N Engl J Med. 2005;353:392–9. https://doi.org/10.1056/NEJMcp043887.
9. Puttlitz CM, DiAngelo DJ. Cervical spine arthroplasty biomechanics. Neurosurg Clin N Am. 2005;16:589–594, v. https://doi.org/10.1016/j.nec.2005.07.002.
10. Ames CP, Blondel B, Scheer JK, Schwab FJ, Le Huec J-C, Massicotte EM, et al. Cervical radiographical alignment: comprehensive assessment techniques and potential importance in cervical myelopathy. Spine. 2013;38:S149–60. https://doi.org/10.1097/BRS.0b013e3182a7f449.
11. Smith JS, Klineberg E, Shaffrey CI, Lafage V, Schwab FJ, Protopsaltis T, et al. Assessment of surgical treatment strategies for moderate to severe cervical spinal deformity reveals marked variation in approaches, osteotomies, and fusion levels. World Neurosurg. 2016;91:228–37. https://doi.org/10.1016/j.wneu.2016.04.020.
12. Karadimas SK, Erwin WM, Ely CG, Dettori JR, Fehlings MG. Pathophysiology and natural history of cervical spondylotic myelopathy. Spine. 2013;38:S21–36. https://doi.org/10.1097/BRS.0b013e3182a7f2c3.
13. Rhee JM, Shamji MF, Erwin WM, Bransford RJ, Yoon ST, Smith JS, et al. Nonoperative management of cervical myelopathy: a systematic review. Spine. 2013;38:S55–67. https://doi.org/10.1097/BRS.0b013e3182a7f41d.
14. Fehlings MG, Wilson JR, Kopjar B, Yoon ST, Arnold PM, Massicotte EM, et al. Efficacy and safety of surgical decompression in patients with cervical spondylotic myelopathy: results of the AOSpine North America prospective multi-center study. J Bone Joint Surg Am. 2013;95:1651–8. https://doi.org/10.2106/JBJS.L.00589.
15. Choi G, Arbatti NJ, Modi HN, Prada N, Kim JS, Kim HJ, et al. Transcorporeal tunnel approach for unilateral cervical radiculopathy: a 2-year follow-up review and results. Minim Invasive Neurosurg MIN. 2010;53:127–31. https://doi.org/10.1055/s-0030-1249681.
16. Hacker RJ, Miller CG. Failed anterior cervical foraminotomy. J Neurosurg. 2003;98:126–30.
17. Lawrence BD, Jacobs WB, Norvell DC, Hermsmeyer JT, Chapman JR, Brodke DS. Anterior versus posterior approach for treatment of cervical spondylotic myelopathy: a systematic review. Spine. 2013;38:S173–82. https://doi.org/10.1097/BRS.0b013e3182a7eaaf.
18. Liu W-J, Hu L, Chou P-H, Wang J-W, Kan W-S. Comparison of anterior cervical discectomy and fusion versus posterior cervical foraminotomy in the treatment of cervical radiculopathy: a systematic review. Orthop Surg. 2016;8:425–31. https://doi.org/10.1111/os.12285.
19. Bono CM, Ghiselli G, Gilbert TJ, Kreiner DS, Reitman C, Summers JT, et al. An evidence-based clinical guideline for the diagnosis and treatment of cervical radiculopathy from degenerative disorders. Spine J. 2011;11:64–72. https://doi.org/10.1016/j.spinee.2010.10.023.
20. Fraser JF, Härtl R. Anterior approaches to fusion of the cervical spine: a metaanalysis of fusion rates. J Neurosurg Spine. 2007;6:298–303. https://doi.org/10.3171/spi.2007.6.4.2.
21. Jiang L, Tan M, Dong L, Yang F, Yi P, Tang X, et al. Comparison of anterior decompression and fusion with posterior laminoplasty for multilevel cervical compressive myelopathy: a systematic review and meta-analysis. J Spinal Disord Tech. 2015;28:282–90. https://doi.org/10.1097/BSD.0000000000000317.
22. Fehlings MG, Smith JS, Kopjar B, Arnold PM, Yoon ST, Vaccaro AR, et al. Perioperative and delayed complications associated with the surgical treatment of cervical spondylotic myelopathy based on 302 patients from the AOSpine North America Cervical Spondylotic Myelopathy Study. J Neurosurg Spine. 2012;16:425–32. https://doi.org/10.3171/2012.1.SPINE11467.
23. Liu B, Ma W, Zhu F, Guo C, Yang W. Comparison between anterior and posterior decompression for cervical spondylotic myelopathy: subjective evaluation and cost analysis. Orthop Surg. 2012;4:47–54. https://doi.org/10.1111/j.1757-7861.2011.00169.x.
24. Ghogawala Z, Martin B, Benzel EC, Dziura J, Magge SN, Abbed KM, et al. Comparative effectiveness of ventral vs dorsal surgery for cervical spondylotic myelopathy. Neurosurgery. 2011;68:622–630–631. https://doi.org/10.1227/NEU.0b013e31820777cf.
25. Whitmore RG, Schwartz JS, Simmons S, Stein SC, Ghogawala Z. Performing a cost analysis in spine outcomes research: comparing ventral and dorsal approaches for cervical spondylotic myelopathy. Neurosurgery. 2012;70:860–7; discussion 867. https://doi.org/10.1227/NEU.0b013e3182367272.
26. Sasso RC, Ruggiero RA, Reilly TM, Hall PV. Early reconstruction failures after multilevel cervical corpectomy. Spine. 2003;28:140–2. https://doi.org/10.1097/01.BRS.0000041590.90290.56.
27. Vaccaro AR, Falatyn SP, Scuderi GJ, Eismont FJ, McGuire RA, Singh K, et al. Early failure of long segment anterior cervical plate fixation. J Spinal Disord. 1998;11:410–5.
28. Shamji MF, Massicotte EM, Traynelis VC, Norvell DC, Hermsmeyer JT, Fehlings MG. Comparison of anterior surgical options for the treatment of multilevel cervical spondylotic myelopathy: a systematic review. Spine. 2013;38:S195–209. https://doi.org/10.1097/BRS.0b013e3182a7eb27.

29. Kasliwal MK, Traynelis VC. Motion preservation in cervical spine: review. J Neurosurg Sci. 2012;56:13–25.
30. Turel MK, Kerolus MG, Adogwa O, Traynelis VC. Cervical arthroplasty: what does the labeling say? Neurosurg Focus. 2017;42:E2. https://doi.org/10.3171/2016.11.FOCUS16414.
31. Sasso WR, Smucker JD, Sasso MP, Sasso RC. Long-term clinical outcomes of cervical disc arthroplasty: a prospective, randomized, controlled trial. Spine. 2016. https://doi.org/10.1097/BRS.0000000000001746.
32. Shamji MF, Cook C, Pietrobon R, Tackett S, Brown C, Isaacs RE. Impact of surgical approach on complications and resource utilization of cervical spine fusion: a nationwide perspective to the surgical treatment of diffuse cervical spondylosis. Spine J. 2009;9:31–8. https://doi.org/10.1016/j.spinee.2008.07.005.
33. Kaptain GJ, Simmons NE, Replogle RE, Pobereskin L. Incidence and outcome of kyphotic deformity following laminectomy for cervical spondylotic myelopathy. J Neurosurg. 2000;93:199–204.
34. Edwards CC, Riew KD, Anderson PA, Hilibrand AS, Vaccaro AF. Cervical myelopathy. Current diagnostic and treatment strategies. Spine J. 2003;3:68–81.
35. Suda K, Abumi K, Ito M, Shono Y, Kaneda K, Fujiya M. Local kyphosis reduces surgical outcomes of expansive open-door laminoplasty for cervical spondylotic myelopathy. Spine. 2003;28:1258–62. https://doi.org/10.1097/01.BRS.0000065487.82469.D9.
36. Iwasaki M, Okuda SY, Miyauchi A, Sakaura H, Mukai Y, Yonenobu K, et al. Surgical strategy for cervical myelopathy due to ossification of the posterior longitudinal ligament: Part 2: advantages of anterior decompression and fusion over laminoplasty. Spine. 2007;32:654–60. https://doi.org/10.1097/01.brs.0000257566.91177.cb.
37. Highsmith JM, Dhall SS, Haid RW, Rodts GE, Mummaneni PV. Treatment of cervical stenotic myelopathy: a cost and outcome comparison of laminoplasty versus laminectomy and lateral mass fusion. J Neurosurg Spine. 2011;14:619–25. https://doi.org/10.3171/2011.1.SPINE10206.
38. Leckie S, Yoon ST, Isaacs R, Radcliff K, Fessler R, Haid R, et al. Perioperative complications of cervical spine surgery: analysis of a prospectively gathered database through the association for collaborative spinal research. Global Spine J. 2016;6:640–9. https://doi.org/10.1055/s-0035-1570089.
39. Goel A, Shah A. Facetal distraction as treatment for single- and multilevel cervical spondylotic radiculopathy and myelopathy: a preliminary report. J Neurosurg Spine. 2011;14:689–96. https://doi.org/10.3171/2011.2.SPINE10601.
40. Tan LA, Straus DC, Traynelis VC. Cervical interfacet spacers and maintenance of cervical lordosis. J Neurosurg Spine. 2015;22:466–9. https://doi.org/10.3171/2014.10.SPINE14192.
41. Heller JG, Edwards CC, Murakami H, Rodts GE. Laminoplasty versus laminectomy and fusion for multilevel cervical myelopathy: an independent matched cohort analysis. Spine. 2001;26:1330–6.
42. Manzano GR, Casella G, Wang MY, Vanni S, Levi AD. A prospective, randomized trial comparing expansile cervical laminoplasty and cervical laminectomy and fusion for multilevel cervical myelopathy. Neurosurgery. 2012;70:264–77. https://doi.org/10.1227/NEU.0b013e3182305669.
43. Woods BI, Hohl J, Lee J, Donaldson W, Kang J. Laminoplasty versus laminectomy and fusion for multilevel cervical spondylotic myelopathy. Clin Orthop. 2011;469:688–95. https://doi.org/10.1007/s11999-010-1653-5.
44. Mummaneni PV, Haid RW, Rodts GE. Combined ventral and dorsal surgery for myelopathy and myeloradiculopathy. Neurosurgery. 2007;60:S82–9. https://doi.org/10.1227/01.NEU.0000215355.64127.76.

Utility of Intraoperative Neuromonitoring

14

Randy S. D'Amico and Peter D. Angevine

Abbreviations

ACDF	Anterior cervical discectomy and fusion
CSM	Cervical spondylotic myelopathy
IONM	Intraoperative neurophysiological monitoring
MAP	Mean arterial pressure
MEP	Motor evoked potential
MR	Magnetic resonance
SCI	Spinal cord injury
S-EMG	Spontaneous electromyography
SSEP	Somatosensory evoked potential
tcMEP	Transcranial motor evoked potential
TIVA	Total intravenous anesthesia

Pearls

1. Mostly useful in two situations:
   (a) With very tight stenosis, with turning a patient prone (with pre-turn and post-turn monitoring) to ensure adequate head position
   (b) With deformity correction
2. Consider using monitoring with an arterial line, as these patients may be very sensitive to MAP and spinal perfusion.

Pitfalls

1. Lack of communication among the surgeons, the neurophysiologist, and the anesthesia teams. Notably with anesthesia turnover during the case. Excellent communication among all members is essential.

Key Points

- The purpose of intraoperative neurophysiological monitoring (intraoperative neuromonitoring, IONM) is to try to detect neurological irritation or injury during high-risk spine surgery.

R. S. D'Amico · P. D. Angevine (✉)
Department of Neurological Surgery, Columbia University Medical Center, New York, NY, USA
e-mail: pda9@cumc.columbia.edu

M. G. Kaiser et al. (eds.), *Degenerative Cervical Myelopathy and Radiculopathy*,
https://doi.org/10.1007/978-3-319-97952-6_14

- Several intraoperative neuromonitoring modalities are currently available including somatosensory evoked potentials (SSEP), transcranial motor evoked potentials (tcMEP), and spontaneous electromyography (S-EMG).
- Surgeons should have a plan or checklist for review in the event of compelling neuromonitoring alerts to allow a prompt and appropriate response.
- Multimodal monitoring is routinely used during cervical spine surgery to maximize diagnostic efficacy as it offers a more comprehensive assessment of the spinal cord as compared with unimodal applications.
- Controversy exists in the utility of the routine use of intraoperative neuromonitoring for "low-risk" anterior cervical discectomy and fusion (ACDF) for degenerative conditions without associated deformity.
- The utility of intraoperative neuromonitoring (IONM) in decompressive surgery for cases of severe cervical myelopathy and/or radiculopathy where nerve conduction pathways may already be dysfunctional is controversial.
- The utility of neuromonitoring to detect delayed C5 palsy is questionable.

Introduction

The prevention of neurological injury is a central tenet of spine surgery. Unfortunately, the surgical treatment of spine disease may place the spinal cord or spinal nerve roots at some risk of injury. As a result, postoperative neurological deficits due to intraoperative injury may occur in up to 4% of anterior cervical discectomy and fusion (ACDF) cases and in up to 30% (average 4.7%) of posterior procedures [19, 22, 46, 53]. Etiologies of intraoperative irritation of, or injury to, the spinal cord or nerve roots include systemic causes such as hypoperfusion of the spinal cord due to hypotension or anemia, reperfusion injuries following decompression, neck manipulation during positioning, surgical decompressive maneuvers, instrumentation during fusion cases, and distraction during deformity correction [2, 9, 19, 46]. In the cervical spine, spinal cord injury (SCI) can have significant negative consequences.

Intraoperative neurophysiological monitoring (intraoperative neuromonitoring, IONM) enables the evaluation of the functional integrity of the spinal cord and nerve roots during surgery and may allow the early detection and possibly the reversal of neurological injury during high-risk spine surgery. Since its inception, IONM has demonstrated an ability to detect neurological deficits due to traction, compression, or ischemia of the spinal cord in thoracolumbar deformity surgery [9, 47, 69]. As a result of these successes, IONM has become adopted as an adjunct in the surgical treatment of other conditions, including degenerative cervical myelopathy and radiculopathy. However, debate exists over the use of IONM in the management of degenerative diseases of the cervical spine as the evidence for its utility for predicting and mitigating postoperative neurological deficits following anterior or posterior cervical spine surgery remains limited (Table 14.1) [2, 13, 18, 43].

Intraoperative Neuromonitoring Modalities

Monitoring plans are determined after consultation between the operating neurosurgeon, neurophysiologists, and anesthesiologists. In creating a monitoring plan, consideration must be given to preoperative neurological deficits, relevant anatomy, planned procedure, relevant comorbidities, planned anesthetic, and previous electrophysiological testing, when available, as all of these factors may influence the methodology and reliability of IONM. Each technique described below has its own advantages and disadvantages, and the choice of one or a combination of several should be carefully considered on a case-by-case basis.

Table 14.1 Key points

The purpose of intraoperative neurophysiological monitoring (intraoperative neuromonitoring, IONM) is to detect and possibly reverse neurological injury during high-risk spine surgery
Several IONM modalities are currently available for spinal surgeries including somatosensory evoked potentials (SSEP), transcranial motor evoked potentials (tcMEP), and spontaneous electromyography (S-EMG)
Surgeons should have a checklist for review in the event of compelling IONM alerts to allow prompt and aggressive detection and possibly reversal of neurological injury
Multimodal monitoring is routinely used during cervical spine surgery to maximize diagnostic efficacy as it offers a more comprehensive assessment of the spinal cord as compared with unimodal applications
Controversy exists in the utility of the routine use of intraoperative neuromonitoring for "low-risk" anterior cervical discectomy and fusion (ACDF) for degenerative conditions without deformity
The utility of IONM in decompressive surgery for cases of severe cervical myelopathy and/or radiculopathy where nerve conduction pathways may already be dysfunctional is not established
The utility of IONM to detect delayed C5 palsy is questionable

Somatosensory Evoked Potentials

Prior to 1977, the gold standard for detecting intraoperative neurological insults involved waking a patient intraoperatively to assess voluntary lower extremity function [68]. Known as the Stagnara wake-up test, this method was uncomfortable for the patient, difficult to perform repetitively during complicated surgeries, and often failed to identify the surgical step responsible for any witnessed deficit and did little to prevent reversible injury.

In 1977 the development of somatosensory evoked potential (SSEP) monitoring significantly advanced the capabilities of IONM. Measured SSEPs reflect the sequential activation of neural structures along somatosensory pathways. Decrements in SSEP amplitude or latency imply damage to the posterior columns of the spinal cord rostral to nerve root levels, where afferent somatosensory activity enters the cord. As a result, SSEP monitoring enables the surgeon to evaluate the functional integrity of ascending sensory pathways travelling from peripheral nerves through the dorsal roots and dorsal columns of the spinal cord and onto the sensory cortex [35, 47]. Typically, stimulation needle electrodes are placed in standard locations including the median and ulnar nerves in the upper extremity and the posterior tibial nerve in the lower extremity. Recording electrodes are placed following set standards, such as the International 10–20 system, and measurements are taken at anatomically accessible sites [37]. Abnormal findings are typically suggested by a 30–60% drop in the SSEP wave amplitude or a 10% delay in the SSEP latency (Fig. 14.1a, b), although thresholds vary according to institutional guidelines and no defined criteria exist [2].

A number of studies have examined the efficacy of SSEP monitoring in cervical spine surgery. For posterior cervical procedures, the sensitivity and specificity of SSEP monitoring range from 21% to 25% and 94% to 100%, respectively, suggesting that greater utility may lie in the negative predictive value of SSEP monitoring [27, 51]. In comparison, the utility of SSEP monitoring for anterior cervical spine surgery remains unclear as outcomes of surgery using intraoperative SSEP monitoring during anterior cervical discectomy and fusion (ACDF) surgery in non-myelopathic patients have not proven superior to unmonitored cases [59, 64].

While SSEP monitoring provides easy setup, monitoring is limited to the afferent tracts of the ascending dorsal column-medial lemniscus pathway and does not provide information about the descending efferent motor fibers of the corticospinal tract or the spinal cord gray matter. Furthermore, recorded SSEPs are summed responses which are filtered to remove artifacts and require averaging over multiple stimulation pulse trains occurring over time to improve the signal-to-noise ratio. As a result, abnormal findings or significant changes may significantly lag behind clinically important changes.

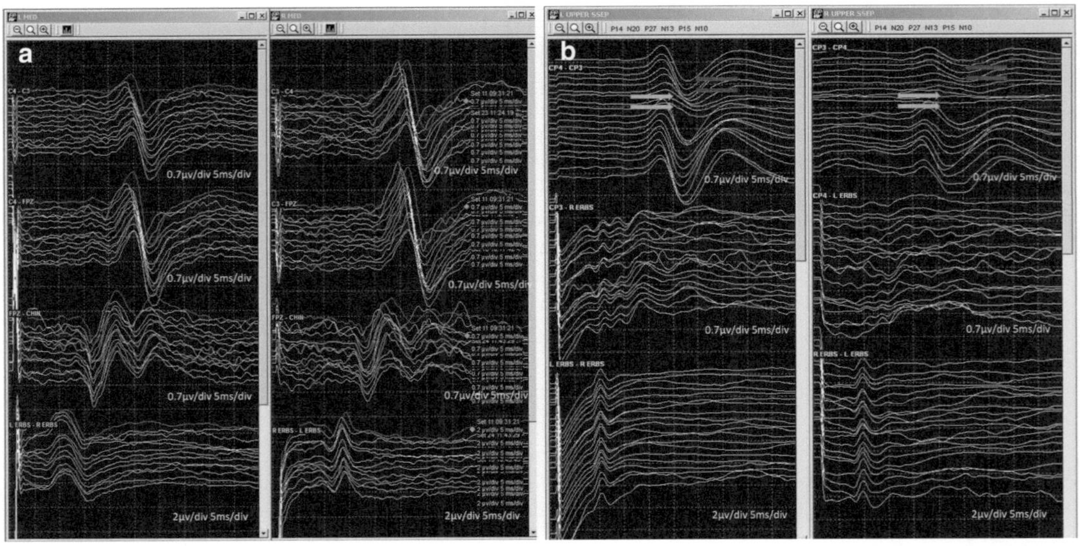

Fig. 14.1 Intraoperative somatosensory evoked potential (SSEP) recordings. (**a**) Representative cases demonstrating reliable SSEP recording. Stimulation electrodes were placed along the median nerve, and bipolar stimulation was used to propagate repetitive action potentials along the peripheral nerves to the dorsal column pathways of the spinal cord and eventually to the contralateral sensory cortex. Bilateral SSEPs were reliably recorded at anatomically accessible sites including Erb's point (ERBS), the Fpz-CHIN region, the C4-Fpz region, and the C4-C3 region according to the International 10–20 system [37]. (**b**) Representative case demonstrating loss and subsequent return of bilateral SSEPs. Bilateral SSEPs were reliably recorded at ERBS, the CP3-R ERBS region, and the C4-C3 regions. Loss (green arrows) and subsequent spontaneous return (red arrows) of SSEP signal amplitudes became apparent during surgery suggesting loss and return of dorsal column conductivity (left greater than right). No new postoperative deficit was encountered

Transcranial Motor Evoked Potentials

In response to concerns over the low sensitivity of SSEP monitoring in detecting postoperative motor deficits, a technique of monitoring neurogenic evoked motor potentials was initially developed to measure peripheral nerve signals elicited from spinal cord stimulation cephalad to levels of interest [50]. However, subsequent neurophysiologic studies demonstrated that this technique likely measured retrograde signals transmitted via the dorsal columns with inaccurate representation of the descending corticospinal motor tracts [66]. Consequently, a method of measuring transcranial motor evoked potentials (tcMEP) was developed to reliably monitor the descending corticospinal motor tract [10].

The technique of tcMEP monitoring involves using electrical scalp stimulation to produce an electrical current within the motor cortex of the brain which then progresses through the descending corticospinal motor pathways. These motor pathways primarily comprise the lateral corticospinal tract and are located within the lateral and the ventral funiculi of the spinal cord. Recording needle electrodes are placed in the muscles of interest throughout the four extremities including the abductor pollicis brevis, first dorsal interosseous, extensor carpi radialis, triceps, biceps, deltoid, abductor hallucis, and anterior tibialis [2]. Muscle motor evoked potentials (MEPs) are then recorded. Measurements are taken as a baseline before surgery and then during intervals during the surgery, following the approach and critical portions of the procedure, and during the surgical closure. During surgery, signal amplitude, duration, and latency are monitored for significant changes (Fig. 14.2a). In general, tcMEPs are described as an "all-or-none" phenomenon, but accepted thresholds vary by institutional protocols, and no strictly defined criteria exist. Commonly, rapid and reproducible loss of

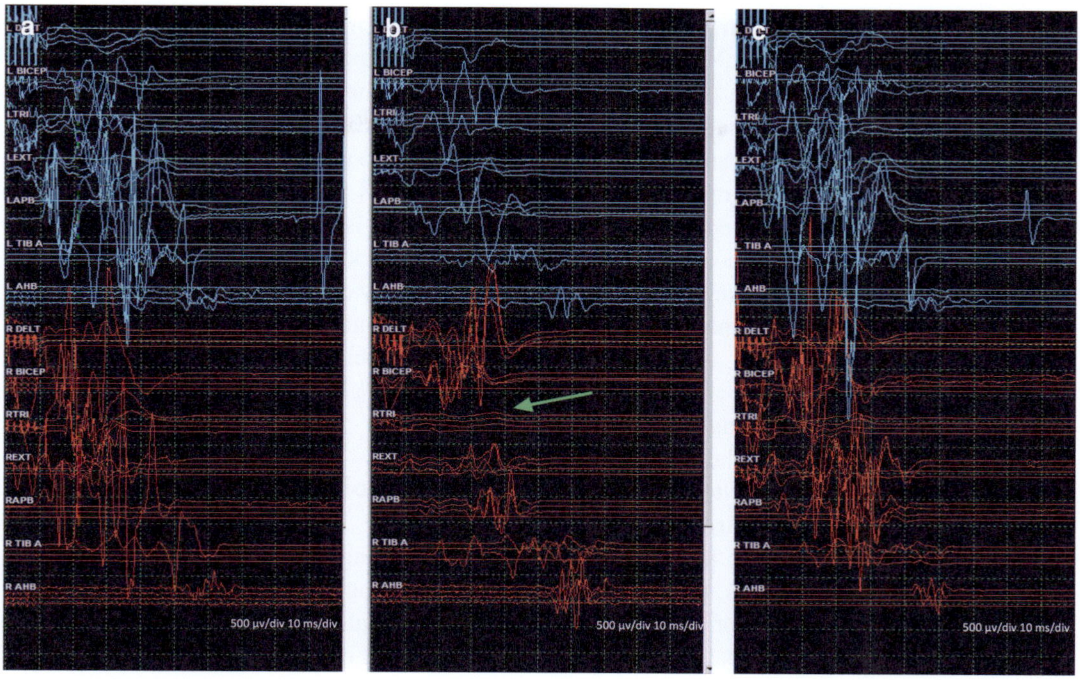

Fig. 14.2 Intraoperative transcranial motor evoked potential (tcMEP) recordings. (**a**) Bilateral upper and lower extremity tcMEPs were recorded at the deltoid (DELT), bicep, triceps (TRI), extensor carpi radialis (EXT), abductor pollicis brevis (APB), tibialis anterior (TIB A), and abductor hallucis (APB). The excellent amplitude and reproducibility provided a baseline for intraoperative monitoring. (**b**) A decrement in the right triceps tcMEPs (green arrow) prompted surgical pause and prompt and aggressive management of its source. (**c**) A modest return of right triceps tcMEP signal was measured prior to wound closure. This signal was less robust and lacking in complexity compared with other tcMEPs measured in other muscles on that side. Notably, the patient awoke without evidence of a postoperative neurological deficit

50–80% tcMEP amplitude is considered to represent a significant monitoring change (Fig. 14.2b, c) [2, 13, 40, 41]. However, even partial attenuation may actually represent injury within the cervical spine as associated muscles have multiple innervations at the level of both the gray matter and the nerve roots which can mask clinically relevant changes [4].

Limitations to tcMEPs exist, and successful baseline tcMEP recording can be influenced by patient age, lesion location, and preoperative neurological deficits as nerve conduction pathways may already be dysfunctional in some patients [12, 41]. As a result, identified changes require a careful appraisal to gauge representation of potential injury. Elicitation of tcMEPs can cause significant patient movement, thus limiting their use during critical portions of some procedures. Finally, the intermittent nature of tcMEP monitoring only reflects events since the last recording and may make differential identification of a specific etiology of intraoperative injury difficult.

Despite these limitations, studies have demonstrated tcMEP monitoring provides earlier detection of neurological injury and is a more sensitive indicator of neurological injury than SSEP monitoring alone, with associated sensitivity and specificity in cervical spine cases ranging from 75% to 100% and 92% to 100%, respectively [13, 27, 38, 56]. However, tcMEP monitoring also produces a rate of false-positive alerts approaching 5.8% and a rate of false-negative alerts approaching 5.0%, in particular with regard to monitoring for C5 palsy, precluding consensus on its true clinical value [42, 52, 63].

Spontaneous Electromyography

Spontaneous electromyography (S-EMG) is an additional IONM modality routinely used to monitor and alert the surgical team to nerve root irritation occurring in a specific myotomal distribution [5, 48, 49]. As S-EMG does not require stimulation, it provides continuous, "real-time" monitoring of nerve action potentials induced by various types of manipulation, including stretch, blunt trauma, compression, and ischemia. Typically, recording electrodes are placed in or near the muscles corresponding to the nerve roots at risk during surgery. The most reliably sampled muscles include the deltoid, biceps, triceps, thenar and hypothenar muscles, the vasti, anterior tibialis, gastrocnemius, abductor hallucis, and first dorsal interosseous, with the trapezius employed for C4 nerve root coverage [55]. In contrast to other IONM modalities, a lack of significant myogenic activity is interpreted as evidence of functionally intact nerve roots, whereas the occurrence of spontaneous spike activity and/or sustained bursting or train activity of S-EMG waves may represent true neurophysiologic changes (Fig. 14.3a, b) [40]. S-EMG is particularly useful in surgeries with risk of radicular injury.

Artefactual S-EMG activity can be produced by irrigation, metal-metal contact within the surgical field, or movement of the surgeon's body weight or equipment against a limb. In addition, ensuring adequate sampling within a monitored muscle is critical as activity in each muscle may reflect injury to a number of nerve roots innervating it. While S-EMG is relatively insensitive to anesthetics, it is profoundly affected by neuromuscular blockade. Historically, S-EMG has high sensitivity and low specificity for predicting postoperative neurological deficits and is best used in combination with other monitoring modalities [24].

Evaluation of Signal Changes

Persistent changes in any IONM modality may signal neurological irritation or impending or established injury. Surgeons should have a plan in place or a checklist for review in the event of a major alert to allow prompt and aggressive management of its source (Fig. 14.4) [20]. Routine considerations include adjusting stimulation parameters and checking electrode placement to rule out technical error; analyzing administered anesthetics to rule out the use of inhalational agents, large bolus injections, or long-acting muscle relaxants; ensuring a mean arterial pressure (MAP) >90 mmHg, temperature >36.5 °C, and hemoglobin >10 g/dL;

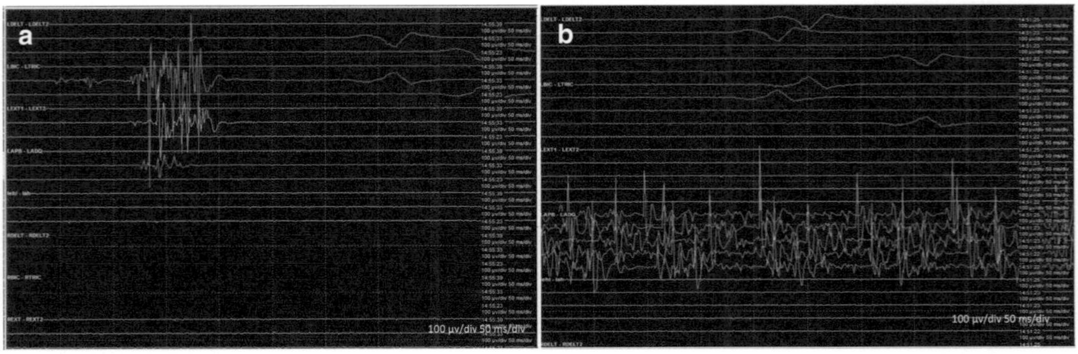

Fig. 14.3 Spontaneous electromyography (S-EMG) recordings of the bilateral upper extremities demonstrating activity in multiple nerve roots as a result of irritation. Sampled muscles include deltoids (DELT), biceps (BIC), triceps (TRI), extensor carpi radialis (EXT), and abductor pollicis brevis (APB). (**a**) Intraoperative S-EMG demonstrates irritation in the region of the left BIC-TRI, EXT, and APB. (**b**) S-EMG demonstrating persistent irritation in the region of the left APB. In comparison to other IONM modalities, a lack of significant myogenic activity is interpreted as evidence of functionally intact nerve roots

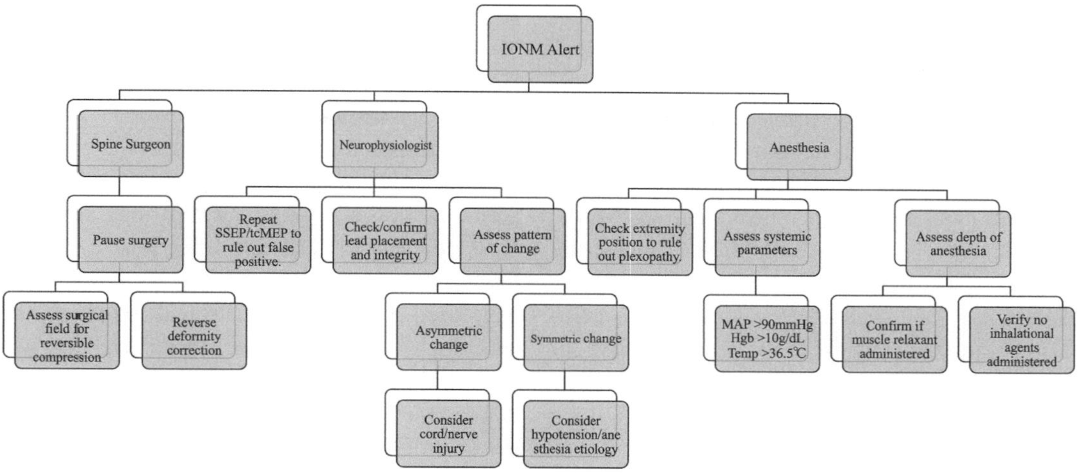

Fig. 14.4 Algorithm for response to IONM alert. IONM intraoperative neuromonitoring, SSEP somatosensory evoked potential, tcMEP transcranial motor evoked potential, MAP mean arterial pressure, Hgb hemoglobin. (Modified from Vitale et al. [69]. and Ziewacz et al. [72])

and evaluating possible position changes such as removing tape from the shoulders, repositioning the neck, releasing deformity corrections, or removing implants. When possible, multiple IONM modalities should be correlated to confirm injury [23, 28, 58, 69]. Consideration should always be given to the fact that false-positive alerts can occur and that some subsequent interventions may actually cause harm.

In the setting of persistent evidence of injury, and dependent on the postoperative neurological exam, consideration should be given to admitting the patient to an intensive care unit where the need for optimization of spinal cord perfusion can be evaluated. Additionally, for new postoperative deficits, consideration should be given to treatment with intravenous steroids. Magnetic resonance (MR) imaging may be considered to evaluate for compression of neurological elements when clinical suspicion is high (Table 14.2). It is important to note that challenging clinical conditions, such as severe myelopathy, spinal cord tumors, obesity, or peripheral neuropathy, can make interpretation of neuromonitoring difficult or at times impossible [13].

Table 14.2 Checklist for the management of persistent IONM changes with corresponding neurological deficit

Consider aborting the surgery and staging procedure
Consider admission to neurological intensive care unit
Evaluate benefit of optimizing spinal cord perfusion (ensure MAP >90 mmHg and Hgb >10 g/dL)
Consider IV steroid therapy
Consider MRI

Modified from Vitale et al. [69] and Ziewacz et al. [72]
IONM intraoperative neuromonitoring, *MAP* mean arterial pressure, *Hgb* hemoglobin, *IV* intravenous, *MRI* magnetic resonance imaging

Utility of Neuromonitoring

The routine use of IONM has reduced the risk of neurological injury in deformity surgery [56, 65]. Extrapolation of these data has resulted in the routine incorporation of IONM in the surgical management of degenerative cervical myelopathy and radiculopathy [1, 27]. However, while the utility of IONM during spinal deformity surgery is considered established [15, 56, 69], the efficacy of IONM in cervical spine surgery is still debated [14, 27, 34, 43, 63, 67]. Reservations are primarily grounded in the evidence of high false-positive rates, low efficiency, and lack of established reliable warning criteria for current IONM modalities. Furthermore, the role of neuromonitoring in patients without severe deformity or with already irreversible preoperative neurological deficits is unknown and carries large economic implications [14, 67]. As a result, the use of IONM may be of limited value in routine, nontraumatic, or non-severe deformity cases in the cervical spine. Importantly, IONM requires multidisciplinary cooperation between neurophysiologists, anesthesiologists, and neurosurgeons to properly and efficiently use these technologies.

Multimodality Neuromonitoring

In general, multimodality monitoring—with a combination of tcMEP, SSEP, and S-EMG—is used to improve the overall sensitivity and maximize the diagnostic efficacy of the individual modalities as it is believed to offer a more comprehensive assessment of the spinal cord as compared with unimodal applications [17, 19, 29, 34, 35, 43, 44, 54, 61, 62]. Sensitivity of multimodal IONM ranges from 50% to 83.3%, with a specificity of 99–100% during cervical spine surgery [18, 40]. However, increased sensitivity carries with it the risk of increased false positives that may not necessarily manifest as a new postoperative neurologic deficits and may result in aborted procedures or potentially harmful alterations in standard surgical techniques [42]. As a result, some continue to argue that unimodal intraoperative monitoring has higher specificity than multimodal monitoring and may minimize subclinical intraoperative alerts [2], which can significantly influence surgical decision-making [42].

Preoperative Deficits

In the presence of significant preoperative weakness, nerve conduction pathways may already be dysfunctional and the utility of IONM in decompressive surgery for cases of severe cervical myelopathy [15, 36, 67] and/or radiculopathy is not well established [15, 36, 41, 67]. In particular, the presence of preoperative myelopathy may be a strong risk factor for IONM changes in cases of cervical spondylotic myelopathy [45]. However, severe preoperative spinal cord dysfunction is associated with worsened baseline tcMEP amplitude, duration, and latency making intraoperative interpretation complicated. In addition, the sensitivity of IONM may also vary based on patient comorbidities and age [13]. Regardless, decreased intraoperative tcMEPs have been shown to correlate with postoperative neurological deficits in cases of cervical myelopathy [13]. While more studies are necessary to better understand and further establish significant alarm thresholds in cases of myelopathy, interpretation of worsened tcMEP monitoring should always be evaluated relative to preoperative baselines specific to each individual case [70].

Recent evidence suggests that tcMEP use may be limited in patients with preoperative motor deficits consistent with radiculopathy causing Medical Research Council (MRC) grades less than 3 as the frequency of successful recordings diminishes substantially [41]. However, if a baseline tcMEP or SSEP can be recorded successfully, the utility of intraoperative neuromonitoring can actually increase [13]. In such cases, attempts to increase stimulus intensity, duration, or interval may improve the success rate of tcMEP monitoring despite a higher risk of seizure, tongue biting, cardiac arrhythmias, and scalp burns with high voltage tcMEP stimulation [3, 32, 33, 57]. Additional techniques for improving the reliability of IONM have been described for patients with severe neuromuscular weakness, impaired spinal cord function, Duchenne muscular atrophy, or Rett syndrome with some success [33]. These techniques involve preconditioning stimulation preceding multiple transcranial electrical stimuli to elicit a larger MEP and facilitate a weak response. In the setting of preoperative weakness of a given muscle, S-EMG monitoring may demonstrate baseline activity in that muscle which then dissipates with decompression [6, 48]. In comparison, chronically compressed motor nerve roots may not fire spontaneously or with stimulus, and a quiet S-EMG does not necessarily mean that the root is not undergoing injury [15].

Anterior Versus Posterior Surgical Procedures

Symptomatic cervical spine disease may be treated by anterior, posterior, or combination (360°) approaches with the degree of surgical complexity varying with approach, surgical goals, anatomic variants, and patient clinical status. Multimodality IONM has become routinely incorporated in cervical spine surgery for symptomatic spondylosis. However, documented rates of neurological injury following anterior and posterior cervical spine surgery for degenerative disease are low, ranging from 0% to 18% in monitored cases [18, 42, 67], with a slightly higher risk in cases involving corpectomies. As a result, there has been debate over the utility and cost-efficacy of routine IONM for these "low-risk" procedures [2]. Unfortunately, studies examining the utility of IONM in cervical spine surgery remain limited by the heterogeneity of procedures and perceived risks. As a result, sensitivity and specificity of the various monitoring techniques differ depending on the patient's diagnosis and the procedure performed [15, 52].

In general, the limited available evidence suggests that multimodal IONM is useful for detecting neurological injury in posterior cervical operations, in particular in the high cervical region [40]. However, IONM may be of limited value in routine, nontraumatic, or non-severe deformity cases as these cases are thought to have lower rates of iatrogenic neurological injury.

Similar controversy exists over the routine use of IONM for anterior cervical spine surgeries for degenerative conditions without deformity. Early proponents of IONM for anterior cervical spine surgery touted improved outcomes due to early detection of impending neurological injury [19]. However, the utility of IONM with, or without, multimodal monitoring in anterior cervical spine surgery has since been found to be of limited value for limiting the frequency of neurological injuries [8, 59, 64]. This is in part due to the low risk of neurological injury with anterior cervical approaches for symptomatic spondylosis and in particular, the low risk of neurological injury in non-myelopathic patients [59].

As a result of these data, a national practice guideline in 2009 gave no recommendation in support of the routine use of IONM for anterior cervical spine surgery for degenerative conditions due to a lack of specificity, a lack of demonstrated clinical improvement, and conflicting class I evidence of monitoring parameters [52]. A recent systematic review further showed that IONM specifically did not influence the risk of neurological injury after anterior cervical discectomy and fusion (ACDF) procedures [2]. Importantly, while these authors did note that procedures involving a corpectomy may carry a higher risk of neurological injury, insufficient data were available to perform a comparative statistical analysis between ACDF alone and procedures involving corpectomies. As a result, no formal recommendation was given regarding the use of IONM in procedures involving a corpectomy. No similar guidelines exist for the use of IONM in posterior cervical spine surgery. Consequently, the decision to use IONM remains guided by surgeon choice and experience, with critical attention paid to the perceived risk of neurological injury.

C5 Palsy

C5 nerve root palsy is a rare, debilitating, often transient complication following both anterior and posterior decompression surgery in the cervical spine [7, 11, 21, 25, 39, 53]. Suggested etiologies of iatrogenic C5 palsies include chronic cord ischemia secondary to compression with reperfusion injury following decompression, posterior migration of the spinal cord resulting in nerve root tethering, thermal damage due to nearby drilling, vascular compromise, or direct injury during screw insertion. Interestingly, C5 palsies often present in a delayed fashion following surgery confusing its etiology.

Neuromonitoring using SSEP, tcMEP, and S-EMG recordings from the deltoids and biceps has been used to detect intraoperative injury to the C5 nerve root [7, 21, 31, 34, 45], with at least one study citing a dramatic reduction in the incidence of C5 palsies [31]. However, while some have reported success with IONM monitoring for the detection of intraoperative C5 nerve injury [40], other studies have shown that delayed C5 palsy without IONM alerts is possible [18, 60, 63]. Unfortunately, as C5 palsies often present in a delayed fashion, the efficacy of multimodal IONM may be restricted in its utility for detection and prevention to injuries occurring during surgery [40, 60]. Similarly, identification and reporting on delayed C5 palsies may also contribute to lower-than-expected reported sensitivities with multimodal IONM recording [40].

Cervical Deformity

Cervical spine realignment through screw and rod systems is a widely accepted, safe, and efficacious surgical technique for the treatment of craniocervical, mid-cervical, or cervicothoracic deformity. However, the utility of IONM in cervical deformity has not been adequately defined as the majority of data is from small retrospective series and case reports. Similar to the efficacy of IONM in degenerative cervical myelopathy and radiculopathy, the presumed benefits in cervical deformity have been extrapolated from the successes in thoracolumbar deformity surgery [9, 47, 69].

Lateral mass and pedicle screw instrumentation of the cervical spine has evolved as a primary construct used in the posterior correction of cervical alignment. Stimulus-evoked pedicle screw EMG is a method used to detect a screw breach with the hopes of preventing or reversing injury of neural or vascular elements [16, 30, 71]. For each screw, the lowest current at which the first stimulus-evoked EMG response is observed and recorded. Low EMG thresholds have been shown to correlate to medial screw placement and as such may be an effective means to rule out medial placement of lateral mass screws [71]. The possibility of screw malposition warrants exploration, repositioning, or possibly removal depending on the pretest probability of a potentially dangerous screw placement [16].

Economics

The addition of neuromonitoring to degenerative cervical surgery has important financial implications. To date, cost-benefit analysis has not demonstrated significant benefits [19, 38, 64, 67]. As a result, some authors have argued that IONM for degenerative anterior cervical spine surgery has little utility when examined from a medical, cost-benefit, or medicolegal standpoint [1, 26, 67].

Traynelis et al. [67] reported no persistent postoperative neurological deficits in patients undergoing cervical spine surgery for symptomatic spondylosis without IONM in their economic analysis of 720 patients and estimated that they saved an hourly rate of $633.32 and a total of $1,024,754 in 2011 US dollars for reimbursement at the 2011 Medicare rate. The authors concluded that decompression and reconstruction/fusion for symptomatic cervical spine disease without IONM may reduce the cost of treatment without adversely impacting patient safety. This rationale stemmed from low rates of postoperative neurological deficits in combination with a million dollars of estimated additional costs.

Conclusion

Intraoperative neurophysiological monitoring (IONM) permits the evaluation of the functional integrity of the spinal cord and nerve roots and provides an opportunity to detect and possibly reverse neurological injury during high-risk spine surgery. As a result, IONM has become commonly used as a surgical adjunct in cases of degenerative cervical myelopathy and radiculopathy. In general, multimodality monitoring is preferred to maximize diagnostic potential, and current evidence suggests that this technique may improve detection of intraoperative neurological injury and outcomes. However, the efficacy of IONM may be restricted in "low-risk" anterior cervical spine surgery, cases of significant preoperative myelopathy and/or radiculopathy, and in the detection and prevention of delayed-onset C5 palsies. To date, data regarding the use of IONM have been primarily derived from retrospective studies of low methodological quality that are further limited by the heterogeneity that exists among various surgical procedures and their associated risks, the heterogeneity of IONM modalities and techniques, and availability of criteria for defining a significant alert. Furthermore, all studies to date suffer from strong selection bias, as election to use IONM is more strongly considered in patients with severe myelopathy and complex pathology where there is an intrinsic higher risk of neurologic injury. Consequently, there is no sufficient body of evidence in the literature to provide definitive answers regarding the utility of IONM in cervical spinal surgery.

References

1. Ajiboye RM, D'Oro A, Ashana AO, Buerba RA, Lord EL, Buser Z, et al. Routine use of intraoperative neuromonitoring during ACDFs for the treatment of Spondylotic myelopathy and radiculopathy is questionable: a review of 15,395 cases. Spine (Phila Pa 1976). 2017;42:14–9.
2. Ajiboye RM, Zoller SD, Sharma A, Mosich GM, Drysch A, Li J, et al. Intraoperative neuromonitoring for anterior cervical spine surgery: what is the evidence? Spine (Phila Pa 1976). 2017;42(6):385–93.
3. Andersson G, Ohlin A. Spatial facilitation of motor evoked responses in monitoring during spinal surgery. Clin Neurophysiol. 1999;110:720–4.
4. Appel S, Korn A, Biron T, Goldstein K, Rand N, Millgram M, et al. Efficacy of head repositioning in restoration of electrophysiological signals during cervical spine procedures. J Clin Neurophysiol. 2017;34(2):174–8.
5. Balzer JR, Rose RD, Welch WC, Sclabassi RJ. Simultaneous somatosensory evoked potential and electromyographic recordings during lumbosacral decompression and instrumentation. Neurosurgery. 1998;42:1318–24; discussion 1324–1315.
6. Beatty RM, McGuire P, Moroney JM, Holladay FP. Continuous intraoperative electromyographic recording during spinal surgery. J Neurosurg. 1995;82:401–5.
7. Bose B, Sestokas AK, Schwartz DM. Neurophysiological detection of iatrogenic C-5 nerve deficit during anterior cervical spinal surgery. J Neurosurg Spine. 2007;6:381–5.
8. Bose B, Sestokas AK, Schwartz DM. Neurophysiological monitoring of spinal cord function during instrumented anterior cervical fusion. Spine J. 2004;4:202–7.
9. Bridwell KH, Lenke LG, Baldus C, Blanke K. Major intraoperative neurologic deficits in pediatric and adult spinal deformity patients. Incidence and etiology at one institution. Spine (Phila Pa 1976). 1998;23:324–31.
10. Burke D, Hicks R, Stephen J, Woodforth I, Crawford M. Assessment of corticospinal and somatosensory conduction simultaneously during scoliosis surgery. Electroencephalogr Clin Neurophysiol. 1992;85:388–96.
11. Bydon M, Macki M, Kaloostian P, Sciubba DM, Wolinsky JP, Gokaslan ZL, et al. Incidence and prognostic factors of c5 palsy: a clinical study of 1001 cases and review of the literature. Neurosurgery. 2014;74:595–604; discussion 604–595.
12. Chen X, Sterio D, Ming X, Para DD, Butusova M, Tong T, et al. Success rate of motor evoked potentials for intraoperative neurophysiologic monitoring: effects of age, lesion location, and preoperative neurologic deficits. J Clin Neurophysiol. 2007;24:281–5.
13. Clark AJ, Ziewacz JE, Safaee M, Lau D, Lyon R, Chou D, et al. Intraoperative neuromonitoring with MEPs and prediction of postoperative neurological deficits in patients undergoing surgery for cervical and cervicothoracic myelopathy. Neurosurg Focus. 2013;35:E7.
14. Cole T, Veeravagu A, Zhang M, Li A, Ratliff JK. Intraoperative neuromonitoring in single-level spinal procedures: a retrospective propensity score-matched analysis in a national longitudinal database. Spine (Phila Pa 1976). 2014;39:1950–9.
15. Devlin VJ, Schwartz DM. Intraoperative neurophysiologic monitoring during spinal surgery. J Am Acad Orthop Surg. 2007;15:549–60.
16. Djurasovic M, Dimar JR 2nd, Glassman SD, Edmonds HL, Carreon LY. A prospective analysis of intraoperative electromyographic monitoring of posterior cervical screw fixation. J Spinal Disord Tech. 2005;18:515–8.
17. Eager M, Shimer A, Jahangiri FR, Shen F, Arlet V. Intraoperative neurophysiological monitoring (IONM): lessons learned from 32 case events in 2069 spine cases. Am J Electroneurodiagnostic Technol. 2011;51:247–63.
18. Eggspuehler A, Sutter MA, Grob D, Jeszenszky D, Porchet F, Dvorak J. Multimodal intraoperative monitoring (MIOM) during cervical spine surgical procedures in 246 patients. Eur Spine J. 2007;16(Suppl 2):S209–15.
19. Epstein NE, Danto J, Nardi D. Evaluation of intraoperative somatosensory-evoked potential monitoring during 100 cervical operations. Spine (Phila Pa 1976). 1993;18:737–47.
20. Epstein NE, Stecker MM. Intraoperative neuromonitoring corner editorial: the need for preoperative sep and mep baselines in spinal surgery: why can't we and our monitoring colleagues get this right? Surg Neurol Int. 2014;5:S548–51.
21. Fan D, Schwartz DM, Vaccaro AR, Hilibrand AS, Albert TJ. Intraoperative neurophysiologic detection of iatrogenic C5 nerve root injury during laminectomy for cervical compression myelopathy. Spine (Phila Pa 1976). 2002;27:2499–502.

22. Flynn TB. Neurologic complications of anterior cervical discectomy in Louisiana. J La State Med Soc. 1984;136:6–8.
23. Garcia RM, Qureshi SA, Cassinelli EH, Biro CL, Furey CG, Bohlman HH. Detection of postoperative neurologic deficits using somatosensory-evoked potentials alone during posterior cervical laminoplasty. Spine J. 2010;10:890–5.
24. Gunnarsson T, Krassioukov AV, Sarjeant R, Fehlings MG. Real-time continuous intraoperative electromyographic and somatosensory evoked potential recordings in spinal surgery: correlation of clinical and electrophysiologic findings in a prospective, consecutive series of 213 cases. Spine (Phila Pa 1976). 2004;29:677–84.
25. Guzman JZ, Baird EO, Fields AC, McAnany SJ, Qureshi SA, Hecht AC, et al. C5 nerve root palsy following decompression of the cervical spine: a systematic evaluation of the literature. Bone Joint J. 2014;96-B:950–5.
26. Harel R, Knoller N, Regev G, Anekstein Y, Zaaroor M, Leitner J, et al. The value of neuromonitoring in cervical spine surgery. Surg Neurol Int. 2014;5:120.
27. Hilibrand AS, Schwartz DM, Sethuraman V, Vaccaro AR, Albert TJ. Comparison of transcranial electric motor and somatosensory evoked potential monitoring during cervical spine surgery. J Bone Joint Surg Am. 2004;86-A:1248–53.
28. Houlden D. Immediate detection of somatosensory evoked potential loss is necessary to prevent neurological deficits. Clin Neurophysiol. 2013;124:836.
29. Hyun SJ, Rhim SC, Kang JK, Hong SH, Park BR. Combined motor- and somatosensory-evoked potential monitoring for spine and spinal cord surgery: correlation of clinical and neurophysiological data in 85 consecutive procedures. Spinal Cord. 2009;47:616–22.
30. Isley MR, Zhang XF, Balzer JR, Leppanen RE. Current trends in pedicle screw stimulation techniques: lumbosacral, thoracic, and cervical levels. Neurodiagn J. 2012;52:100–75.
31. Jimenez JC, Sani S, Braverman B, Deutsch H, Ratliff JK. Palsies of the fifth cervical nerve root after cervical decompression: prevention using continuous intraoperative electromyography monitoring. J Neurosurg Spine. 2005;3:92–7.
32. Journee HL, Polak HE, De Kleuver M. Conditioning stimulation techniques for enhancement of transcranially elicited evoked motor responses. Neurophysiol Clin. 2007;37:423–30.
33. Journee HL, Polak HE, de Kleuver M, Langeloo DD, Postma AA. Improved neuromonitoring during spinal surgery using double-train transcranial electrical stimulation. Med Biol Eng Comput. 2004;42:110–3.
34. Kelleher MO, Tan G, Sarjeant R, Fehlings MG. Predictive value of intraoperative neurophysiological monitoring during cervical spine surgery: a prospective analysis of 1055 consecutive patients. J Neurosurg Spine. 2008;8:215–21.
35. Khan MH, Smith PN, Balzer JR, Crammond D, Welch WC, Gerszten P, et al. Intraoperative somatosensory evoked potential monitoring during cervical spine corpectomy surgery: experience with 508 cases. Spine (Phila Pa 1976). 2006;31:E105–13.
36. Kim DH, Zaremski J, Kwon B, Jenis L, Woodard E, Bode R, et al. Risk factors for false positive transcranial motor evoked potential monitoring alerts during surgical treatment of cervical myelopathy. Spine (Phila Pa 1976). 2007;32:3041–6.
37. Klem GH, Luders HO, Jasper HH, Elger C. The ten-twenty electrode system of the International Federation. The International Federation of Clinical Neurophysiology. Electroencephalogr Clin Neurophysiol Suppl. 1999;52:3–6.
38. Lall RR, Lall RR, Hauptman JS, Munoz C, Cybulski GR, Koski T, et al. Intraoperative neurophysiological monitoring in spine surgery: indications, efficacy, and role of the preoperative checklist. Neurosurg Focus. 2012;33:E10.
39. Lawrence BD, Jacobs WB, Norvell DC, Hermsmeyer JT, Chapman JR, Brodke DS. Anterior versus posterior approach for treatment of cervical spondylotic myelopathy: a systematic review. Spine (Phila Pa 1976). 2013;38:S173–82.
40. Lee HJ, Kim IS, Sung JH, Lee SW, Hong JT. Significance of multimodal intraoperative monitoring for the posterior cervical spine surgery. Clin Neurol Neurosurg. 2016;143:9–14.
41. Lee JM, Kim DH, Kim HS, Choi BK, Han IH. The applicability of intraoperative neuromonitoring in patients with preoperative motor weakness during spine surgery. Korean J Spine. 2016;13:9–12.
42. Lee JY, Hilibrand AS, Lim MR, Zavatsky J, Zeiller S, Schwartz DM, et al. Characterization of neurophysiologic alerts during anterior cervical spine surgery. Spine (Phila Pa 1976). 2006;31:1916–22.
43. Li F, Gorji R, Allott G, Modes K, Lunn R, Yang ZJ. The usefulness of intraoperative neurophysiological monitoring in cervical spine surgery: a retrospective analysis of 200 consecutive patients. J Neurosurg Anesthesiol. 2012;24:185–90.
44. MacDonald DB, Al Zayed Z, Khoudeir I, Stigsby B. Monitoring scoliosis surgery with combined multiple pulse transcranial electric motor and cortical somatosensory-evoked potentials from the lower and upper extremities. Spine (Phila Pa 1976). 2003;28:194–203.
45. May DM, Jones SJ, Crockard HA. Somatosensory evoked potential monitoring in cervical surgery: identification of pre- and intraoperative risk factors associated with neurological deterioration. J Neurosurg. 1996;85:566–73.
46. Nanda A, Sharma M, Sonig A, Ambekar S, Bollam P. Surgical complications of anterior cervical diskectomy and fusion for cervical degenerative disk disease: a single surgeon's experience of 1,576 patients. World Neurosurg. 2014;82:1380–7.
47. Nash CL Jr, Lorig RA, Schatzinger LA, Brown RH. Spinal cord monitoring during operative

treatment of the spine. Clin Orthop Relat Res. 1977:(126);100–5.
48. Nichols GS, Manafov E. Utility of electromyography for nerve root monitoring during spinal surgery. J Clin Neurophysiol. 2012;29:140–8.
49. Owen JH, Kostuik JP, Gornet M, Petr M, Skelly J, Smoes C, et al. The use of mechanically elicited electromyograms to protect nerve roots during surgery for spinal degeneration. Spine (Phila Pa 1976). 1994;19:1704–10.
50. Owen JH, Laschinger J, Bridwell K, Shimon S, Nielsen C, Dunlap J, et al. Sensitivity and specificity of somatosensory and neurogenic-motor evoked potentials in animals and humans. Spine (Phila Pa 1976). 1988;13:1111–8.
51. Pease M, Gandhoke GS, Kaur J, Thirumala P, Balzer J, Crammond D, et al. 319 predictive value of intraoperative neurophysiological monitoring during spine surgery: a prospective analysis of 4489 consecutive patients. Neurosurgery. 2016;63(Suppl 1):192–3.
52. Resnick DK, Anderson PA, Kaiser MG, Groff MW, Heary RF, Holly LT, et al. Electrophysiological monitoring during surgery for cervical degenerative myelopathy and radiculopathy. J Neurosurg Spine. 2009;11:245–52.
53. Sakaura H, Hosono N, Mukai Y, Ishii T, Yoshikawa H. C5 palsy after decompression surgery for cervical myelopathy: review of the literature. Spine (Phila Pa 1976). 2003;28:2447–51.
54. Sala F, Palandri G, Basso E, Lanteri P, Deletis V, Faccioli F, et al. Motor evoked potential monitoring improves outcome after surgery for intramedullary spinal cord tumors: a historical control study. Neurosurgery. 2006;58:1129–43; discussion 1129–1143.
55. Schirmer CM, Shils JL, Arle JE, Cosgrove GR, Dempsey PK, Tarlov E, et al. Heuristic map of myotomal innervation in humans using direct intraoperative nerve root stimulation. J Neurosurg Spine. 2011;15:64–70.
56. Schwartz DM, Auerbach JD, Dormans JP, Flynn J, Drummond DS, Bowe JA, et al. Neurophysiological detection of impending spinal cord injury during scoliosis surgery. J Bone Joint Surg Am. 2007;89: 2440–9.
57. Schwartz DM, Sestokas AK, Dormans JP, Vaccaro AR, Hilibrand AS, Flynn JM, et al. Transcranial electric motor evoked potential monitoring during spine surgery: is it safe? Spine (Phila Pa 1976). 2011;36:1046–9.
58. Schwartz DM, Sestokas AK, Hilibrand AS, Vaccaro AR, Bose B, Li M, et al. Neurophysiological identification of position-induced neurologic injury during anterior cervical spine surgery. J Clin Monit Comput. 2006;20:437–44.
59. Smith PN, Balzer JR, Khan MH, Davis RA, Crammond D, Welch WC, et al. Intraoperative somatosensory evoked potential monitoring during anterior cervical discectomy and fusion in nonmyelopathic patients--a review of 1,039 cases. Spine J. 2007;7:83–7.
60. Spitz S, Felbaum D, Aghdam N, Sandhu F. Delayed postoperative C5 root palsy and the use of neurophysiologic monitoring. Eur Spine J. 2015;24:2866–71.
61. Sutter M, Eggspuehler A, Grob D, Jeszenszky D, Benini A, Porchet F, et al. The diagnostic value of multimodal intraoperative monitoring (MIOM) during spine surgery: a prospective study of 1,017 patients. Eur Spine J. 2007;16(Suppl 2):S162–70.
62. Sutter M, Eggspuehler A, Grob D, Jeszenszky D, Benini A, Porchet F, et al. The validity of multimodal intraoperative monitoring (MIOM) in surgery of 109 spine and spinal cord tumors. Eur Spine J. 2007;16(Suppl 2):S197–208.
63. Tanaka N, Nakanishi K, Fujiwara Y, Kamei N, Ochi M. Postoperative segmental C5 palsy after cervical laminoplasty may occur without intraoperative nerve injury: a prospective study with transcranial electric motor-evoked potentials. Spine (Phila Pa 1976). 2006;31:3013–7.
64. Taunt CJ Jr, Sidhu KS, Andrew SA. Somatosensory evoked potential monitoring during anterior cervical discectomy and fusion. Spine (Phila Pa 1976). 2005;30:1970–2.
65. Thirumala PD, Huang J, Thiagarajan K, Cheng H, Balzer J, Crammond DJ. Diagnostic accuracy of combined multimodality somatosensory evoked potential and transcranial motor evoked potential intraoperative monitoring in patients with idiopathic scoliosis. Spine (Phila Pa 1976). 2016;41:E1177–84.
66. Toleikis JR, Skelly JP, Carlvin AO, Burkus JK. Spinally elicited peripheral nerve responses are sensory rather than motor. Clin Neurophysiol. 2000;111:736–42.
67. Traynelis VC, Abode-Iyamah KO, Leick KM, Bender SM, Greenlee JD. Cervical decompression and reconstruction without intraoperative neurophysiological monitoring. J Neurosurg Spine. 2012;16:107–13.
68. Vauzelle C, Stagnara P, Jouvinroux P. Functional monitoring of spinal cord activity during spinal surgery. Clin Orthop Relat Res. 1973;93:173–8.
69. Vitale MG, Skaggs DL, Pace GI, Wright ML, Matsumoto H, Anderson RC, et al. Best practices in intraoperative neuromonitoring in spine deformity surgery: development of an intraoperative checklist to optimize response. Spine Deform. 2014;2:333–9.
70. Wang S, Tian Y. Exploration of the intraoperative motor evoked potential. Spine (Phila Pa 1976). 2016;41:470–5.
71. Wilson B, Curtis E, Hirshman B, Oygar A, Chen K, Gabel BC, et al. Lateral mass screw stimulation thresholds in posterior cervical instrumentation surgery: a predictor of medial deviation. J Neurosurg Spine. 2016:26(3):346–52. doi 10.3171.2016.8.SPINE16580. Epub 2016 Dec 9.
72. Ziewacz JE, Berven SH, Mummaneni VP, Tu TH, Akinbo OC, Lyon R, et al. The design, development, and implementation of a checklist for intraoperative neuromonitoring changes. Neurosurg Focus. 2012;33:E11.

Factors Predictive of Operative Outcome

15

Jerry Ku and Jefferson R. Wilson

Pearls/Pitfalls Outline

- On average, patients with degenerative cervical myelopathy (DCM) seem to experience clinical deterioration over time.
- At a patient level, there is variability in the clinical course. As a result there is a need to identify patient-specific features that predict long-term postoperative outcomes for DCM patients.
- With respect to clinical variables, there is consistency throughout the literature that increased age, worsened preoperative functional status, longer duration of preoperative symptoms, smoking, and the presence of psychiatric comorbidities are associated with reduced potential for postoperative functional recovery.
- The literature surrounding the predictive importance of MRI and electrophysiological tests is less consistent; specific variables and tests are discussed in detail.
- A combination of important clinical variables has been used to create a well-validated clinical prediction rule, enabling clinicians and researchers to estimate postoperative outcomes for DCM patients undergoing surgery.

J. Ku · J. R. Wilson (✉)
Division of Neurosurgery, St. Michael's Hospital, University of Toronto, Toronto, ON, Canada
e-mail: wilsonjeff@smh.ca

Introduction

Thenatural history of degenerative cervical myelopathy (DCM) is usually one of a slow, stepwise decline, with a minority of patients experiencing periods of quiescence or even subtle clinical improvement with nonoperative treatment over time [1]. Surgical intervention, on average, has convincingly shown to improve neurological outcomes, functional status, and quality of life in DCM patients, regardless of the severity of preoperative functional status [2]. As a result, surgery remains the preferred treatment approach for this patient population. That said, at the individual patient level, postoperative outcomes continue to be variable. As such, surgeons should be aware of the factors which predict operative outcome; such knowledge is essential to aid preoperative communications and to manage patient expectations for recovery in the short and long term.

M. G. Kaiser et al. (eds.), *Degenerative Cervical Myelopathy and Radiculopathy*,
https://doi.org/10.1007/978-3-319-97952-6_15

Based on current studies, the preoperative factors found predictive of postoperative outcome include age, duration and severity of symptoms, gait and sexual dysfunction, smoking history, psychiatric history, sensory evoked potentials (SEPs), and certain magnetic resonance imaging (MRI) findings. The evidence and rationale for each of these will be described in detail in this chapter. Factors which have not been found to be predictive of postoperative outcome, or those of unclear significance, include gender, race, other specific signs and symptoms, other comorbid conditions, and motor evoked potentials (MEPs).

Age

Age has been a commonly investigated predictive factor for patients with DCM undergoing surgical intervention. Unfortunately, inconsistencies in study design make inter-study comparisons and generalizations difficult, including different thresholds for age dichotomization (e.g., 40 versus 60 versus 70) and differences in outcome measures considered and in the duration of follow-up. Recently, Tetreault et al. [3] found that increasing age was associated with reduced odds of an optimal postsurgical neurologic outcome at 1 year postoperatively, as defined as mJOA score greater or equal to 16 (OR 0.96, 95% CI 0.94–0.99). Additionally, patients with increasing age were also found to be less likely to experience a minimally clinically important difference, as seen as an improvement on the mJOA score at 2 years postoperatively of 3 points for severe myelopathy, 2 for moderate myelopathy, and 1 for mild myelopathy (RR = 0.924, 95% CI 0.889–0.960) [4]. Similarly, Morio et al. [5] found that increasing age was inversely related with recovery rate, as defined by the change in JOA score at mean follow-up of 3.4 years postoperatively. Overall, systematic reviews have demonstrated that the majority of studies have shown a negative relationship between age and postoperative functional and neurological outcome as measured by the change in Nurick, JOA, or mJOA score pre- and postoperatively, with the strength of association in these studies ranging from weak to moderate, with R-values between −0.28 and − 0.65 [6, 7].

As such, surgeons should be aware that advancing age may negatively affect postoperative functional outcomes in patients. Elderly patients may not be able to translate neurological recovery to functional improvements as well as the younger population. Age-related changes in the spinal cord, including a decrease in c-motor neurons, the number of anterior horn cells, and the number of myelinated fibers in the cortical spinal tracts and posterior columns, may be the anatomical and pathophysiological correlates behind this clinical observation [6]. Furthermore, the presence of unassociated comorbidities may affect outcome or their ability to conduct all activities on a certain functional scale [6]. Lastly, in addition to its impact on functional outcomes, increasing age has also been found to be associated with higher risk of perioperative complications [8].

Duration and Severity of Symptoms

Other commonly investigated predictive variables include the duration and severity of symptoms. Tetreault et al. [3] found that longer duration of symptoms was associated with reduced odds of an optimal postsurgical outcome at 1 year postoperatively, as defined as mJOA score greater or equal to 16 (OR 0.76, 95% CI 0.59–0.99). Similarly, patients with longer duration of symptoms were also less likely to experience a minimally clinically important difference on their mJOA score at 2 years postoperatively (RR 0.943) [4]. Kusin et al. [9] found that the duration of symptoms greater than 2 years had a negative influence on the change in Nurick score at 2 years postoperatively. Systematic reviews have also confirmed this relationship, as multiple studies have noted that longer duration of symptoms is related to worse functional postsurgical outcome as measured by the Nurick, JOA, or mJOA score, with the strength of the relationship ranging from weak to strong in various studies, with R-values between −0.225 and − 0.82 [6, 7]. Study designs have varied from assessing the duration of preoperative symptoms as a continuous variable, separating duration into discrete time groups (<3 months, 3–6 months, 6–12 months, 12–24 months, >24 months), or dichotomizing patients to symptom duration greater or lesser than 1 or 2 years [7].

The severity of DCM symptoms on presentation has also been found to be a negative predictor of postoperative functional outcome. Tetreault et al. [3] also found that higher mJOA score was associated with increased odds of an optimal postsurgical outcome at 1 year postoperatively, as defined as mJOA score greater or equal to 16 (OR 1.21, 95% CI 1.07–1.37). Similarly, Alafifi et al. [10] found that higher preoperative impairment, as measured by the Nurick score, was associated with a lower likelihood of improving on the Nurick score postoperatively, with a mean follow-up of 2.5 years. Systematic reviews have also found that preoperative severity of symptoms as demonstrated by mJOA, JOA, or Nurick scores had a weak to strong relationship with functional outcome, with R-values ranging from 0.22 to 0.93 [6, 7].

Pathological studies have shown that severe and/or chronic, long-standing DCM leads to demyelination of white matter and necrosis of both gray and white matter [1]. This likely limits the potential for recovery following operative intervention as these changes may not be fully reversible despite surgical correction of the compression. Given that worse severity and longer duration of symptoms are related to unfavorable postoperative functional outcomes, surgeons should keep these clinical factors in mind when deciding to offer a surgical versus watchful waiting approach to management for patients with DCM.

Specific Signs and Symptoms

There has also been some research interest in determining whether the presence of specific signs or symptoms may be predictive of operative outcome. One such variable is gait impairment. One analysis of a multicenter cohort study found that preoperative gait dysfunction was associated with a decreased likelihood of attaining an mJOA score greater or equal to 16 at 1 year postoperatively, with an odds ratio of 2.48 (95% CI 1.10–5.57) [3]. Similarly, Alafifi et al. [10] found that the presence of leg spasticity was associated with a lower likelihood of improving on the Nurick score postoperatively, with a mean follow-up of 2.5 years. In addition, patients who presented with a broad-based unstable gait were less likely to experience a minimally clinically important difference on their mJOA score at 2 years postoperatively (RR 0.869) [4]. A systematic review also found the presence of gait or leg spasticity was predictive of worse functional outcome in three out of four studies, with the other study not finding a significant relationship [6]. This review also found four cohort studies which showed that the presence of sexual dysfunction is also a negative predictor of postoperative functional outcome as measured by Nurick, JOA, or neurosurgical spine scale [6]. It is plausible that gait and sexual dysfunction are markers of more severe or long-standing DCM, which is the major underlying predictive factor.

Conversely, no strong evidence exists that supports the relationship between other specific signs or symptoms and operative outcome. Most have been found to have unclear significance, or there have been conflicting results in different studies. These include lower extremity dysfunction, upper extremity dysfunction, bowel/bladder dysfunction, Hoffman's sign, Babinski sign, clonus, atrophy, radicular pain, cervical range of motion, and long tract signs [6]. More research is required to determine whether specific signs and symptoms may be predictive of operative outcome and whether any associations are indeed independent variables or merely a reflection of the severity or duration of disease.

Comorbid Conditions

Certain comorbid conditions have also been found to be predictive of operative outcome. One multicenter cohort study found that a patient who smokes is less likely to have a successful postoperative functional outcome than a nonsmoker, as defined by mJOA score of 16 or more at 2 years postoperatively (OR 0.50, 95% CI 0.22–1.14) [3]. In addition, smokers were less likely to experience a minimally clinically important difference on their mJOA score at 2 years postoperatively (RR 0.837) [4]. Kusin et al. [9] also found that on average, smokers improved by 0.6 points on the Nurick score at 2 years postoperatively, whereas nonsmokers improved by 1.53 points. This study also demonstrated a negative association between packs per day and change in Nurick score, as well as pack years and change in Nurick score [9]. Smoking has been correlated with lower rates of bony fusion and higher rates of wound infections and may also have a directly toxic effect on the intrinsic healing capability of the spinal cord [9].

Arnold et al. [11] found that there was no difference in surgical complication rates or in the level of improvement in mJOA and Nurick scores at 1 and 2 years postoperatively between patients with diabetes and patients without diabetes, though diabetic patients experienced less improvement in the SF36v2 physical functioning scale. On the other hand, Kim et al. [12] found that the presence of diabetes was a significant risk factor for a poor postoperative outcome (OR 2.92, 95% CI 1.32–6.12), as defined by lack of improvement in JOA score at 2 years postoperatively, and that the interaction of diabetes with smoking or with age increased that risk even further. Kusin et al. [9] also found that the presence of diabetes had a negative influence on the postoperative functional outcome, as defined by improvement in Nurick score 2 years postoperatively.

Tetreault et al. [3] found that the presence of psychiatric comorbidities was associated with a decreased likelihood of an optimal postsurgical outcome at 1 year postoperatively, as defined as mJOA score greater or equal to 16 (OR 0.33, 95% CI 0.15–0.69). A systematic review showed that the presence of any comorbid condition has not been found to be related to a worse postoperative functional outcome and that there is conflicting evidence whether the number of comorbid conditions would predict worse postoperative functional outcomes [6].

Currently, the evidence states that smoking status is a negative predictive factor of postoperative functional outcome, whereas the evidence surrounding diabetes is conflicting. In terms of complications, a systematic review did not find smoking status, diabetes, or other comorbidities to be associated with increased risk for perioperative complications [8]. Again, this is an area that requires more research, but surgeons should be aware that certain comorbid conditions may have an effect on operative outcome.

Neurophysiologic Testing

Neurophysiological techniques such as sensory evoked potentials (SEPs), motor evoked potentials (MEPs), and electromyography (EMG) may be used during the workup of DCM in assessing the level and severity of disease, supplementing clinical examination and neuroimaging findings [13]. There has also been research interest as to whether these neurophysiologic tests may be predictive of postoperative outcome as well.

Lyu et al. [14] found that normal median nerve SEPs preoperatively were correlated with an increased recovery rate, as defined by the change in mJOA at 6 months postoperatively. Additionally, a systematic review found three studies that showed that in patients with preoperative median nerve abnormalities, early postoperative normalization of SEPs within 1 or 2 weeks also predicted postoperative functional improvement [7]. Interestingly, this relationship was only true for median nerve SEPs, as tibial nerve SEPs have not been found to be correlated with operative outcome [7]. MEPs and EMGs, on the other hand, are well correlated with clinical and neuroimaging findings and may be used in predicting the development of myelopathy in minimally symptomatic patients or to quantify clinical improvement, but there is no supporting evidence for their predictive value in operative outcome [7, 13].

MEPS are more sensitive than SEP in detecting myelopathy [13, 14], likely due to the anatomical positioning of the ventrolateral versus the dorsal columns. In DCM, the most common pathology involves cervical disks bulging posteriorly into the spinal canal causing reduction in the anteroposterior diameter of the spinal cord and decreased vascular supply due to compression of the anterior spinal artery [14]. As such, abnormal SEPs may indicate a more severe compression of the spinal cord in comparison to abnormal MEPs alone and thus would subsequently lead to less favorable functional outcomes postoperatively.

Magnetic Resonance Imaging

Magnetic resonance imaging (MRI) is a ubiquitous imaging modality utilized in the assessment of DCM. In addition to its diagnostic utility, certain MRI parameters may also play a role in predicting postoperative outcome. These fall into the categories of measurements of canal/spinal cord dimensions or assessment of T1 and/or T2 signal change and have been widely studied for the potential predictive utility.

The degree of spinal cord compression may be assessed through various methods, including qualitative measures such as canal flattening or narrowing or the shape of the spinal cord on cross-sectional or midsagittal views, but these have not been found to hold predictive value [15]. More recently, there has been greater focus on quantitative techniques via the measurement of the anteroposterior diameter, transverse area (TA), or compression ratio of the spinal cord [15]. It was initially reported by Fukushima et al. [16] that a preoperative MRI finding of TA of the spinal cord less than 45 mm^2 at the site of maximum compression was associated with worse recovery rate, as defined by the change in JOA score with a mean follow-up of 1 year and 5 months, despite morphologic restoration of the spinal canal following decompressive surgery. Conversely, Morio et al. [5] did not find a significant relationship between TA and recovery rate, as defined by the change in JOA score at mean follow-up of 3.4 years postoperatively. Systematic reviews have found that most subsequent studies have agreed that TA is predictive of postoperative functional outcome, although other studies have found no significant relationship [15, 17, 18]. It is possible that this discrepancy is secondary to the limitations of TA, as it is a measure of single point of maximal compression, whereas DCM is a multilevel disease with varying degrees of compression at different levels. Another measurement is maximum canal compromise (MCC), as defined by measuring the greatest reduction of spinal canal diameter on midsagittal views compared to nonreduced diameters from above and below, and greater MCC has been shown by Nouri et al. [19] to be predictive of a poorer postsurgical functional outcome, as defined by mJOA score not improving to 16 or more at 6 months postoperatively. Other quantitative techniques have not been shown to be predictive factors [15, 17, 18].

Assessment of signal intensity change within the spinal cord on T1- and/or T2-weighted imaging has also been evaluated as a possible prognostic indicator. These changes are thought to indicate severity of compression, chronicity of disease, and irreversibility. There are conflicting studies as to whether the presence of T2 hyperintensity by itself is a predictive factor of postoperative functional recovery [15, 17]. T2 signal changes are non-specific and may be seen in reversible edema or ischemia but may also reflect irreversible changes. Diffuse borders of T2 signal change indicate milder changes such as edema, demyelination, or Wallerian degeneration, whereas sharper borders are associated with more severe histological changes of necrosis, microcavitation, or spongiform changes [15]. Unfortunately, there is no current standard in grading or classifying the degree of T2 signal change [18]. Specifically, the MRI finding of irreversible gray matter necrosis, or "snake-eye appearance," is associated with poorer postoperative functional outcome, as defined by JOA score recovery rate [20]. Fernandez de Rota et al. [21] found that while focal T2 signal change was not significantly associated with mJOA recovery rate at mean follow-up of 39 months, the presence of multi-segmental T2 hyperintensity changes was predictive of a poorer postoperative functional outcome.

Systematic reviews have found that most studies have agreed that T1 hypointensity signal change, on the other hand, is correlated with poorer postoperative functional outcome [15, 17]. Specifically, Nouri et al. [19] also found T1 hypointensity to be predictive of a poorer postsurgical functional outcome, as defined by mJOA score not improving to greater or equal to 16 at 6 months postoperatively (OR 0.242, 95% CI 0.068–0.866). Similarly, Alafifi et al. [10] found that low intramedullary signal on T1 imaging was predictive of a lower likelihood of improving on the Nurick score postoperatively, with a mean follow-up of 2.5 years. Morio et al. [5] also found that T1 low signal intensity changes on preoperative MRI were predictive of a poorer recovery rate, as defined by the change in JOA score at mean follow-up of 3.4 years postoperatively. T1 signal changes are thought to reflect more severe and irreversible damage to neural tissue, infarction, and cavitation, leading to a less favorable clinical outcome [22].

Overall, given the routine use of MRI in the diagnosis of DCM, careful review and assessment of specific parameters including TA, MCC, and signal change can provide some insight into operative outcome. Specifically, signal changes within the cord that reflect more severe or irreversible damage to the spinal cord are unsurprisingly predictive of poorer postsurgical functional recovery.

Clinical Prediction Rule

There has been some interest in the development of clinical prediction rules to determine operative outcome. A recent study done on an international level utilized clinical factors (see Table 15.1) to develop a clinical prediction tool (see Fig. 15.1). This tool was found to have good ability to discriminate between patients who will have optimal outcome and those who will not, with strong internal and external validity, using clinical factors alone [3]. The addition of MRI parameters did not significantly improve the prediction model [23].

Table 15.1 Odds ratio of clinical factors predictive of operative outcome, defined as attainment of mJOA score 16 or greater at 1 year postoperatively

Predictor	Odds ratio	95% Confidence interval
Age	0.96	0.94–0.99
Baseline mJOA score	1.21	1.07–1.37
Duration of symptoms	0.76	0.59–0.99
Impaired gait	2.48	1.10–5.57
Smoking status	0.50	0.22–1.14
Psychiatric disorder	0.44	0.22–0.88

Adapted from Tetreault et al. [3]
OR odds ratio

$$P=\frac{e^{1.59+(-0.81)P+(0.19)\mathrm{mJOA}+(-0.036)A+(0.91)\mathrm{IG}+(-0.69)S+(-0.27)\mathrm{DS}}}{1+e^{1.59+(-0.81)P+(0.19)\mathrm{mJOA}+(-0.036)A+(0.91)\mathrm{IG}+(-0.69)S+(-0.27)\mathrm{DS}}},$$

Fig. 15.1 Clinical prediction rule adapted from Tetreault et al. [3] of the probability of a postoperative mJOA score greater or equal to 16. Abbreviations: A age in years, DS duration of symptoms (1, ≤3 months; 2, >3, ≤6 months; 3, >6, ≤12 months; 4, >12, ≤24 months; 5, >24 months), IG impaired gait (1, present; 2, absent), mJOA0 baseline modified Japanese Orthopaedic Association score (0–18), Ps depression or bipolar disorder (1, absent; 2, present), S smoking status (1, nonsmoker; 2, smoker)

Case Presentations

Below is excerpted with permission from Tetreault et al. [24].

The following two cases demonstrate how predicting outcome before surgery can aid in managing expectations.

- Case 1: A 49-year-old nonsmoking man presented with moderate myelopathy (mJOA = 14) secondary to spondylosis, disk herniation, and congenital stenosis. This patient had numb and clumsy hands, muscular weakness, corticospinal motor deficits, hyperreflexia, and upgoing plantar responses. The duration of symptoms was 2 months. The patient also had coexisting moderate hypertension, mild respiratory disease, and mild diabetes.
- Case 2: A 69-year-old nonsmoking man presented with moderate myelopathy (mJOA = 13) secondary to spondylosis, disk herniation, and

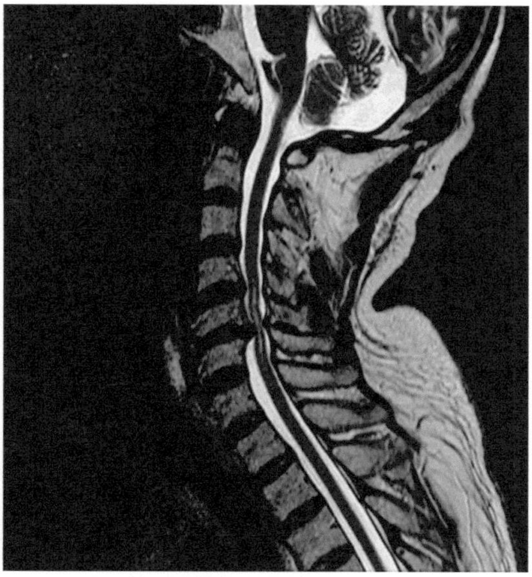

Fig. 15.2 Sagittal T2-weighted MRI of case 2 [24]

hypertrophied ligamentum flavum (Fig. 15.2). This patient had numb and clumsy hands, an impaired gait, muscular weakness, corticospinal distribution motor deficits, hyperreflexia, a positive Hoffman sign, upgoing plantar responses, and a broad-based unstable gait. The duration of symptoms was 120 months. The patient had a mild stroke.

Table 15.2 Case examples and applications of the clinical prediction rule [24]

Case no.	Patient information to be entered into Eq. 1	Probability of achieving an mJOA score ≥ 16 (%)
1	mJOA0 = 14, *DS* = 1, *S* = 1, *Ps* = 1, *IG* = 2, *A* = 49	92.7
2	mJOA0 = 13, *DS* = 5, *S* = 1, *Ps* = 1, *IG* = 1, *A* = 69	41.0
3	mJOA0 = 17, *DS* = 2, *S* = 1, *Ps* = 1, *IG* = 2, *A* = 53 versus **mJOA0 = 15**, ***DS* = 4**, *S* = 1, *Ps* = 1, *IG* = 2, ***A* = 54** versus mJOA0 = 15, *DS* = 4, *S* = 1, *Ps* = 1, ***IG* = 1**, *A* = 54	93.6 85.0 69.6
4	mJOA0 = 15, *DS* = 5, *S* = 1, *Ps* = 1, *IG* = 2, *A* = 62	76.4

Note: **Bolded** values indicate a change from the patient's original information

Abbreviations: A, age in years; *DS* duration of symptoms (1, ≤3 months; 2, >3, ≤6 months; 3, >6, ≤12 months; 4, >12, ≤24 months; 5, >24 months), *IG* impaired gait (1, present; 2, absent), *mJOA0* baseline modified Japanese Orthopaedic Association score (0–18), *Ps* depression or bipolar disorder (1, absent; 2, present), *S* smoking status (1, nonsmoker; 2, smoker)

Based on estimates computed by Eq. 1, case 1 has a 92.7% chance of improving to an mJOA score ≥16, whereas case 2 only has a 41.0% chance of achieving this outcome (see Table 15.2). These patients should be managed differently during the surgical consent process. The attending surgeon should inform both patients that they are likely to improve following surgery but should notify case 2 that he will still have substantial residual neurologic deficit and may require assistance with activities of daily living. This information will help manage case 2's expectations of outcome and, in turn, help to improve his overall satisfaction. With respect to the observed outcome, case 1 was neurologically normal postoperatively (mJOA = 18), whereas case 2 improved from 13 to 15 but did not reach a score ≥16.

Case 3 provides an example how a CPR can be used to facilitate shared decision-making and to counsel concerned patients as to potential options.

- Case 3: A 53-year-old nonsmoking man presented with mild myelopathy (mJOA = 17) secondary to spondylosis and disk herniation (Fig. 15.3). This patient had numb and clumsy hands, bilateral arm paresthesia, muscular weakness, and atrophy of intrinsic hand muscles. The duration of symptoms was 4 months. The patient had unspecified endocrine comorbidities.

This case is an example of a patient with mild myelopathy and a short preoperative duration of symptoms. This patient has an excellent surgi-

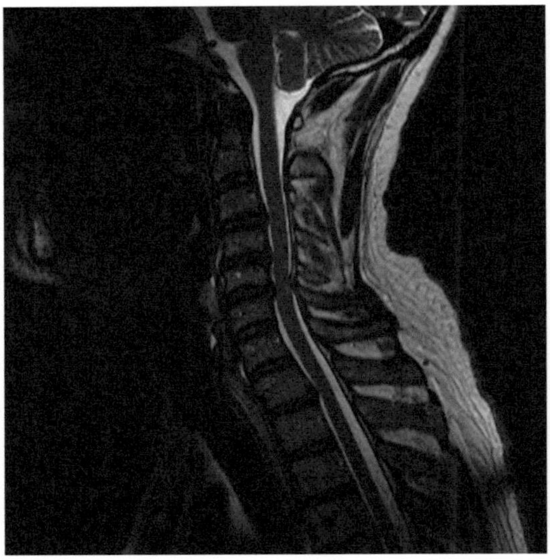

Fig. 15.3 Sagittal T2-weighted MRI of case 3 [24]

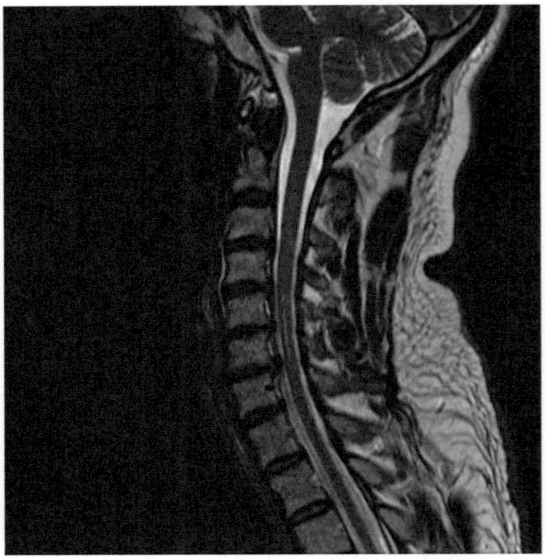

Fig. 15.4 Sagittal T2-weighted MRI of case 4 [24]

cal prognosis; however, he may be reluctant to consent to neurosurgery for such mild upper limb symptoms. This CPR can help surgeons counsel this patient and inform him that if he is operated on early and at his current disease state, he will achieve a better outcome than if he were to wait (see Table 15.2). We assumed that if the patient waits 1 year before surgery, he will exhibit a 2-point decline on his preoperative mJOA score, will be 1 year older, and will have a significantly longer duration of symptoms. As a result, his probability of achieving a score ≥16 on the mJOA decreases from 93.6 to 85.0%. Furthermore, if he starts to exhibit signs and symptoms of gait dysfunction, this estimate further decreases to 69.6%. These figures would be valuable to help clinicians counsel their patients and to enable shared decision-making.

Case 4: A 62-year-old nonsmoking man presented with mild myelopathy (mJOA = 15) secondary to spondylosis, disk herniation, and congenital stenosis (Fig. 15.4). This patient had numb hands, Lhermitte phenomena, weakness, atrophy of intrinsic hand muscles, and a positive Hoffmann sign. The duration of symptoms was 36 months. The patient had coexisting mild gastrointestinal (stomach/intestine) disorders.

For each participant of the study, the surgeon was asked to predict how the subject would fare following surgical intervention: improve from baseline status, remain the same, or worsen. For case 4, the surgeon believed the subject would be the same as baseline. However, the CPR predicted a 76.4% chance the patient would achieve a score ≥16 and therefore improve by at least 1 point on the mJOA (see Table 15.2). The patient did indeed improve following surgery and was neurologically normal at 1-year follow-up (mJOA = 18). This example demonstrates how a CPR can help align surgeons' perceptions with more objective evidence.

Discussion/Conclusion

Knowledge of factors predictive of operative outcome, summarized in Table 15.3, helps surgeons predict who will benefit most surgical intervention. In degenerative cervical myelopathy, these factors include age, duration and severity of symptoms, the specific signs/symptoms of gait and sexual dysfunction, smoking history, and psychiatric history. Other clinical factors have not been shown to be of prognostic utility. Neurophysiologic testing may also be utilized in DCM assessment, and median nerve SEPs are also predictive of operative outcome, whereas MEP and EMG are not. MRI findings of transverse area, area of maximal cord compression, and cord signal changes signifying significant

Table 15.3 Summary of predictive factors of operative outcomes

Predictive factor	Operative outcome
Age	Increasing age is associated with poorer functional and neurologic outcome Increasing age is associated with increased risk of perioperative complications
Duration and severity of symptoms	Duration and severity of symptoms are associated with poorer functional and neurological outcome
Specific signs/ symptoms	Gait and sexual dysfunction are associated with poorer functional and neurological outcome Other specific signs and symptoms have not been found to be predictive
Comorbid conditions	Smoking status and psychiatric history are associated with poorer functional and neurological outcome There is conflicting evidence on the predictive value of diabetes Comorbid conditions are not associated with increased risk of perioperative complications
Neurophysiologic testing	Normal median nerve SEPs or early postoperative normalization of median nerve SEPs are associated with better functional and neurological outcome EMG and MEPs are not predictive of operative outcome
MRI compression measures	Increased maximal canal compromise is associated with poorer functional and neurological outcome There is conflicting evidence regarding the relationship between transverse area and functional outcome Other measures have not been found to be predictive
MRI signal change	T1 signal hypointensity is associated with poorer functional and neurological outcome T2 "snake-eye appearance" and multi-segmental hyperintensities are associated with poorer functional and neurological outcome There is conflicting evidence regarding the relationship between T2 hyperintensity signal change and operative outcome

disease are also predictive of operative outcome; however further evidence is needed to clarify the predictive importance of imaging-related variables. It is anticipated that the predictive utility will improve with technological advances expected in the coming years. Surgeons should keep in mind these factors when assessing and offering surgical interventions for patients suffering from DCM. When in doubt, clinical prediction rules may aid in predicting long-term surgical outcomes for DCM patient.

Key Recommendations

- For purposes of aiding preoperative communication and managing expectations for the future, it is essential that surgeons develop a sound understanding of the key variables which predict long-term outcomes for DCM patients undergoing surgery.

Bibliography

1. Matz PG, Anderson PA, Holly LT, et al. The natural history of cervical spondylotic myelopathy. J Neurosurg Spine. 2009;11(2):104–11.
2. Fehlings MG, Wilson JR, Kopjar B, et al. Efficacy and safety of surgical decompression in patients with cervical spondylotic myelopathy: results of the AOSpine North America prospective multi-center study. J Bone Joint Surg Am. 2013;95(18):1651–8.
3. Tetreault LA, Côté P, Kopjar B, Arnold P, Fehlings MG, Network ANAaICTR. A clinical prediction model to assess surgical outcome in patients with cervical spondylotic myelopathy: internal and external validations using the prospective multicenter AOSpine North American and international datasets of 743 patients. Spine J. 2015;15(3):388–97.
4. Tetreault L, Wilson JR, Kotter MR, et al. Predicting the minimum clinically important difference in patients undergoing surgery for the treatment of degenerative cervical myelopathy. Neurosurg Focus. 2016;40(6):E14.
5. Morio Y, Teshima R, Nagashima H, Nawata K, Yamasaki D, Nanjo Y. Correlation between operative outcomes of cervical compression myelopathy and MRI of the spinal cord. Spine (Phila Pa 1976). 2001;26(11):1238–45.
6. Tetreault LA, Karpova A, Fehlings MG. Predictors of outcome in patients with degenerative cervical

spondylotic myelopathy undergoing surgical treatment: results of a systematic review. Eur Spine J. 2015;24(Suppl 2):236–51.
7. Holly LT, Matz PG, Anderson PA, et al. Clinical prognostic indicators of surgical outcome in cervical spondylotic myelopathy. J Neurosurg Spine. 2009;11(2):112–8.
8. Tetreault L, Ibrahim A, Côté P, Singh A, Fehlings MG. A systematic review of clinical and surgical predictors of complications following surgery for degenerative cervical myelopathy. J Neurosurg Spine. 2016;24(1):77–99.
9. Kusin DJ, Ahn UM, Ahn NU. The effect of smoking on spinal cord healing following surgical treatment of cervical myelopathy. Spine (Phila Pa 1976). 2015;40(18):1391–6.
10. Alafifi T, Kern R, Fehlings M. Clinical and MRI predictors of outcome after surgical intervention for cervical spondylotic myelopathy. J Neuroimaging. 2007;17(4):315–22.
11. Arnold PM, Fehlings MG, Kopjar B, et al. Mild diabetes is not a contraindication for surgical decompression in cervical spondylotic myelopathy: results of the AOSpine North America multicenter prospective study (CSM). Spine J. 2014;14(1):65–72.
12. Kim HJ, Moon SH, Kim HS, et al. Diabetes and smoking as prognostic factors after cervical laminoplasty. J Bone Joint Surg Br. 2008;90(11):1468–72.
13. Nardone R, Höller Y, Brigo F, et al. The contribution of neurophysiology in the diagnosis and management of cervical spondylotic myelopathy: a review. Spinal Cord. 2016;54(10):756–66.
14. Lyu RK, Tang LM, Chen CJ, Chen CM, Chang HS, Wu YR. The use of evoked potentials for clinical correlation and surgical outcome in cervical spondylotic myelopathy with intramedullary high signal intensity on MRI. J Neurol Neurosurg Psychiatry. 2004;75(2):256–61.
15. Karpova A, Arun R, Cadotte DW, et al. Assessment of spinal cord compression by magnetic resonance imaging--can it predict surgical outcomes in degenerative compressive myelopathy? A systematic review. Spine (Phila Pa 1976). 2013;38(16):1409–21.
16. Fukushima T, Ikata T, Taoka Y, Takata S. Magnetic resonance imaging study on spinal cord plasticity in patients with cervical compression myelopathy. Spine (Phila Pa 1976). 1991;16(10 Suppl):S534–8.
17. Mummaneni PV, Kaiser MG, Matz PG, et al. Preoperative patient selection with magnetic resonance imaging, computed tomography, and electroencephalography: does the test predict outcome after cervical surgery? J Neurosurg Spine. 2009;11(2):119–29.
18. Tetreault LA, Dettori JR, Wilson JR, et al. Systematic review of magnetic resonance imaging characteristics that affect treatment decision making and predict clinical outcome in patients with cervical spondylotic myelopathy. Spine (Phila Pa 1976). 2013;38(22 Suppl 1):S89–110.
19. Nouri A, Tetreault L, Zamorano JJ, et al. Role of magnetic resonance imaging in predicting surgical outcome in patients with cervical spondylotic myelopathy. Spine (Phila Pa 1976). 2015;40(3):171–8.
20. Mizuno J, Nakagawa H, Inoue T, Hashizume Y. Clinicopathological study of "snake-eye appearance" in compressive myelopathy of the cervical spinal cord. J Neurosurg. 2003;99(2 Suppl):162–8.
21. Fernández de Rota JJ, Meschian S, Fernández de Rota A, Urbano V, Baron M. Cervical spondylotic myelopathy due to chronic compression: the role of signal intensity changes in magnetic resonance images. J Neurosurg Spine. 2007;6(1):17–22.
22. Karpova A, Arun R, Kalsi-Ryan S, Massicotte EM, Kopjar B, Fehlings MG. Do quantitative magnetic resonance imaging parameters correlate with the clinical presentation and functional outcomes after surgery in cervical spondylotic myelopathy? A prospective multicenter study. Spine (Phila Pa 1976). 2014;39(18):1488–97.
23. Nouri A, Tetreault L, Côté P, Zamorano JJ, Dalzell K, Fehlings MG. Does magnetic resonance imaging improve the predictive performance of a validated clinical prediction rule developed to evaluate surgical outcome in patients with degenerative cervical myelopathy? Spine (Phila Pa 1976). 2015;40(14):1092–100.
24. Tetreault L, Le D, Côté P, Fehlings M. The practical application of clinical prediction rules: a commentary using case examples in surgical patients with degenerative cervical myelopathy. Global Spine J. 2015;5(6):457–65.

The Cost-Effectiveness of Various Surgical Procedures in the Cervical Spine

16

Blake N. Staub and Todd J. Albert

Introduction

As the cost of healthcare in the United States continues to grow, a focus on the value of the actual healthcare provided has intensified. To determine the value, many cost-effectiveness analysis (CEA) studies are being employed to help guide practitioners to provide safe, economically viable care.

The cost of spine surgery is rising exponentially as are most aspects of healthcare in the United States. It was recently reported that the overall expenditures on degenerative spine care in the United States will exceed $85 billion dollars in a single year [1]. Without question, this yearly figure has risen since the time of that report.

Marked improvements in the care of the degenerative cervical spine pathologies have occurred over the last few decades. There are multiple approaches to the treatment of cervical spine pathology, each of which provides a similar clinical result. To be responsible providers of healthcare, it is imperative that spine surgeons not only assess the quality of each of these interventions but also determine the value the procedure brings to the patient and to society.

B. N. Staub
Texas Back Institute, Plano, TX, USA

T. J. Albert (✉)
Hospital for Special Surgery, New York, NY, USA

Value

Value is defined as the overall quality of a good or service divided by the cost. In healthcare, value is commonly described as the health outcomes achieved per dollar spent [2].

$$\text{Value} = \frac{\text{Quality}}{\text{Cost}}$$

It is important to note that the actual value of healthcare increases with either an increase in quality or a decrease in cost. In surgical specialties, the cost of the procedure itself is not the only variable in the denominator of the value equation. Rather, all inpatient and outpatient preoperative, perioperative, and postoperative costs need to be included in the denominator to truly understand value. Utilizing a less expensive or less efficacious surgical procedure at the expense of higher direct and indirect perioperative costs does not actually realize any savings for the healthcare economy.

To quantify the quality of an intervention, researches utilize quality-adjusted life years (QALY) as a standard unit of measure. Researches use QALYs to measure the impact a specific procedure has on overall health. A single QALY gained implies 1 year of perfect health. Death equates with zero QALYs. These values are typically derived from the common HRQOL forms, such as the SF-36, EQ-5D, or PROMIS, that are often found in spine clinics today.

Two principal means of value analysis in healthcare are cost-effectiveness analysis and

M. G. Kaiser et al. (eds.), *Degenerative Cervical Myelopathy and Radiculopathy*,
https://doi.org/10.1007/978-3-319-97952-6_16

cost-utility analysis. Cost-effectiveness studies rely on a fixed outcome and cannot quantify the subjectivity of different patients that have a similar clinical outcome. Cost-utility analysis, alternatively, relies on QALYs to impart a patient-centric view on the outcome of an intervention.

In spine surgery, it is not only important to perform the procedure that gives your patient the best outcome. Surgeons also need to realize the overall value of the procedures they are performing. With simple, degenerative cervical spine surgery, there are often at least two surgical approaches for each problem – an anterior or posterior approach. Researchers rely on the incremental cost-effectiveness ratio (ICER) to help delineate between the utility of two interventions for the same underlying diagnosis. The ICER utilizes a ratio comparing the cost of a given intervention to the quality of life years gained. In essence, it is comparing the value of two interventions.

$$\text{ICER} = \frac{\text{Cost of surgery A} - \text{Cost of surgery B}}{\text{QALY of surgery A} - \text{QALY of surgery B}}$$

This formula reflects the actual cost of the additional QALYs provided by one procedure in comparison to another. For example, there are three different surgical procedures for treating cervical radiculopathy: foraminotomy, ACDF, and cervical disc replacement.

Intervention	QALY gained (all hypothetical)	Cost (all hypothetical)
Foraminotomy	2	$1000
ACDF	2.2	$1500
Cervical disc replacement	2.5	$2000

To calculate the ICER, we want to determine the incremental cost of an ACDF compared to a foraminotomy.

$$\text{ICER} = \frac{\text{Cost of surgery A}\left(\$1500\right) - \text{Cost of surgery B}\left(\$500\right)}{\text{QALY of surgery A}\left(2.2\right) - \text{QALY of surgery B}\left(2\right)}$$

$$\text{ICER} = \frac{\$500}{0.2}$$

$$\text{ICER} = \$2500$$

The incremental cost, in this example, of utilizing an ACDF versus a foraminotomy is $2500 per QALY. Using the same idea and calculations, the incremental cost of a cervical disc replacement versus an ACDF is $1666 per QALY. Utilization of this type of analysis allows for healthcare dollars to be spent on the most efficient and valuable interventions.

Once the value of a medical intervention is determined, it is then important to determine whether that cost/QALY is within the societal threshold. In the United States, $50,000 is generally the value placed on a single QALY [3].

Ambulatory Surgery Centers and Outpatient Surgery

As healthcare continues to evolve, the economics of medicine are one of the overwhelming drivers of change. Medical treatment in large, tertiary hospitals is not always the most efficient for the patient and is frequently more expensive than potential alternatives. Both surgeons and payers are always looking for medically equivalent, yet less expensive, alternatives.

Over the past decade, the advent of specialized, ambulatory surgery centers (ASCs) has provided an alternative surgical avenue for indicated surgical procedures compared to the traditional hospital-centric paradigm. The goal of an ASC is to take outpatient surgical procedures out of the hospital setting to save on both time and costs. These centers are said to both increase efficiency while maintaining the high level of quality seen in a traditional hospital.

As spine surgery has become less invasive, the opportunity to utilize ASCs has increased. There is ample evidence in the lumbar spine literature suggesting that lumbar discectomies and decompressions can be done safely in an outpatient setting while also providing close to a 30% cost savings [4]. The overall complication rate of cervical surgery done in ambulatory care centers has also been studied and found to be quite low [4–6]. In one large study detailing outpatient one- and two-level anterior cervical discectomy and fusion (ACDF) procedures, the overall complication rate was less than 1%. Out of 1000 patients, only two patients developed prevertebral hematomas which were both managed safely [4]. Overall, outpatient anterior cervical discectomies have very low readmission and complication rates [6]. Based on these cost-saving studies, it has been suggested that moving applicable ACDFs to an outpatient setting could save the total healthcare economy more than $100 million annually [5]. Considering that the cost is in the denominator of the value equation, any decrease in the cost will result in an inversely proportional increase in value.

Cost is clearly associated with the specific physical location a procedure is performed. Location on a more global scale also plays a role in the overall cost-value relationship. Throughout the United States, cost varies significantly by the geographic location. At the state level, costs can vary by up to 129% from the least to the most expensive state [7]. Consequently, the geographical location of a study cannot be ignored as a 100% difference in price would clearly skew the overall value calculated for a given intervention.

Radiculopathy

There are two surgical approaches to the treatment of cervical radiculopathy: anterior or posterior. A posterior cervical foraminotomy was the gold standard in the treatment of degenerative cervical radiculopathy for many years. Over the past few decades, the anterior cervical discectomy and subsequent fusion has become the most utilized procedure for cervical radiculopathy. The cervical artificial disc was conceived and developed as literature began to accumulate detailing possible adjacent segment degeneration/disease potentially originating from motion segment loss after an ACDF. If each of these interventions is considered to have a relative clinical equipoise, then the overall cost of the respective surgical technique will be of great importance in determining its value.

Both ACDF and CDR procedures are cost-effective [8–12]. Both procedures have a cost/QALY ratio of less than $50,000 [8]. There are numerous studies comparing the cost-effectiveness and overall value of these surgical interventions. As previously mentioned, all of the published reports conclude that both procedures are cost-effective and efficacious; however, there are conflicting conclusions as to which procedure actually provides the most value to the patient and to society.

Qureshi et al. reviewed the cost-effectiveness of single-level ACDF versus single-level CDR for the treatment of cervical radiculopathy. They assumed a 5% rate of pseudoarthrosis and hardware failure in the ACDF group as well as a 3% rate of adjacent segment degeneration. They utilized a 1.5% hardware failure rate in their model for the CDR cohort. Interestingly, even if a 5% rate of pseudoarthrosis and a 3% rate of adjacent segment degeneration are accurate estimates, most of the patients with these complications are neither symptomatic nor need further surgical intervention, thus complicating this analysis. Utilizing previous studies of CDR and ACDF, each procedure was given a specific utility value (a value of 1 is perfect health and a value of 0 equates to death). An ACDF was given the value of 0.8, and a CDR was given the value of 0.9. In this study, the total lifetime cost of a CDR was $4836 less than an ACDF. A CDR was seen to generate 3.94 QALYs, while an ACDF only provided 2.02 over a patient's lifetime. Given this data, the overall cost-effectiveness ratio of a CDR in this specific clinical scenario was $3042 per QALY, while an ACDF required $8760 per QALY. In this instance, the ICER is -$2394 in favor of the CDR, implying that CDR is both less costly and more effective than the alternative.

Warren et al. studied a randomized patient population undergoing either a single-level ACDF or a single-level CDR. They found that, while both an ACDF and CDR are cost-effective procedures, the cost/QALY analysis in their study favored the ACDF even though the ACDF was a more costly procedure. Interestingly, there were no revisions in this ACDF cohort, which would cause the data to vary greatly when compared to studies that are assuming a 5% reoperation rate [13].

Another study from McAnany et al. reviewed the 5-year cost-effectiveness of ACDFs and cervical disc replacements. Their data revealed a cost per QALY difference of nearly 7000 dollars favoring CDR. Per their report, as long as complication rates can be kept below a threshold value of 4.4%, then CDR is the dominant technique for a single-level radiculopathy. Interestingly, the QALYs gained are not statistically different. However, the overall cost is nearly 20,000 dollars higher over 5 years in the ACDF subgroup [10].

Ament et al. studied 330 patients with two-level degenerative disc disease randomized to either undergo a two-level CDR or a two-level ACDF with 5-year follow-up. They attempted to calculate QALYs for each cohort. In terms of direct cost, the CDR costs $1687 more than a comparable ACDF over a 5-year period. However, the CDR cohort had significantly less productivity loss, $34,377, when compared to the ACDF group given a markedly different return to work rate. In this study, the ICER for a CDR is -$165,103 per QALY from a societal perspective and $8518 from a health systems perspective [14].

Given the upfront costs of a cervical disc replacement and the cost of a revision, it has been shown that for a CDR to be cost-effective it must last more than 7 years [9]. In addition, the reoperation rate must stay below 10.5%. Most of the current literature shows the overall reoperation rate for CDR to be much less than this cutoff value of 10.5% [15]. However, in patients over 65 years old, the reoperation rate after a CDR rises to 13% [15]. In this patient population, both an ACDF and a foraminotomy would seem to be a more cost-effective intervention.

In addition to the anterior decompression of neural elements, posterior decompressive surgery is a viable option for the treatment of radicular pain. Anecdotally, many surgeons deride the posterior cervical foraminotomy (PCF) option when evaluating a patient for surgical intervention. However, ACDFs are much more expensive than a single-level foraminotomy for the treatment of cervical radiculopathy yet provide a very similar clinical outcome [16]. The increased operative costs of the ACDF are chiefly driven by the cost of instrumentation and the difference in length of stay [16].

Tumialan et al. studied the cost-effectiveness of the PCF compared to a single-level anterior cervical discectomy and fusion in a military population. In this study, both the direct and indirect costs of the foraminotomy were far less than the ACDF [17]. The direct surgical costs for the ACDF were $6508 more than the PCF. The indirect costs were calculated to be between $13,585 and $24,045 greater in the ACDF group. Again, similar to the CDR data, the patients undergoing the arthrodesis were kept out of work for an average of 14.8 weeks longer than the patients in the PCF group. Cleary this will skew the overall value equation. In regard to long-term costs, the reoperation rates for ACDF and PCFs are very similar [18]. Another recent study showed ACDFs to cost $11,757 more than a PCF for the actual index procedure itself and another $11,420 over the first 30 postoperative days [19].

Myelopathy

There is no question that the surgical treatment of degenerative cervical myelopathy (DCM) is cost-effective [19, 20]. Regardless of the severity of the disease, surgical decompression of the spinal cord results in improved function and quality of life. It has been shown that without surgery, 20–62% of patients worsen over a 3–6-year period. Surgery has been shown to provide a long-lasting, significant improvement for the patient at an acceptable cost [19]. All the accepted treatments of CSM (anterior cervical corpectomy and fusion, laminoplasty, laminectomy with fusion) have been found to have similar neurologic outcomes [21].

Compared to radiculopathy data, there is a paucity of data examining the value of anterior versus posterior surgery for CSM. Ghogawala et al. undertook a small pilot study looking at 50 patients with CSM treated with either anterior or posterior decompression and arthrodesis. As expected, both groups had a similar improvement in neurological function after surgery. However, the hospital costs for the posterior fusion group were significantly higher, $29,465 versus $19,245. No indirect costs or direct costs relating to postoperative care were calculated in this study, limiting its overall usefulness [22].

Whitmore et al. conducted a similar study. They used two different models to assess the value of each intervention. One method revealed overall direct hospital costs were $27,942 ± 14,220 versus $21,563 ± 8721 for the posterior cervical fusion and the ACDF, respectively. Using a different mechanism of assessing direct costs, there appeared to be no difference in overall hospital costs between the two procedures [23]. However, even with similar costs, given the slightly improved outcomes in the anterior group, the overall ICER is in favor of ACDF.

Laminoplasty has been shown to have equivalent outcomes to ACDF in the treatment of CSM [24]. Unfortunately, given the overall rarity of cost-effectiveness data on cervical spine interventions, no studies to date have been performed examining the actual value of a laminoplasty compared to other possible interventions in the cervical spine.

Discussion

As the US government and payers move from a fee-for-service payment schedule to a more value-driven system, the need for cost-effectiveness analyses will increase greatly. Although much data exists comparing the efficacy of specific surgical interventions, little data actually exists showing the value of these interventions in the cervical spine.

Much of the cost-effectiveness debate in the cervical spine literature focuses on the cost and value difference between an anterior cervical discectomy and fusion and a cervical disc replacement. There is literature supporting the superior value of each technique over the other.

Much of the literature advocating the superior value of the CDR over the ACDF comes from the initial, randomized clinical trials sponsored by the device companies and administrated by the physicians who helped design the devices and who may be investors in the companies themselves. This obviously imposes a potential source of bias on all of the data. In addition, the patients in these studies were perfectly screened. As new products make their way out into the community and away from these stringent surgical requirements, the initial excellent results may not be reproduced. This might be the case with CDRs. Recent research outside the realm of the IDE studies seems to indicate increased rates of heterotopic ossification than previously reported and equivalent levels of adjacent segment disease when compared to ACDFs [25–29]. In one study, the rates of surgical revision were actually higher in the CDR group [30]. This would greatly confound the value data that currently suggests a CDR is a more valuable procedure than an ACDF. As much of the data on CDRs originates from IDE studies that employ ideal indications for surgery, the studies themselves favor successful results.

There are other confounding variables within the CDR studies that could possibly alter the results of a cost/value analysis. Some of the data suggesting that the CDR is a more valuable procedure relies on the fact that the surgeon's fees for this procedure are markedly lower than for an ACDF [15].

In addition, the speed at which patients return to work appears to be one of the more important variables affecting the overall value of these procedures. CDR patients had a much higher return to work rate when compared to ACDF patients [14]. One study even showed that CDR patients returned to work 38 days quicker than ACDF patients [31]. A quicker return to work leads to markedly lower indirect costs. Interestingly, this phenomenon appears to be completely surgeon generated as there is no good data regarding the appropriate timing for return to work after either of these procedures. One could argue that surgeons are iatrogenically inflating the long-term costs of an ACDF by requiring the use of rigid collars and keeping patients out of work for extended periods of time. The use of a rigid collar is a significant impediment to return to work after an ACDF, and current literature does not support the use of a collar in one-level fusions [32].

A foraminotomy has been shown to be much more cost-effective in a population of people with a physically demanding job. Aside from the difference in cost between a foraminotomy and any instrumented procedure, much of the cost savings revolve around the quicker return to work. In cases of single-level cervical radiculopathy, a foraminotomy demonstrates clinical equipoise to an ACDF (and thus a CDR) while providing improved short-term (due to lack of instrumentation) and long-term costs given the similar revision rates and quicker returns to work.

Conclusion

Given the state of modern healthcare, it is imperative that all medical interventions not only be scrutinized for their success rates but also for the overall value. ACDFs, CDRs, and PCFs are all viable options for the treatment of one-level cervical radiculopathy. Currently, both a CDR and PCF appear to be more valuable interventions for properly indicated patients. However, newer research does seem to question the initial value improvement espoused by CDR supporters. Overall, there is a dearth of literature looking at the value of cervical spine surgery. The few papers that exist contain potentially significant bias and also do not portend a consistent means of measuring value. As with all academic endeavors, more research needs to be done.

References

1. Martin BI, Deyo RA, Mirza SK, et al. Expenditures and health status among adults with back and neck problems. JAMA. 2008;299(6):656–64.
2. Nwachukwu BU, Hamid KS, Bozic KJ. Measuring value in orthopaedic surgery. JBJS Rev. 2013;1(1) https://doi.org/10.2106/JBJS.RVW.M.00067.
3. Grosse SD. Assessing cost-effectiveness in healthcare: history of the $50,000 per QALY threshold. Expert Rev Pharmacoecon Outcomes Res. 2008;8(2):165–78.
4. Adamson T, Godil SS, Mehrlich M, Mendenhall S, Asher AL, McGirt MJ. Anterior cervical discectomy and fusion in the outpatient ambulatory surgery setting compared with the inpatient hospital setting: analysis of 1000 consecutive cases. J Neurosurg Spine. 2016;24(6):878–84.
5. Silvers HR, Lewis PJ, Suddaby LS, Asch HL, Clabeaux DE, Blumenson LE. Day surgery for cervical microdiscectomy: is it safe and effective? J Spinal Disord. 1996;9(4):287–93.
6. McClelland S 3rd, Oren JH, Protopsaltis TS, Passias PG. Outpatient anterior cervical discectomy and fusion: a meta-analysis. J Clin Neurosci. 2016;34:166–8.
7. Goz V, Rane A, Abtahi AM, Lawrence BD, Brodke DS, Spiker WR. Geographic variations in the cost of spine surgery. Spine (Phila Pa 1976). 2015;40(17):1380–9.
8. Carreon LY, Anderson PA, Traynelis VC, Mummaneni PV, Glassman SD. Cost-effectiveness of single-level anterior cervical discectomy and fusion five years after surgery. Spine (Phila Pa 1976). 2013;38(6):471–5.
9. Qureshi SA, McAnany S, Goz V, Koehler SM, Hecht AC. Cost-effectiveness analysis: comparing single-level cervical disc replacement and single-level anterior cervical discectomy and fusion: clinical article. J Neurosurg Spine. 2013;19(5):546–54.
10. McAnany SJ, Overley S, Baird EO, et al. The 5-year cost-effectiveness of anterior cervical discectomy and fusion and cervical disc replacement: a markov analysis. Spine (Phila Pa 1976). 2014;39(23):1924–33.
11. Radcliff K, Zigler J, Zigler J. Costs of cervical disc replacement versus anterior cervical discectomy and fusion for treatment of single-level cervical disc disease: an analysis of the blue health intelligence database for acute and long-term costs and complications. Spine (Phila Pa 1976). 2015;40(8):521–9.
12. Ament JD, Yang Z, Nunley P, Stone MB, Kim KD. Cost-effectiveness of cervical total disc replacement vs fusion for the treatment of 2-level symptomatic degenerative disc disease. JAMA Surg. 2014;149(12):1231–9.
13. Warren D, Andres T, Hoelscher C, Ricart-Hoffiz P, Bendo J, Goldstein J. Cost-utility analysis modeling at 2-year follow-up for cervical disc arthroplasty versus anterior cervical discectomy and fusion: a single-center contribution to the randomized controlled trial. Int J Spine Surg. 2013;7:e58–66.
14. Ament JD, Yang Z, Nunley P, Stone MB, Lee D, Kim KD. Cost utility analysis of the cervical artificial disc vs fusion for the treatment of 2-level symptomatic degenerative disc disease: 5-year follow-up. Neurosurgery. 2016;79(1):135–45.
15. Ghori A, Konopka JF, Makanji H, Cha TD, Bono CM. Long term societal costs of anterior discectomy and fusion (ACDF) versus cervical disc arthroplasty (CDA) for treatment of cervical radiculopathy. Int J Spine Surg. 2016;10:1.
16. Mansfield HE, Canar WJ, Gerard CS, O'Toole JE. Single-level anterior cervical discectomy and fusion versus minimally invasive posterior cervical

foraminotomy for patients with cervical radiculopathy: a cost analysis. Neurosurg Focus. 2014;37(5):E9.
17. Tumialan LM, Ponton RP, Gluf WM. Management of unilateral cervical radiculopathy in the military: the cost effectiveness of posterior cervical foraminotomy compared with anterior cervical discectomy and fusion. Neurosurg Focus. 2010;28(5):E17.
18. Bydon M, Mathios D, Macki M, et al. Long-term patient outcomes after posterior cervical foraminotomy: an analysis of 151 cases. J Neurosurg Spine. 2014;21(5):727–31.
19. Witiw CD, Tetreault LA, Smieliauskas F, Kopjar B, Massicotte EM, Fehlings MG. Surgery for degenerative cervical myelopathy: a patient-centered quality of life and health economic evaluation. Spine J. 2016;16:S231.
20. Fehlings MG, Jha NK, Hewson SM, Massicotte EM, Kopjar B, Kalsi-Ryan S. Is surgery for cervical spondylotic myelopathy cost-effective? A cost-utility analysis based on data from the AOSpine north america prospective CSM study. J Neurosurg Spine. 2012;17(1 Suppl):89–93.
21. Cunningham MR, Hershman S, Bendo J. Systematic review of cohort studies comparing surgical treatments for cervical spondylotic myelopathy. Spine (Phila Pa 1976). 2010;35(5):537–43.
22. Ghogawala Z, Martin B, Benzel EC, et al. Comparative effectiveness of ventral vs dorsal surgery for cervical spondylotic myelopathy. Neurosurgery. 2011;68(3):622–30; discussion 630-1.
23. Whitmore RG, Schwartz JS, Simmons S, Stein SC, Ghogawala Z. Performing a cost analysis in spine outcomes research: comparing ventral and dorsal approaches for cervical spondylotic myelopathy. Neurosurgery. 2012;70(4):860–7; discussion 867.
24. Liu T, Yang HL, Xu YZ, Qi RF, Guan HQ. ACDF with the PCB cage-plate system versus laminoplasty for multilevel cervical spondylotic myelopathy. J Spinal Disord Tech. 2011;24(4):213–20.
25. Nunley P, Kerr E, et al. Clinical implications of heterotopic ossification after cervical disc arthroplasty. In: Forty-fourth annual meeting of the Cervical Spine Research Society. 2016.
26. Marques C, MacDowall A, et al. Unintended fusion in cervical artifical disc replacement: a prospective study on heterotopic ossification with 5 years follow-up. In: Forty-fourth annual meeting of the Cervical Spine Research Society. 2016.
27. Zhou F, Ju K, et al. Progressive bone formation after cervical disc replacement: a 5-year follow-up. In: Forty-fourth annual meeting of the Cervical Spine Research Society. 2016.
28. Skeppholm M. Elevated risk for repeated surgery after ADR compared to ACDF in a cohort of 715 patients – a retrospective study with minimum five-year follow-up. In: Forty-fourth annual meeting of the Cervical Spine Research Society. 2016.
29. Alvin MD, Qureshi S, Klineberg E, et al. Cervical degenerative disease: systematic review of economic analyses. Spine (Phila Pa 1976). 2014;39(22 Suppl 1):S53–64.
30. Campbell MJ, Carreon LY, Traynelis V, Anderson PA. Use of cervical collar after single-level anterior cervical fusion with plate: is it necessary? Spine (Phila Pa 1976). 2009;34(1):43–8.
31. Miller J, Sasso R, et al. Adjacent-level degeneration after Bryan cervical disc arthroplasty compared with anterior discectomy and fusion. In: Forty-fourth annual meeting of the Cervical Spine Research Society. 2016.
32. MacDowall A, Canto Moreia N, et al. Artifical disc replacements do not prevent adjacent segment degeneration in the cervical spine. In: Forty-fourth annual meeting of the Cervical Spine Research Society. 2016.

An Overview of Various Surgical Approaches

17

Matthew J. Tormenti and Mark R. McLaughlin

Pitfalls

- Multilevel ACDF produces better lordosis than corpectomy/corpectomies.
- Approaching centrally located anterior pathology through a posterior approach can lead to inferior outcomes.
- Posterior approaches are typically inferior for patients with fixed kyphosis.
- Failure to recognize ossified anterior pathology can lead to increased risk of morbidity.

Pearls

- Failure to preserve/restore sagittal alignment leads to less favorable outcomes.
- Differentiating myelopathy, radiculopathy, and myeloradiculopathy is essential to developing a treatment paradigm.
- Maintaining cervical lordosis can improve patient-reported outcomes.
- Natural history of the disease process should come into play in surgical decision-making.

M. J. Tormenti
Princeton Brain and Spine, Langhorne, PA, USA

M. R. McLaughlin (✉)
Princeton Brain and Spine Care, LLC,
Princeton, NJ, USA
e-mail: m.mclaughlin@princetonbrainandspine.com

Introduction

Degenerative cervical myelopathy and radiculopathy are a leading cause of disability in the aging population. The two conditions are distinct but related and can often be seen in tandem. Myelopathy refers to damage to the spinal cord and central nervous system itself. This differs from radiculopathy which is damage or irritation of a nerve root that is part of the peripheral nervous system. In treating degenerative disease of the cervical spine, surgeons often can observe myeloradiculopathy which has characteristics of both central and peripheral nervous system dysfunctions.

Nonsurgical options for the treatment of cervical myelopathy include physical therapy and a cervical collar brace and are of limited value. Surgery is often necessary to alleviate compression of the spinal cord and halt the progression of the disease. Widening of the spinal canal (laminoplasty) can be a motion-sparing option for

M. G. Kaiser et al. (eds.), *Degenerative Cervical Myelopathy and Radiculopathy*,
https://doi.org/10.1007/978-3-319-97952-6_17

some patients. Others may benefit from spinal decompression surgery with or without spinal fusion, which stabilizes the spine after herniated discs, bone spurs, or ossified ligaments are fully or partially removed. These surgeries can be performed posteriorly or anteriorly [4].

Degenerative Cervical Myelopathy

Degenerative cervical myelopathy is often termed cervical spondylotic myelopathy. Spondylotic myelopathy results from compression of the cervical spinal cord by a combination of degenerative disc disease and osteophytes anteriorly and ligamentous hypertrophy posteriorly. The location of the pathology will often dictate the surgical approach. Myelopathy can present with a multitude of symptoms referable to dysfunction of the cervical spinal cord. This includes numbness and tingling in the hands and feet, loss of fine motor skills, and gait dysfunction. Late manifestations of this disease include progressive spastic quadriparesis and bowel and bladder dysfunction. On physical examination, patients will often have weakness in their extremities, atrophy of hand intrinsic musculature, as well as evidence of long tract findings such as hyperreflexia or pathologic reflexes. The natural history of the disease usually follows a stepwise pattern of deterioration but may include long periods of quiescence [41].

Degenerative Cervical Radiculopathy

Cervical radiculopathy usually results from injury or irritation to a single nerve root and presents as unilateral symptoms in a specific nerve root distribution. Among younger patients, cervical radiculopathy is a result of a disc herniation or an acute injury causing foraminal impingement of an exiting nerve [2]. Disc herniation accounts for 20–25% of the cases of cervical radiculopathy. In older patients, this condition is often a result of foraminal narrowing from osteophyte formation, decreased disc height, and degenerative changes of the uncovertebral joints anteriorly and of the facet joints posteriorly. Symptoms include pain, sensory dysfunction, or motor weakness in the structures innervated by the affected nerve root. Physical examination will often reveal sensory disturbance or muscular weakness in a specific nerve root distribution with preservation or diminution of reflexes.

The natural history of radiculopathy can be quite varied. Often patients will have acute symptomatic episodes followed by asymptomatic periods. Chronic constant radiculopathy is another manifestation of the disease.

Myeloradiculopathy

Often patients will present with a combination of myelopathic and radicular symptoms. These patients are said to have myeloradiculopathy. Myeloradiculopathy results from compression of both the spinal cord and peripheral nerve by the offending pathology. Physical examination will show a combination of peripheral and central nervous system findings. Typically the treatment paradigm for patients with myeloradiculopathy will follow a trajectory based on the myelopathic symptoms. Posterior cervical approaches were first utilized for cervical myelopathy over 100 years ago as described by Sir Victor Horsley [5]. In the 1930s, Byron Stookey performed the first posterior cervical foraminotomy for radiculopathy.

Since these first treatments were described, various approaches and techniques have been employed to treat patients with these diseases.

In the 1950s, surgery for cervical radiculopathy was revolutionized by Ralph Cloward and Smith and Robinson [6]. They popularized the highly successful technique of anterior cervical discectomy and fusion that is still utilized today (Fig. 17.1).

Posterior cervical foraminotomy is another effective option for motion preservation and symptom relief in patients with cervical radiculopathy [7]. Newer developments in cervical arthroplasty and posterior cervical facet joint replacement will be discussed later in this chapter.

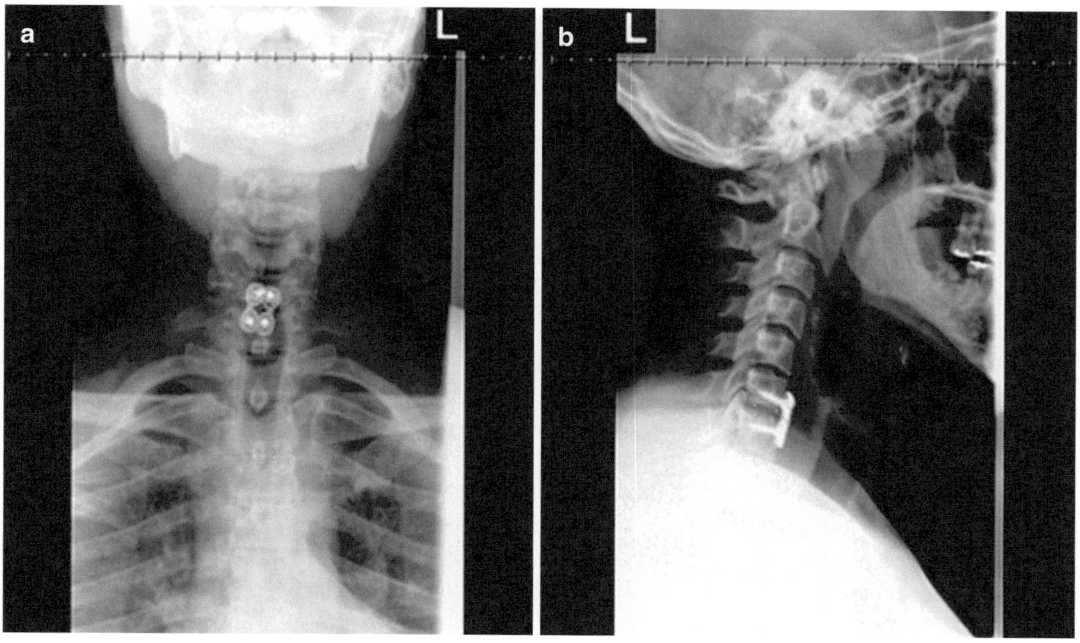

Fig. 17.1 (**a**, **b**) Postoperative X-ray of a single-level anterior cervical discectomy and fusion

Laminectomy continues to be an option for treatment of cervical myelopathy in the elderly with minimal or no neck pain and a stiff spine, but our knowledge of post-laminectomy kyphosis as discussed by Magerl and others has added cervical fusion to prevent post-laminectomy kyphosis [8].

Laminoplasty, championed by Heller et al. [9], is an additional technique for treating cervical myelopathy. Newer techniques for treating these very common diseases have improved outcomes and decreased morbidity.

Degenerative Cervical Radiculopathy and Myelopathy Background and Indications

Indications for surgical treatment include intractable pain, progressive motor or sensory deficit, or refractory symptoms after a reasonable period of non-operative therapy. When symptoms and signs correlate with radiographic evidence of nerve root compression, there is a strong likelihood of a favorable outcome with either anterior or posterior approaches to surgery [10].

The goals of surgical treatment are to decompress the nerves, restore sagittal balance, and, if necessary, stabilize the spine. Consequently, the treatment of cervical degenerative disease can be divided into decompression alone, fixation alone, or a combination of both. In addition, it can be divided into anterior or posterior procedures in terms of approach to the cervical spine.

Surgical Treatment of Degenerative Cervical Myelopathy and Radiculopathy

Surgical Technique Options

Posterior Cervical Foraminotomy

This procedure is perhaps the oldest spine surgery known to neurosurgeons and orthopedic spine surgeons. First performed by Stookey and championed by Fager and others, posterior cervical laminoforaminotomy remains an important modality in addressing osteophytes and lateral disc herniations that do not compress the spinal cord and cause isolated arm pain, with minimal neck pain. The patient is placed in a Mayfield three-point head fixation device and positioned with the affected side and level prepped and draped. An incision is made approximately 1 centimeter off midline and carried down to the posterior cervical fascia. The soft tissue is dissected and a self-retaining retractor is placed. We prefer to use a tubular retractor or a slender blade Ducker type retractor.

The appropriate level is identified radiographically, and then the operating microscope is brought into the field. A small semihemilaminectomy is performed with either a high-speed drill or a Kerrison 2MM or 1MM rongeur. The nerve root is identified and then skeletonized. As documented in many studies, care must be taken to preserve approximately 50% of the facet joint.

Once the nerve root is identified, a generous decompression is performed to relieve pressure on the nerve root. Although the authors have had limited success in performing a discectomy for soft disc herniations using this approach, many advocate performing a discectomy for soft disc herniations [11] to decompress the nerve root.

Once the nerve root has been decompressed—either by foraminotomy with or without discectomy—the area is irrigated and packed with a hemostatic agent. The wound is closed in routine fashion.

Over the years, many approaches have been utilized to decrease epidural blood loss from this procedure. Some authors advocate the sitting position for the procedure [12], but we have found the prone position to be a more effective option [12]. With the use of the Floseal hemostatic matrix, epidural bleeding can be kept to a minimum.

Published results for this procedure are favorable, including a success rate of approximately 90–95% with preservation of motion [7]. Because motion is preserved, the biomechanical factors which led to the osteophyte/disc complex are still active, so, as expected, the recurrence rate can be as high as 6.5–7% [7].

The authors prefer to use this technique for single-level, unilateral nerve root compression in patients with minimal neck pain.

Anterior Cervical Discectomy and Fusion

Most neurosurgeons and orthopedic surgeons utilize the anterior cervical discectomy and fusion approach to treat cervical radiculopathy. This procedure yields high success rates, minimal postoperative neck pain, and fast recovery [13].

For this procedure, patients are placed in a supine position in gentle extension, and their shoulders are taped inferiorly to allow good radiographic visualization of all levels. The level appropriate to anterior cervical crease is opened, either in a transverse or longitudinal fashion, and the avascular plane between the carotid sheath laterally and the trachea and esophagus medially is dissected.

The prevertebral fascia is identified and opened. The affected level is identified, and distraction pins are placed, and distraction is applied to open the disc space. An interoperative microscope is brought into position. A generous discectomy and a bilateral foraminotomy are performed, with drilling of the medial uncinate process and supplemented with 2MM and 1MM Kerrison rongeurs.

In all cases, it is our practice to completely remove the posterior longitudinal ligament. Our philosophy is that we prefer to have direct visualization of the spinal cord and the affected nerve root [14].

Once decompression of the spinal cord and nerve root is completed, a customized graft is placed, and either autograft, allograft, titanium, or a PEEK spacer of appropriate size is tamped and secured into position with an anterior cervical plate. We prefer to utilize a hybrid plate, using variable screws superiorly and fixed screws inferiorly to allow for graft compression promoting bone growth via Wolff's law. Some surgeons prefer the use of integral spacers with screws, although there are few studies to evaluate long-term efficacy of this device for single-level and particularly multilevel fusions.

Meticulous carpentry is an important part of this procedure with proper mortising of the graft. It is important to create effective parallel end plate planes that allow good visualization of the nerve roots and the spinal cord for placement of the appropriate customized graft under compression.

Another proven option is cervical arthroplasty [15]. The appropriate patient population for this option will be discussed later in this chapter.

Posterior Cervical Laminectomy for Myelopathy

Some have argued that posterior cervical laminectomy and/or fusion for cervical myelopathy is the procedure of choice for patients with multilevel (more than three levels) disc disease [16]. Others favor posterior cervical laminectomy and fusion for the elderly, as they are more prone to dysphagia with anterior approaches (Fig. 17.2).

For this procedure, the patient is placed in a prone position in a Mayfield three-point head fixation device and in good cervical lordosis. The incision is carried down, the posterior elements and the lamina are exposed, and if a fusion is needed, the lateral masses are exposed.

Once the affected levels are identified, they are decompressed using a Horsley bone cutter, a Leksell rongeur, and a Midas Rex drill. Even when severe stenosis exists, the authors generally utilize a Midas Rex B-5 footplate to perform the laminectomy; we have found that this approach is the least traumatic and efficient and decreases the frequency introducing small instruments into the narrowed spinal canal. Some surgeons prefer a technique to use the Midas AM 8 matchstick to drill troughs on each side of the lamina and then lift the lamina off en bloc.

Once the affected lamina has been drilled, it is removed, and the lateral gutters are trimmed with Kerrison 1MM and 2MM rongeurs.

If lateral mass fixation is required, pilot holes are marked and drilled prior to the laminectomy. In our experience, marking and predrilling the lateral mass screw holes provide the surgeon with more reliable landmarks and protection of the spinal cord. This provides a safeguard for the surgeon in case the drill chatters off course. Lateral mass fusion is performed using the technique of placing the screws in a 30-degree lateral and 20-degree cephalad direction.

We typically reserve cervical fusions after laminectomy for patients with straightening or reversal of cervical lordosis, severe neck pain, or other unstable cervical spine diseases, which present the possibility of progression of disease [17]. If the facet joints and lordosis are preserved, however, cervical fusion is not necessary in all cases, and laminectomy alone is a treatment option.

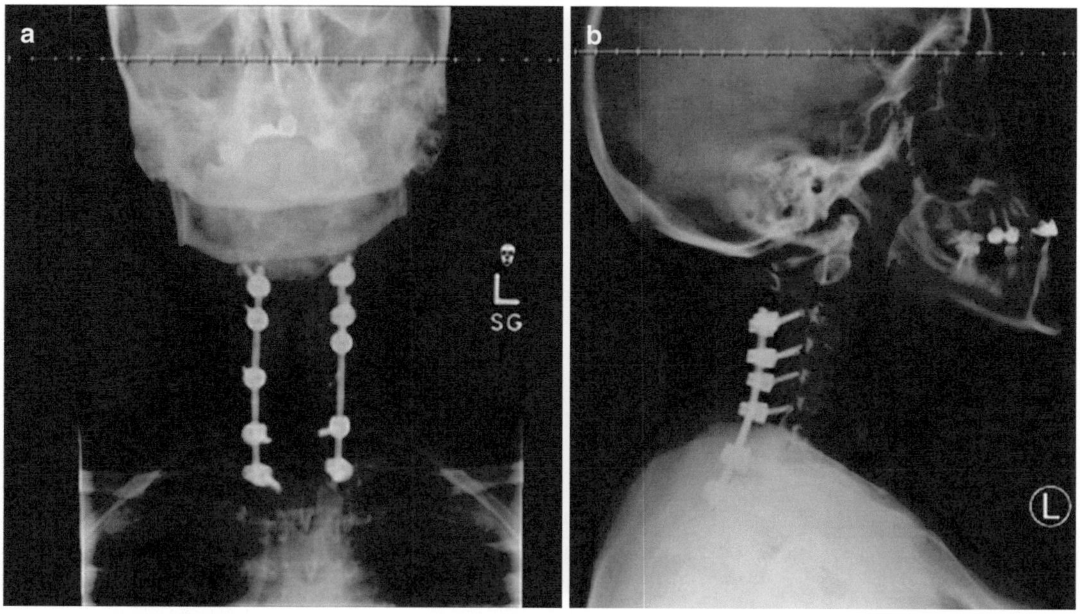

Fig. 17.2 (**a**, **b**) Postoperative X-ray of a multilevel posterior cervical laminectomy and lateral mass fixation incorporating the thoracic junctional level

Cervical Arthroplasty

The exposure techniques for cervical arthroplasty are identical to those for cervical fusion. Typically, the distraction pin is placed in the mid-vertebral body, but when performing arthroplasty, we tend to place it a millimeter or 2 above the mid portion of the cephalic body and a millimeter or 2 below the mid portion of the caudal body. This allows for good visualization when deploying the arthroplasty device.

When considering a patient for arthroplasty, preoperative radiographs of the cervical spine in flexion and extension must rule out instability, and imaging must demonstrate that the facet joints are without degeneration and therefore amenable to arthroplasty.

When preparing the end plates for cervical arthroplasty, avoid drilling of the end plate using only light curettage and decompress with Kerrison rongeurs to prevent bone dust formation. Care is taken to preserve as much of the end plate as possible with proper removal of the superior and inferior apophyseal ring.

When performing an arthroplasty, we favor more curettage rather than drilling the end plates. Once the end plates have been prepared, an appropriate size of artificial disc device can be placed. There are six cervical arthroplasty devices on the market at this time and only two (Mobi-C and Prestige LP) with FDA approval for two-level implantation [18].

Laminoplasty

The technique for cervical laminoplasty was introduced in the late 1970s [19]. This procedure was first popularized by Japanese neurosurgeons in their treatment of ossification of the posterior longitudinal ligament, a disease with a high prevalence in the Asian population. Due to severe ossification, anterior approaches can lead to significant complications and generally were not well-suited for this disease.

Laminoplasty was utilized prior to the development of posterior cervical instrumentation techniques to help prevent post-laminectomy kyphosis [20]. Two prototype techniques were developed nearly simultaneously: Hirabayashi's open-door laminoplasty [21] and Kurokawa's spinous process-splitting (double-door) laminoplasty [22]. Over time, variations of these procedures were developed utilizing different osteotomy and reattachment techniques.

The selection of patients for cervical laminoplasty is based on several factors. Similar to cervical laminectomy, patients with mostly anterior disease or kyphotic deformity that would best be addressed via an anterior approach should be excluded. Likewise, patients who display overt instability on dynamic radiographs would be better treated with either anterior or posterior decompression with adjunctive fusion.

For cervical laminectomy, the patient is usually in a prone position in a Mayfield headrest to stabilize the spine in a lordotic position while alleviating stress on the patient's eyes. The skin is then prepared and draped using sterile technique. A midline incision is made at the appropriate surgical levels, and subcutaneous dissection is carried out with electrocautery. Every attempt should be made to remain in the midline avascular plane to minimize blood loss. Care taken to leave the supraspinous and interspinous ligaments intact will help prevent postoperative deformity.

The paraspinous musculature is then dissected, and localizing X-rays are obtained to verify the appropriate surgical level. Using a surgical microscope may help with visualization. Though various surgical techniques can be used to disconnect the lamina, the authors prefer to drill bilateral troughs utilizing a high-speed burr or footplate.

The disconnected laminae are then reflected superiorly and out of the field with the uppermost ligamentum flavum as a hinge. The intercanalicular portion of the surgery (e.g., spondylotic decompression, tumor resection) can then be performed. Small microfixation plates are attached to the lamina. The lamina is then re-approximated to the microfixation plates and in contact with the lateral masses. The plates should be spaced far enough apart to avoid restenosis and attached to the lateral masses with screws.

Complications

Posterior Cervical Foraminotomy

This procedure is used for decompression of the nerve root to treat foraminal stenosis or remove soft disc fragments. It retains motion in the affected segment and does not cause major instability [23]. Due to the nature of the approach, it also has a lower complication rate compared to anterior procedures [24]. The shorter duration of the operation compared to anterior surgery is a major advantage. However, complications of this technique include neurological damage, infection, and recurrence of symptoms [25]. A major limitation of the procedure is that it does not allow removal of offending lesions located medioventral to the nerve root [26]. The incidence of C5 palsy has been documented to be higher in a posterior approach.

Anterior Cervical Discectomy and Fusion

Anterior cervical discectomy and fusion (ACDF) of one to three levels is an effective and safe method for alleviating pressure on spinal nerves. Applying this procedure to more than three levels, however, can result in complications, including graft extrusion, subsidence, fracture, and pseudoarthrosis [27]. The type of plate fixation remains a controversial issue. In multilevel ACDFs, studies show that rigid plate fixation dramatically increased fusion rates [28], but some studies advocate better fusion rates with dynamic plating [29]. Plating may also lead to complications including adjacent level degeneration, soft tissue injury, and implant failure [30].

Posterior Cervical Laminectomy for Myelopathy

Laminectomy is proven to be a safe and effective technique for multilevel decompression for cervical spondylotic myelopathy [31]. Laminectomy without fusion has achieved comparable postoperative results to laminoplasty and anterior procedures. There is a body of evidence, however, demonstrating late deterioration, with rates as high as 40% [32]. Neurologic injury is a rare but serious complication of this procedure. The incidence of spinal cord injury is from 0% to 3%, whereas injury to an individual nerve root can be as high as 15% [33]. Nerve root injury occurs due to direct manipulation of the spinal cord after decompression [34]. Despite the increased stability provided by the procedure, adding instrumentation can lead to complications such as hardware failure with loss of alignment and neurological damage from misplaced lateral mass screws [35].

Another complication the authors have experienced in their own practice and is well described in the literature is junctional instability at the cervicothoracic region due to not incorporating T1 or T2 in long segment cervical fixation.

Cervical Arthroplasty

Cervical disc arthroplasty has emerged as a promising potential alternative to anterior cervical discectomy and fusion (ACDF) in appropriately selected patients [15]. Adverse events associated with cervical disc arthroplasty include implant failure/wear, bone implant failures, iatrogenic deformity, segmental kyphosis, failed kinematics, neurologic injury, and infection. Although the goal of cervical arthroplasty is to maintain normal range of motion and biomechanics, some patients develop postoperative segmental kyphosis. Troyanovich et al. argued that adjacent levels compensate for the kyphotic level, but undue stress at these interspaces accelerates adjacent segment degeneration [36]. Appropriate modifications in surgical techniques that address these two major issues have shown that adverse outcomes are avoidable [37].

Laminoplasty

Laminoplasty was developed to allow spinal cord decompression while preserving motion with less substantial alteration to the natural biomechanics of the cervical spine. Multiple studies using the Japanese Orthopaedic Association (JOA) scale have demonstrated its effectiveness, with approximately 55–65% achieving recovery [38]. Frequently reported complications are decreased range of movement and axial neck pain. Ratliff and Cooper determined that the overall incidence of postoperative axial neck pain ranged from 6% to 60% regardless of the specific variation of laminoplasty [39]. Other authors have reported that preservation of subaxial deep extensor muscles, including the semispinalis cervicis groups, reduces these adverse effects after laminoplasty [40] (Fig. 17.3).

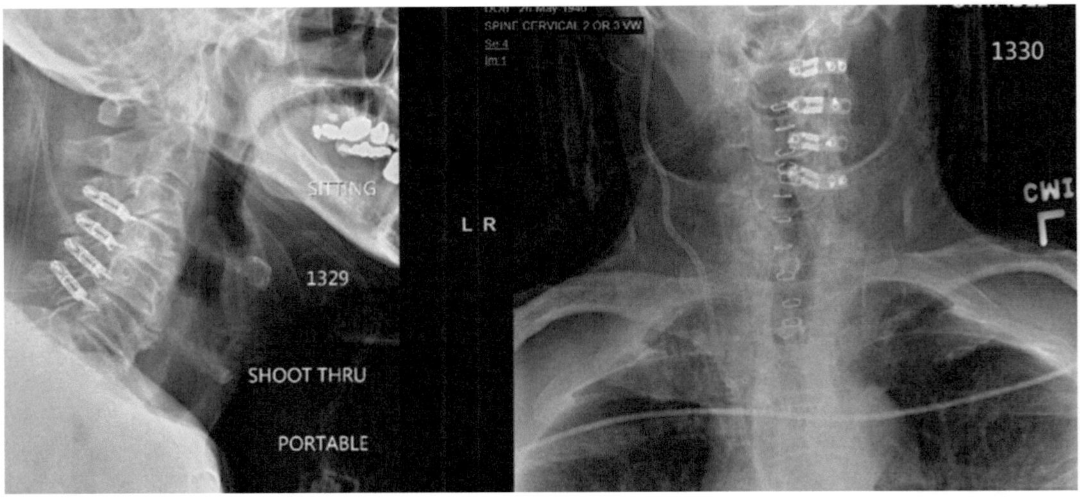

Fig. 17.3 (**a**, **b**) Postoperative AP and lateral X-ray of a posterior cervical laminoplasty

Discussion/Conclusion

Degenerative cervical radiculopathy and myelopathy, extremely common conditions, will certainly increase in incidence as the leading edge of the baby boomers enters their later decades of life. Spine surgeons should maintain proficiency in as many of the techniques described in this chapter to better serve patients with this condition. It has been our experience that these diseases cannot be treated with a one-size-fits-all approach. Patients and surgical interventions must be individualized based upon the patient's history, radiographic studies, medical status, and goals for surgical outcome.

Key Recommendations

- Cervical degenerative disease resulting in radiculopathy and myelopathy can be treated with many different surgical approaches, and patients are best served when their treating surgeon is facile in all techniques such that an appropriate plan can be tailored to suit the patient's unique needs and goals.
- Motion preservation technology and techniques continue to evolve. The data on its impact related to diminishing adjacent level disease is still not available at this time.
- Generally, surgical success rates and long-term outcomes for the treatment of cervical degenerative disease are higher than for the treatment of thoracic and lumbar disease.

Bibliography

1. Ellenberg MR, Honet JC, Treanor WJ. Cervical radiculopathy. Arch Phys Med Rehabil. 1994; 75(3):342–52.
2. Murphey F, Simmons JC, Brunson B. Ruptured cervical discs, 1939 to 1972. Clin Neurosurg. 1973;20:9–17.
3. Shelerud RA, Paynter KS. Rarer causes of radiculopathy: spinal tumors, infections, and other unusual causes. Phys Med Rehabil Clin N Am. 2002 Aug;13(3):645–96.
4. Johns Hopkins Medicine Health Library. Myelopathy. Available from: http://www.hopkinsmedicine.org/healthlibrary/conditions/nervous_system_disorders/myelopathy_22,Myelopathy/

5. Boos N, Aebi M, editors. Spinal disorders: fundamentals of diagnosis and treatment. New York: Springer; 2008. p. 457.
6. Aronson N, Filtzer D, Bagan M. Anterior cervical fusion by the Smith-Robinson approach. J Neurosurg. 1968;29:397–404.
7. Galbraith JG, Butler JS, Dolan AM, O'Byrne JM. Operative outcomes for cervical myelopathy and radiculopathy. Adv Orthop. 2011:1–5.
8. Heller JG, Raich AL, Dettori JR, Riew KD. Comparative effectiveness of different types of cervical laminoplasty. Evid Based Spine Care J. 2013;4(2):105–15.
9. Bydon M, Mathios D, Macki M, de la Garza-Ramos R, Sciubba DM, Witham TF, et al. Long-term patient outcomes after posterior cervical foraminotomy: an analysis of 151 cases. J Neurosurg Spine. 2014;21(5):727–31.
10. Kishner S. Degenerative disc disease treatment & management. Medscape. 2017. http://emedicine.medscape.com/article/1265453-treatment
11. Kim CH, Kim KT, Chung CK, Park SB, Yang SH, Kim SM, et al. Minimally invasive cervical foraminotomy and discectomy for laterally located soft disc herniation. Eur Spine J. 2015;24(12):3005–12.
12. Rozet I, Vavilala MS. Risks and benefits of patient positioning during neurosurgical care. Anesthesiol Clin. 2007;25(3):631.
13. Lied B, Roenning PA, Sundseth J, Helseth E. Anterior cervical discectomy with fusion in patients with cervical disc degeneration: a prospective outcome study of 258 patients (181 fused with autologous bone graft and 77 fused with a PEEK cage). BMC Surg. 2010;10:10.
14. Wang X, Chen Y, Chen D, Yuan W, Zhao J, Jia L, et al. Removal of posterior longitudinal ligament in anterior decompression for cervical spondylotic myelopathy. J Spinal Disord Tech. 2009;22(6):404–7.
15. Moatz B, Tortolani PJ. Cervical disc arthroplasty: pros and cons. Surg Neurol Int. 2012;3(Suppl 3):S216–24.
16. Phan K, Scherman DB, Xu J, Leung V, Virk S, Mobbs RJ. Laminectomy and fusion vs laminoplasty for multi-level cervical myelopathy: a systematic review. Eur Spine J. 2017;26(1):94–103.
17. Ain MC, Shirley ED. Spinal fusion for kyphosis in achondroplasia. J Pediatr Orthop. 2004;24(5):541–5.
18. Goldstein J. Cervical artificial disc replacement technologies. Deerfield: Spine-Health; 2015. Available from: https://www.spine-health.com/treatment/artificial-disc-replacement/cervical-artificial-disc-replacement-technologies
19. Derenda M, Kowalina I. Cervical laminoplasty—review of surgical techniques, indications, methods of efficacy evaluation, and complications. Neurol Neurochir Pol. 2006;40(5):422–32.
20. Steinmetz M, Resnick D. Cervical laminoplasty. Spine J. 2006;6:274S–81S.
21. Hirabayashi K, Watanabe K, Wakano K, Suzuki N, Satomi K, Ishii Y. Expansive open-door laminoplasty for cervical spinal stenotic myelopathy. Spine. 1983;8(7):693–9.
22. Hirabayashi S. Surgical technique and results of double-door laminoplasty at the cervical spine (Kurokawa's method)—focusing on the change of sagittal alignment. Int J Surg Surgical Porced. 2017;2:118.
23. Zdeblick TA, Zou D, Warden KE, McCabe R, Kunz D, Vanderby R. Cervical stability after foraminotomy. A biomechanical in vitro analysis. J Bone Joint Surg Am. 1992;74(1):22–7.
24. Herkowitz HN, Kurz LT, Overholt DP. Surgical management of cervical soft disc herniation: a comparison between the anterior and posterior approach. Spine. 1990;15(10):1026–30.
25. Kumar GRV, Maurice-Williams RS, Bradford R. Cervical foraminotomy: an effective treatment for cervical spondylotic radiculopathy. Br J Neurosurg. 1998;12(6):563–8.
26. Korinth MC, Kruger A, Oertel MF, Gilsbach JM. Posterior foraminotomy or anterior discectomy with polymethyl methacrylate interbody stabilization for cervical soft disc disease: results in 292 patients with monoradiculopathy. Spine. 2006;31(11):1207–14.
27. Bolesta MJ, Rechtine GR, Chrin AM. Three- and four-level anterior cervical discectomy and fusion with plate fixation: a prospective study. Spine. 2000;25(16):2040–4.
28. Kaiser MG, Haid RW, Subach BR, Barnes B, Rodts GE. Anterior cervical plating enhances arthrodesis after discectomy and fusion with cortical allograft. Neurosurgery. 2002;50:229–36.
29. Hong SW, Lee SH, Khoo LT. A comparison of fixed-hole and slotted-hole dynamic plates for anterior cervical discectomy and fusion. J Spinal Disord Tech. 2010;23(1):22–6.
30. Vaccaro AR, Balderston RA. Anterior plate instrumentation for disorders of the subaxial cervical spine. Clin Orthop Relat Res. 1997;(335):112–21.
31. Fehlings MG, Cooper PR, Errico TJ. Posterior plates in the management of cervical instability: long-term results in 44 patients. J Neurosurg. 1994;81(3):341–9.
32. Ebersold MJ, Pare MC, Quast LM. Surgical treatment for cervical spondylotic myelopathy. J Neurosurg. 1995;82(5):745–51.
33. Yonenobu K, Hosono N, Iwasaki M, Asano M, Ono K. Neurologic complications of surgery for cervical compression myelopathy. Spine. 1991;16(11):1277–82.
34. Saunders RL, Pikus HJ, Ball P. Four-level cervical corpectomy. Spine. 1998;23(22):2455–61.
35. Heller JG, Silcox DH, Sutterlin CE. Complications of posterior cervical plating. Spine. 1995;20(22):2442–8.
36. Troyanovich SJ, Stroink AR, Kattner KA, Dornan WA, Gubina I. Does anterior plating maintain cervical lordosis versus conventional fusion techniques? A retrospective analysis of patients receiving

single-level fusion. J Spinal Disord Tech. 2002;15: 69–74.
37. Cao JM, Zhang YZ, Shen Y, Xu JX, Ding WY, Yang DL, et al. Clinical and radiological outcomes of modified techniques in Bryan cervical disc arthroplasty. J Clin Neurocsci. 2011;18:1308–12.
38. Wada E, Suzuki S, Kanazawa A, Matsuoka T, Miyamoto S, Yonenobu K. Subtotal corpectomy versus laminoplasty for multilevel cervical spondylotic myelopathy: a long-term follow-up study over 10 years. Spine. 2001;26(13):1443–7.
39. Ratliff JK, Cooper PR. Cervical laminoplasty: a critical review. J Neurosurg. 2003;98(3):230–8.
40. Shiraishi T, Fukuda K, Yato Y, Nakamura M, Ikegami T. Results of skip laminectomy—minimum 2-year follow-up study compared with open-door laminoplasty. Spine. 2003;28(24):2667–762.
41. Matz PG, Anderson PA, Holly LT, Groff MW, Heary RF, Kaiser MG, Mummaneni PV, Ryken TC, Choudhri TF, Vresilovic EJ, Resnick DK, Joint Section on Disorders of the Spine and Peripheral Nerves of the American Association of Neurological Surgeons and Congress of Neurological Surgeons. The natural history of cervical spondylotic myelopathy. J Neurosurg Spine. 2009;11(2):104–11. https://doi.org/10.3171/2009.1.SPINE08716.

Part IV

Motion Preservation Surgery for Cervical Degenerative Disorders

Posterior Laminoforaminotomy for Radiculopathy

18

James S. Harrop and John L. Gillick

Pitfalls

- Midline pathology is a relative contraindication as it can be difficult to address via a foraminotomy.
- Neck pain as the predominant symptom also represents a relative contraindication as this procedure has its best results in unilateral radiculopathy.
- Localization in this procedure is of paramount importance, and since intraoperative imaging of the subaxial cervical spine can be difficult, especially below C5, anteroposterior and lateral localizing X-rays should be taken. These films may even be repeated during key steps in the case in order to avoid wrong-level surgery.
- At the C4–C5 level, the C5 root motor fibers can be very sensitive. Therefore, when performing a foraminotomy at this level, one should minimize manipulation of the root. Take extra note of this in patients with bony stenosis, and an external osseous decompression may be beneficial.

Pearls

- Placing the patient in slight reverse Trendelenburg, or in the seated position, can help reduce epidural venous oozing.
- If it proves to be difficult to elevate the ligamentum flavum laterally, one can expand the decompression medially to further develop a plane superficial to the dura.
- During the partial facetectomy, the surgeon must keep the junction of the inferior articular process and superior articular process in the center of the field in order to perform a balanced removal of the cephalad and caudad processes.
- For a soft disc herniation, once a wide foraminotomy is completed, gently retract the nerve root with a microinstru-

J. S. Harrop (✉)
Department of Neurological and Orthopedic Surgery, Division of Spine and Peripheral Nerve Surgery, Delaware Valley SCI Center, Thomas Jefferson University, Philadelphia, PA, USA
e-mail: James.Harrop@jefferson.edu

J. L. Gillick
Department of Neurosurgery, Thomas Jefferson University, Philadelphia, PA, USA

Department of Neurosurgery, Rutgers-New Jersey Medical School, Newark, NJ, USA

M. G. Kaiser et al. (eds.), *Degenerative Cervical Myelopathy and Radiculopathy*,
https://doi.org/10.1007/978-3-319-97952-6_18

ment, and while palpating, the free fragment can often be found in the axilla. Occasionally, gentle pressure on the disc itself will deliver the fragment. One should define both the ventral (motor) and dorsal (sensory) nerve divisions.

Introduction

Cervical spondylosis is a commonly encountered degenerative condition and represents one of the most frequently treated diagnoses in neurosurgery. Its prevalence has recently been demonstrated as 89.7% in patients with a mean age of 56.4 [1]. Patients with this condition may present with neck pain or asymptomatically. In fact, approximately 50–80% of these patients have at least one episode of neck pain with or without associated radicular component annually [2]. Additionally, these patients may have more severe symptoms from nerve root or spinal cord compression, resulting in radicular pain or myelopathy, possibly causing a neurological deficit.

Posterior cervical laminoforaminotomy (PCLF) was first described by Spurling and Scoville in 1944 and represents a safe and effective surgical technique by which to treat cervical radiculopathy in patients who have failed conservative therapy [3]. The aim of this chapter is to describe the indications, contraindications, technique, and complications of PCLF, while providing a review of the current literature regarding this approach.

Cervical Radiculopathy Epidemiology and Natural History

Cervical radiculopathy results from compression of a nerve root due to a disc herniation, cervical spondylosis, or a combination of the two. In a landmark epidemiological study of cervical radiculopathy, Radhakrishnan and colleagues found an annual age-adjusted incidence of 107.3 for males and 63.5 for females per 100,000. The authors also found that a monoradiculopathy involving the C7 nerve root was most frequent, followed by C6. In addition, 21.9% of patients demonstrated a disc herniation alone, whereas 68.4% of patients' symptoms were due to spondylosis alone or in combination with a disc protrusion [4]. Cervical radiculopathy can be the end result of the degenerative cascade, which is the product of disc desiccation, followed by reactive osteophyte formation, leading to ligamentous hypertrophy and/or buckling. All of these processes can result in nerve root impingement, which leads to ischemia secondary to vascular compression. In addition, when foraminal stenosis is present, the nerve root may be subjected to repeated local trauma and traction, resulting in inflammation. These patients may exhibit numbness, weakness, pain, or a combination of these symptoms in a distribution referable to the compressed nerve root.

Once the symptoms of cervical radiculopathy occur, most patients will exhibit a self-limited course, not requiring surgery. In 1963, Lees and Turner found that in 57 cervical radiculopathy patients followed up to 19 years, 75% exhibited a single pain episode without recurrence, while 25% had persistent pain with worsening symptoms [4]. More recently, Radhakrishnan et al. had found that at 4-year follow-up, almost 90% of patients with cervical radiculopathy were either asymptomatic or had only mild symptoms [5, 6]. In addition, a systematic review by Wong et al. found that substantial improvement in radiculopathy symptoms tends to occur within 4–6 months after onset, with 83% of patients experiencing complete recovery within 24–36 months [7].

In patients with persistent symptoms, a course of nonoperative treatment may be initially pursued, as a significant proportion of these patients may improve without requiring surgery. One longitudinal cohort study found that 24/26 patients improved without surgery. Patients included in the study had a cervical disc <4 mm on MRI with extremity pain consistent with cervical radiculopathy. Patients with severe canal stenosis or symptomatic cervical myelopathy were excluded. Nonoperative management consisted of cervical traction, specific physical therapy exercises, oral anti-inflammatory medication, and patient education [8]. However, patients that display persistent radicular symptoms despite conservative treatment, or a progressive or profound neurological deficit, may require surgery. Surgical options for the treatment of cervical radiculopathy include anterior cervical discectomy and fusion (ACDF), cervical arthroplasty, and PCLF.

Posterior Cervical Laminoforaminotomy (PCLF) Background, Indications, and Contraindications

PCLF allows direct decompression of the affected nerve root, without the need for fusion, thereby preserving a motion segment [9–12]. This procedure is usually performed for one- or two-level unilateral cervical radiculopathy due to a disc herniation, disc-osteophyte complex, cervical spondylosis, or a combination of these pathologies. Some authors also have described a three-level procedure [8, 13]. One of the biggest advantages of PCLF is the ability to decompress the nerve root without subjecting the patient to a fusion by preserving the disc space and minimizing facet removal. However, in order to confer this benefit, the surgeon must take care to resect less than 50% of the joint capsule in order to avoid future instability [14].

When determining if a patient would benefit from PCLF, several considerations must be made to ensure the procedure is properly indicated. The indications for PCLF are similar to ACDF and cervical arthroplasty in the sense that the patient should have a progressive or profound neurological deficit or persistent radicular symptoms despite conservative treatment. However, for patients undergoing PCLF, the symptoms must be unilateral. PCLF may also be indicated in the setting of persistent unilateral radiculopathy after a previous ACDF or a prior cervical arthroplasty due to failed decompression of the symptomatic root (particularly after arthroplasty). The posterior approach allows the surgeon to decompress the nerve root, without the associated risks of the anterior approach in a revision case such as dysphagia, dysphonia, esophageal perforation, or recurrent laryngeal nerve injury [9]. Above all else, the most important indication for PCLF is that the patient exhibits clinical findings that correlate with imaging.

Ideally, the patient undergoing this procedure is young (less than 60 years of age) and has a lateral, "soft" disc herniation on MRI [9]. However, this procedure can also be performed in cases of cervical disc-osteophyte disease [15]. Preoperatively, the disc herniation can be best visualized with a T2-weighted MRI, which should also demonstrate compression of the exiting nerve root. Other imaging modalities that may be pursued are a CT scan to evaluate if the disc is calcified or "soft" and a flexion/extension X-ray to rule out any instability. If significant cervical instability is observed, PCLF is contraindicated.

Other contraindications to PCLF include myelopathy or midline pathology. Unfortunately, the decompression provided in this procedure is not sufficient to address any ventral pathology, which may be more appropriately treated from an anterior or more extensive posterior approach. Patients with neck pain alone should not be offered this procedure. In addition, patients with significant neck pain and radiculopathy should be carefully selected prior to undergoing this procedure as this population has been shown to have a higher risk of reoperation and a shorter time to reoperation [16]. Also, bilateral radiculopathies are a relative contraindication as bilateral foraminotomies may result in instability due to disruption of both facets. Previous foraminotomy and lateral mass hypoplasia also represent contraindications as instability may be introduced with further facetectomy [8]. It is also worth noting that PCLF can be a technically difficult procedure as the visualization is small, and a thorough understanding of this unfamiliar anatomy is essential. It is therefore necessary that the primary surgeon have sufficient experience in order to maximize postoperative patient outcomes.

PCLF Planning

Prior to undergoing PCLF, the patient should have all the necessary preoperative imaging. As stated previously, it is the authors' practice to obtain a preoperative MRI, CT, and flexion/extension X-rays. These studies serve the purpose to not only characterize the disc and the type of compression it is subjected to but also evaluate the anatomy of the facet joints and rule out any instability. This surgery is usually performed as an outpatient procedure or in the setting of a 23-h stay. This procedure can be performed using the traditional open method or a minimally invasive technique with the aid of a microscope or endoscope. In addition, patient positioning can depend on surgeon preference. The surgeon can opt for the traditional prone position, but this procedure can also be performed in the seated position. Zeidman and Ducker found that in 172 patients undergoing open PCLF in the seated position, 97% had improvement in pain, while 93% had improved strength, with no wound infections reported, 4 air emboli, and 1 patient with postoperative central cord syndrome [17]. Therefore, when considering seated position, special anesthetic considerations should be made. The patient's body habitus and cardiovascular status should be evaluated preoperatively. Intraoperatively, a precordial Doppler should be placed in order to screen for air embolus. Whether the seated or prone position is chosen, the fundamentals of the operation are the same.

Surgical Technique

Once the patient has been induced by anesthesia, the head is secured using a three-point Mayfield headrest, and the patient is positioned either prone or sitting. Next, the correct cervical level is localized. This can either be accomplished with a lateral X-ray or fluoroscopic image. If the lower cervical levels (i.e., below C6) cannot be visualized adequately, an AP image may be obtained. Once the correct level has been identified, the skin incision is made based on the approach used.

In the traditional, open approach, a midline incision is made, and the posterior cervical musculature is divided and elevated using subperiosteal dissection and Bovie electrocautery until the superior and inferior facets of the correct foramen are exposed. If one is using the minimally invasive (MIS) approach, a 1.5-cm vertical incision is made, 2-cm lateral to the midline on the side of the radiculopathy. During the exposure, the surgeon must meticulously ensure that no more than 50% of the facet capsule is disrupted. A retractor or tube is then inserted depending on whether the approach is open or MIS. In the MIS approach, a series of dilators is used to create the operative corridor. With either approach, a microscope can be used to aid visualization. In the MIS approach, an endoscope may also be used.

After the correct facet joint is exposed, a keyhole foraminotomy is performed using a high-speed burr. First, the inferior articular process of the cephalad facet is drilled (Fig. 18.1), followed by the superior articular process of the caudad facet (Fig. 18.2). Once the partial facetectomy is performed, the exiting nerve root is identified. Utilizing a Kerrison rongeur, the foraminotomy is expanded. Three dimensionally, the superior border of the foramen is the pedicle of the cephalad vertebrae, and the inferior border is the pedicle of the caudad vertebrae. The floor of the foramen is bound by the disc and the uncovertebral joint. A discectomy can sometimes be performed is intermittently inserted into the foramen to ensure that pedicle to pedicle, superior to inferior, the foramen has been decompressed (Fig. 18.3). In addition, the foraminotomy is also extended in a medial-to-lateral direction, just lateral to the pedicles. During this part of the procedure, the Kerrison rongeur should be used in a superolateral trajectory, similar to the course of the exiting nerve root. If a soft disc herniation was identified preoperatively, some surgeons will attempt a discectomy at this time.

A discectomy can be performed by carefully retracting the exiting nerve root in a superior direction and tracing it to its axilla at the thecal sac. Using a no. 15 scalpel blade, an annulotomy can be performed. Once this is accomplished, any compressive disc material or osteophyte can be removed. Since the operating corridor is typically small, and one is working with motor roots, care is taken to minimize retraction and only

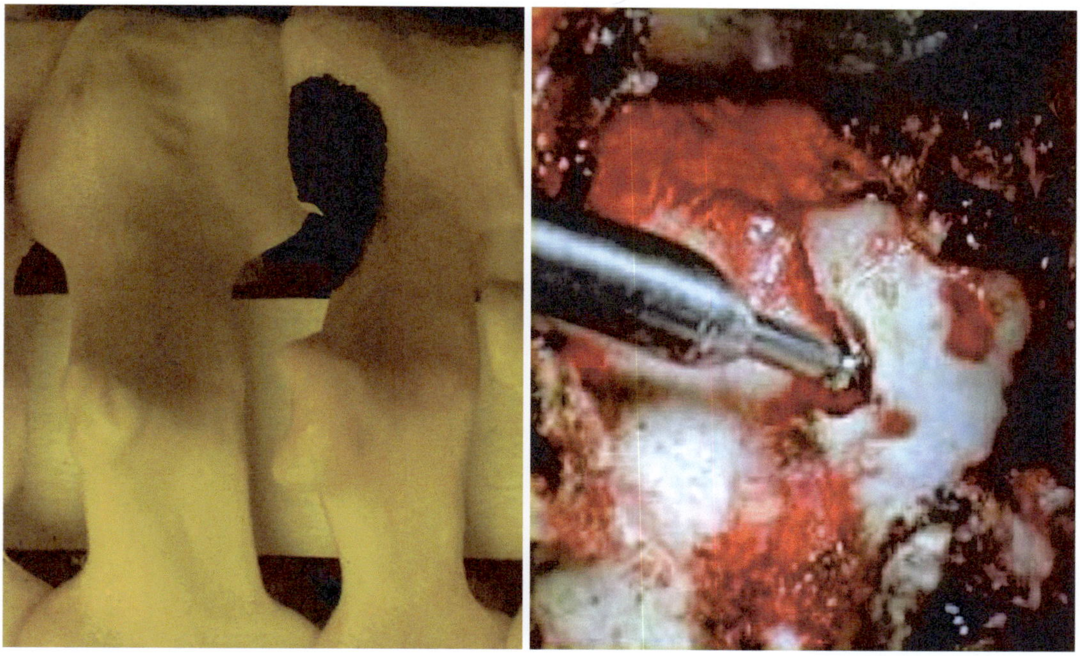

Fig. 18.1 The keyhole foraminotomy begins by using a high-speed burr to remove the medical half of the inferior articular process (IAP) as depicted in by a model (left) and intraoperative photograph (right)

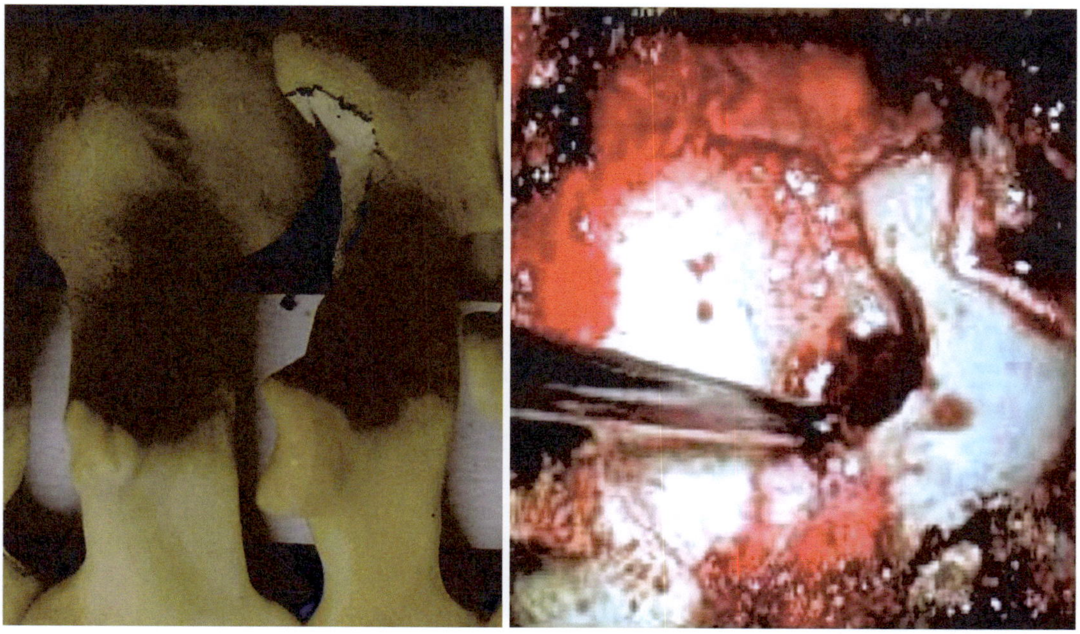

Fig. 18.2 Following removal of the medial half of the IAP, the medial half of the superior articular process (SAP) is removed as depicted by a bone model (left) and intraoperative photograph (right)

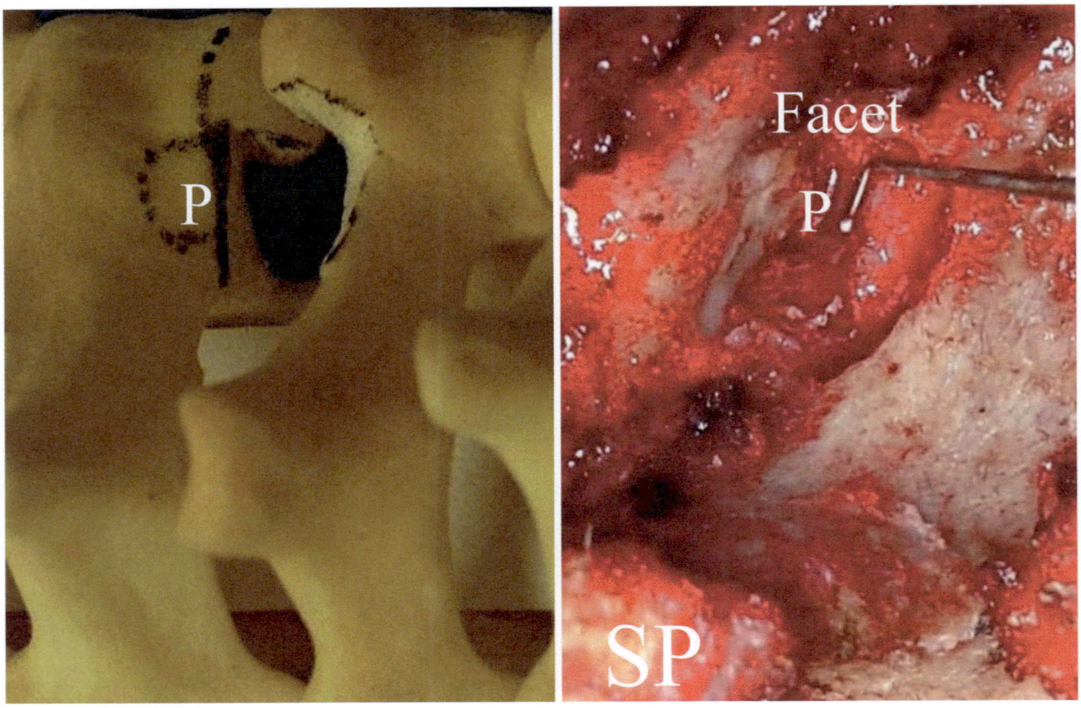

Fig. 18.3 Once the foraminotomy is completed, a nerve hook is passed medial to lateral and cranial to caudal to ensure adequate decompression. Demonstrated by the intraoperative photograph (right) (P, pedicle; SP, spinous process)

remove disc material that can easily be excised. Lastly, a Woodson elevator or nerve hook can be used to palpate the entire foramen, in order to ensure adequate neural decompression. Once this is accomplished, the wound is closed in standard fashion. Patients who undergo this procedure can either be discharged on the day of surgery or the following morning. Physical therapy can usually begin several days after surgery. The patients will then follow up at 2 weeks, 6 weeks, and 3 months.

Open Versus MIS Technique

Some surgeons will advocate a MIS approach and justify it based on a smaller incision size, less blood loss, and possibly a shorter in-hospital stay. Several studies have compared these techniques side by side. Fessler and Khoo performed one of the first of these, comparing microendoscopic foraminotomy (MEF) with traditional, open PCLF. Although the clinical outcomes of the two groups were comparable in terms of radiculopathy, the MEF group experienced less blood loss during surgery, a shorter hospitalization, and lower postoperative pain requirement [18]. These results were further substantiated in a systematic review performed by Clark et al. The authors found, in a review of 19 publications, MIS foraminotomy was associated with lower intraoperative blood loss, shorter surgical time, less inpatient analgesic use, and shorter hospital stay [19]. Although the MIS approach may result in the above-stated benefits, the clinical outcomes of the patients in each of these studies were comparable in both the MIS and the traditional open group [18, 19]. In fact, a meta-analysis performed by McAnany et al. demonstrated a pooled clinical success rate of 92.7% for open PCLF and 94.9% for MIS foraminotomy [20]. Therefore, although the MIS has demonstrable benefit in the short term, the long-term clinical course of the patient is similar in both procedures.

Complications

The most common complications from PCLF include dural tear, nerve root injury, infection, worsening neck pain, and neurologic injury. In a review of 1085 PCLFs, Church et al. found 36 overall complications, representing 3.3% of procedures. Out of these complications, there were 19 surgical site infections (14 requiring operation), 7 dural tears (5 of which resulted in CSF leak and 3 required reoperation to repair), 6 patients with a new focal sensory disturbance, and 3 patients with new focal weaknesses. There was also one patient who had a scalp laceration due to the application of the Mayfield head holder [10]. Overall, the rate of immediate complications with this procedure is relatively low with a published range of 1.5–5.5% [9, 10, 15, 21, 22]. The other complications encountered with this procedure occurred in a delayed fashion. These include a lack symptomatic improvement or recurrence, adjacent segment disease, and cervical instability.

Although PCLF can be quite an effective surgery, the patient must be preoperatively counseled regarding the possibility that their symptoms may not improve. In the large case series of Church et al., out of 630 30-day visits, 20 (3.2%) had persistent arm pain, 26 (4.1%) had residual weakness, and 3 (0.5%) had persistent pain and weakness [10]. These authors also found that patients with soft disc herniations versus those with osteophyte pathologies had significantly higher rates of improved pain postoperatively, improved weakness, and improved function. However, Church et al. were still able to conclude that radiculopathy due to osteophyte disease is still an "excellent" indication for PCLF [10], as their results in the osteophyte group was comparable to prior studies [22].

In a study of 151 retrospectively reviewed PCLFs, Bydon et al. found that at final follow-up (average time 4.15 years), there was an overall improvement of 85%, with 91.4% experiencing improvement within the first month. However, 16.1% of this subgroup experienced symptom recurrence at an average of 7.3 years after the initial surgery. The overall reoperation rate was 9.9% (15 patients), and the second operation was most commonly performed at the index level compared to a distant or adjacent level. In addition, the reoperation rate increased to 18.3% after 2 years of follow-up and 24.3% after 10 years [16]. These patients were treated mostly with ACDF, followed by cervical laminectomy and fusion, and redo PCLF. When evaluating symptom recurrence, the surgeon should rule out adjacent segment disease or iatrogenic instability as the etiology.

One of the benefits of PCLF is that it avoids subjecting the patient to a fusion. Since fusion can predispose a patient to adjacent segment disease (ASD), one may hypothesize that the incidence of ASD in PCLF may be lower when compared to ACDF. In a landmark paper by Hilibrand et al. in 374 patients, totaling 409 ACDFs, ASD occurred at a rate of 2.9% per year during 10 years [23]. The authors further demonstrated that 10 years after the operation 25.6% of patients who had an ACDF would have ASD [23]. In a retrospective study of ASD in 303 patients undergoing PCLF, Clarke et al. found that the annual risk of developing symptomatic ASD was 0.7% with a cumulative risk at 10 years of 6.7% [24]. Additionally, by not fusing the index level, the patient is also subject to breakdown at that level, same level disease. These authors found that the 5- and 10-year risk rate of developing disease at the index level were 3.2% and 5.0%, respectively [24].

Another potential risk assumed by not fusing is the development of postsurgical instability and deformity. In a retrospective review of 162 patients undergoing PCLF, Jagannathan et al. found postoperative instability at the surgical level in 8 patients (4.9%). Of these, eight were asymptomatic, but one required fusion. Loss of cervical lordosis defined as segmental Cobb angle <10° was observed in 30 patients (18.5%), of which 9 had symptoms [15]. The authors also found that among the significant predictors of developing a postoperative deformity were age >60 years, preoperative segmental lordosis <10°, and previous cervical laminectomy [15]. Therefore, patients that exhibit these characteristics may necessitate a more aggressive radiographic follow-up in order to identify the development of deformity postoperatively.

Case Presentations

A 52-year-old female presented with 6 weeks of left shoulder pain and left arm weakness. On physical examination, she was noted to have 3/5 strength in her left triceps and no evidence of myelopathy. She had undergone physical therapy and epidural steroid injections with no symptomatic improvement. An MRI of the cervical spine demonstrated a left-sided C6–C7 disc herniation with impingement upon the exiting left C7 nerve root (Fig. 18.4). She was taken to the operating room for a microscopic left C6/C7 PCLF.

A 56-year-old male with a previous history of a C3–C7 laminectomy and fusion for myelopathy presented with 10 weeks of right-sided arm pain with radiation to his hand. He had received an epidural steroid injection with transient improvement, but his symptoms recurred. He had also noted some difficulty with fine motor control in his right hand and was found to have 4/5 weakness in his right hand intrinsics on physical exam. An MRI of the cervical spine revealed a large right-sided C7–T1 disc herniation (Fig. 18.5). Due to his lack of

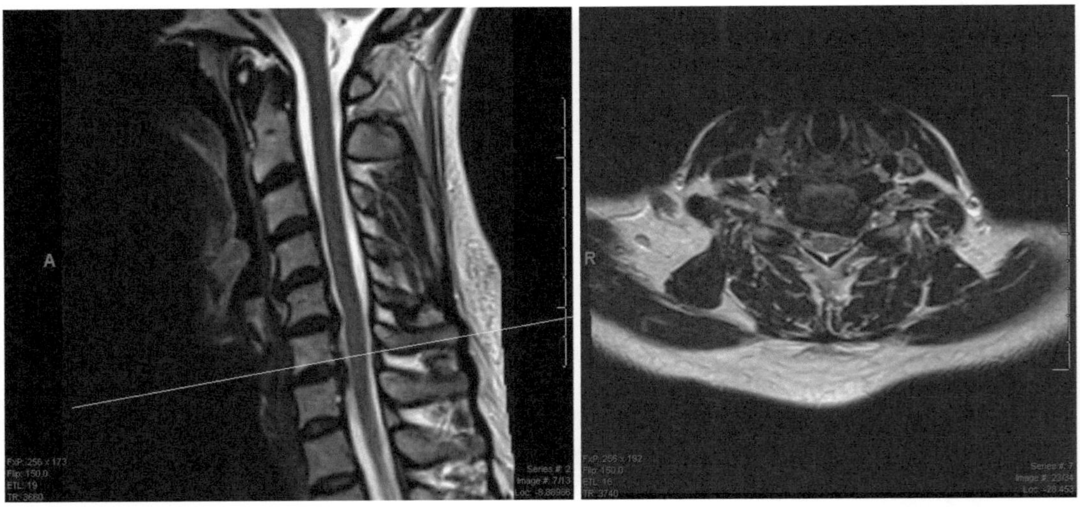

Fig. 18.4 Left-sided C6–C7 disc herniation in a 52-year-old female with radiculopathy and triceps weakness

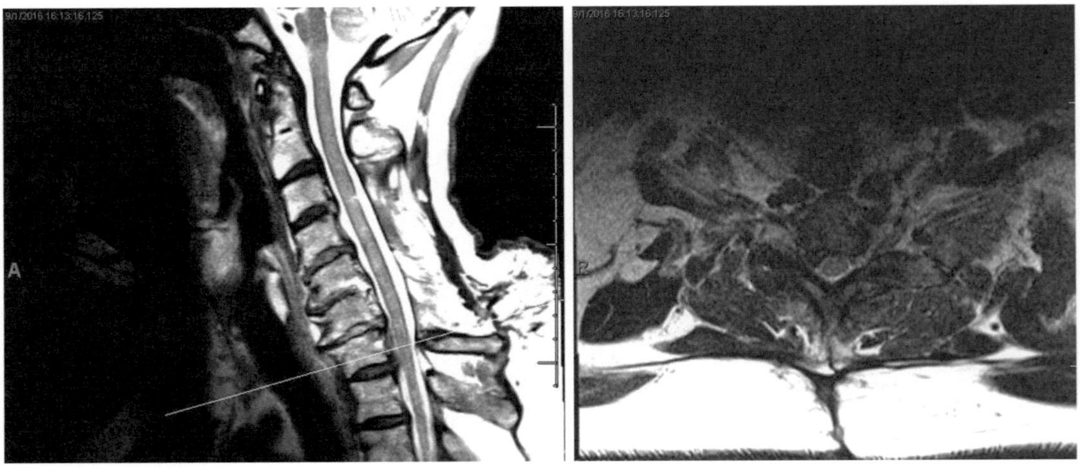

Fig. 18.5 Right-sided C7–T1 disc herniation in a 56-year-old male with right arm pain and hand weakness

improvement with nonoperative care, a right C7–T1 microscopic PCLF was performed.

Discussion/Conclusion

When considering PCLF as a treatment option for cervical radiculopathy, one typically also evaluates if ACDF would be an effective procedure. Although the pathologies that are treated with these two procedures may differ in terms of neck pain and cervical instability, either can accomplish the goal of nerve root decompression. For the treatment of cervical radiculopathy, Liu et al. performed a systematic review including three prospective randomized trials and seven retrospective comparative studies. The authors found mean complication rate of 7% in the ACDF group and 6% in the PCLF group. In addition, the risk of reoperation was 4% in the ACDF group and 6% in the PCLF group. The authors concluded that ACDF and PCLF were equally safe and effective, with PCLF inducing a lower medical cost. As healthcare in the United States shifts to value-based reimbursement and bundle payments, the concept of cost-effectiveness becomes ever more applicable.

In a study of cost-effectiveness for the treatment of cervical radiculopathy in the military, Tumialán et al. found the direct cost of ACDF to be $10,078 compared to $3570 for PCLF and the indirect cost (based on a 14.8-week difference in time to return to active duty) to range from $13,586 to $30,553 greater for the ACDF group [20]. Therefore, from a cost-effective analysis, it appears PCLF may have a slight benefit when compared to ACDF.

When considering operative approaches to the management of cervical radiculopathy, PCLF is an appropriate option in cases of "soft" disc herniation, disc-osteophyte complex, cervical spondylosis, or a combination of these. Whether to approach the cases sitting or prone, MIS or open, the surgeon should use the technique with which he or she is most comfortable. Regardless of the approach chosen, the long-term results of PCLF are comparable to that of ACDF for the right indications.

Key Recommendations

- Localization is of the utmost importance during this procedure; therefore AP and lateral X-rays should be used in order to confirm levels.
- Disrupting 50% of the facet at most is key in order to avoid introduction of instability.
- The best results are achieved in patients with unilateral radiculopathy and foraminal stenosis whose symptoms have persisted despite conservative management in which the imaging matches the clinical findings.

References

1. Nouri A, Martin A, Tetreault L, Nater A, Kato S, Nakashima H, Nagoshi N, Reihani-Kermani H, Fehlings MG. MRI analysis of the combined prospectively collected AOSpine North America and International Data: the prevalence and spectrum of pathologies in a global cohort of patients with degenerative cervical myelopathy. Spine (Phila Pa 1976). 2017;42(14):1058–67.
2. Hult L. The Munkfors investigation; a study of the frequency and causes of the stiff neck-brachialgia and lumbago-sciatica syndromes, as well as observations on certain signs and symptoms from the dorsal spine and the joints of the extremities in industrial and forest workers. Acta Orthop Scan Suppl. 1954;16:1–76.
3. Spurling RG, Scoville WB. Lateral rupture of the cervical intervertebral disks: a common cause of shoulder and arm pain. Surg Gynecol Obstet. 1944;78:350–8.
4. Lees F, Turner JW. Natural history and prognosis of cervical spondylosis. Br Med J. 1963;2(5373):1607–10.
5. Radhakrishnan K, Litchy WJ, O'Fallon WM, Kurland LT. Epidemiology of cervical radiculopathy. A population-based study from Rochester, Minnesota, 1976 through 1990. Brain. 1994;117(Pt 2):325–35. https://doi.org/10.1093/brain/117.2.325.
6. Iyer S, Kim HJ. Cervical radiculopathy. Cur Rev Musculoskelet Med. 2016;9(3):272–80.
7. Wong JJ, Cote P, Quesnele JJ, Stern PJ, Mior SA. The course and prognostic factors of symptomatic cervical disc herniation with radiculopathy: a systematic review of the literature. Spine J. 2014;14:1781–9. https://doi.org/10.1016/j.spinee.2014.02.032.
8. Saal JS, Saal JA, Yurth EF. Nonoperative management of herniated cervical intervertebral disc with radiculopathy. Spine (Phila Pa 1976). 1996;21(16):1877–83.

9. Dodwad SJ, Dodwad SN, Prasam ML, Savage JW, Patel AA, Hsu WK. Posterior cervical foraminotomy: indications, technique, and outcomes. Clin Spine Surg. 2016;29(5):177–85.
10. Church EW, Halpern CH, Faught RW, Balmuri U, Attiah MA, Hayden S, Kerr M, Maloney-Wilensky E, Bynum J, Dante SJ, Welch WC, Simeone FA. Cervical laminoforaminotomy for radiculopathy: symptomatic functional outcomes in a large cohort with long-term follow-up. Surg Neurol Int. 2014;5(Suppl 15):S536–43.
11. Woods BI, Hilibrand AS. Cervical radiculopathy: epidemiology, etiology, diagnosis, and treatment. J Spinal Disord Tech. 2015;28:E251–9.
12. Albert TJ, Murrell SE. Surgical management of cervical radiculopathy. J Am Acad Orthop Surg. 1999;7:368–76.
13. Skovrlj B, Gologorsky Y, Haque R, Fessler RG, Qureshi SA. Complications, outcomes, and need for fusion after minimally invasive posterior cervical foraminotomy and microdiscectomy. Spine J. 2014;14(10):2405–11.
14. Zbeblick TA, Abitbol JJ, Kunz DN, McCabe RP, Garfin S. Cervical stability after sequential capsule resection. Spine (Phila Pa 1976). 1993;18(14):2005–8.
15. Jagannathan J, Sherman JH, Szabo T, Shaffrey CI, Jane JA. The posterior cervical foraminotomy in the treatment of cervical disc/osteophyte disease: a single-surgeon experience with a minimum of 5 years' clinical radiographic follow-up. J Neurosurg Spine. 2009;10:347–56.
16. Bydon M, Mathios D, Macki M, de la Garza-Ramos R, Sciubba DM, Witham TF, Wolinsky JP, Gokasalan ZL, Bydon A. Long-term patient outcomes after posterior cervical foraminotomy: an analysis of 151 cases. J Neurosurg Spine. 2014;21(5):727–31.
17. Zeidman SM, Ducker TB. Posterior cervical laminoforaminotomy for radiculopathy: review of 172 cases. Neurosurgery. 1993;33(3):356–62.
18. Fessler RG, Khoo LT. Minimally invasive cervical microendoscopic foraminotomy: an initial clinical experience. Neurosurgery. 2002;51(5 Suppl):S37–45.
19. Clark JG, Abdullah KG, Steinmetz MP, Benzel EC, Mroz TE. Minimally invasive versus open cervical foraminotomy: a systematic review. Global Spine J. 2011;1(1):9–14.
20. Tumialán LM, Ponton RP, Gluf WM. Management of unilateral cervical radiculopathy in the military: the cost effectiveness of posterior cervical foraminotomy compared with anterior cervical discectomy and fusion. Neurosurg Focus. 2010;28(5):E17.
21. Henderson CM, Hennessy RG, Shuey HM, Shackelford EG. Posterior-lateral foraminotomy as an exclusive operative technique for cervical radiculopathy: a review of 846 consecutively operated cases. Neurosurgery. 1983;13(5):504–12.
22. Kumar GR, Maurice-Williams RS, Bradford R. Cervical foraminotomy: an effective treatment for cervical spondylotic radiculopathy. Br J Neurosurg. 1998;12(6):563–8.
23. Hilibrand AS, Carlson GD, Palumbo MA, Jones PK, Bohlman HH. Radiculopathy and myelopathy at segments adjacent to the site of a pervious anterior cervical arthrodesis. J Bone Joint Surg Am. 1999;81(4):519–28.
24. Clarke MJ, Ecker RD, Krauss WE, McClelland RL, Dekutoski MB. Same-segment and adjacent-segment disease following posterior cervical foraminotomy. J Neurosurg Spine. 2007;6(1):5–9.

19 Cervical Laminoplasty

Lionel N. Metz, Grigoriy Arutyunyan, Deeptee Jain, Lee A. Tan, and K. Daniel Riew

Introduction

Cervical laminoplasty is an effective and well-established treatment for cervical myelopathy and myeloradiculopathy. The original laminoplasty technique was described by Tsuji in 1982 in a series of 12 patients, where the cervical laminae were cut bilaterally at the affected levels and the resultant "lamina flap" was left to "float" on top of the spinal cord [1]. Many different laminoplasty methods have been developed over the last 35 years since the original technique, including open-door laminoplasty, French-door laminoplasty, dome-shaped laminoplasty, and many other variations. Various methods for stabilization and fixation techniques following laminoplasty have also been developed including the mini-plate fixation, ceramic plate stabilization, suture-anchor stabilization, tension-band laminoplasty, etc. [2–4].

The open-door laminoplasty, which was first described by Hirabayashi et al. in 1983, is the most popular laminoplasty technique today [5]. This technique expands the dorsal spinal canal by opening the lamina on one side, while hinging the lamina on the other side, thus creating more space for the spinal cord. Laminoplasty is most effective in a lordotic cervical spine, which allows the spinal cord to drift dorsally to indirectly alleviate ventral compression. However, the procedure can still be effective in patients with neutral or slightly kyphotic (<10°) cervical alignment. Suda et al. reviewed a series of 114 patients and found that when local cervical kyphosis is greater than 13°, patients had worse clinical outcome after laminoplasty [6]. In addition, newer concepts such as "K-line" and "modified K-line" can also help spine surgeons to predict if adequate spinal cord decompression can be achieved with laminoplasty [7–9]. Furthermore, a recent study demonstrated that increased C2–C7 SVA and higher T1 slope are correlated with loss of cervical lordosis after laminoplasty [10].

Indications

Cervical laminoplasty with posterior foraminotomy can be an effective treatment for many patients with progressive myelopathy or myeloradiculopathy due to multilevel cervical stenosis. The etiology of multilevel cervical stenosis may include cervical spondylosis, congenital spinal stenosis, or ossification of the posterior longitudinal ligament (OPLL). Although lami-

L. N. Metz · G. Arutyunyan · D. Jain
Department of Orthopedic Surgery, UCSF Medical Center, San Francisco, CA, USA

L. A. Tan · K. D. Riew (✉)
The Spine Hospital, Columbia University Medical Center, New York, NY, USA
e-mail: kr2637@cumc.columbia.edu

M. G. Kaiser et al. (eds.), *Degenerative Cervical Myelopathy and Radiculopathy*,
https://doi.org/10.1007/978-3-319-97952-6_19

noplasty with posterior foraminotomy can improve or halt symptoms of myelopathy and myeloradiculopathy, its effect on axial neck pain is unpredictable. Specifically, axial neck pain related to cervical spondylosis and facet arthropathy typically does not improve. Therefore, patients who have severe axial neck pain as a major part of the overall symptomatology may not be ideal candidates for laminoplasty. Nonetheless, a more recent study demonstrated that patients may have substantial improvements of total Neck Disability Index (NDI) score, as well as the NDI pain score after laminoplasty [11]. Thus, we believe that in patients with only mild to moderate neck pain, who desire preservation of cervical motion, laminoplasty may still be a good option as long as there are realistic expectations and clear understandings of the surgical goals.

Compared to laminectomy and fusion, cervical laminoplasty offers several significant advantages. First, since laminoplasty is a motion-preserving procedure, it does not reduce the range of motion in the cervical spine after surgery, and it does not carry the risk of pseudoarthrosis. Second, laminoplasty preserves the posterior bony elements, which prevents soft-tissue scarring on to the dura (extremely beneficial during revision surgery) and prevents soft-tissue buckling into the spinal cord during neck extension. In addition, compared to laminectomy alone, there is a decreased risk of postoperative kyphosis following laminoplasty, and it restores the soft-tissue tension band through the preservation of bony attachments for paraspinal muscles [12]. Furthermore, laminoplasty requires less instrumentation and is less morbid compared to laminectomy and fusion, which may lead to a more expedited recovery [13].

In patients with cervical myeloradiculopathy, the radiculopathy component can often be addressed by nerve root decompression via posterior foraminotomies. However, in patients with severe radiculopathy with neurologic deficits, especially those with bilateral disease, we have found a higher rate of failure with posterior decompression than with the anterior approach.

Contraindication

Cervical kyphosis in the region of planned posterior decompression is generally a contraindication for laminoplasty. The kyphotic segment does not allow for the spinal cord to drift back, and there is a high risk for persistent ventral compression after laminoplasty. However, for patients who wish to preserve their range of motion and/or are not good medical candidates for a fusion procedure, laminoplasty can still be a good treatment option in setting of mild kyphosis and circumferential stenosis.

Conversely, for myelopathic patients with kyphotic alignment and anterior compression yet adequate cerebrospinal fluid behind the cord, a laminoplasty is unlikely to be successful. Fujiyoshi et al. used the "K-line," which is a line drawn by connecting the midpoint of the spinal canal at C2 and C7 on standing lateral cervical X-rays, to predict clinical outcome after laminoplasty in patients with OPLL [7]. They found that neurological recovery rate was much lower in patients with anterior compression exceeding the "K-line." Taniyama et al. demonstrated that patients with <4-mm space between the anterior compression factor and the modified "K-line" (K-line drawn on sagittal MRI instead of on upright lateral X-rays) had much higher risk for persistent anterior spinal cord compression after laminoplasty [8]. In select cases with multilevel stenosis and kyphotic deformity, laminoplasty can be combined with an instrumented posterior fusion as an alternative to laminectomy and fusion, as to preserve protective bony elements and increase surface area for fusion mass. Although the potential benefits of combining a posterior-based fusion with laminoplasty may seem intuitive, this concept has not been studied extensively.

Although cervical laminoplasty is a very effective option for treating myelopathy due to compression of neurologic elements in setting of cervical spine stenosis, debilitating axial neck pain is a relative contraindication to laminoplasty. Hosono et al. reported postoperative axial neck pain prevalence to be 60% following laminoplasty as compared to 19% following anterior fusion operations [14]. Contrastingly, Yoshida et al. found that French-door laminoplasty had no effect on either the development or resolution of neck or shoulder pain [15]. Though preoperative neck pain is not an absolute contraindication, it is an important factor to discuss with the patient during surgical planning to set appropriate expectations.

Degenerative spondylolisthesis is also not an absolute contraindication to laminoplasty. Shigematsu et al. investigated the comorbidity of degenerative spondylolisthesis in elderly patients with cervical spondylotic myelopathy and found that spondylolisthesis was not a negative prognostic indicator for laminoplasty, which has also been our experience [16]. In addition, interscapular and upper trapezius pains are often results of radiculopathy due to foraminal stenosis, and they usually improve after posterior foraminotomies at the corresponding levels.

Preoperative Evaluation

A comprehensive evaluation of the patient should be performed prior to performing laminoplasty. The evaluation should include a detailed clinical questionnaire, a thorough physical examination, and appropriate diagnostic imaging modalities. A detailed review should include the documentation of all cervical spine-related symptoms, especially symptoms indicating progressive spinal cord compression. Timing, onset, chronicity, exacerbating factors, the overall course and trajectory, history of falls, changes and bowel and bladder function, the presence of axial neck pain, and the distribution of arm pain are essential to document. Physical exam should document range of motion of the neck, gait pattern, muscle weakness in upper or lower extremities, and signs of upper motor neuron dysfunction such as hyperreflexia and Hoffmann's or Babinski reflex. The radiographic evaluation of patients for whom laminoplasty may be considered includes standard anterior-posterior (AP) and lateral radiographs, flexion and extension lateral radiographs, and oblique radiographs (to visualize the neural foramen) of the cervical spine. These are used to assess cervical alignment, ROM, degenerative changes, instability and spondylolisthesis, underlying congenital stenosis, foraminal stenosis, autofusions, and other pathologies of the cervical spine.

Magnetic resonance imaging (MRI) is used to evaluate the severity and craniocaudal extent of stenosis as well as study contributing etiologies such as disk bulging, uncovertebral and facet arthrosis, hypertrophy and infolding of the ligamentum flavum, underlying congenital stenosis, deformity, or ossification of the posterior longitudinal ligament (OPLL). Computed tomography (CT) of the cervical spine is indicated for the evaluation of bony or calcified causes of stenosis, including OPLL and uncovertebral or facet arthrosis causing foraminal stenosis. CT myelography is indicated when MRI is contraindicated or cannot be obtained. If a CT scan is obtained, a topographic reconstruction of the posterior cervical spine may provide reference landmarks that supplement intraoperative fluoroscopic examination.

Surgical Technique

Patient Positioning

The patient undergoing cervical laminoplasty is positioned on a Jackson table with four bolsters in the prone position. Proximally, pads are placed at the level of the sternum, and the arms are tucked at the sides. Distally, pads are placed at the anterior superior iliac spine, and the lower extremities are supported in a well-padded sling. Special attention should be given during the intubation of the patient with cervical myelopathy; chin-lift and jaw-thrust maneuvers should be avoided to minimize risk of spinal cord injury. Mean arterial pressure (MAP) should be maintained at an adequate level (usually >70 mmHg) to ensure cord perfusion. Upon securing the endotracheal tube, Gardner-Wells tongs are placed. Transcranial motor-evoked potentials and somatosensory-evoked potentials are used for all procedures. The patient is then rotated into the prone position, and approximately 15 lbs. of traction is applied to the Gardner-Wells tongs on the flexion rope of a bivector traction system in

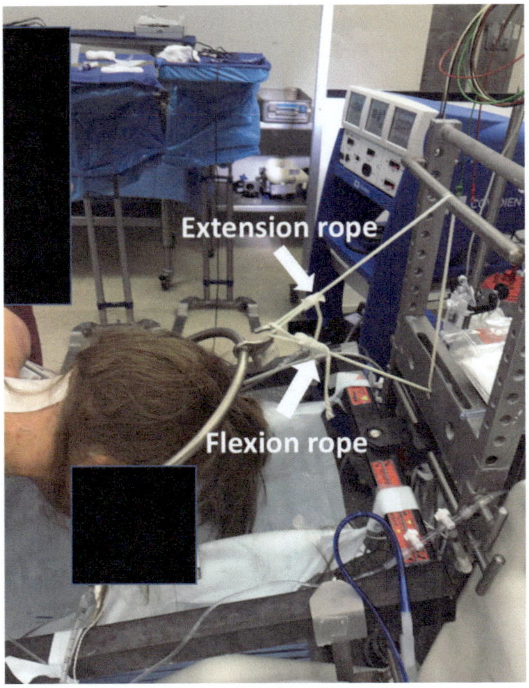

Fig. 19.1 A photograph demonstrating the bivector cervical traction setup with Gardner-Wells tongs

order to obtain optimal surgical exposure (Fig. 19.1). Bivector traction consists of traction applied through two ropes. The flexion rope is in line with the external auditory meatus and cranial vertex for positioning the cervical spine in slight flexion; the extension rope is placed over an elevated crossbar at the head of the Jackson frame, providing an extension vector to extend the neck intraoperatively when necessary. The head is positioned using the flexion rope from the time of surgical exposure of the spine through fixation with a laminoplasty plate and then extended using the extension rope to test ROM and check for bony block before closure.

All bony prominences should be well padded, the abdomen should hang freely in the midline, and the patient is belted securely to the frame. Slight reverse Trendelenburg is used to reduce venous pressure at the wound, to decrease facial and laryngeal swelling, and to reduce intraorbital pressure and the risk of blindness associated with prone positioning. A forced-air warming blanket is placed beneath the patient and Jackson frame, since most thermal losses occur at the patient's ventral surface. Placement of the warming blanket beneath the patient also prevents the air blanket from interfering with the drapes when the blanket is inflated. The cervical area undergoing surgery is then prepped and draped in the appropriate sterile fashion, providing skin exposure from the occiput proximally to the upper thoracic spine distally, as well as sufficient skin exposure on either side of the wound for the lateral passage of drains at the distal edges of the wound.

Surgical Exposure

We prefer to use the operating microscope for the entire procedure from skin incision to wound closure. Using the microscopic not only provides much better visualization and illumination of the surgical field, it also provides the most ergonomic posture for the surgeon throughout the case.

An incision is made with a blade from C3 through C7 in the midline centered over the spinous processes. Electrocautery is used to perform subcutaneous dissection through avascular cervical raphe without violating the muscle sheath on either side. The spinous processes should be frequently palpated to ensure that dissection remains precisely in the midline without injuring the adjacent muscles (Fig. 19.2). There should be very minimal blood loss during this stage of surgery if the dissection is done meticulously. When deep to the fascia, a combination of Metzenbaum scissors and electrocautery may be used to spread in line with muscle fibers to identify and develop the relatively avascular midline raphe. Meticulous dissection and attention to the tissue planes help optimize closure, reduce bleeding, and maximize potential for wound healing. In addition, mindful handing of the soft-tissue envelope may decrease postoperative pain associated with the procedure.

After the paraspinal muscles are separated in the midline down to the level of the spinous processes, the bifid spinous processes are palpated with a finger to correlate intraoperatively anatomic landmarks to the anatomical features noted on preoperative imaging studies. Cautery is used

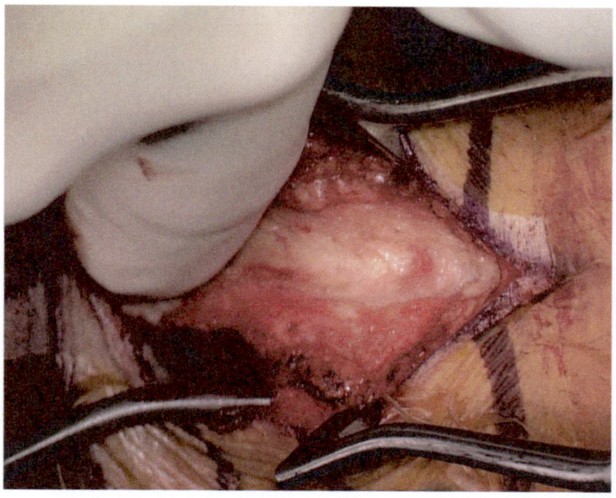

Fig. 19.2 The spinous processes are frequently palpated to ensure that the dissection remains precisely in the midline

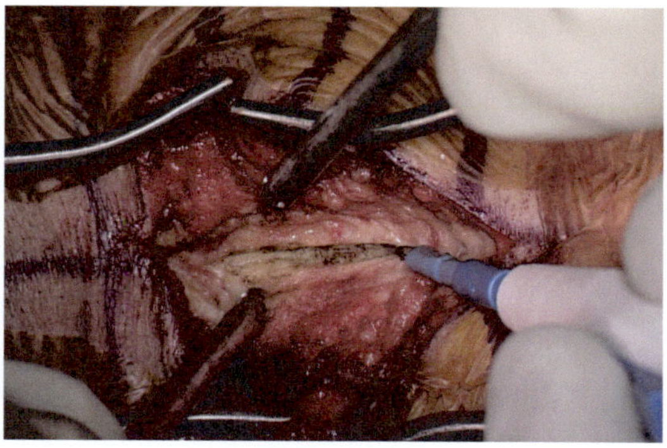

Fig. 19.3 Electrocautery is used to dissect down to the bifid spinous processes dorsally, leaving muscle attachments at the dorsal tips and lateral edges intact

along the midline sulcus of the bifid spinous processes dorsally, leaving muscle attachments at the dorsal tips and lateral edges of these processes (Fig. 19.3). In monofid spinous processes of C7 and often C6, the midline of the dorsal process is exposed with electrocautery. The most ventral paraspinal muscles are bluntly dissected along the midline, in an atraumatic fashion. Muscle fibers tethered on the lamina above and below the spinous processes are released through electrocautery while leaving the dorsal and lateral muscle attachments to each bifid spinous process as the only remaining midline muscle attachment.

Next, a small bone cutter is used to cut each bifid process at the level of the sulcus (Fig. 19.4).

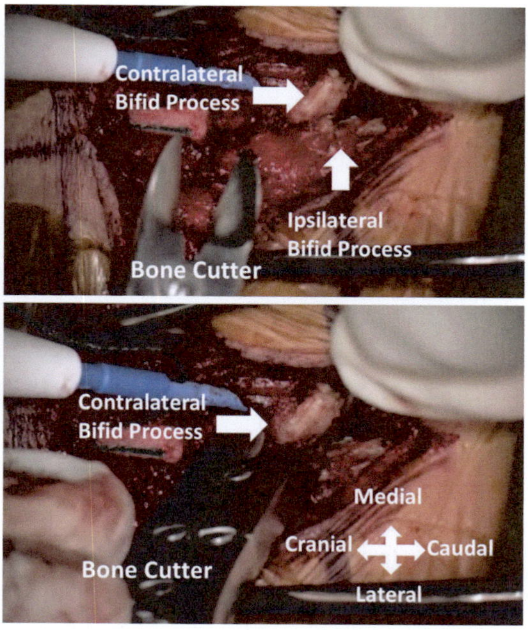

Fig. 19.4 A small bone cutter is used to cut the tip of each bifid process at each level

When performing the osteotomy, the instrument should be held horizontally to the wound and moved in a midline-to-lateral direction so as not to risk cutting ventrally into the lamina or entering the spinal canal. Because only the bifid tips of the spinous processes are cut, the bases are left for manipulation during open hinging of the lamina. Alternatively, a half-inch osteotome can be used to perform the osteotomy of the spinous processes as described originally by Shiraishi et al. [17]. Cutting the bifid spinous processes allows better visualization of the surgical field with the broad, bifid processes removed and aids in subperiosteal dissection and in reapproximation of the paraspinal muscles at the time of wound closure. Our technique has been slightly modified as compared to original description whereby we use a small bone cutter rather than an osteotome for the osteotomies, as to avoiding percussion over an often myelopathic spinal cord. To facilitate closure, the bony fragments are tagged with sutures at the time of osteotomy; these sutures can be used to reapproximate the bony fragment at each corresponding level at the time of wound closure.

If a CT scan is available, a surface reconstruction of the posterior aspect of the spine can be an especially useful map of the intraoperative anatomy of posterior elements. Specifically, the spinous processes can function as a confirmatory adjunct to fluoroscopic localization. Completion of the osteotomies at each level requiring exposure substantially facilitates subperiosteal dissection, and soft tissue can be elevated in an atraumatic fashion. A small Cobb elevator can be then used to mobilize the paraspinal muscles laterally, taking care to stay superficial to the facet joint capsule, to a point a few millimeters past the medial portion of the undisturbed, underlying joint. Surgical dissection lateral to the lateral masses should be avoided to prevent bleeding from the lateral periarticular venous plexus. Meticulous hemostasis in conjunction with an atraumatic dissection will maximize the efficiency and safety of the operation. Various agents are used for hemostasis, but it is paramount that agents that inhibit bone healing not be used on bony surfaces that are intended to heal, such as the hinge region when performing laminoplasty. It is important to place all self-retaining retractors with only gentle force; aggressive retractor placement may increase bleeding and postoperative soft-tissue pain. In addition, only blunt-tipped retractors should be used; sharp retractors can easily penetrate the muscle sheath and cause unnecessary bleeding and soft-tissue trauma. After dissection is carried to the lateral mass, self-retaining McCulloch retractors of the appropriate depth are placed at either end of the incision with their blades oriented in a parasagittal fashion; this blade arrangement can aid in orienting the subsequent opening and hinging laminoplasty cuts.

Foraminotomy

Foraminotomy is always performed using the operating microscope by the senior author. Alternatively, loupe magnification can be used for this part of the procedure if a microscope is not available. It is no longer our routine practice to perform prophylactic bilateral foraminotomies at C4–C5 to prevent C5 nerve palsy, as we found that it made no difference in the risk of C5 palsy. However, we perform foraminotomies at all the symptomatic levels in which preoperative imaging clearly demonstrates foraminal stenosis. In this chapter, we intentionally outline a posterior foraminotomy in detail since it is frequently performed with laminoplasty to address foraminal stenosis posteriorly and may expand the efficacy of laminoplasty in patients with myeloradiculopathy. Furthermore, we believe that some postoperative neck pain is actually a manifestation of radiculopathy related to residual foraminal stenosis. Thus, having an understanding of anatomic boundaries to neural foramina and performing a critical assessment of the foramen on preoperative imaging are essential to performing this procedure safely.

The cervical neural foramen is bound ventrally by the intervertebral disk and uncovertebral joint, dorsally by the superior articular process of the caudal vertebra (e.g., the superior articular process of C6 at the C5–C6 foramen) (Fig. 19.5), and cranial-caudally by the adjacent pedicles. Posterior foraminotomy relieves nerve root compression by unroofing the dorsal boundary of the foramen with removal of the superior articular process of the caudal vertebra from its medial aspect up to the lateral margins of the pedicles, thereby allowing the nerve root to drift dorsally away from the ventral disk bulge/fragment or uncinate bone spur. Because the pedicles form the cranial and caudal borders of the neural foramen, adequate decompression entails resection

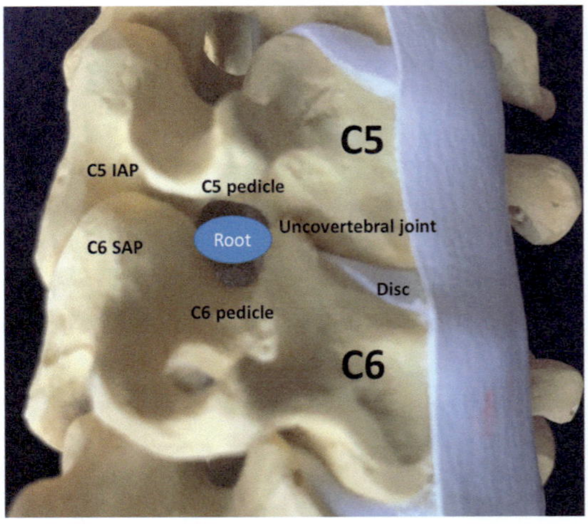

Fig. 19.5 The boundaries of the neural foramen are demonstrated on a Sawbones model

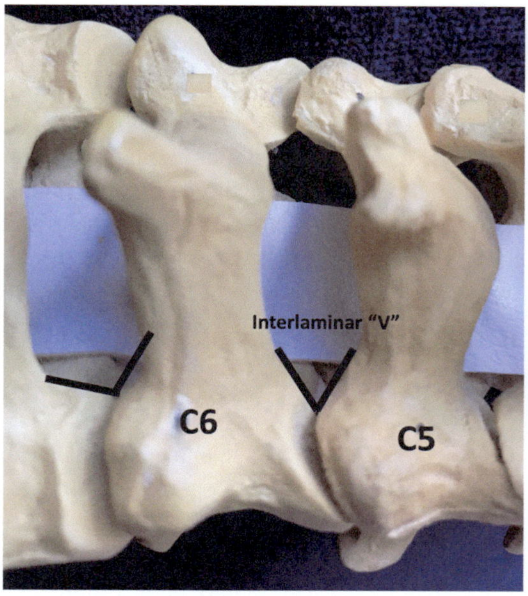

Fig. 19.6 The interlaminar "V," a key landmark for both foraminotomy and laminoplasty, is delineated by the distal aspect of the cranial lamina intersecting the leading edge of the caudal lamina

of the superior articular process up to the lateral margins of the pedicles. It is important to note that under-resection of the superior articular process leads to residual foraminal stenosis; however, overaggressive resection may lead to facet joint instability. A key landmark both for foraminotomy and subsequent laminoplasty is the interlaminar "V," which is the point at which the distal aspect of the cranial lamina intersects the leading edge of the caudal lamina (Fig. 19.6).

The foraminotomy begins with the distal-medial resection of the overlying inferior articular process (IAP) until the cranial edge of the superior articular process is visualized. This can be accomplished quickly by using a high-speed burr (Fig. 19.7). No more than 50% of the mediolateral width of the facet should be removed to ensure stability. Flexion of the neck can help to uncover the underlying superior articular process as the inferior articular process translates cranially. Next, the exposed medial aspect of the superior articular process (SAP) is removed with a burr by cutting an L-shaped trough (Fig. 19.8), with the vertical limb of the "L" cut along the lateral border of the pedicle, and the horizontal

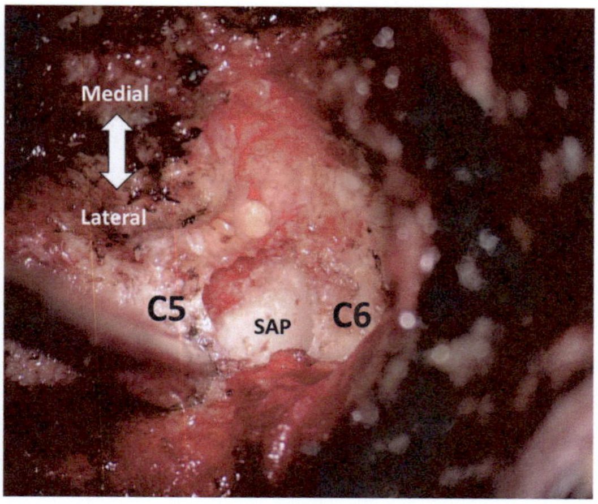

Fig. 19.7 An intraoperative photograph demonstrating the removal of the medial half of the C5 inferior articular process and visualization of the underlying medial half of the C6 superior articular process (SAP)

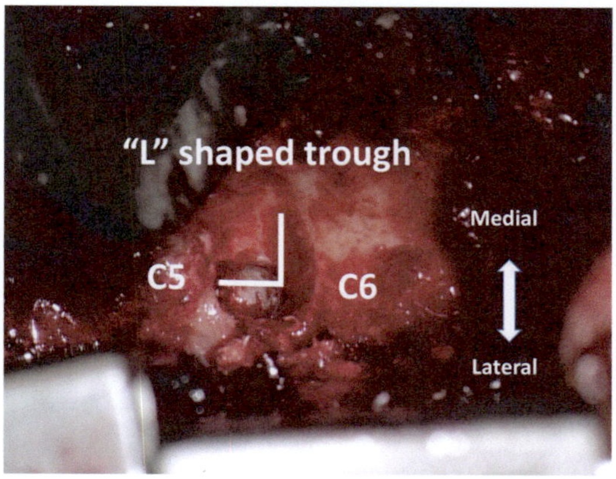

Fig. 19.8 An intraoperative photograph showing the "L"-shaped trough, with the vertical cut along the lateral border of the pedicle and the horizontal cut just cranial to the caudal pedicle

cut just cranial to the caudal pedicle. If the cranial border of the C6 superior articular facet is not exposed, it can easily lead to "sickle-shaped" decompression with persistent nerve root compression (Fig. 19.9). To avoid this scenario, the cranial border of the C6 facet should be exposed before the decompression begins. Adequate visualization can be achieved by maximal flexion of the neck and using interlaminar spreader for additional distraction if needed. Generous irrigation using an 18-gauge flexible angiocatheter on a 20-cc syringe should be used to avoid thermal injury to the nerve and to enhance visualization by constantly washing away the bone dust.

We prefer using a high-speed burr rather than a Kerrison rongeur to avoid introducing space-occupying instruments into an already stenotic foramen. Once most of the foramen has been unroofed, a 1-mm Kerrison punch or a small curette (Codman 1B or 2B curette) is used to clean up any overhanging bone (Fig. 19.10). At the conclusion of the foraminotomy, the lateral walls of the cranial and caudal pedicles should be readily palpable with a nerve hook or a small curette (Fig. 19.11). There should be no overhanging bone at the medial or cranial aspects of the caudal pedicle. After completing the foraminotomy, meticulous hemostasis is obtained with local hemostatic agents such as powdered thrombin or Gelfoam (Pfizer).

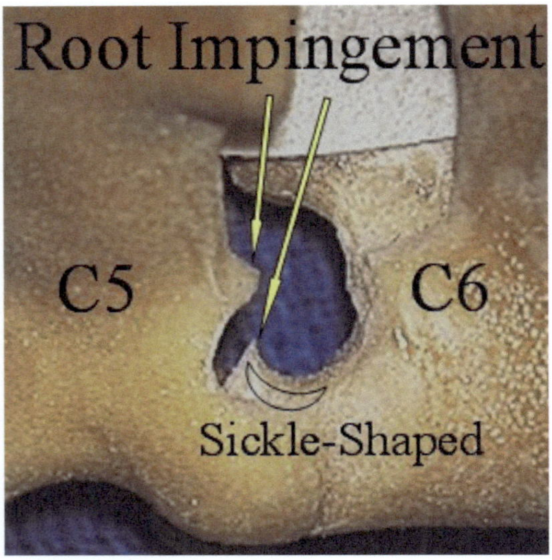

Fig. 19.9 Failure to visualize the cranial border of the superior articular process can result in a "sickle-shaped" decompression, which leads to persistent nerve root compression

Laminoplasty

This section describes a C3 laminectomy and C4, C5, and C6 open-door laminoplasty for the treatment of multilevel spondylotic stenosis from C2–C3 to C6–C7 causing myelopathy (Fig. 19.12). The steps outlined below may be in conjunction with a partial C2 dome laminectomy and/or partial C7 laminectomy, depending on the proximal and distal extents of the stenosis. The levels addressed during the decompression depend on the pathology unique to each patient.

First, a C3 laminectomy is performed with a high-speed burr using a controlled side-to-side sweeping motion. The ligamentum flavum lies deep to the distal two thirds of the lamina and protects the underlying dura. Extra precaution should be taken if the proximal third of the lamina must be removed, as there is no underlying

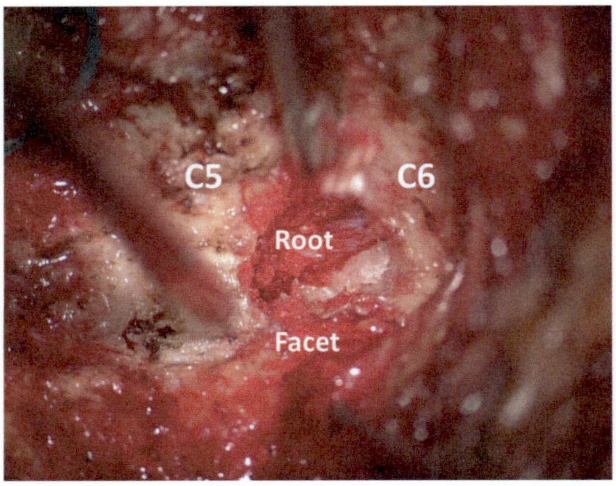

Fig. 19.10 An intraoperative photograph demonstrating adequate removal of superior articular process with decompression of the exiting nerve root

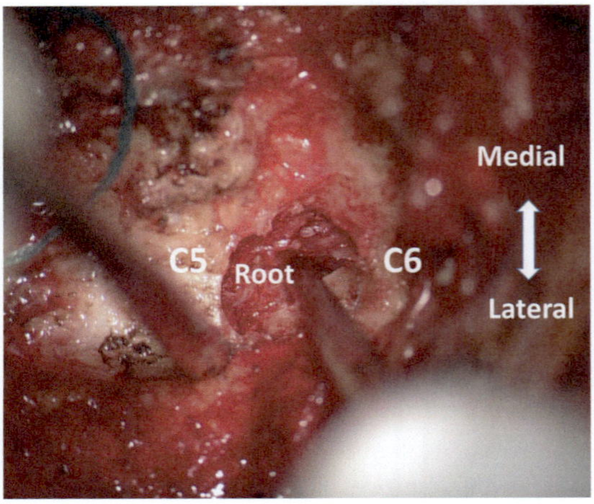

Fig. 19.11 The lateral walls of the cranial and caudal pedicles should be readily palpable with a nerve hook or a small curette at the completion of the foraminotomy

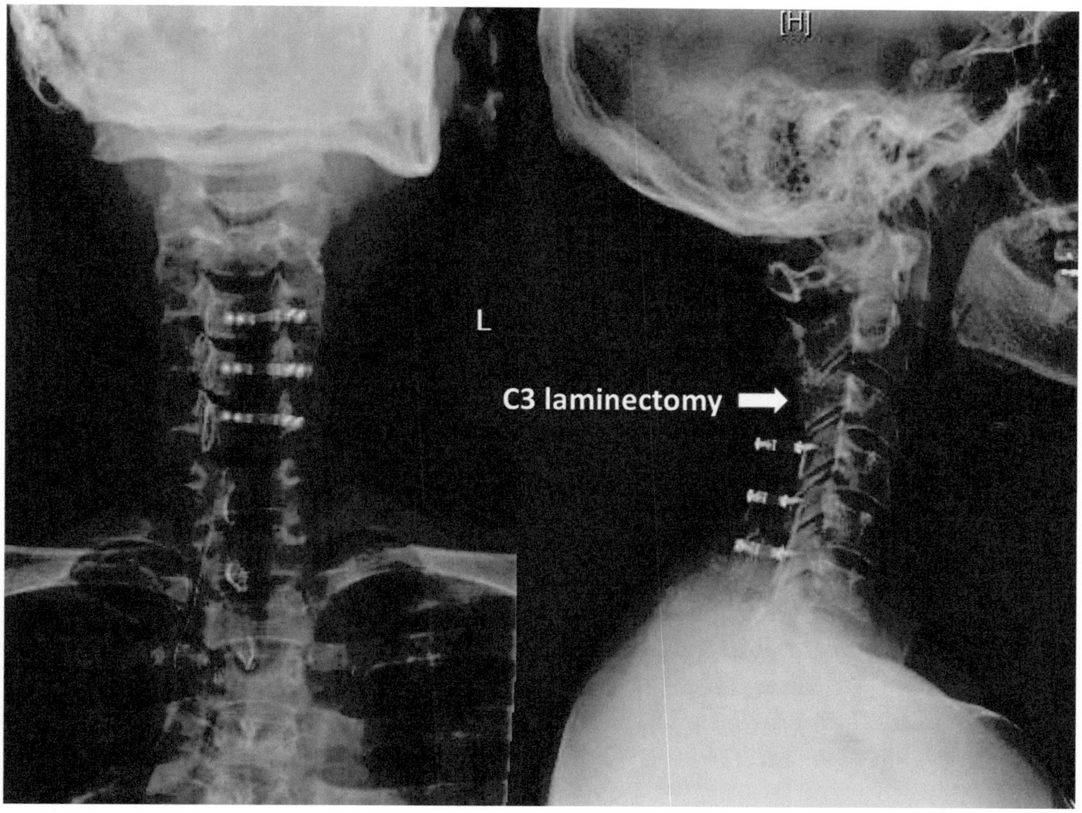

Fig. 19.12 AP and lateral X-rays illustrating the typical radiographic appearance after C3 laminectomy; C4, C5, and C6 laminoplasty; and partial C7 laminectomy

ligamentum flavum and there is increased risk for incidental durotomy. If complete laminectomy is necessary, the cranial third of the lamina can be thinned down to the ventral cortex with a burr, and the remaining thin shell of bone can be removed with a curette or Kerrison rongeur. The ligamentum flavum is then detached from the cranial portion of the dorsal C4 lamina with a burr or curette without transmitting excessive force to the spinal cord.

Next, the complete cut through the lamina is made using the high-speed burr on the open side of the open-door laminoplasty, which is usually the side with more severe cord compression or the side that requires one or more foraminotomies. The cutline of the open side is first defined with electrocautery, which is the line that delineates the lamina-facet junction by connecting the interlaminar Vs at the corresponding level. The first pass using the burr should be at depth that removes the dorsal cortical bone along with much of the underlying cancellous bone. The second pass removes the remaining cancellous bone and thins the ventral cortical lamina to a shell (Fig. 19.13). Both of these passes can be safely completed quickly with some practice. Bone wax placed on a cottonoid patty can be used to effectively stop bone bleeding from the trough. The final pass with the burr completes the cut at each lamina, as evidenced by movement across the cut at each level with gentle pressure on the spinous process. If there is uncertainty regarding the completion of the cut through the ventral cortex, a curette can be used to verify the presence of remaining bony bridges.

When the lamina cuts are completed on the open side, the high-speed burr is used to detach the ligamentum flavum from the cranial portion of the dorsal C7 lamina. In similar fashion to the C3 segment, the cranial portion of C7 can be

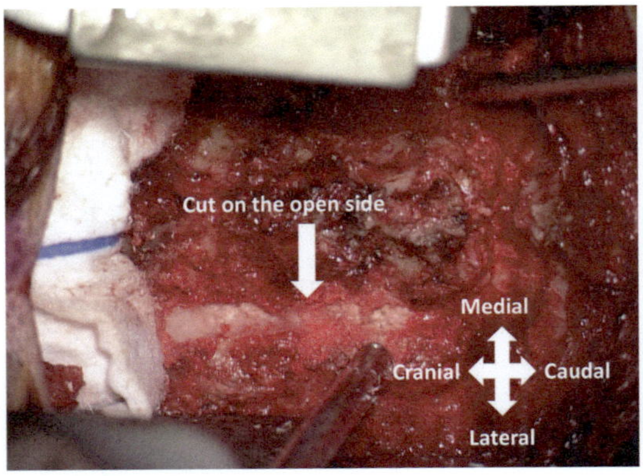

Fig. 19.13 An intraoperative photograph showing the cut on the open side after second pass with the high-speed burr leaving only a thin shell of ventral cortical bone; bone wax is applied with a small cottonoid patty for hemostasis before a final pass with the high-speed burr to complete the cut

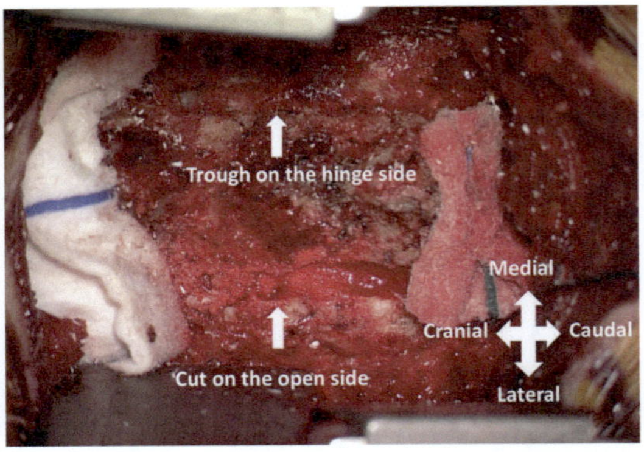

Fig. 19.14 The trough on the hinge side is completed by first creating two notches at the adjacent interlaminar "V"s and then connecting these notches with high-speed burr to remove the dorsal cortical bone while leaving an adequate amount of cancellous bone and the ventral cortical bone intact

thinned with a burr and resected if necessary depending on the extent of stenosis. The ligamentum flavum is thinned with the burr and released between C6 and C7 with a curette or Kerrison rongeur. Next, attention is directed to the hinge side of the laminoplasty. The safest and most efficient way to complete this step is as follows: (1) the burr is used to notch the cranial and caudal edges of each lamina through its full thickness along the planned hinge line, since these regions of the lamina are tricortical and therefore provide the greatest resistance to hinging, and (2) a trough is then made by removing the dorsal cortex and a small amount of the underlying cancellous bone between the two previously made laminar notches (Fig. 19.14). If done appropriately, upon completing burring through the cancellous bone, hinging of the lamina should be easily achievable with gently pressure.

Hinging of the lamina requires great care and finesse. If done too forcefully, the lamina can easily fracture off on the hinge side. In addition, sudden recoil of the lamina during hinging can potentially cause intragenic spinal cord injury with possible devastating neurological sequelae. Therefore, this part of the procedure should be done with both hands, with the thumb of one hand pushing on the stump of the spinous process toward the hinge side while the other hand gently lifting the lamina up with a small curette under the lamina (Fig. 19.15). Several factors may complicate this step of the procedure: (1) residual ligamentum flavum attachments to bony elements, (2) adhesions to the underlying dura, or (3) an inadequately thinned ventral cortex on the hinge side prevents easy opening of the lamina. Because bone is viscoelastic, the lamina should be hinged slowly and gradually. It is our routine practice to start distally, first hinging C6 and then C5 and C4 sequentially, repeating this process in a distal to proximal orientation three or more times, to achieve the maximum desired amount of laminar opening/hinging.

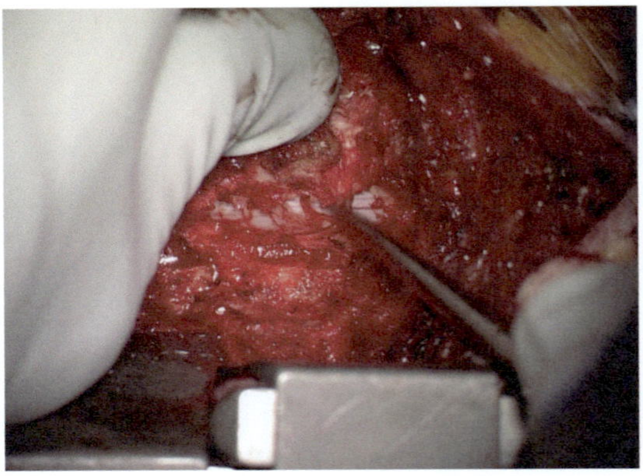

Fig. 19.15 Hinging of the lamina should be completed with the thumb pushing on the stump of the spinous process toward the hinge side while the other hand gently lifting the lamina up with a small curette on the open side

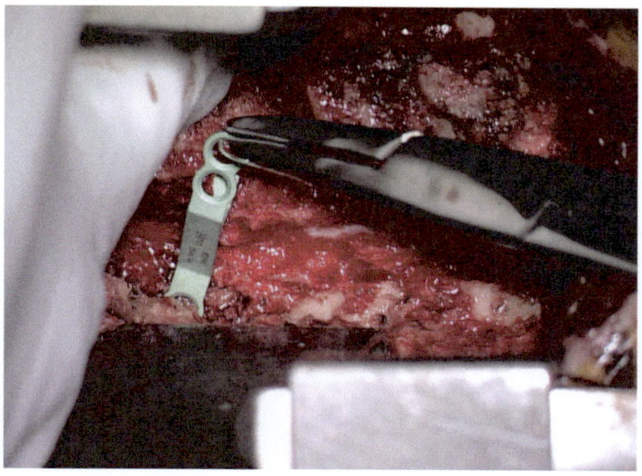

Fig. 19.16 The laminoplasty plate is introduced onto the lamina on the tip of a long-handled, fine-tipped hemostat as shown in the photograph

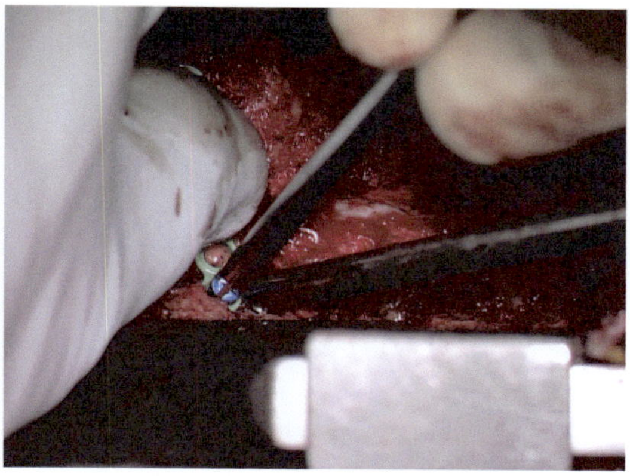

Fig. 19.17 Two 7-mm-deep holes are drilled through the plate into the lateral mass, and two 7-mm-long screws are inserted to secure the laminoplasty plates onto the lateral mass

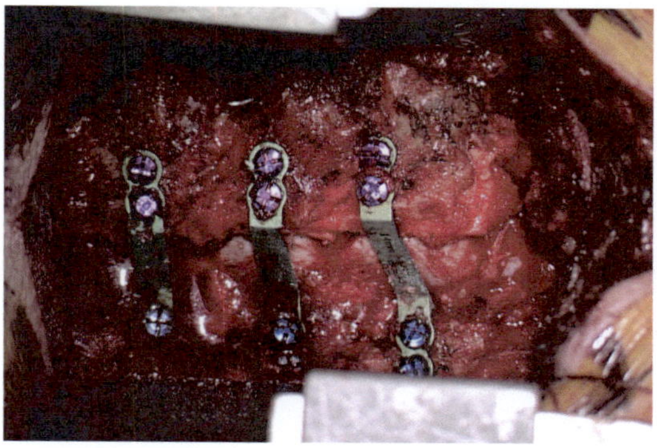

Fig. 19.18 The plates are secured to the lamina by two 5-mm-long screws at each level

If all the laminae hinge successfully, they are secured unilaterally using screw-plate fixation. The plate is introduced onto the lamina on the tip of a long-handled, fine-tipped hemostat (Fig. 19.16). The plate is held straddling the dorsal and ventral edges of the lamina with a thumb by the surgeon and with a curette or by the assistant at the lateral mass. A 7-mm-deep hole is then drilled through the plate into the lateral mass, and a 7-mm-long screw is inserted (Fig. 19.17). A second screw is then inserted through the plate and into the lateral mass in parallel to the first screw. The holes are drilled and the upper 1/3 of the lateral mass in a trajectory similar to lateral mass screws to minimize the risk of facet joint violation. Subsequently, two 5-mm-long screws are placed through the plate into the lamina (Fig. 19.18). If the lamina breaks off during the hinging process, the lamina can be reattached to the lateral mass on the hinged side using a small plate and a screw. These steps are repeated at each segment. After plate fixation, the spinous processes are removed with the burr to allow improved motion and to aid in wound closure (Fig. 19.19).

After completing the plate fixation, an important step is to check for bony block/impingement during neck extension. This can be achieved by asking the anesthesia team to switch the Gardner-Wells tong traction from flexion rope to extension rope. If bony impingement is identified, additional bone is removed, and the ligamentum flavum is thinned as necessary until the laminae can move freely during neck extension (Fig. 19.20). If range of motion is appropriate, the Gardner-Wells tongs are reattached to the flexion rope for the remainder of the procedure to facilitate wound closure. The dura is once again thoroughly interrogated for compression; dural pulsations are noted as indicators of adequate decompression, and final hemostasis is achieved. The wound should be generously irrigated with normal saline until all bone dust and debris are removed. This minimizes the risk for unintended fusion in this motion-preserving procedure [18].

Prior to closure, we routinely apply epidural methylprednisolone acetate (40 mg in 1 cc solu-

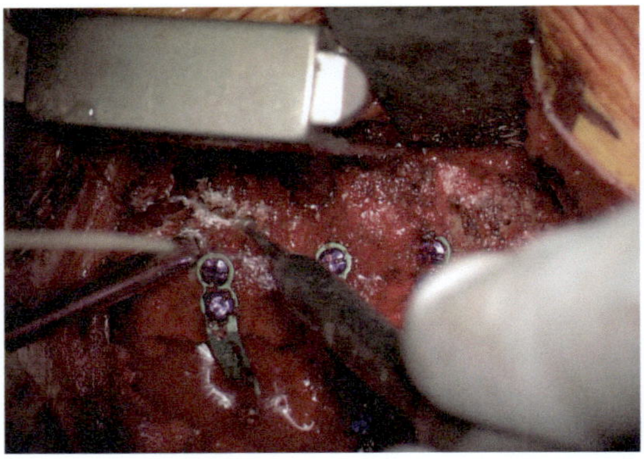

Fig. 19.19 The spinous processes are removed with the burr to prevent bony block and facilitate wound closure

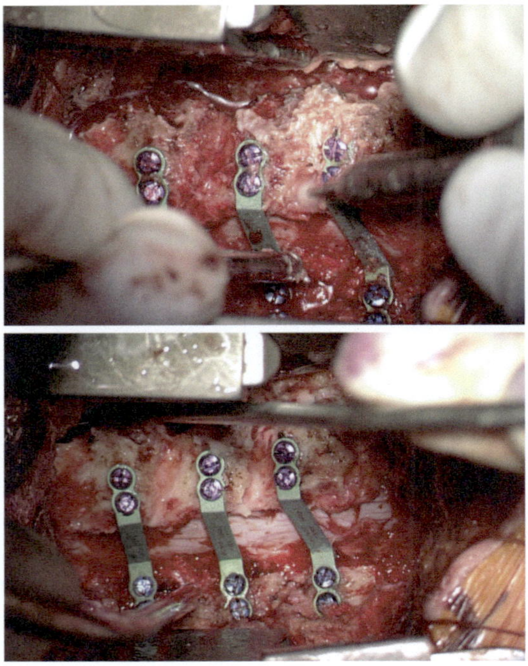

Fig. 19.20 If bony impingement is identified with extension of the neck, additional bone is removed (top), and the ligamentum flavum is thinned at each level until the laminae can move freely (bottom)

tion) using an 18-gauge angiocatheter under the most caudal lamina (Fig. 19.21). Another dose of methylprednisolone acetate (40 mg in 1 cc solution) is injected into the subcutaneous fat to provide pain relief for the first 1–2 weeks of the postoperative recovery. A deep drain is then placed, and vancomycin powder 1 g is sprinkled into the wound before closure. Once again, hemostatic agents can be used to facilitate meticulous hemostasis. We routinely place a thrombin-soaked Gelfoam over the laminoplasty levels to facilitate hemostasis (Fig. 19.22). However, Gelfoam should not be placed over exposed spinal cord as it can cause cord compression as it expands. Using such hemostatic techniques, most patients have minimal drainage and are able to be discharged the next day [19].

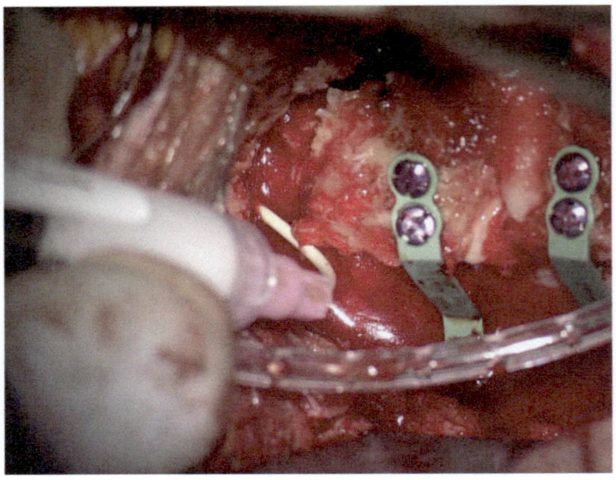

Fig. 19.21 Prior to closure, epidural methylprednisolone acetate (40 mg/cc solution) is applied using an 18-gauge angiocatheter under the most caudal lamina to decrease postoperative pain

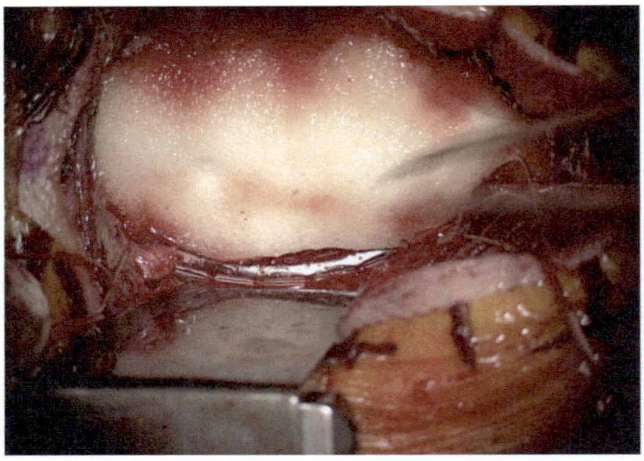

Fig. 19.22 A thrombin-soaked Gelfoam is applied over the laminoplasty levels to facilitate hemostasis; however, it should not be placed over exposed spinal cord as it can cause cord compression when it expands

Closure

Closure, as the rest of the operation, should be done meticulously with great care. Meticulous dissection at the time of exposure renders closure much easier with readily identifiable anatomic planes. First, the previously osteotomized bone fragments are re-approximated with the tagging sutures; because the bone fragments are still attached to the muscles laterally, the paraspinal muscles are also brought together as the bone fragments are re-approximated. Additional "figure-of-eight" #1 Vicryl sutures are used at each level to reinforce the re-approximation of the bony fragments in addition to the initial tagging sutures. Next, the remaining paraspinal muscles are re-approximated in eight to ten layers, minimizing potential dead space after wound closure. Only the muscle sheath and a minimal amount of muscle are captured with each stitch. Large bites of tissue or overtightening of suture knots during muscle approximation can lead to muscle necrosis. The fascia is closed with interrupted #1 Vicryl sutures (Ethicon) in a watertight fashion. The wound is then again irrigated. If the subcutaneous fatty layer is greater than 2 cm, we place a superficial drain above the fascia, after which the subcutaneous tissue is closed in layers with 2–0 interrupted and buried Vicryl sutures, again leaving no dead space. The skin is closed with a subcuticular 3–0 Monocryl suture (Ethicon) followed by the application of a dressing of the surgeon's choice.

We routinely use over 120 sutures to close an incision from C3 to C7, and this practice has dramatically decreased the incidence of infection or any other wound-related issues. In fact, with the muscle-sparing dissection and these meticulous closure techniques, we find posterior cervical procedures have the same low risk of infection as the anterior cervical procedures. In addition, postoperative pain is dramatically less, and our patients routinely go home on postoperative day 1 or 2 with minimal pain.

Postoperative Care

Postoperative care is unique to each institution and surgeon. In our practice patients are placed in a soft collar for comfort. This collar can be removed for sleep and should be discontinued as soon as the patient is able to wean him or herself out of it. Typically, several criteria should be met prior to disposition home: wound drainage less than 20 cc per 8 h, pain control with oral medications, and return of bowel/bladder function to baseline. This typically requires an overnight admission. Patients do not have any restrictions on range of motion or with any activities and are counseled to avoid only those activities that cause them excessive pain. Patients are discharged with an oral pain medication and instructed to return to the clinic for routine follow-up at 6 weeks after their surgery. A rapid return to activities of daily living and aerobic exercise is encouraged.

References

1. Tsuji H. Laminoplasty for patients with compressive myelopathy due to so-called spinal canal stenosis in cervical and thoracic regions. Spine. 1982;7(1):28–34.
2. Hase H, Watanabe T, Hirasawa Y, et al. Bilateral open laminoplasty using ceramic laminas for cervical myelopathy. Spine. 1991;16(11):1269–76.
3. O'brien MF, Peterson D, Casey AT, Crockard HA. A novel technique for laminoplasty augmentation of spinal canal area using titanium miniplate stabilization: a computerized morphometric analysis. Spine. 1996;21(4):474–83.
4. Tsuzuki N, Abe R, Saiki K, Iizuka T. Tension-band laminoplasty of the cervical spine. Int Orthop. 1996;20(5):275–84.
5. Hirabayashi K, Watanabe K, Wakano K, Suzuki N, Satomi K, Ishii Y. Expansive open-door laminoplasty for cervical spinal stenotic myelopathy. Spine. 1983;8(7):693–9.
6. Suda K, Abumi K, Ito M, Shono Y, Kaneda K, Fujiya M. Local kyphosis reduces surgical outcomes of expansive open-door laminoplasty for cervical spondylotic myelopathy. Spine. 2003;28(12):1258–62.
7. Fujiyoshi T, Yamazaki M, Kawabe J, et al. A new concept for making decisions regarding the surgical approach for cervical ossification of the posterior longitudinal ligament: the K-line. Spine. 2008;33(26):E990–E3.
8. Taniyama T, Hirai T, Yamada T, et al. Modified K-line in magnetic resonance imaging predicts insufficient decompression of cervical laminoplasty. Spine. 2013;38(6):496–501.
9. Taniyama T, Hirai T, Yoshii T, et al. Modified K-line in magnetic resonance imaging predicts clinical outcome in patients with nonlordotic alignment after laminoplasty for cervical spondylotic myelopathy. Spine. 2014;39(21):E1261–E8.
10. Zhang JT, Li JQ, Niu RJ, Liu Z, Tong T, Shen Y. Predictors of cervical lordosis loss after laminoplasty in patients with cervical spondylotic myelopathy. Eur Spine J. 2017;26(4):1205–10.

11. Mesfin A, Park M-S, Piyaskulkaew C, et al. Neck pain following laminoplasty. Global Spine J. 2015;5(01):017–22.
12. Nowinski GP, Visarius H, Nolte LP, Herkowitz HN. A biomechanical comparison of cervical laminaplasty and cervical laminectomy with progressive facetectomy. Spine. 1993;18(14):1995–2004.
13. Lau D, Winkler EA, Than KD, Chou D, Mummaneni PV. 169 laminoplasty vs laminectomy with posterior spinal fusion for multilevel cervical spondylotic myelopathy: matched cohorts of regional sagittal balance. Neurosurgery. 2016;63:167–8.
14. Hosono N, Yonenobu K, Ono K. Neck and shoulder pain after laminoplasty: a noticeable complication. Spine. 1996;21(17):1969–73.
15. Yoshida M, Tamaki T, Kawakami M, et al. Does reconstruction of posterior ligamentous complex with extensor musculature decrease axial symptoms after cervical laminoplasty? Spine. 2002;27(13):1414–8.
16. Shigematsu H. Degenerative spondylolisthesis does not influence surgical results of laminoplasty in elderly cervical spondylotic myelopathy patients. Eur Spine J. 2010;19(5):720–5.
17. Shiraishi T, Fukuda K, Yato Y, Nakamura M, Ikegami T. Results of skip laminectomy—minimum 2-year follow-up study compared with open-door laminoplasty. Spine. 2003;28(24):2667–72.
18. Hyun S-J, Riew KD, Rhim S-C. Range of motion loss after cervical laminoplasty: a prospective study with minimum 5-year follow-up data. Spine J. 2013;13(4):384–90.
19. Cho SK, Yi J-S, Park MS, et al. Hemostatic techniques reduce hospital stay following multilevel posterior cervical spine surgery. J Bone Joint Surg Am. 2012;94(21):1952–8.

Cervical Disc Arthroplasty

20

Jau-Ching Wu, Praveen V. Mummaneni, and Regis W. Haid

Introduction

Cervical disc arthroplasty (CDA) has gained tremendous popularity in recent years because of its preservation of segmental motion and the potential to reduce adjacent segment disease (ASD) [1–5]. There are several US Food and Drug Administration (US FDA) prospective randomized control trials comparing CDA to anterior cervical discectomy and fusion (ACDF) with 5–8 years of data published [6–12]. For one- and two-level cervical disc disease (causing radiculopathy) without facet arthropathy, the results of these FDA trials indicate that CDA is at least similar or even superior to ACDF in the relief of neurological symptoms [6–8, 13]. These studies have also clearly demonstrated that CDA is effective in preservation of segmental motion. The average range of motion during cervical flexion-extension is preserved by most of the CDA devices at approximately 7–9 degrees for each treated segment [10, 14–16]. Long-term follow-up is necessary to determine the effect of CDA on adjacent segment disease. It is suggested that CDA can actually lower the incidence of adjacent segment disease, which reportedly ranges from 0.8% to 2.9% per year after ACDF [3, 17].

Appropriate patient selection is the key to a successful CDA [5]. Cervical arthroplasty should be best reserved for patients with one- or two-level cervical disc disease with radiculopathy or early myelopathy who have no other arthropathy or deformity. Moreover, the CDA only replaces the degenerated and herniated disc that caused radiculopathy and is unlikely to alter or decelerate the natural course of degeneration of both the facet joints at the index level or other adjacent segments.

Indications and Contraindications

The FDA arthroplasty trials included adult patients of one- or two-level cervical disc disease, including herniated nucleus pulposus and spondylosis, ,at C3–C7 that caused medically refractory radiculopathy, myelopathy, or both [2, 5, 18]. In general, CDA might not be recommended for elderly patients because of preexisting facet arthropathy. The FDA trials did not enroll patients more than 75 years old, and there is little data on CDA in the elderly. The best candidate for CDA is a young patient who has

J.-C. Wu
Department of Neurosurgery, Taipei Veteran's General Hospital, Taipei, Taiwan

School of Medicine, National Yang-Ming University, Taipei, Taiwan

P. V. Mummaneni
Department of Neurological Surgery, University of California, San Francisco, CA, USA

R. W. Haid (✉)
Atlanta Brain and Spine Care, Atlanta, GA, USA
e-mail: RHaid@AtlantaBrainandSpine.com

M. G. Kaiser et al. (eds.), *Degenerative Cervical Myelopathy and Radiculopathy*,
https://doi.org/10.1007/978-3-319-97952-6_20

radicular symptoms caused by a herniated cervical disc without any facet incompetence.

Relative contraindications of CDA are cervical kyphosis, facet arthropathy (incompetence), instability (i.e., more than 2–3 mm translation/subluxation on dynamic flexion/extension lateral radiographs), ossification of posterior longitudinal ligament (OPLL), ankyloses, or osteoporosis (Table 20.1).

Clinical Considerations

The design ,rationale of CDA is to replace the diseased disc which is causing radiculopathy while preserving the segmental motion at the index level. The artificial disc aims to preserve normal physiological motion, including bending, rotation, translation, and buffering axial loading, after decompression of neural tissue. The current CDA devices are successful in preserving motion after surgery but cannot restore cervical alignment or lost motion due to facet disease.

Fusion surgery eliminates motion, which is advocated by some authors in the management of cervical spondylotic myelopathy (CSM). However, there is some evidence showing that CDA is also effective in management of early one- or two-level CSM [19–21]. The FDA-IDE trials also enrolled patients with cervical myelopathy and demonstrated similar improvement of myelopathy in both CDA and ACDF patients. Although it is reasonable to use CDA for multiple-level cervical disc diseases causing CSM, the true effect of CDA in management of cervical myelopathy requires further investigation.

Table 20.1 Indications and contraindications of cervical disc arthroplasty

Indications of CDA	Relative contraindications of CDA
One- or two-level cervical disc disease, including herniated nucleus pulposus and spondylosis	Cervical kyphosis
	Facet arthropathy (incompetence)
	Segmental instability
	Ossification of posterior longitudinal ligament
	Ankylosis
	Osteoporosis

In theory, CDA surgery is more demanding than ACDF because of the more precise localization required for the implant to preserve motion. The bone graft inserted during ACDF is intended to increase disc height as well as enlarge the neuroforamen indirectly. Thus, ACDF is capable of increasing cervical lordosis and correcting preexisting deformity. Moreover, by alleviation of segmental mobility between the vertebral bodies fused, ACDF immobilizes the facets, which could be a pain generator in some patients. Therefore, patients of advanced age or severe spondylosis, whose facets are frequently degenerated, are better candidates for ACDF rather than CDA.

Preoperative Evaluation

Both MRI and computed tomography (CT) are typically used to evaluate patients in preparation for CDA surgery.MRI is useful for evaluation of spinal canal stenosis as well as foraminal stenosis. Obtaining a CT scan preoperatively is helpful in detection of ossification of the posterior longitudinal ligament (OPLL), calcified discs, or osteophytes. In patients with such problems (i.e., segmental OPLL or a large calcified disc), anterior discectomy may be associated with the unnecessary higher risk of durotomy and nerve injury. In particular, OPLL has been listed as a relative contraindication to CDA in most published literature. Moreover, preoperative CT scans are particularly useful for detection of facet arthropathy prior to CDA surgery. If a patient's facets are severely degenerated or fused, there is little chance of motion preservation even after successful CDA insertion.

Both anterior-posterior and lateral radiographs, including lateral dynamic views, should be obtained preoperatively for evaluation and documentation of segmental mobility and cervical spinal alignment. Patients with preexisting cervical kyphosis are not considered candidates for CDA surgery, because it is not likely CDA could correct the cervical alignment. Instrumented

ACDF is a well-accepted surgical procedure to ameliorate kyphosis by supporting the anterior column with lordotic interbody bone grafts. In contrast, CDA is unlikely to change the cervical alignment [22].

The most commonly performed level of CDA is C5–C6, followed by C6–C7 and C4–C5. The FDA-IDE trials included any level from C3 to C7. Patients with a large mandible or short neck may make CDA surgery more challenging, since the artificial disc needs to be centered precisely. There was a retrospective study by Chang et al. addressing the differences between levels of CDA performed and demonstrating more development of heterotopic ossification in CDA at C3–C4 with uncertain cause [23]. There were also a few case reports on CDA at C7–T1, which is technically feasible but rarely indicated. To date, there has been no case report on CDA at C2–C3.

Like ACDF, most right-handed spine surgeons use a right-sided approach for all levels of subaxial cervical spine access when attempting CDA. For patients who have undergone prior anterior cervical discectomy or thyroid surgery, a preoperative evaluation of the vocal cords should be considered. An approach from the virgin side would thus be suggested if both vocal cords are fine. On the other hand, the same side approach must be taken when there is unilateral vocal cord palsy in order to avoid the risk of bilateral vocal cord deficit and requirement for tracheostomy after surgery.

Surgical Techniques

General anesthesia with either a nasal or an oral endotracheal tube and prophylactic antibiotics are usually recommended for all patients of CDA. Intraoperative neuromonitoring and perioperative steroids are options that may be considered. After positioning of the patient, a lateral fluoroscopy of the cervical spine is necessary prior to CDA surgery to ensure that the index level is clearly visualized.

Appropriate positioning of the patient's neck is the first step to a successful CDA surgery. The patient's neck should be placed straight, without head rotation, and in neutral or slightly lordotic alignment. The targeted level of the disc space must be well visualized on lateral fluoroscopy, and ideally the two end plates are parallel. Sometimes, chin or shoulder retraction is useful in obese patients or those with a short neck. Similar to ACDF, an adequate cushion placed underneath the neck is helpful during surgery to achieve appropriate alignment. An anterior-posterior fluoroscopy is sometimes useful to assure the head and neck are placed in the orthogonal position.

The surgical approach for CDA is very similar to the standard ACDF approach. A transverse skin incision along one of the preexisting skin creases is adequate for exposure up to two disc levels. Sharp dissection between the carotid sheath and strap muscles, which is anterior-medial to the sternocleidomastoid muscle, leads to entry into an avascular plane. By retracting the trachea and esophagus medially with blunt dissection, the prevertebral retropharyngeal space can be exposed. After retraction of the longus colli muscle insertion sites around the disc level, self-retaining retractor blades can be inserted underneath the muscle for protection of the esophagus medially and large vessels laterally. Caution should be taken during dissection to avoid injury to the superior and recurrent laryngeal nerves, which could be associated with post-operative hoarseness and dysphagia. Thus, typically a sharp dissection medial to the carotid sheath would be suggested.

After confirmation of the targeted level of disc by intraoperative fluoroscopy, anterior cervical discectomy begins. The authors preferred the use of distraction pins placed into the vertebral bodies to facilitate discectomy with gentle retraction. For CDA, resection of the posterior longitudinal ligament is recommended for confirmation of adequate decompression of the dural sac [24]. Moreover, the authors also recommended removal of bilateral uncovertebral joints, even in the asymptomatic side, to ensure decompression of the nerve roots [24]. Since CDA aims at preservation of segmental motion, there is greater necessity to ensure an effective decompression of the neuronal tissue so that nerve impingement during neck movement is avoided. Unlike the conventional ACDF surgery, which partially relies on indirect decompression through distraction of the disc space, CDA is solely dependent on direct decompression. The enlarged neuroforamen is subjected to movement during neck motion. Therefore, generous decompression is warranted to prevent recurrence of radicular symptoms during extreme range of motion (e.g., flexion/extension, axial rotation, and lateral bending) of the neck.

To achieve the optimal outcome of CDA surgery, each of the artificial discs must be installed precisely, including sizing, centering, and positioning. The appropriately centered device has the best chance to achieve physiologic range of motion similar to that of an intact disc. Therefore, end plate preparation in CDA is more critical than that in ACDF because it directly affects the primary stability of the artificial disc device installed. During the process of decompression, care must be undertaken not to violate too much of the cortical end plate; otherwise the risk of device subsidence or migration is increased.

There are many designs of artificial discs currently available on the market. Each of the CDA devices has a specialized fixation mechanism, such as keel-, teeth-, or dome-shaped designs, with or without screws, requiring specific installation to ensure best integration into the vertebral bodies. There is no study that demonstrates superiority of one device over another or if one device is more durable. Therefore, surgeons should follow the specific instructions for each device and select the largest footprint that would fit and the proper height that is closest to physiologically functioning disc. Moreover, precise midline acquisition and a proper insertion trajectory cannot be overemphasized. Thus, visual confirmation and use of both anterior-posterior and lateral fluoroscopy are typically required during surgery.

The most essential foundation of CDA surgery consists of generous decompression and precise installation, which yields neurological relief and restoration of joint function. In the authors' opinion, thorough decompression including removal of the PLL and bilateral foraminal decompression is absolutely necessary. Given CDA aims to restore joint function rather than arthrodesis, tailor-made installation of the most-fit artificial disc allows the best chance to maintain mobility for the long term.

Postoperative Management and Complications

General postoperative management of CDA is very similar to that of ACDF, except that CDA patients need not wear a neck collar and nonsteroidal anti-inflammatory drugs (NSAIDs) are often prescribed to CDA patients to reduce the chances of heterotopic ossification around the artificial disc [25]. The incidence of heterotopic ossification varied tremendously depending on the method of detection. Common suggestions to lower the chance of developing heterotopic ossification included copious irrigation during the drilling to minimize bone dust deposition and waxing the exposed surfaces of the cancellous bone. The incidences of complications and adverse events of CDA surgery in the literature are as low as or even lower than that of conventional ACDF. In most reported series of CDA, the devices had very few problems and seldom required reoperations [4, 5, 10, 12, 13, 22, 26, 27].

Most of the FDA-IDE trials used NSAIDs perioperatively and reported very low incidence rate (less than 5%) of heterotopic ossification in their follow-up reports. Heterotopic ossification refers to the undesired ectopic bone formation around the artificial disc implanted. In the authors' opinion, the heterotopic ossification should not be considered as one of the complications of CDA surgery. The heterotopic ossification is more likely the consequence of continuously ongoing degeneration, similar to those marginal osteophytes, that develops as a physiological reaction to stabilize the spine. However, more evidence is required to support this theory. The CDA surgery only replaces the diseased disc itself and can only, for the best, postpone the process of degeneration. For the same reasons, the continuous degeneration, as a natural process of aging, is likely the cause of adjacent segment disease, rather than the indexed level surgery. It is reasonable to anticipate reduction of adjacent segment degeneration after CDA, but it is impossible to stop the aging process across uninvolved spinal segment, beyond the site of either CDA or ACDF.

State-of-the-Art Applications

There are many CDA devices now on the market with various materials and articulating designs. Each of these designs features in biomechanical characteristics, and the implant choice for each patient should be individually considered. However, there has not been enough evidence to demonstrate superiority of any device so far. Also, there is lack of standardized classification or concordant nomenclature used to describe these implants. Most of them can be simply categorized into non-, uni-, and biarticulating, per its mechanism of motion allowed [28]. Furthermore, according to the material used in the contact surfaces of articulation, they can be further divided into metal on metal, metal on polymer, and polymer on polymer or ceramics (Fig. 20.1).

The best currently available data of CDA are the published FDA-IDE trials, which enrolled patients with one- and two-level cervical disc herniation, degenerative disc disease, or spondylosis, and demonstrated similar results for both CDA and ACDF for up to 8 years [6, 8, 10–12, 14–16]. These trials demonstrated that CDA yielded similar clinical outcomes to ACDF in relief of neurological symptoms and was associated with less or at least equal reoperations or adverse events compared to ACDF. However, the possibility of selection bias or lack of clinical equipoise between cohorts exists, and those patients enrolled could have slightly different pathologies, degrees of degeneration, or severity of symptoms. For example, it was not clear that patients with unilateral radiculopathy have similar results as those with spondylotic myelopathy after CDA, since these clinical trials did not separate these patients a priori or provide subgroup analysis. There were a few retrospective series that demonstrated similar results in patients who underwent CDA for different indications [4, 20, 29]. In general, patients who had the least arthritic degeneration preoperatively should have the best long-term outcome after CDA. One would agree that a patient with prolapsed disc fragment causing root irritation had far less degeneration than a patient with a calcified spur causing severe myelopathy [4, 26]. Therefore, the best outcome of CDA can be anticipated in young patients who had a herniated disc causing cervical radiculopathy.

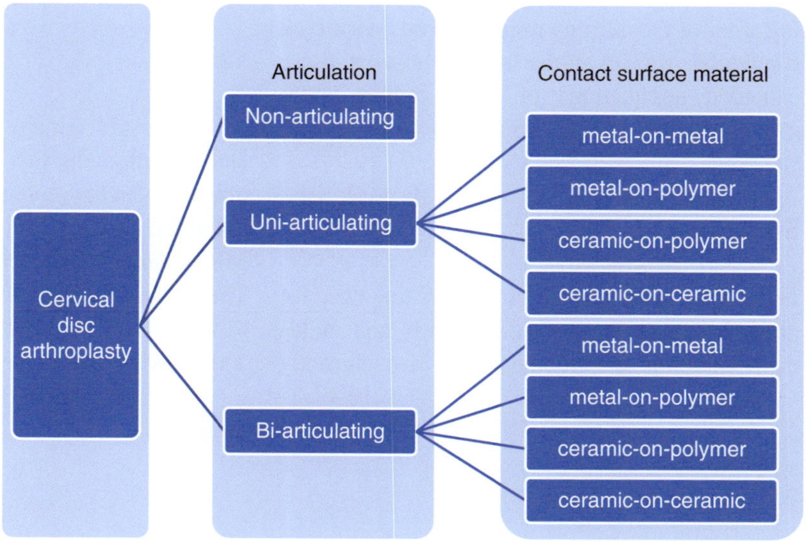

Fig. 20.1 Classification of cervical disc arthroplasty devices

Cervical arthroplasty merits more in management for multilevel disc degeneration. For each level of disc replaced, many clinical trials have demonstrated persistent preservation of range of motion at 7–9 degrees during flexion and extension by CDA. On the other hand, the loss of 7–9 degrees after single-level ACDF does not significantly affect daily activities and is seldom noticed by the patient. However, two- or three-level ACDF inevitably limits more neck mobility and may cause noticeable hindrances to the patients. Thus, CDA is theoretically more advantageous than ACDF in multiple levels of disc diseases requiring surgery. There were a few reports of clinical series utilizing CDA for multilevel (i.e., more than two) degenerative disease causing radiculopathy, myelopathy, or both [19–21, 23, 26, 27, 29, 30]. These reports demonstrate satisfactory clinical outcomes of CDA in up to three levels of discs treated. However, more long-term follow-up is still needed, including those with hybrid constructs combining fusion and arthroplasty. Also, still it remains unclear whether CDA for management of cervical spondylotic myelopathy is as effective as fusion, despite results from several clinical series [19, 21].

The future application of CDA might include patients with more than two levels of DDD and combined use of ACDF or corpectomy with CDA. Patients of traumatic disc herniation but no facet disruption or other causes of stenosis requiring anterior discectomy might also be considered candidates of CDA in the future. However, these extended applications of CDA require more investigation with long-term follow-up.

Summary

In selected patients, CDA spares the need of arthrodesis after anterior discectomy and yields excellent clinical outcomes. The best currently available data supports the use of CDA in one and two levels of cervical DDD causing radiculopathy or myelopathy that is refractory to medical management. Further study may expand the application of CDA for cervical stenosis caused by different pathologies or multiple-level disease.

Case Illustrations

A 53-year-old female presented with neck pain and left-sided radiculopathy that was refractory to medical management for more than 5 months. The symptoms were aggravated during neck extension. There were also mild symptoms of cervical myelopathy, which were referable to a disc herniation at C4–C5 demonstrated by MRI. The preoperative CT scan also confirmed the stenosis at C4–C5 and ruled out ossification of posterior longitudinal ligament. The preoperative lateral flexion and extension radiographs demonstrated a normal range of motion.

The patient then underwent one-level CDA with ProDisc-C Vivo (DePuy Synthes Spine, MA). The surgery went smoothly, and her symptoms were completely relieved after surgery. The postoperative radiographs taken at 6 months post-operation demonstrated good mobility (Fig. 20.2). There were no complications and reoperations to date.

Case #2

A 45-year-old female presented with neck pain and radiculopathy that was refractory to medical management for more than 3 months. There were herniated discs C4–C5–C6 demonstrated by MRI, which could be correlated to her symptoms. The patient underwent two-level CDA with ProDisc-C Nova (DePuy Synthes Spine, MA). The surgery went smoothly, and her symptoms

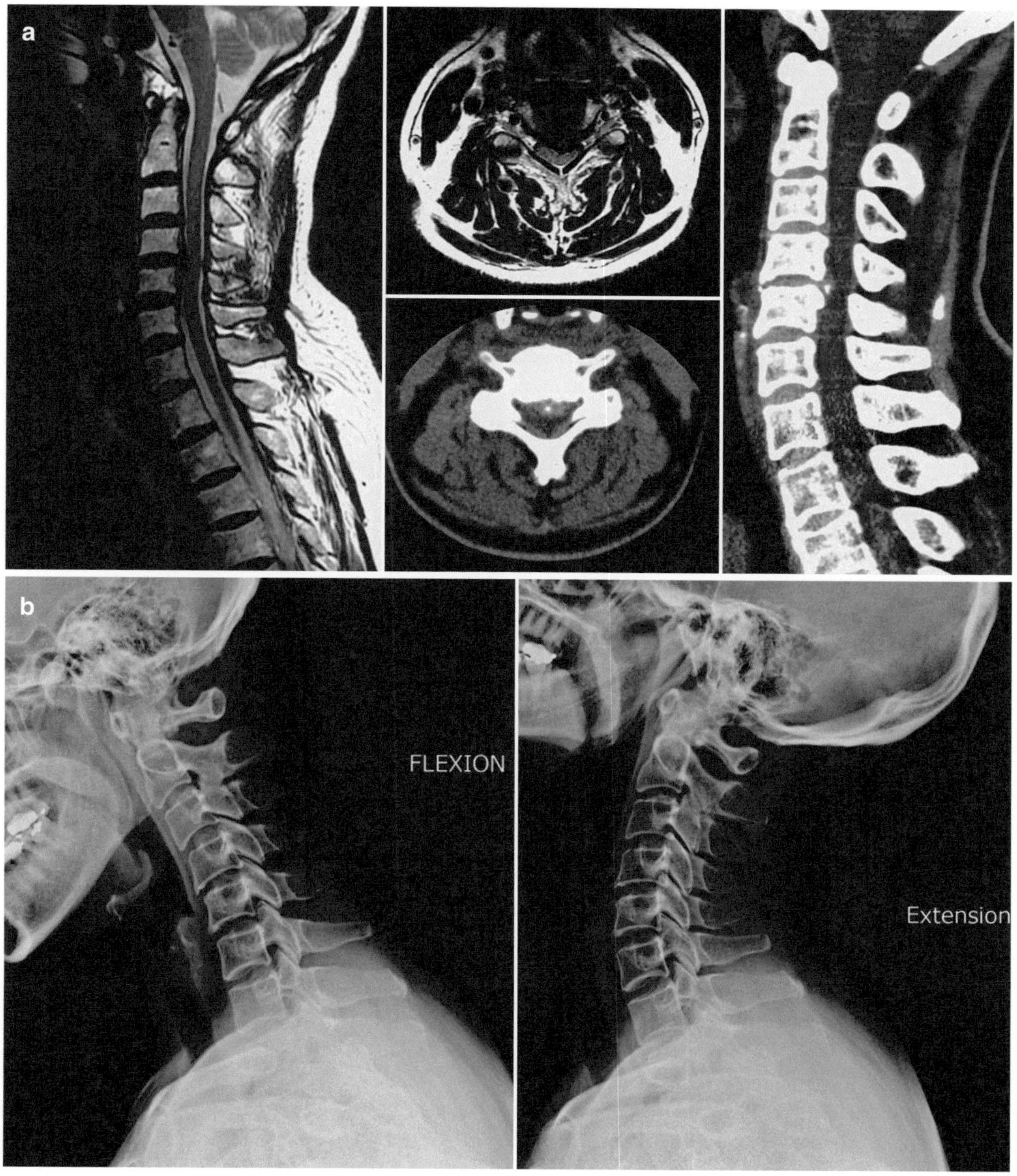

Fig. 20.2 (**a**) Preoperative T2-weighted magnetic resonances images (MRI) and computed tomography (CT) scans demonstrated a large C4–C5 disc herniation with slight calcification causing compression to the thecal sac that required a cervical discectomy. (**b**) The lateral flexion and extension radiographs demonstrated good segmental mobility throughout the subaxial cervical spine. (**c**) The postoperative lateral flexion and extension radiographs demonstrated preservation of the segmental mobility at C4–C5 by the cervical disc arthroplasty (ProDisc-C Vivo)

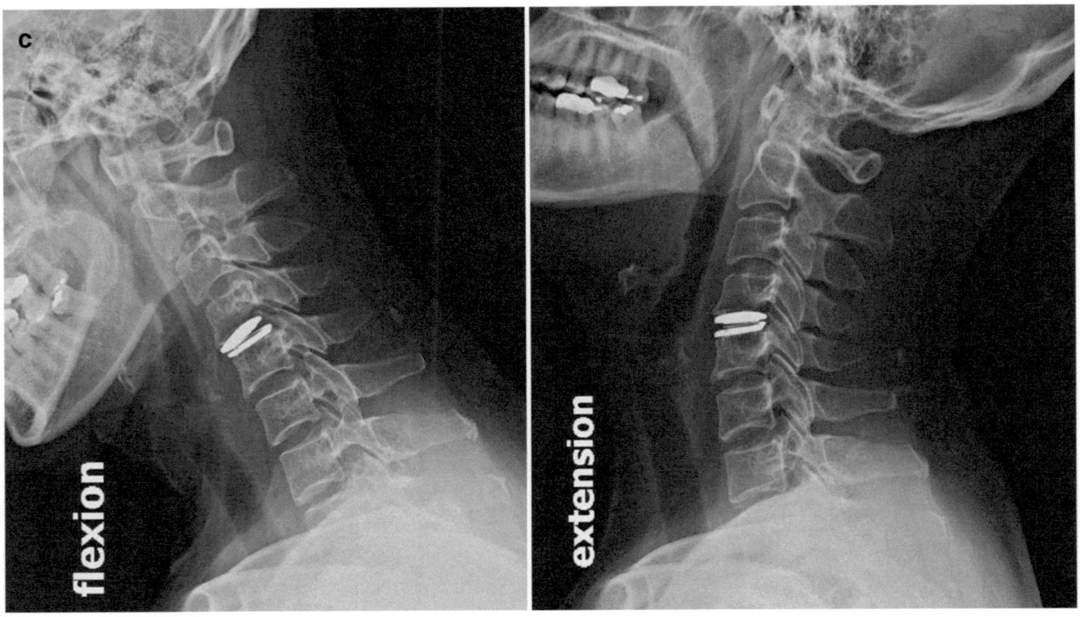

Fig. 20.2 (continued)

were completely relieved after surgery. The 12-month postoperative radiographs demonstrated good mobility (Fig. 20.3). There were no complications and reoperations to date.

Case #3

A 46-year-old female presented with cervical myeloradiculopathy caused by disc herniation at the levels of C4–C5 and C5–C6. There were retrolisthesis and instability at C5–C6 which would preclude a successful cervical disc arthroplasty. The lateral flexion and extension radiographs demonstrated possible instability at C4–C5 and marked deformity at C5–C6, which indicated that the cervical disc arthroplasty was unlikely to restore the alignment. The preoperative computed tomography also demonstrated severe spondylosis and segmental kyphosis at C5–C6. The patient underwent anterior cervical discectomy and fusion (ACDF) for C4–C5–C6. The two-level ACDF successfully restored the lordotic alignment, and the patient was free of symptoms after the surgery (Fig. 20.4).

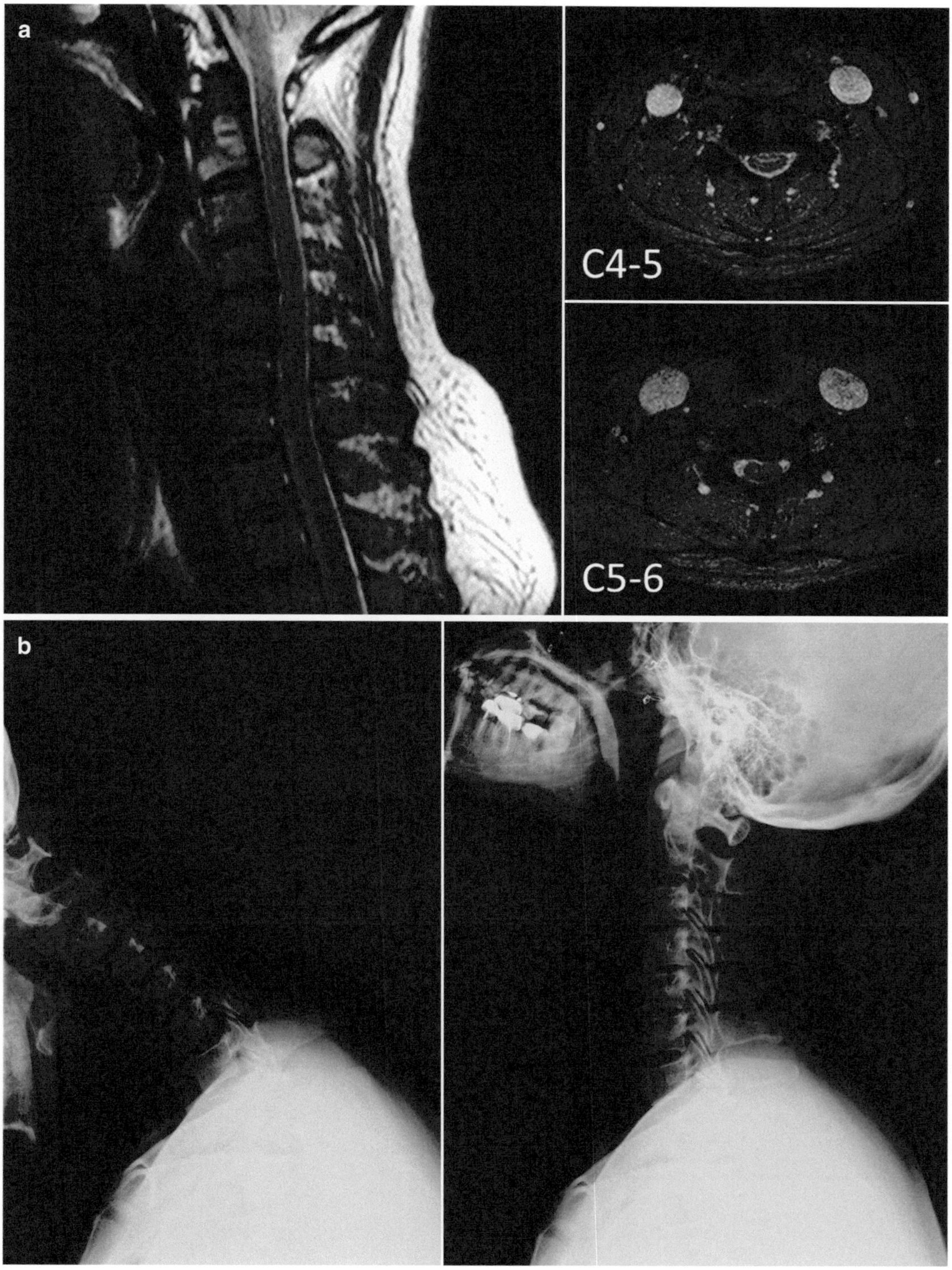

Fig. 20.3 (**a**) Preoperative T2-weighted magnetic resonances images (MRI) demonstrated a herniated disc causing foraminal stenosis at C4–C5 and thecal sac compression at C5–C6. (**b**) The disc heights of C4–C5 and C5–C6 were decreased. However, the lateral flexion and extension radiographs demonstrated good segmental mobility throughout the subaxial cervical spine. (**c**) The postoperative anterior-posterior and lateral radiographs of the two-level cervical disc arthroplasty with ProDisc-C Nova. (**d**) The postoperative lateral flexion and extension radiographs demonstrated preserved range of motion with the two-level cervical disc arthroplasty (ProDisc-C Nova) at 12-month post-operation

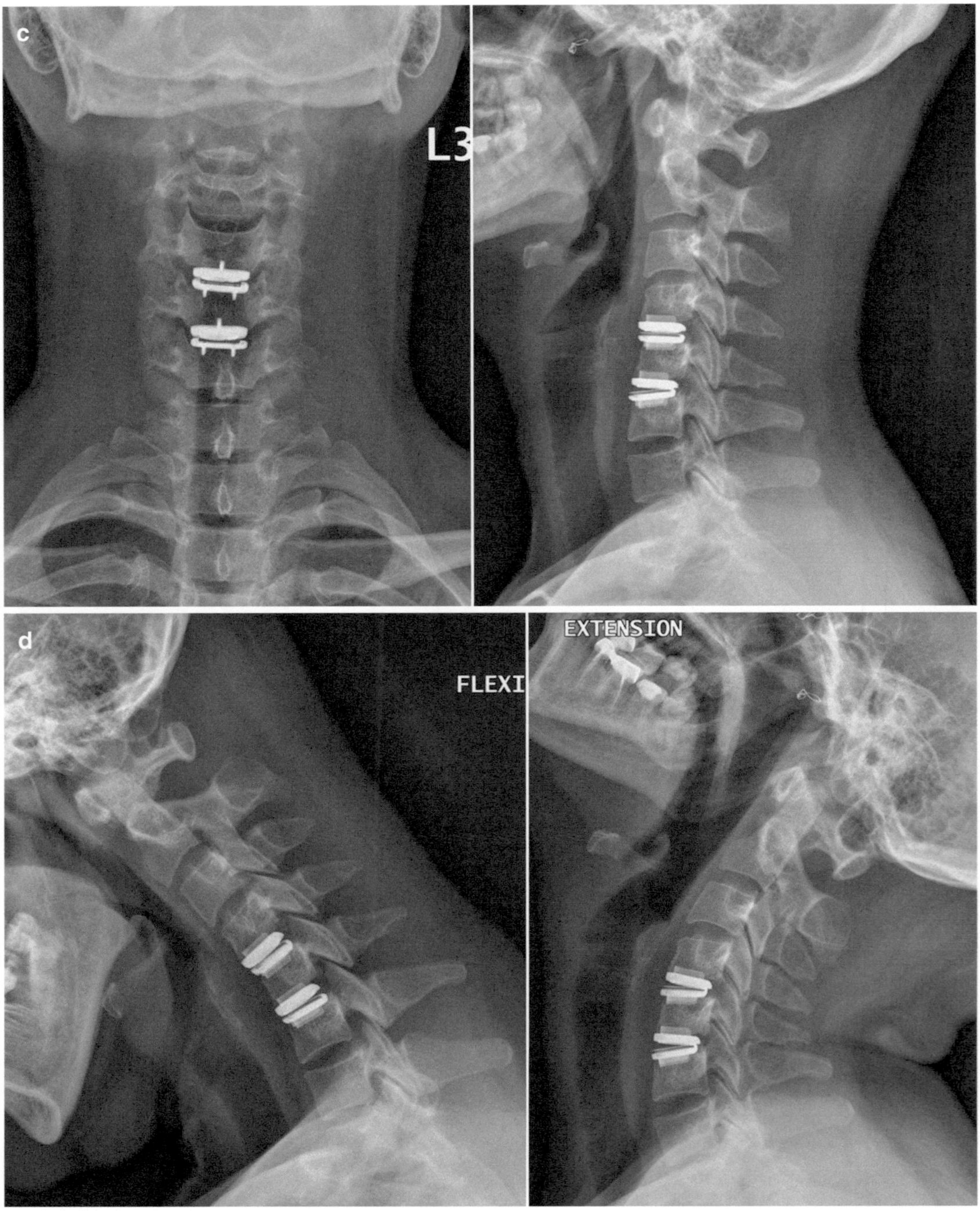

Fig. 20.3 (continued)

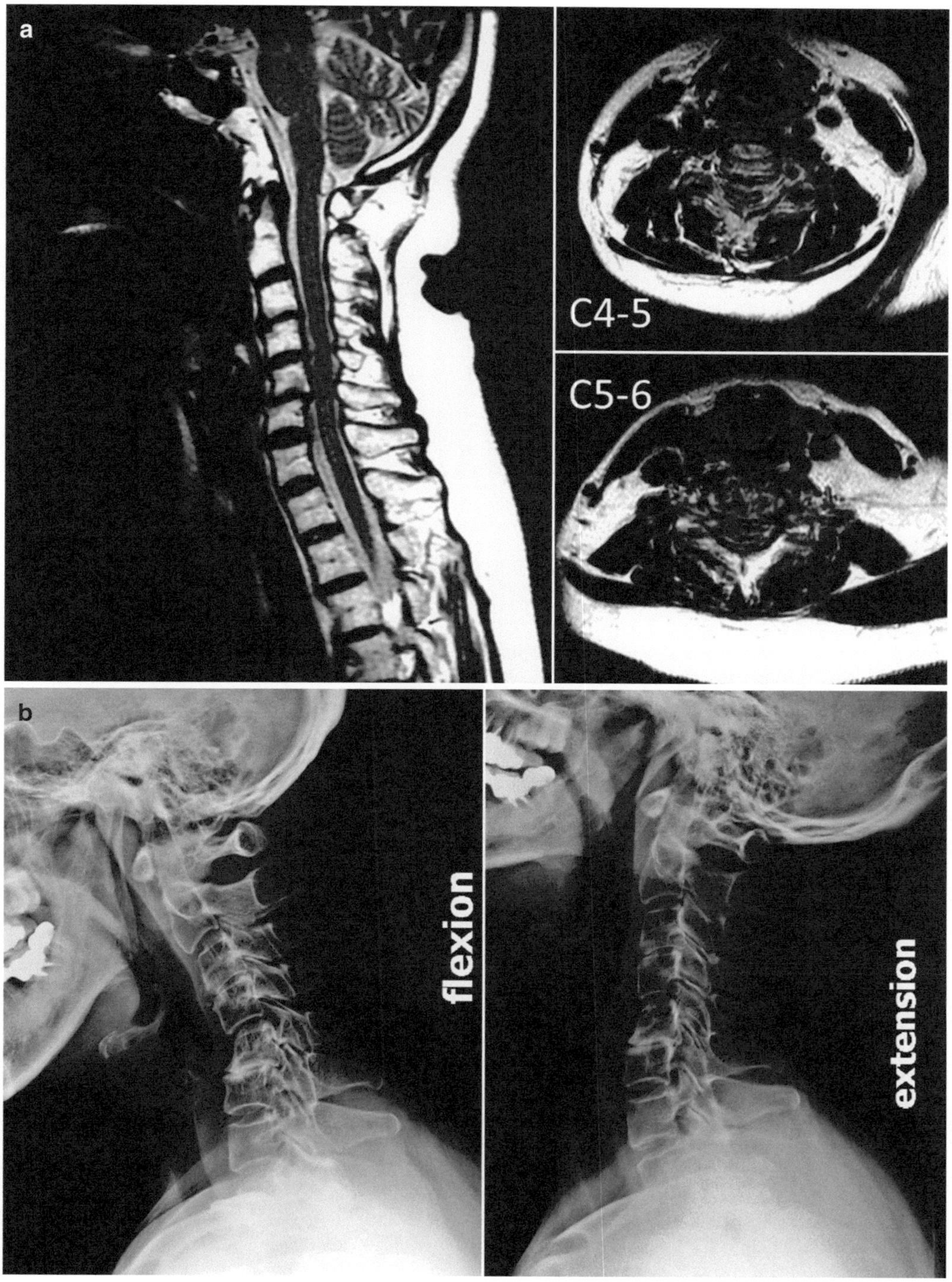

Fig. 20.4 (**a**) A 46-year-old female presented with cervical myeloradiculopathy caused by disc herniation at the levels of C4–C5 and C5–C6. There were retrolisthesis and instability at C5–C6 which would preclude a successful cervical disc arthroplasty. (**b**) The lateral flexion and extension radiographs demonstrated possible instability at C4–C5 and marked deformity at C5–C6, which indicated that the cervical disc arthroplasty was unlikely to restore the alignment. (**c**) The preoperative computed tomography also demonstrated severe spondylosis and segmental kyphosis at C5–C6. (**d**) The patient underwent anterior cervical discectomy and fusion (ACDF) for C4–C5–C6. The two-level ACDF successfully restored the lordotic alignment, and the patient was free of symptoms after the surgery

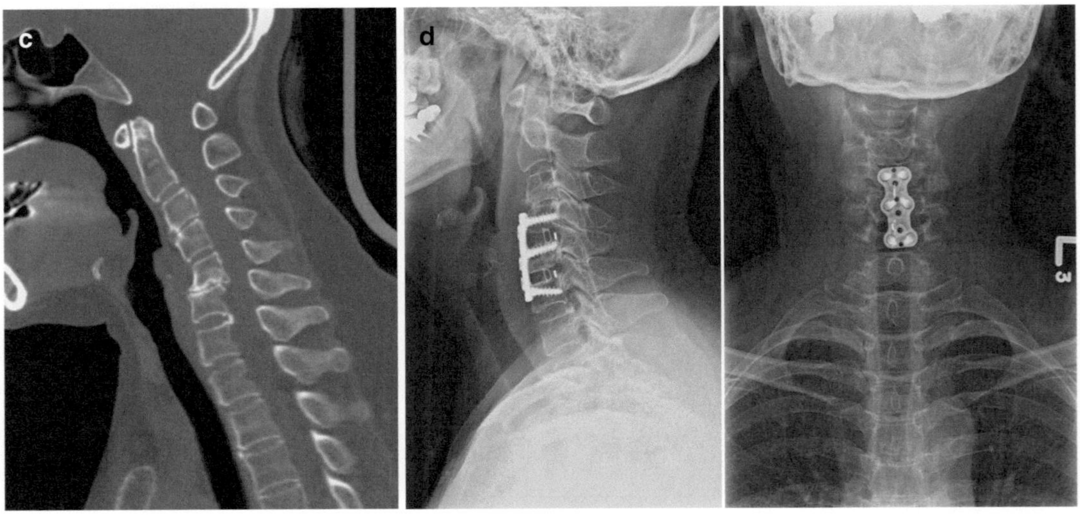

Fig. 20.4 (continued)

References

1. Wu JC, Hsieh PC, Mummaneni PV, Wang MY. Spinal motion preservation surgery. BioMed Res Int. 2015;2015:372502. PubMed PMID: 26881197. Pubmed Central PMCID: PMC4736217.
2. Wu JC, Meyer SA, Gandhoke G, Mummaneni PV. PRESTIGE cervical arthroplasty: past, present, and future. Semin Spine Surg. 2012: Elsevier.
3. Wu JC, Liu L, Wen-Cheng H, Chen YC, Ko CC, Wu CL, et al. The incidence of adjacent segment disease requiring surgery after anterior cervical diskectomy and fusion: estimation using an 11-year comprehensive nationwide database in Taiwan. Neurosurgery. 2012;70(3):594–601. PubMed PMID: 22343790.
4. Wu JC, Huang WC, Tu TH, Tsai HW, Ko CC, Wu CL, et al. Differences between soft-disc herniation and spondylosis in cervical arthroplasty: CT-documented heterotopic ossification with minimum 2 years of follow-up. J Neurosurg Spine. 2012;16(2):163–71. PubMed PMID: 22136390.
5. Mummaneni PV, Amin BY, Wu JC, Brodt ED, Dettori JR, Sasso RC. Cervical artificial disc replacement versus fusion in the cervical spine: a systematic review comparing long-term follow-up results from two FDA trials. Evid Based Spine Care J. 2012;3(S1):59–66. PubMed PMID: 23236315. Pubmed Central PMCID: 3519406.
6. Radcliff K, Coric D, Albert T. Five-year clinical results of cervical total disc replacement compared with anterior discectomy and fusion for treatment of 2-level symptomatic degenerative disc disease: a prospective, randomized, controlled, multicenter investigational device exemption clinical trial. J Neurosurg Spine. 2016;25:1–12. PubMed PMID: 27015130.
7. Gornet MF, Burkus JK, Shaffrey ME, Argires PJ, Nian H, Harrell FE Jr. Cervical disc arthroplasty with PRESTIGE LP disc versus anterior cervical discectomy and fusion: a prospective, multicenter investigational device exemption study. J Neurosurg Spine. 2015;31:1–16. PubMed PMID: 26230424.
8. Burkus JK, Traynelis VC, Haid RW Jr, Mummaneni PV. Clinical and radiographic analysis of an artificial cervical disc: 7-year follow-up from the Prestige prospective randomized controlled clinical trial: clinical article. J Neurosurg Spine. 2014;21(4):516–28. PubMed PMID: 25036218.
9. Davis RJ, Kim KD, Hisey MS, Hoffman GA, Bae HW, Gaede SE, et al. Cervical total disc replacement with the Mobi-C cervical artificial disc compared with anterior discectomy and fusion for treatment of 2-level symptomatic degenerative disc disease: a prospective, randomized, controlled multicenter clinical trial: clinical article. J Neurosurg Spine. 2013;19(5):532–45. PubMed PMID: 24010901.
10. Upadhyaya CD, Wu JC, Trost G, Haid RW, Traynelis VC, Tay B, et al. Analysis of the three United States Food and Drug Administration investigational device exemption cervical arthroplasty trials. J Neurosurg Spine. 2012;16(3):216–28. PubMed PMID: 22195608.
11. Quan GM, Vital JM, Hansen S, Pointillart V. Eight-year clinical and radiological follow-up of the Bryan cervical disc arthroplasty. Spine. 2011;36(8):639–46. PubMed PMID: 21178838.
12. Burkus JK, Haid RW, Traynelis VC, Mummaneni PV. Long-term clinical and radiographic outcomes of cervical disc replacement with the Prestige disc: results from a prospective randomized controlled clinical trial. J Neurosurg Spine. 2010;13(3):308–18. PubMed PMID: 20809722.

13. Coric D, Kim PK, Clemente JD, Boltes MO, Nussbaum M, James S. Prospective randomized study of cervical arthroplasty and anterior cervical discectomy and fusion with long-term follow-up: results in 74 patients from a single site. J Neurosurg Spine. 2013;18(1):36–42. PubMed PMID: 23140129.
14. Murrey D, Janssen M, Delamarter R, Goldstein J, Zigler J, Tay B, et al. Results of the prospective, randomized, controlled multicenter food and drug administration investigational device exemption study of the ProDisc-C total disc replacement versus anterior discectomy and fusion for the treatment of 1-level symptomatic cervical disc disease. Spine J. 2009;9(4):275–86. PubMed PMID: 18774751.
15. Heller JG, Sasso RC, Papadopoulos SM, Anderson PA, Fessler RG, Hacker RJ, et al. Comparison of BRYAN cervical disc arthroplasty with anterior cervical decompression and fusion: clinical and radiographic results of a randomized, controlled, clinical trial. Spine. 2009;34(2):101–7. PubMed PMID: 19112337.
16. Mummaneni PV, Burkus JK, Haid RW, Traynelis VC, Zdeblick TA. Clinical and radiographic analysis of cervical disc arthroplasty compared with allograft fusion: a randomized controlled clinical trial. J Neurosurg Spine. 2007;6(3):198–209. PubMed PMID: 17355018.
17. Hilibrand AS, Carlson GD, Palumbo MA, Jones PK, Bohlman HH. Radiculopathy and myelopathy at segments adjacent to the site of a previous anterior cervical arthrodesis. J Bone Joint Surg Am. 1999;81(4):519–28. PubMed PMID: 10225797.
18. Wu JC. Cervical total disc replacement. Formosan J Surg. 2014;47:49–52.
19. Chang PY, Chang HK, Wu JC, Huang WC, Fay LY, Tu TH, et al. Is cervical disc arthroplasty good for congenital cervical stenosis? J Neurosurg Spine. 2017;10:1–9. PubMed PMID: 28291414.
20. Chang HK, Huang WC, Wu JC, Chang PY, Tu TH, Fay LY, et al. Should cervical disc arthroplasty be done on patients with increased intramedullary signal intensity on magnetic resonance imaging? World Neurosurg. 2016;89:489–96. PubMed PMID: 26893039.
21. Chang HC, Tu TH, Chang HK, Wu JC, Fay LY, Chang PY, et al. Hybrid corpectomy and disc arthroplasty for cervical spondylotic myelopathy caused by ossification of posterior longitudinal ligament and disc herniation. World Neurosurg. 2016;95:22–30. PubMed PMID: 27474455.
22. Chang HK, Chang CC, Tu TH, Wu JC, Huang WC, Fay LY, et al. Can segmental mobility be increased by cervical arthroplasty? Neurosurg Focus. 2017;42(2):E3. PubMed PMID: 28142280.
23. Chang PY, Chang HK, Wu JC, Huang WC, Fay LY, Tu TH, et al. Differences between C3-4 and other subaxial levels of cervical disc arthroplasty: more heterotopic ossification at the 5-year follow-up. J Neurosurg Spine. 2016;24(5):752–9. PubMed PMID: 26824584.
24. Tu TH, Chang CC, Wu JC, Fay LY, Huang WC, Cheng H. Resection of uncovertebral joints and posterior longitudinal ligament for cervical disc arthroplasty. Neurosurg Focus. 2017;42(VideoSuppl1):V2. PubMed PMID: 28042720.
25. Tu TH, Wu JC, Huang WC, Chang HK, Ko CC, Fay LY, et al. Postoperative nonsteroidal antiinflammatory drugs and the prevention of heterotopic ossification after cervical arthroplasty: analysis using CT and a minimum 2-year follow-up. J Neurosurg Spine. 2015;22(5):447–53. PubMed PMID: 25723121.
26. Wu JC, Huang WC, Tsai HW, Ko CC, Fay LY, Tu TH, et al. Differences between 1- and 2-level cervical arthroplasty: more heterotopic ossification in 2-level disc replacement: clinical article. J Neurosurg Spine. 2012;16(6):594–600. PubMed PMID: 22443547.
27. Wu JC, Huang WC, Tsai TY, Fay LY, Ko CC, Tu TH, et al. Multilevel arthroplasty for cervical spondylosis: more heterotopic ossification at 3 years of follow-up. Spine. 2012;37(20):E1251–9. PubMed PMID: 22739672.
28. Mummaneni PV, Haid RW. The future in the care of the cervical spine: interbody fusion and arthroplasty. Invited submission from the Joint Section Meeting on Disorders of the Spine and Peripheral Nerves, March 2004. J Neurosurg Spine. 2004;1(2):155–9. PubMed PMID: 15347000.
29. Fay LY, Huang WC, Wu JC, Chang HK, Tsai TY, Ko CC, et al. Arthroplasty for cervical spondylotic myelopathy: similar results to patients with only radiculopathy at 3 years' follow-up. J Neurosurg Spine. 2014;21(3):400–10. PubMed PMID: 24926929.
30. Tu TH, Wu JC, Cheng H, Mummaneni PV. Hybrid cervical disc arthroplasty. Neurosurg Focus. 2017;42(VideoSuppl1):V5. PubMed PMID: 28042726.

MIS Approaches for Cervical Spondylotic Disease

21

Mena G. Kerolus and Richard G. Fessler

Pitfalls/Pearls

- Using a K-wire in the cervical spine is ill-advised as it may inadvertently cause direct injury to the spinal cord. The wide interlaminar space in the cervical spine increases the risk of plunging, which can cause a dural or spinal cord injury. The fascia is to be opened under direct vision (in a mini-open fashion), the muscles spread with Metz scissors, and a small or medium single dilator is docked on the facet.
- Positioning is crucial for a safe and smooth operation. When utilizing the sitting position, the head should be slightly flexed and the neck perpendicular to the floor. Further, the skin and musculature should remain loose and should never be kinked.
- In cases of MIS posterior cervical laminoforaminotomy, the tubular dilators should be docked on the laminar-facet junction.
- An angled curette is used to dissect the ligament from the undersurface of the bone to avoid dural tears. A Kerrison or drill is used for bony resection. Partial removal of the facet is necessary for decompression of the nerve root. However, the facet may be destabilized if more than 50% is removed.
- When performing an MIS posterior cervical laminectomy, do not remove the ligamentum flavum until you have medialized the dilator and drilled the contralateral lamina. The ligament provides a protective barrier between the spinal cord and drill bit.
- The cervical spinal cord cannot be manipulated during decompression as can be done with the thecal sac in the lumbar spine, making central or medial paracentral disc herniations a contraindication to MIS posterior laminoforaminotomy.
- MIS posterior cervical techniques have a large learning curve.
- To access a lateral herniated disc, the superomedial pedicle of the caudal level can be drilled.
- The ventral and dorsal nerve root should be palpated with a nerve hook, and the lateral edge of the cervical spinal dura and proximal nerve root should be visualized to confirm a full decompression.

M. G. Kerolus
Department of Neurosurgery, Rush University Medical Center, Chicago, IL, USA

R. G. Fessler (✉)
Department of Neurosurgery, Rush University, Chicago, IL, USA
e-mail: rfessler@rush.edu

M. G. Kaiser et al. (eds.), *Degenerative Cervical Myelopathy and Radiculopathy*,
https://doi.org/10.1007/978-3-319-97952-6_21

Introduction

Cervical spondylotic disease is the most common pathology of the cervical spine [1]. Minimally invasive endoscopic surgery (MIS) was introduced to minimize muscle dissection and soft tissue trauma. Foley et al. introduced the first minimally invasive endoscopic approach for lumbar disc disease; this was later applied to the cervical spine [2–5]. Minimally invasive approaches for the cervical spine have reduced operative times, blood loss, and duration of hospital stays [6–8]. MIS posterior cervical laminoforaminotomy and discectomy are well-described surgical techniques for the cervical spine. MIS posterior cervical laminectomy, laminoplasty, and posterior cervical fixation have been described, but not widely used. Finally, MIS transfacet fixation techniques have been developed to provide stability to the cervical spine. In this chapter, we will discuss the evidence for using MIS techniques in the cervical spine and discuss different approaches, surgical techniques, and limitations of MIS techniques when operating on the cervical spine.

Main Ideas Supported by Relevant Literature and References

Open posterior cervical spine procedures require extensive dissection of the paraspinal muscles, leading to prolonged operative times and increased bleeding. Long-term consequences of the open procedure include worse postoperative pain and severe muscle atrophy. Multilevel laminectomies are associated with an increased risk of postlaminectomy kyphosis which is thought to occur because of a violation to the posterior tension band and aggressive facet resection [9]. Open cervical laminoplasty attempts to diminish this complication, but thus far the results have been inconclusive [10]. Ventral spinal cord pathology can be addressed with open anterior approaches, either discectomy or corpectomy, allowing resection of the ventral spinal cord pathology and maintenance of cervical alignment with excellent clinical outcomes; however, some surgeons are uncomfortable with the anatomy of the neck and the risk of complications associated with the large vessels, the upper aerodigestive tract, and superior and recurrent laryngeal nerves. This is mostly true in the case of elderly patients and when addressing higher cervical levels where the incidence of postoperative dysphagia and airway edema is greater [11, 12].

In patients with cervical spondylotic radiculopathy or myelopathy, several posterior cervical MIS approaches have been developed to address these symptoms. Posterior cervical MIS laminoforaminotomies have been shown to both reduce symptoms of radiculopathy in up to 97% of patients and maintain motion while avoiding complications such as adjacent segment disease often seen in patients undergoing ACDF [2, 4, 6, 7, 13]. Both Fessler et al. and Kim and Kim compared open and MIS cervical foraminotomy and demonstrated similar clinical outcomes and decreased hospitalization, blood loss, and narcotic use in those who underwent the MIS posterior foraminotomy procedures [6, 7]. However, in patients with cervical spondylotic radiculopathy, posterior foraminotomy and ACDF approaches provide no significant difference in patient outcomes with nearly all patients experiencing complete relief [14].

In patients with cervical spondylotic myelopathy, MIS surgical techniques include MIS laminectomy, laminoplasty, and/or fusion, with the treatment goal being adequate spinal cord decompression, maintenance of surgical alignment, and stability. An MIS approach for decompression of the cervical spine preserves the tension band, in the likelihood that cervical alignment remains after surgery. In patients undergoing an MIS laminectomy, the clinical experience has been reported with good results, but given the strict indications for surgery, the number of cases has been limited. Further clinical studies are needed to assess the incidence of postlaminectomy kyphosis [15, 16].

Similar to MIS laminectomy, MIS laminoplasty was developed with the intent to maintain the posterior tension band. The open "French-door" laminoplasty addressed the concern of the posterior tension band, but it is still an open surgical approach with increased soft tissue and muscle dissection. In a cadaveric study, Wang et al. demonstrated the feasibility of performing a minimally invasive laminoplasty [17]. In 2008, the MIS laminoplasty technique was demonstrated on a limited number of patients, but it was found to be technically challenging leading to operative times that were twice as long as in open techniques [17, 18]. In 2016, Zhang et al. reported on a series of 45 patients undergoing MIS laminoplasty, demonstrating short operative times and successful clinical results [8].

MIS posterior cervical instrumentation for arthrodesis can either be done with lateral mass screws or transfacet screws, although application of MIS techniques for these procedures is rare with only a few reported series published [19–21]. One of the first reports of microendoscopic lateral mass fixation on patients was described by Sehati and Khoo in ten patients in the setting of cervical trauma. All instrumentation was placed accurately and easily confirmed with fluoroscopy [20]. However, rod placement remains a common difficulty when using MIS lateral mass fixation. Ahmad et al. reported on a series of over 20 patients who underwent successful placement of percutaneous transfacet fixation in conjunction with an ACDF where further hardware supplementation was desired to aid with fusion. It was not used as a primary means of fusion because the MIS approach provided insufficient bony surface for fusion [21].

Tissue-sparing posterior cervical transfacet fusion cages were developed to treat patients with cervical radiculopathy without kyphosis and without symptomatic central canal stenosis [22]. The goal was to simultaneously provide indirect decompression of a cervical spinal level while providing cervical stability and enhance fusion using a minimally invasive approach [23, 24]. This procedure was first introduced as an open procedure by Goel et al. and later modified by McCormack et al. using a tissue-sparing approach [22, 25]. In their study of 60 patients with cervical radiculopathy, 1- and 2-year follow-up revealed improved NDI, SF-12, and VAS scores [22, 26]. Posterior cervical cages and spacers have also been shown to increase foraminal height, improve VAS scores, and increase lordosis for patients with symptomatic cervical pseudoarthrosis after an ACDF [27, 28]. Recently, its use as a method to treat single-level cervical radiculopathy as a stand-alone treatment was found effective in a prospective randomized control trial [29].

Surgical Techniques

The initial surgical exposure and technique for microendoscopic foraminotomy, discectomy, laminectomy, laminoplasty, and lateral mass fixation are similar. The technique for posterior cervical cages is unique and will be discussed separately. Due to the lack of evidence supporting MIS cervical laminoplasty, MIS cervical lateral mass fixation, and MIS cervical transfacet screws, the surgical steps for these procedures will not be discussed.

Indications/Contraindications (Table 21.1)

MIS Posterior Cervical Laminoforaminotomy and Discectomy

Candidates for MIS posterior cervical foraminotomy and discectomy present with cervical radiculopathy secondary to foraminal stenosis from an osteophyte, facet arthropathy, or lateralized cervical disc herniation. Further, patients who have undergone a prior ACDF with persistent radiculopathy or patients with contraindications to undergoing an ACDF are also candidates. Imaging findings on MRI should correlate with the patient's symptoms. Paracentral disc herniation, medial foraminal disc herniation that may require manipulation of the cervical cord, cervical instability, ventral spinal cord disease, cervical kyphosis, or cervical myelopathy cannot be adequately addressed with MIS posterior cervical foraminotomy or discectomy. As such, MIS posterior cervical foraminotomy or discectomy is contraindicated. This procedure can be done under general anesthesia in either the seated or prone position.

Table 21.1 Indications/contraindications

Indications	Contraindications
Posterior MIS foraminotomy	
Symptoms include cervical radiculopathy	Paracentral disc herniation or medial foraminal disc herniation that would require extensive manipulation of the cervical cord
Foraminal stenosis secondary to osteophyte, facet arthropathy, or lateralized cervical disc herniation	Primary ventral cervical spinal cord compression
Patients who underwent a prior ACDF with persistent radiculopathy	Cervical instability
Contraindication for decompression with an ACDF (e.g., patient with prior neck radiation)	Cervical kyphosis
	+/− cervical myelopathy
Posterior MIS laminectomy	
Symptoms include cervical myelopathy or neck pain	Primary ventral spinal cord compression
Cervical stenosis	Cervical kyphosis
Primarily dorsal spinal cord compression	
Lordotic or straight cervical alignment	
Percutaneous transfacet spacers	
Symptoms include radiculopathy with radiographic findings of foraminal stenosis	Cervical kyphosis
+/− cervical myelopathy	
+/− pseudoarthrosis after prior ACDF with normal cervical alignment	

ACDF anterior cervical discectomy and fusion

MIS Posterior Cervical Laminectomy

Patients with cervical myelopathy secondary to cervical stenosis with maintenance of cervical lordosis are candidates for MIS laminectomy. Additionally, patients with primarily dorsal spinal cord compression involving two or more levels are candidates for MIS posterior cervical decompression if cervical alignment is preserved. In patients with loss of cervical lordosis, the surgeon should avoid the MIS posterior cervical approach alone without prior correction of alignment. Contraindications to MIS posterior cervical laminectomy include cervical instability and primarily ventral spinal cord disease.

Tissue-Sparing Posterior Cervical Transfacet Fusion Cages

Patients with radiculopathy and radiographic findings of foraminal stenosis without cervical kyphosis are candidates for tissue-sparing posterior cervical transfacet fusion cages. There is a debate whether patients with myelopathy or myeloradiculopathy are candidates for interfacet tissue-sparing cages. Goel et al. demonstrated that patients with myelopathy and/or radiculopathy may benefit from open posterior cervical spacers as it can unbuckle the ligament flavum and indirectly decompress the spinal cord; however, cervical stenosis with myelopathy has not been exclusively studied using MIS percutaneous interfacet techniques [22, 25]. Open and tissue-sparing posterior cervical transfacet fusion cages can be placed in conjunction with an anterior cervical procedure or alone in a posterior-only procedure [29, 30]. Additionally, posterior cervical spacers have been shown to statistically improve radiculopathy and VAS neck pain scores in patients that develop pseudoarthrosis after an ACDF [27, 28]. Patients with cervical kyphosis should not undergo posterior cervical transfacet cages without prior correction of cervical alignment.

Positioning

After induction of general anesthesia, the table is turned 180° away from the anesthesia station and the head placed in a Mayfield head clamp. The table is flexed so that the patient is in a semi-

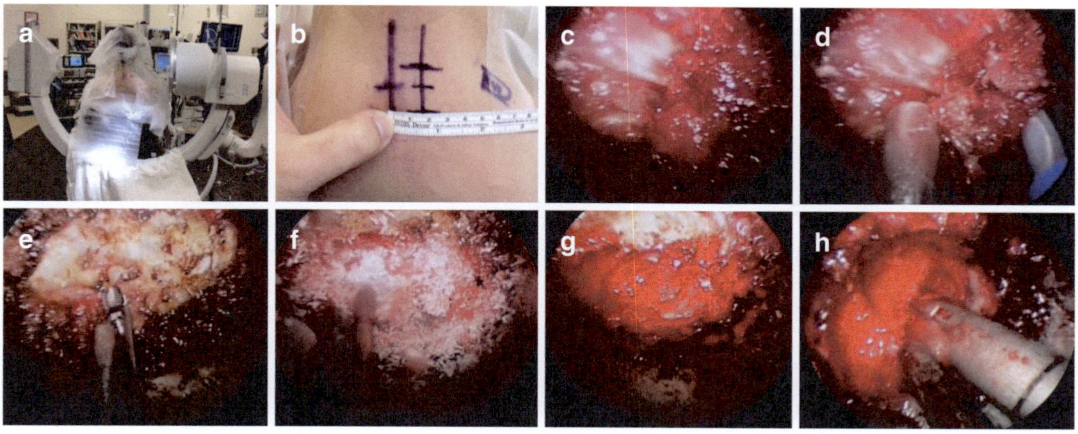

Fig. 21.1 (**a**) The semi-sitting position for a MIS posterior cervical laminoforaminotomy. Note that the head is perpendicular to the floor and the neck slightly flexed. The fluoroscopy is placed under the patient and the base on the right side, which is the same side as the planned incision (**b**) which is 1.5 cm from the midline. This positioning provides an ideal "surgical flow" during the case. (**c**) An endoscopic tubular view of the soft tissue after dilation and (**d**) soft tissue removal with a Bovie and pituitary rongeurs in a lateral to medial direction. (**e**) A Kerrison punch is initially used to remove the bone. Prior to this, an angled curette is used to mobilize the soft tissue from the undersurface of the bone so the Kerrison can be used safely. (**f**) A drill is used to remove bone that is difficult to remove with a Kerrison, completing the laminectomy (**g**). (**h**) The drill can also be used to perform the medial facetectomy in order to expose the proximal nerve root

sitting position with the neck perpendicular to the floor and the head slightly flexed. The head is secured anteriorly to a cross-body bar that is fixated to the Mayo stand in front of the patient's waist (Fig. 21.1a). We advocate a seated position because it reduces blood loss and also minimizes blood in the operative field. Accumulated blood drains out of the operative field providing adequate visibility. The patient's arms are placed at the waist and padded appropriately. Intraoperative lateral fluoroscopy is positioned at the level of the patient's neck with the base of the fluoroscopy on the side of the decompression. Fluoroscopy can be placed above or below the patient's head as long as it is out of the way of the surgeon. The procedure can be done while standing; but if a microscope is needed, it is easier for the surgeon to sit because of the positioning. Intraoperative monitoring using somatosensory evoked potentials and myotomal EMG monitoring are used to monitor the spinal cord.

If the prone position is chosen (for tissue-sparing posterior cervical transfacet fusion cages), the patient is placed on two chest rolls with the head secured in a Mayfield in the standard fashion. A belt is placed around the waist and the patient positioned in the reverse Trendelenburg position. The arms are tucked and padded along the patient's waist. Often simultaneous anteroposterior (AP) and lateral imagings are also used to verify the cervical level and for ease of implantation.

Anesthesia Considerations

In the seated position, the anesthesiologist is able to visualize the face and endotracheal tube. Although rare, the risk of a venous air embolism and hemodynamic instability are complications that may occur while in the seated position. A transesophageal echocardiogram probe or precordial Doppler can be used to help identify an air embolism sooner that can be detected by changes observed with increased endotracheal CO_2 and/or hemodynamic changes. Additionally, the seated position leads to venous pooling in the legs which may also lead to systemic hypotension. Macroglossia can develop secondary to a decrease in venous and lymphatic outflow when the neck is flexed. Finally, unique peripheral nerve injuries can occur while in the seated position, including ulnar and common peroneal nerve compression, and adequate padding of the elbows and legs will minimize this complication.

Technique

A crucial step in performing a minimally invasive spine surgery is planning the incision. Using fluoroscopy, the appropriate level is visualized. The midline is identified, and a paramedian incision about 1.5–2.0 cm is marked (Fig. 21.1a, b). A paramedian incision is preferred to avoid tension along the tubular retractor system. Also, if several levels will be decompressed, we find a paramedian incision allows greater manipulation of the soft tissues. If bilateral decompression is desired in the same operation, a midline incision can be used and the skin retracted laterally for individual dilations. The proposed incision is infiltrated with local anesthetic, and a stab incision approximately 2.0 cm in length is made at the desired level. Under direct vision, the fascia is cut with a Bovie, and a Metz scissors is used to spread the paraspinal muscles to the level of the facets. We avoid forceful dilation of the fascia or musculature as aggressive dilation in the cervical spine increases the risk of "plunging" given the widened, medial interlaminar space. A small or medium dilator is then advanced perpendicular to the bone at the laminofacet junction at the appropriate cervical level. During our initial experience, the Kirschner wire (K-wire) was used to assist with dilation; however, over the last several years, we found that muscle dissection with Metz scissors or small tubular dilators provided adequate access to the bone without the unnecessary and increased risk of dural or spinal cord injury from the K-wire. We typically use 18 mm tubes, but more importantly, the tube should be the same size as the incision to avoid unnecessary movement of the tubular system. Fluoroscopy is positioned in such a manner so that it can be easily used for intraoperative confirmation without getting in the way of the surgical procedure. Fluoroscopy should be used as often as needed during tubular dilation to verify the position of the tube during placement.

MIS Posterior Cervical Laminoforaminotomy and Discectomy

The paramedian incision should be approximately 1.5 cm from the midline. The preoperative MRI can be reviewed to measure the exact distance for the starting position. The ideal position for addressing the cervical foramina and disc space is the laminar facet junction. After docking and securing of the tubular system, monopolar electrocautery and pituitary rongeurs are used to remove the soft tissue in a lateral to medial direction exposing the medial edge of the lateral mass (Fig. 21.1c, d). An upangled curette is used to dissect the ligament from the undersurface of the lamina. Epidural venous bleeding can be controlled using bipolar cautery or thrombin-soaked Gelfoam. Using either a 2.0 mm Kerrison punch or a high-speed drill, the lateral portion of the lamina and medial facet is removed in a medial to lateral and inferior direction along the nerve root foramen (Fig. 21.1e, f). The drill may be used to thin the bone so that a curette or Kerrison punch may be used. We have not encountered complications such as increased C5 sensitivity when using a Kerrison punch. Drilling should continue in the lateral and inferior direction; however, removing too much bone laterally or removing more than 50% of the facet may cause instability of the facet joint. An angled curette should be used frequently to dissect the soft tissue from the bone. When the neural foramen is decompressed, the ligament can be mobilized medially, and the lateral edge of the dura and proximal edge of the nerve root are exposed (Fig. 21.1g, h). In most cases, the nerve can be decompressed after removal of a small part of the laminar facet junction. At this step, the nerve root can be mobilized to palpate the ventral foramen to identify osteophytes or disc fragments. In cases of an osteophyte complex, it can be removed using an angled curette or drill. In the case of a herniated disc, the nerve root can be gently elevated and the disc material removed using a small pituitary. This maneuver can be facilitated by drilling off 2–3 mm of the cephalad portion of the caudal pedicle. Herniated discs that are medial to the neural foramen are a relative contraindication to posterior laminoforaminotomy because of the potential of excessive manipulation of the spinal cord.

MIS Posterior Cervical Laminectomy

In a microendoscopic laminectomy approach, the midline is identified, and a 1.0 cm paramedian incision is preferred to prevent excessive muscle retraction and to provide a preferable 30–45° working angle for the tubular dilators. An incision is made in the standard fashion as described above. The fascia is directly cut and the paraspinal muscles carefully dissected. If multiple adjacent levels are being addressed, the fascia can be cut in a cranial or caudal direction through an extended single incision to allow easy mobility of the tubular dilators. The inferior edge of the lamina is exposed, and then using a high-speed Midas Rex Legend drill with a TDQ bit (Midas Rex, Fort Worth, Tx), the lamina is drilled in a caudal to cranial direction. On the undersurface of the lamina, the ligamentum flavum will appear and should be left intact to provide a barrier during contralateral decompression. After the initial hemilaminectomy is completed, the tubular dilating system should be pointed medially and the drilling continued to decompress the ventral surface of the spinous process and contralateral lamina. The spinous process and portions of the lamina facet junction on the contralateral side should remain intact. After the drilling is complete, a small-angled curette is used to separate the ligament from the dura, and then the ligament is removed using the curette and/or Kerrison punch.

Tissue-Sparing Posterior Cervical Transfacet Fusion Cages

When placing multiple tissue-sparing posterior cervical transfacet fusion cages, two fluoroscopy units are positioned simultaneously for AP and lateral imaging. A midline incision is made using sharp dissection to the level of the cervicodorsal fascia, and a 1 cm incision is made at the cervicodorsal fascial incision at each respective level. In cases of single-level radiculopathy, the incision is made 1 cm off midline 2–3 spinal segments below the intended level, which may vary based on the facet orientation. The dilators will be placed in a medial to lateral trajectory. Using a combination of the tongue chisel, decorticator, guide tube, and rasp, the posterior facet capsule and cartilage are removed (Fig. 21.2a). The implant holder is

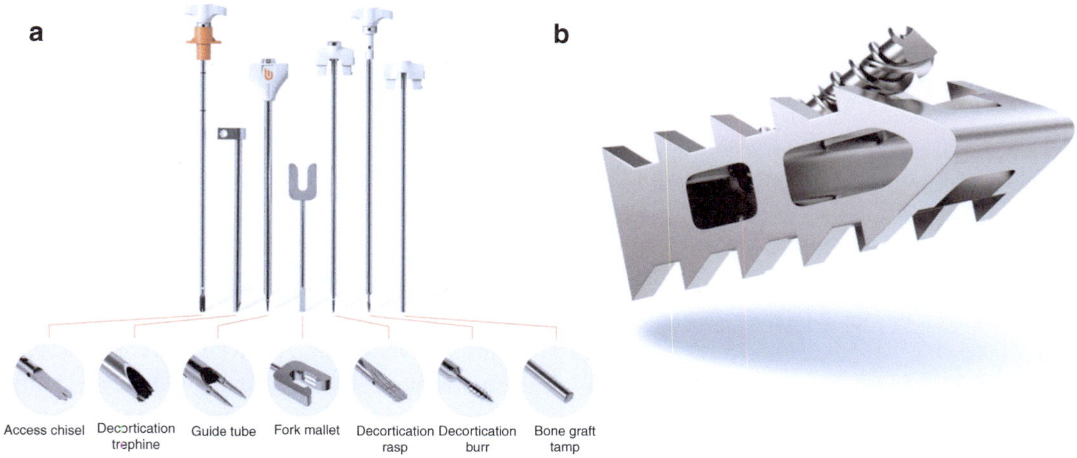

Fig. 21.2 (**a**) Diagram of the instrumentation used during placement of a tissue-sparing posterior cervical transfacet fusion cage. (**b**) Illustration of a posterior cervical transfacet fusion cage with a facet screw which is engaged using a screw handle. (Images provided by Providence Medical Technology)

inserted into the guide tube so that the guide tube abuts the posterior facet margin, and the anterior portion should rest on the superior vertebral body. The round handle advances a facet screw that provides supplemental fixation to the implant (Fig. 21.2b). Lateral and AP fluoroscopy is used to confirm distraction of the facet and implant position. In cases of splaying of the implant or a facet fracture, the screw can be loosened and the implant removed. Allograft is then placed into the transfacet fusion cage and the guide tube removed.

Closure

In cases of tubular decompression, once the ligamentum flavum is removed and the neurologic structures decompressed, the endoscopic tubular system can be removed. When removing the tube, careful hemostasis is achieved by using a "stop and cauterize" approach when withdrawing the tube every few centimeters. The muscle or soft tissue may bleed which can easily be addressed using bipolar electrocautery. Once the tube is completely removed, 2–0 absorbable suture is used to close the fascia, and the skin is closed with 3–0 absorbable suture and glue. When using tissue-sparing posterior transfacet fusion cages, the guide tubes can be removed and the fascia closed in a similar fashion.

Postoperative Care/Concerns

Patients undergoing MIS posterior cervical laminoforaminotomy, discectomy, or laminectomy will generally recover in the post-anesthesia care unit as the anesthesia wears off. Patients ambulate a few hours after surgery and if feeling well, are discharged the same day.

Complication Management/Avoidance

Complications during MIS laminoforaminotomy, discectomy, or laminectomy are rare. However, injury to the nerve root or spinal cord may occur. Docking the tubes and dilating in the appropriate location is a crucial portion of the operation. If dilation occurs a few millimeters from the area of interest, serious neurologic injury, vascular injury, or instability will occur. Understanding the bony anatomy is crucial during drilling and especially if a K-wire is used as the wide interlaminar space provides a route for dura and spinal cord injury.

If a durotomy occurs, the defect can be sealed using a dural sealant. Primary repair in the cervical spine is generally not necessary when using MIS techniques but can be used in large leaks near midline. CSF leak or pseudomeningocele formation is rare but a lumbar drain can be placed if there is concern for persistent leak although we find this unnecessary. Bed restrictions or length of stay is typically not affected, although if patients are symptomatic, we would advocate an additional day of observation. Finally, when decompressing the nerve root using a high-speed drill, as much of the facet complex should be preserved to avoid instability of the joint.

Case Presentations

MIS Posterior Cervical Laminoforaminotomy

A 34-year-old male, with a 4-week history of neck and left arm pain and paresthesia, described radiating pain down his left arm involving his left middle finger and hand. He attempted conservative management including physical therapy, medications, and epidural steroid injections. Neurologic exam was significant for LUE numbness in the C7 nerve distribution and finger extension weakness grade 4/5. There were no signs of myelopathy. A MRI of the cervical spine demonstrated a very large left and central extruded disc at C6/C7 compressing the exiting spinal nerve root and with some compression of his spinal cord (Fig. 21.3a, b). Due to the continued left upper extremity radiculopathy, numbness, and weakness, he elected to proceed with

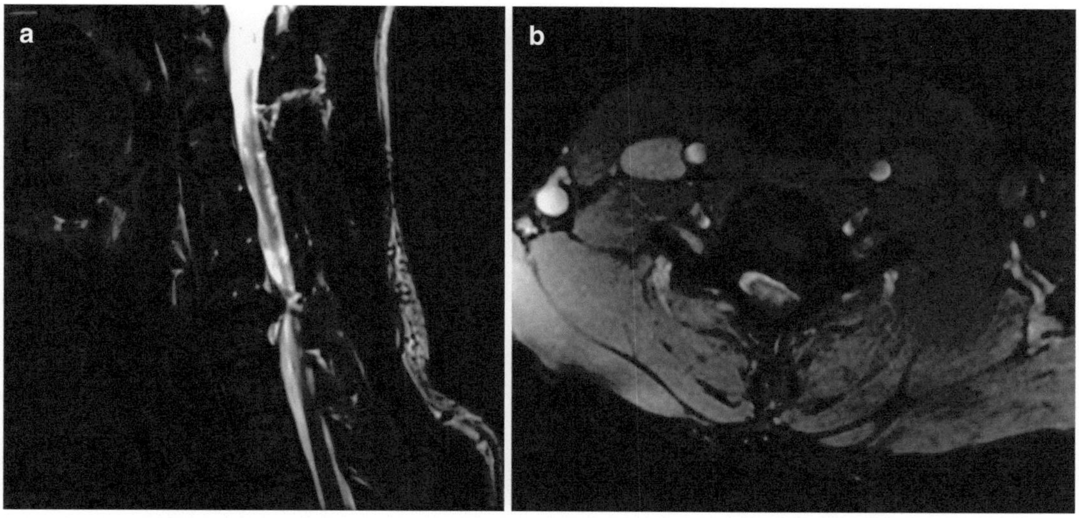

Fig. 21.3 (**a**) Sagittal and (**b**) axial T2-weighted magnetic resonance imaging (MRI) of the left foramina

surgery. He underwent a left MIS posterior C6/C7 discectomy. At 6 weeks postoperatively, his pain was nearly gone and strength improved in his left hand.

Tissue-Sparing Posterior Cervical Transfacet Fusion Cages

The patient is a 59-year-old female with a prior history of a cervical tumor that was resected approximately 8 years ago, who presents with 8/10 neck and right arm pain. She describes posterior midline neck pain and interscapular pain, with progressive difficulty writing and now dropping objects. She has tried conservative management including physical therapy and medications with minimal relief. On neurologic examination, she has a grade 3/5 strength in her right deltoid and 3+ reflexes throughout. Cervical lateral, flexion, and extension radiographs demonstrate multilevel disc degeneration with C3–C6 kyphosis and dynamic instability at C3/C4 (Fig. 21.4a–c). MRI of the cervical spine demonstrated C4/C5 right foraminal stenosis and C5/C6 central canal stenosis and bilateral foraminal stenosis (Fig. 21.4d, e). Due to the patient's continued neck pain and myeloradiculopathy due to a combination of prior C1–C3 myelomalacia from her prior spinal cord tumor but also progressive C3–C6 kyphosis, instability, and stenosis, a C3–C6 ACDF along with posterior transfacet cage placement was performed. Postoperatively, patient recovered well, and at her 3-month follow-up, nearly all her pain was gone. Neutral lateral radiographs demonstrate stable appearance of her instrumentation with correction of her kyphosis (Fig. 21.4f).

Conclusion

MIS techniques to the cervical spine provide an opportunity to minimize blood loss and disruption of the soft tissues as well as decrease the duration of hospitalization. The MIS posterior cervical foraminotomy and discectomy are the most commonly used minimally invasive surgeries for treatment of cervical spondylotic radiculopathy. Surgical techniques have been developed for laminectomy, laminoplasty, and lateral mass fixation, although widespread use of these surgical techniques is limited. There is a large learning curve when performing MIS, especially in the cervical spine. As a surgeon's familiarity with *MIS* instrumentation improves, more surgeries will be performed using minimally invasive techniques.

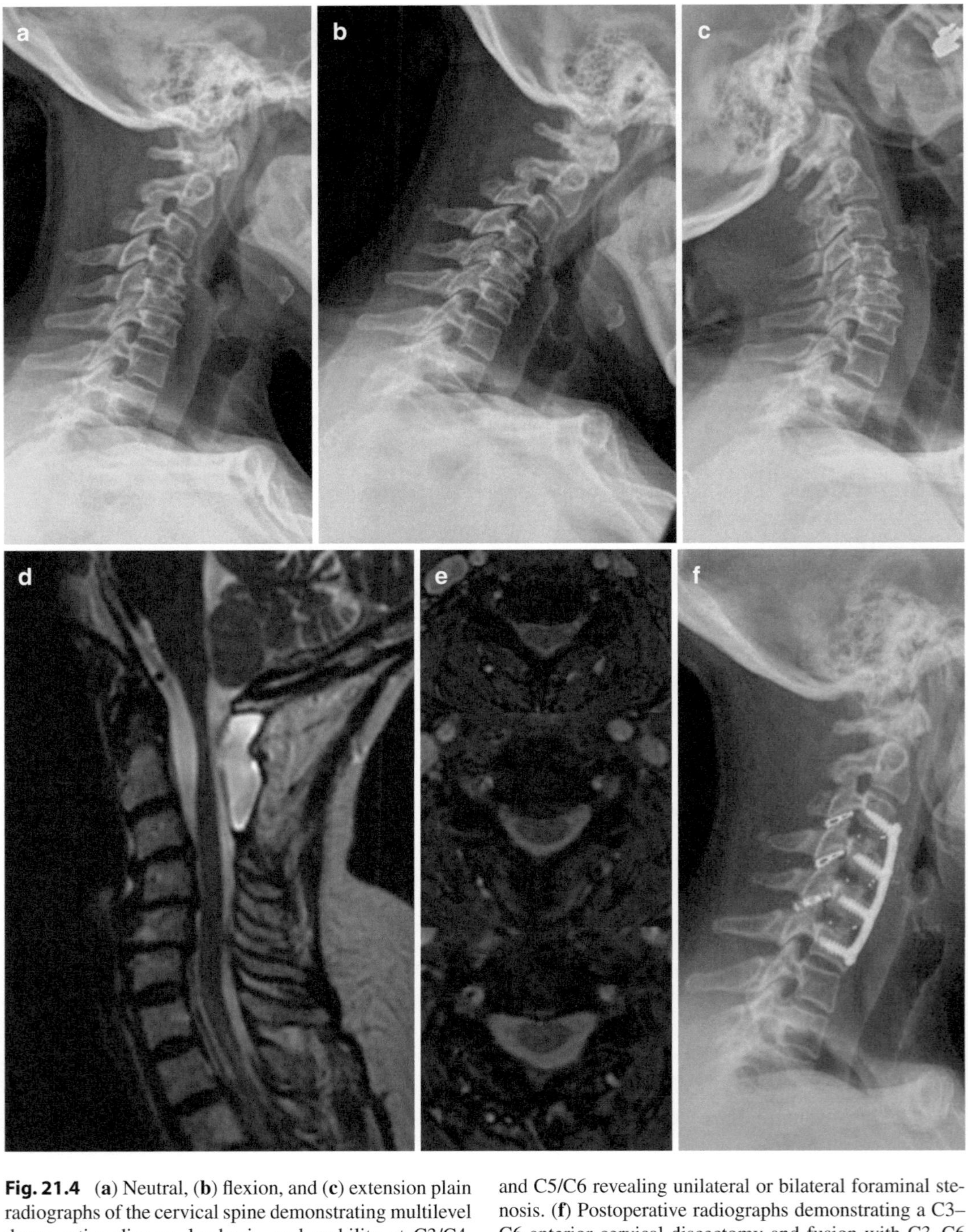

Fig. 21.4 (**a**) Neutral, (**b**) flexion, and (**c**) extension plain radiographs of the cervical spine demonstrating multilevel degenerative disease, kyphosis, and mobility at C3/C4. (**d**) MRI demonstrating multilevel degenerative disease and cervical kyphosis. (**e**) Axial views of C3/C4, C4/C5, and C5/C6 revealing unilateral or bilateral foraminal stenosis. (**f**) Postoperative radiographs demonstrating a C3–C6 anterior cervical discectomy and fusion with C3–C6 posterior interfacet spacers

References

1. Klineberg E. Cervical spondylotic myelopathy: a review of the evidence. Orthop Clin North Am. 2010;41:193–202. https://doi.org/10.1016/j.ocl.2009.12.010.
2. O'Toole JE, Sheikh H, Eichholz KM, Fessler RG, Perez-Cruet MJ. Endoscopic posterior cervical foraminotomy and discectomy. Neurosurg Clin N Am. 2006;17:411–22. https://doi.org/10.1016/j.nec.2006.06.002.
3. Khoo LT, Palmer S, Laich DT, Fessler RG. Minimally invasive percutaneous posterior lumbar interbody fusion. Neurosurgery. 2002;51:S166–81.
4. Roh SW, Kim DH, Cardoso AC, Fessler RG. Endoscopic foraminotomy using MED system in cadaveric specimens. Spine. 2000;25:260–4.
5. Foley KT, Smith MM, Rampersaud YR. Microendoscopic approach to far-lateral lumbar disc herniation. Neurosurg Focus. 1999;7:e5. https://doi.org/10.3171/foc.1999.7.6.6.
6. Fessler RG, Khoo LT. Minimally invasive cervical microendoscopic foraminotomy: an initial clinical experience. Neurosurgery. 2002;51:S37–45.
7. Kim K-T, Kim Y-B. Comparison between open procedure and tubular retractor assisted procedure for cervical radiculopathy: results of a randomized controlled study. J Korean Med Sci. 2009;24:649–53. https://doi.org/10.3346/jkms.2009.24.4.649.
8. Zhang C, Li D, Wang C, Yan X. Cervical endoscopic laminoplasty for cervical myelopathy. Spine. 2016;41(Suppl 19):B44–51. https://doi.org/10.1097/BRS.0000000000001816.
9. Herkowitz HN. A comparison of anterior cervical fusion, cervical laminectomy, and cervical laminoplasty for the surgical management of multiple level spondylotic radiculopathy. Spine. 1988;13:774–80.
10. Chiba K, Ogawa Y, Ishii K, Takaishi H, Nakamura M, Maruiwa H, et al. Long-term results of expansive open-door laminoplasty for cervical myelopathy–average 14-year follow-up study. Spine. 2006;31:2998–3005. https://doi.org/10.1097/01.brs.0000250307.78987.6b.
11. Chung W-F, Liu S-W, Huang L-C, Chang H-K, Wu J-C, Chen L-F, et al. erious dysphagia following anterior cervical discectomy and fusion: long-term incidence in a national cohort. J Neurosurg Sci. 2017; https://doi.org/10.23736/S0390-5616.17.03970-4.
12. Kim SW, Jang C, Yang MH, Lee S, Yoo JH, Kwak YH, et al. The natural course of prevertebral soft tissue swelling after anterior cervical spine surgery: how long will it last? Spine J Off J North Am Spine Soc. 2017;17:1297. https://doi.org/10.1016/j.spinee.2017.05.003.
13. Clark JG, Abdullah KG, Steinmetz MP, Benzel EC, Mroz TE. Minimally invasive versus open cervical foraminotomy: a systematic review. Glob Spine J. 2011;1:9–14. https://doi.org/10.1055/s-0031-1296050.
14. Wirth FP, Dowd GC, Sanders HF, Wirth C. Cervical discectomy. A prospective analysis of three operative techniques. Surg Neurol. 2000;53:340–6. -348.
15. Dahdaleh NS, Wong AP, Smith ZA, Wong RH, Lam SK, Fessler RG. Microendoscopic decompression for cervical spondylotic myelopathy. Neurosurg Focus. 2013;35:E8. https://doi.org/10.3171/2013.3.FOCUS135.
16. Minamide A, Yoshida M, Yamada H, Nakagawa Y, Maio K, Kawai M, et al. Clinical outcomes of microendoscopic decompression surgery for cervical myelopathy. Eur Spine J Off Publ Eur Spine Soc Eur Spinal Deform Soc Eur Sect Cerv Spine Res Soc. 2010;19:487–93. https://doi.org/10.1007/s00586-009-1233-0.
17. Wang MY, Green BA, Coscarella E, Baskaya MK, Levi ADO, Guest JD. Minimally invasive cervical expansile laminoplasty: an initial cadaveric study. Neurosurgery. 2003;52:370–3; discussion 373.
18. Benglis DM, Guest JD, Wang MY. Clinical feasibility of minimally invasive cervical laminoplasty. Neurosurg Focus. 2008;25:E3. https://doi.org/10.3171/FOC/2008/25/8/E3.
19. Wang MY, Prusmack CJ, Green BA, Gruen JP, Levi ADO. Minimally invasive lateral mass screws in the treatment of cervical facet dislocations: technical note. Neurosurgery. 2003;52:444–7. -448.
20. Sehati N, Khoo LT. Minimally invasive posterior cervical arthrodesis and fixation. Neurosurg Clin N Am. 2006;17:429–40. https://doi.org/10.1016/j.nec.2006.06.009.
21. Ahmad F, Sherman JD, Wang MY. Percutaneous trans-facet screws for supplemental posterior cervical fixation. World Neurosurg. 2012;78:716.e1–716.e4. https://doi.org/10.1016/j.wneu.2011.12.092.
22. McCormack BM, Bundoc RC, Ver MR, Ignacio JMF, Berven SH, Eyster EF. Percutaneous posterior cervical fusion with the DTRAX facet system for single-level radiculopathy: results in 60 patients. J Neurosurg Spine. 2013;18:245–54. https://doi.org/10.3171/2012.12.SPINE12477.
23. Voronov LI, Siemionow KB, Havey RM, Carandang G, Patwardhan AG. Biomechanical evaluation of DTRAX(®) posterior cervical cage stabilization with and without lateral mass fixation. Med Devices Auckl NZ. 2016;9:285–90. https://doi.org/10.2147/MDER.S111031.
24. Leasure JM, Buckley J. Biomechanical evaluation of an interfacet joint decompression and stabilization system. J Biomech Eng. 2014;136:071010. https://doi.org/10.1115/1.4026363.
25. Goel A, Shah A. Facetal distraction as treatment for single- and multilevel cervical spondylotic radiculopathy and myelopathy: a preliminary report. J Neurosurg Spine. 2011;14:689–96. https://doi.org/10.3171/2011.2.SPINE10601.
26. Siemionow K, Janusz P, Phillips FM, Youssef JA, Isaacs R, Tyrakowski M, et al. Clinical and radiographic results of indirect decompression and posterior cervical fusion for single-level cervical radiculopathy

using an expandable implant with 2-year follow-up. J Neurol Surg Part Cent Eur Neurosurg. 2016;77:482–8. https://doi.org/10.1055/s-0036-1584210.
27. Kasliwal MK, Corley JA, Traynelis VC. Posterior cervical fusion using cervical interfacet spacers in patients with symptomatic cervical pseudarthrosis. Neurosurgery. 2016;78:661–8. https://doi.org/10.1227/NEU.0000000000001087.
28. Smith W, Gillespy M, Huffman J, Vong V, McCormack BM. Anterior cervical pseudarthrosis treated with bilateral posterior cervical cages. Oper Neurosurg Hagerstown Md. 2017;14:236. https://doi.org/10.1093/ons/opx103.
29. Lenzi J, Nardone A, Passacantilli E, Caporlingua A, Lapadula G, Caporlingua F. Posterior cervical transfacet fusion with facetal spacer for the treatment of single-level cervical radiculopathy: a randomized, controlled prospective study. World Neurosurg. 2017;100:7–14. https://doi.org/10.1016/j.wneu.2016.12.125.
30. Tan LA, Straus DC, Traynelis VC. Cervical interfacet spacers and maintenance of cervical lordosis. J Neurosurg Spine. 2015;22:466–9. https://doi.org/10.3171/2014.10.SPINE14192.

Part V

Fusion Techniques for Cervical Degenerative Disorders

22 Anterior Cervical Discectomy and Fusion

Luis M. Tumialán

Introduction

A seismic shift occurred in the management of cervical radiculopathy and myelopathy with the introduction of an anterior approach to the cervical spine by Smith and Robinson [1] and by Cloward [2]. The patient experience transformed almost immediately from the significant discomfort generated by posterior decompressions of either the foramen or the central canal by laminectomies and foraminotomies to a well-tolerated and highly reliable operation to decompress the cervical spinal cord and cervical nerve roots. Since its inception, the anterior cervical discectomy and fusion (ACDF) has been perhaps the most dependable, reproducible, and effective operation in the spine surgeon's armamentarium. Over the years, refinements to the procedure with cervical plating and interbody graft options have added to that reliability and efficacy. The ACDF has now evolved into a consistently high-quality and low-cost outpatient procedure [3].

The goal of this chapter is to review the indications, contraindications, surgical techniques, and complication avoidance in patients with cervical radiculopathy and/or myelopathy being managed with an anterior approach to the cervical spine. Case presentations at the end of the chapter illustrate and reinforce various key points.

L. M. Tumialán
Department of Neurosurgery, Barrow Neurological Institute, St. Joseph's Hospital and Medical Center, Phoenix, AZ, USA
e-mail: Neuropub@barrowneuro.org

Indications

Cervical Radiculopathy

Patients who present with cervical nerve root compression syndromes or cervical myelopathy primarily from ventral compression are ideal candidates for the ACDF. Cervical disc herniations or disc osteophyte complexes that result in cervical radiculopathy are perhaps the most common indication for an anterior approach to decompress the neural elements (Fig. 22.1). However, special consideration for a minimally invasive posterior cervical foraminotomy should be given to patients who present with unilateral single-level cervical radiculopathy but without compression of the spinal cord or significant collapse or degeneration of the disc space. These patients may be better candidates for a motion-preserving minimally invasive option (Fig. 22.2) [4–6].

Cervical Myelopathy

Patients who present with cervical myelopathy from severe central stenosis at one level or

M. G. Kaiser et al. (eds.), *Degenerative Cervical Myelopathy and Radiculopathy*,
https://doi.org/10.1007/978-3-319-97952-6_22

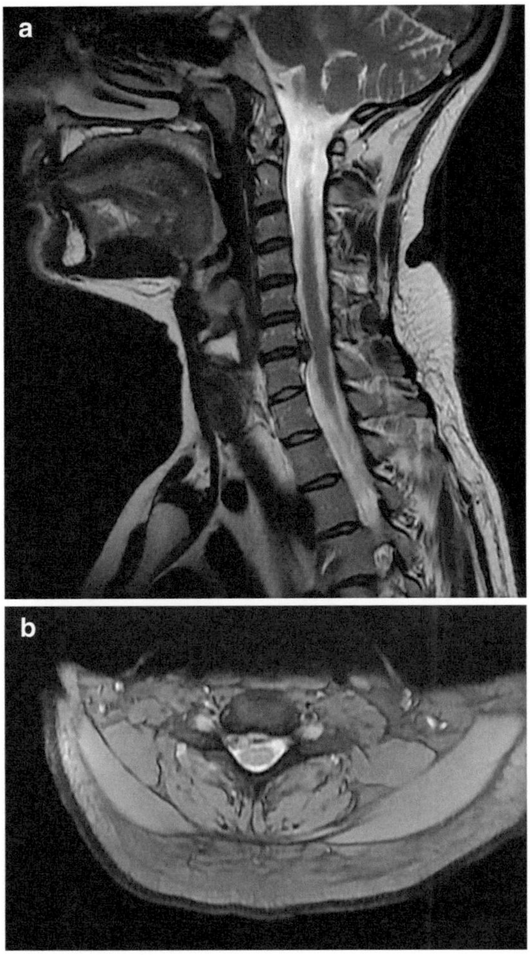

Fig. 22.1 Indications for anterior cervical discectomy and fusion: cervical radiculopathy. A patient with a C6–7 disc herniation causing right-sided nerve root compression and spinal cord compression. (**a**) Sagittal T2-weighted magnetic resonance image (MRI) demonstrating the degree of spinal cord compression. (**b**) Axial T2-weighted MRI demonstrating a broad-based disc herniation compressing the exiting nerve root of C7 on the right and the ventral aspect of the spinal cord. The nature of such compression requires a ventral approach to adequately decompress the entire segment. In this case, a posterior minimally invasive cervical foraminotomy with discectomy would not offer comprehensive decompression of the nerve root and spinal cord, given the degree of ventral compression. (Used with permission from Barrow Neurological Institute, Phoenix, Arizona)

multiple levels have a clear indication for an anterior approach. This indication is especially the case when the source of the compression of

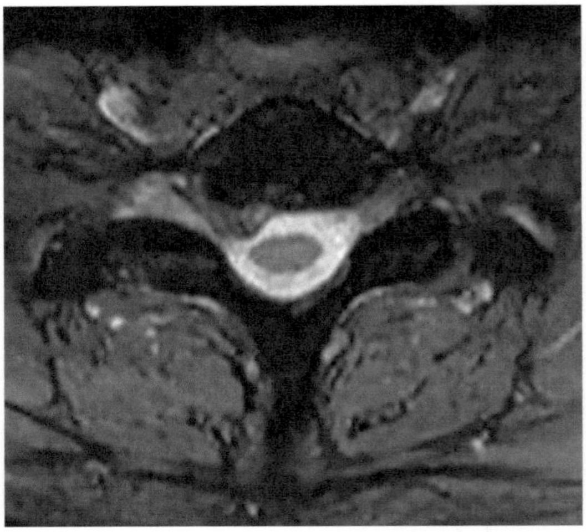

Fig. 22.2 Consideration for a minimally invasive posterior cervical foraminotomy. Axial T2-weighted magnetic resonance image of a C5–6 disc extrusion. In this case, the disc herniation is completely lateral to the spinal cord and limited almost exclusively to the foramen. Although an anterior cervical discectomy and fusion is an acceptable option for addressing the nerve root compression and resolving the radiculopathy, a minimally invasive posterior cervical foraminotomy with discectomy may be a better alternative. *(*Used with permission from Barrow Neurological Institute, Phoenix, Arizona)

the neural elements originates ventrally from the disc space and not from the dorsal elements (Fig. 22.3) [7].

Cervical Spondylosis with Radiculopathy or Myelopathy and Kyphosis

The most unique element of the ACDF is its capacity to restore disc height and reverse a focal cervical kyphosis (Fig. 22.4) in patients with radiculopathy or myelopathy [8, 9]. In these patients, a posterior approach may decompress the nerve root but will not restore disc height or correct kyphosis [10]. In patients with a positive sagittal cervical balance, especially in cases of myelopathy, mounting evidence in the neurosurgical literature suggests that the ACDF is the procedure of choice to restore alignment, namely, sagittal balance, while simultaneously decompressing the neural elements [11, 12].

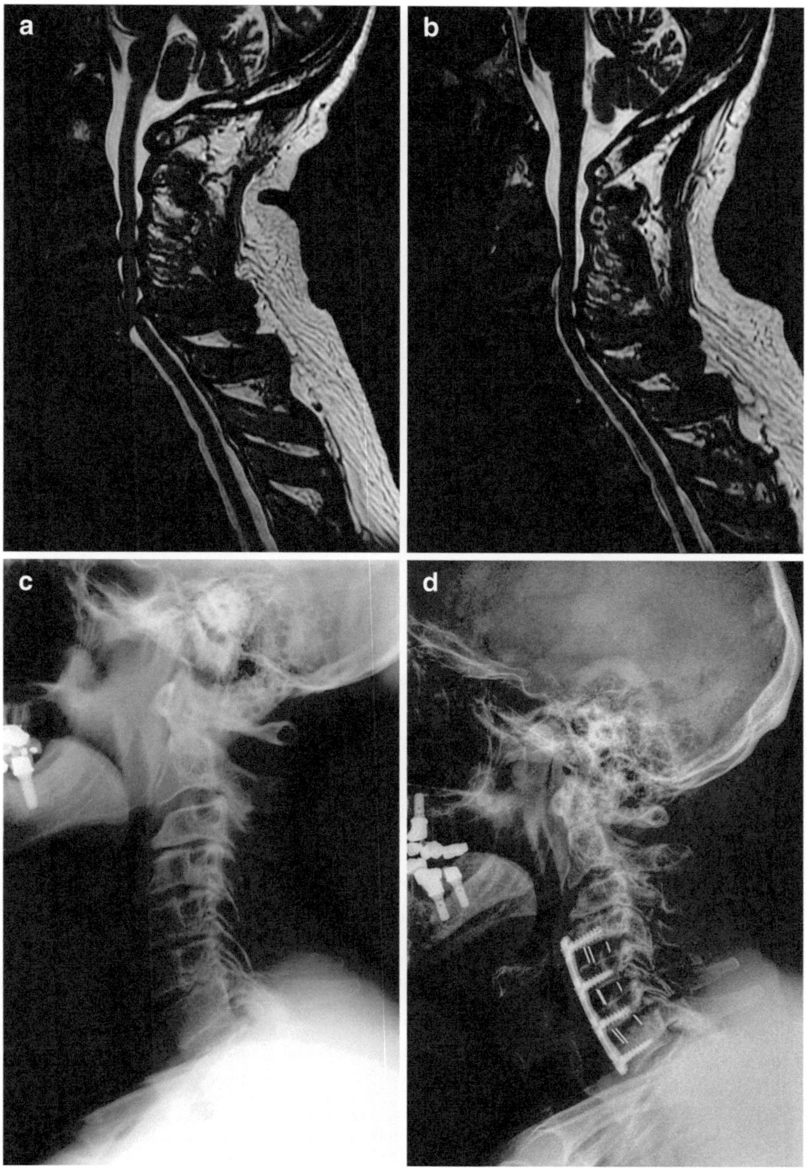

Fig. 22.3 Multiple-level cervical spondylosis with myelopathy. (**a**) Sagittal T2-weighted magnetic resonance image (MRI) of a 67-year-old man who presented with overt signs of myelopathy (positive Romberg sign, incapable of tandem walk, and hyperreflexic) and multiple levels of compression with associated myelomalacia. (**b**) Postoperative sagittal T2-weighted MRI of the cervical spine after a C4–5, C5–6, and C6–7 anterior cervical discectomy and fusion (ACDF) produced improvement in gait and balance. (**c**) Preoperative lateral cervical radiograph demonstrating multiple levels of cervical spondylosis. (**d**) Postoperative lateral cervical radiograph demonstrating a three-level ACDF. (Used with permission from Barrow Neurological Institute, Phoenix, Arizona)

Contraindications

Previous Non-spinal Cervical Surgery

The main relative contraindication for an anterior approach is extensive previous non-spinal surgery in the vicinity of the surgical site. When considering whether to recommend an anterior approach, the clinician should evaluate the patient's history of esophageal or throat cancer with or without irradiation where any surgery was performed. Any radical neck dissection has the potential to make the dissection planes difficult to navigate onto the spine, thereby increasing the risk of esophageal, carotid, and recurrent laryngeal nerve injury. The final decision to recommend an anterior approach for patients in this category should be made jointly with an ears, nose, and throat (ENT) surgeon who is familiar with the procedure and may assist with the exposure.

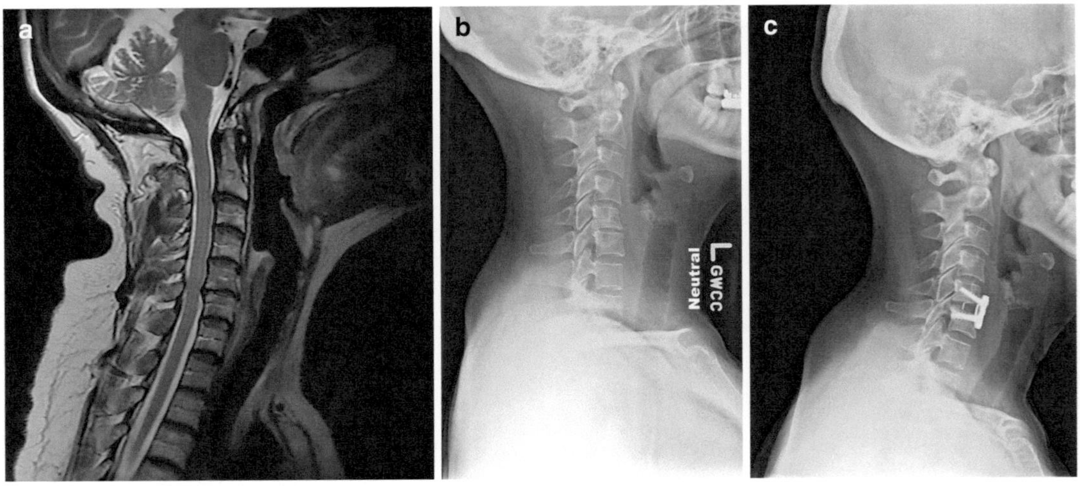

Fig. 22.4 Segmental kyphosis and anterior cervical discectomy and fusion (ACDF). (**a**) Sagittal T2-weighted magnetic resonance image demonstrating a disc osteophyte complex at C5–6. (**b**) Lateral radiograph demonstrating advanced cervical spondylosis at C5–6 with segmental kyphosis. The patient presented with C6 radiculopathy refractory to exhaustive nonoperative management. Although a posterior cervical foraminotomy might decompress the neural foramen, it would not restore disc height or segmental lordosis. (**c**) Postoperative lateral radiograph demonstrating correction of the focal kyphosis and restoration of disc height after a C5–6 ACDF. (Used with permission from Barrow Neurological Institute, Phoenix, Arizona)

Because the thyroid is located a considerable distance from where a cervical incision would be placed, previous thyroidectomies make up a distinct category. I have not encountered any significant difficulty in anterior cervical operations for patients who have undergone previous thyroid surgery without radical neck dissection or irradiation. Nevertheless, the integrity of the laryngeal nerves should be investigated in these patients to help determine the side of the approach (see the following section "Prior ACDF Surgery").

Prior ACDF Surgery

A previous ACDF is not a contraindication for another anterior approach to the cervical spine. However, patients with a previous ACDF should undergo indirect laryngoscopy by an ENT surgeon to determine the functionality of the recurrent laryngeal nerve on the side of the surgery before undergoing repeat anterior cervical surgery. Awareness of partial or complete recurrent laryngeal nerve palsy is crucial before any further surgery. Those patients with recurrent laryngeal nerve palsy must have their operation on the same side of the palsy, as bilateral laryngeal nerve palsy would be a potentially devastating complication. Those patients with intact function of the recurrent laryngeal nerve may have an approach on either side of the cervical spine.

Ankylosing Spondylitis, Diffuse Idiopathic Skeletal Hyperostosis, and Ossified Posterior Longitudinal Ligament

Special consideration should be given to patients with ankylosing spondylitis, diffuse idiopathic skeletal hyperostosis (DISH) (Fig. 22.5), or ossified posterior longitudinal ligament (OPLL). In cases of ankylosing spondylitis or DISH, multiple levels of the cervical spine may have already autofused. Although magnetic resonance imaging (MRI) may demonstrate compression of the neural elements, the anteroposterior (AP) and lateral radiographs will demonstrate the extent of any autofusion. An anterior approach is still feasible, but it is technically more challenging. When multiple levels must be decompressed, a posterior approach may be the more viable option.

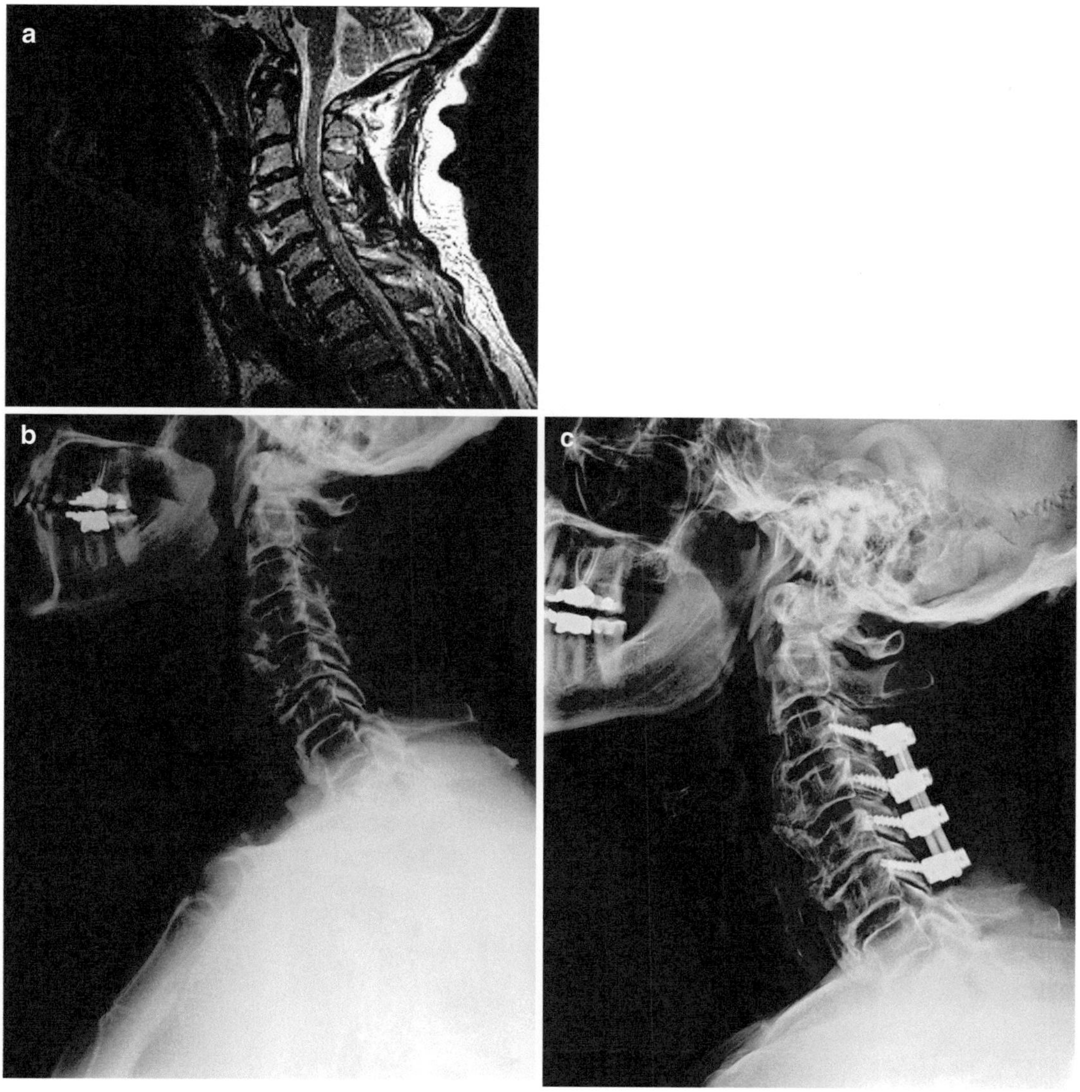

Fig. 22.5 Diffuse idiopathic skeletal hyperostosis. (**a**) Sagittal T2-weighted magnetic resonance image demonstrating multiple levels of stenosis throughout the cervical spine in a patient with overt myelopathy on clinical examination. (**b**) Preoperative lateral radiograph demonstrating bridging osteophytes throughout the entire cervical spine. Although a multiple-level anterior cervical discectomy and fusion might be feasible in this patient, it may not be the preferred approach. (**c**) Postoperative lateral radiograph demonstrating a C3–C6 laminectomy with lateral mass fixation, a procedure that allows for multiple levels of decompression efficiently, thereby avoiding the multiple levels of bridging osteophytes that would be encountered anteriorly. (Used with permission from Barrow Neurological Institute, Phoenix, Arizona)

Patients with OPLL typically have multiple levels involved, so a focal single-level approach is usually not feasible. Determining the extent of the ossification across the various segments is therefore essential. In these circumstances, both MRI and computed tomography (CT) are valuable—MRI determines the extent of compression of the neural elements, whereas CT determines the extent of calcification. In the absence of kyphosis, a posterior approach may be preferable to an anterior approach, thereby avoiding the elevated risk of a durotomy [13]. However, the presence of kyphosis or prominent calcification occupying 60% of the canal may further prompt an anterior approach rather than a posterior approach [14, 15].

Preoperative Planning, Materials, Setup, and Anesthetic Considerations

The operating room is set up to optimize the flow of the surgery. If a microscope is to be used, it is positioned on the side of the incision and draped before the operation starts. The fluoroscope is positioned on the opposite side of the microscope. An alternative to using a fluoroscope is a cross table lateral x-ray, which would require puncture of the presumptive disc with a spinal needle. I prefer to avoid any disruption of the cervical anatomy, including the disc space, until confirming the segment to be operated on. Current evidence suggests that puncturing an annulus that is not the surgical target may begin a degenerative cascade [16].

A Caspar head holder is secured to the head of the bed, which facilitates securing the head of the patient and optimizing cervical lordosis (Fig. 22.6). An alternative to the Caspar head holder is to position the patient on a donut gel pillow with a 1-L bag of intravenous fluid behind the shoulders. The downside to this approach is that it impedes stabilization of the head.

The decision to use electrophysiological monitoring in the non-myelopathic patient depends on the preference of the surgeon. In a review of 1039 consecutive non-myelopathic patients who underwent ACDF with electrophysiological monitoring, Smith et al. [17] observed that an intraoperative neurological deficit is possible despite normal somatosensory evoked potentials. My preference is to reserve electrophysiological monitoring for patients with myelopathy where distracting the disc space with Caspar pins can change the somatosensory evoked potentials or at C7–T1 where significant traction on the shoulders is anticipated to adequately view the segment. The brachial plexus may be stretched in these cases, and electrophysiological monitoring can quickly identify neuropraxia, prompting release of the traction on the shoulder. Before final positioning, baseline somatosensory evoked potentials should be obtained, and the electrophysiology technician and the anesthesiologist should have a clear line of communication to

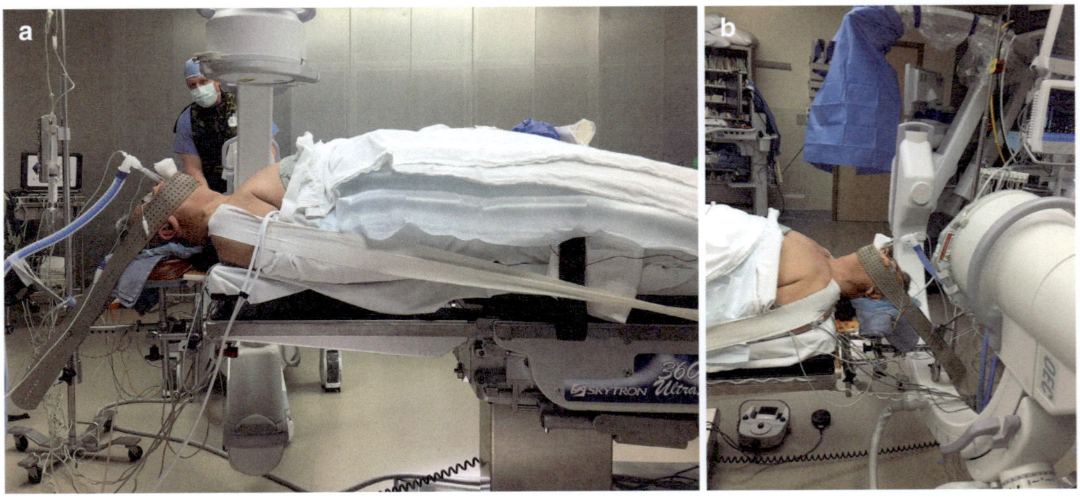

Fig. 22.6 Operating room setup. (**a**) Intraoperative photograph of a patient positioned for an anterior cervical discectomy and fusion. The head is stabilized in a Caspar head holder, which immobilizes the neck and maintains cervical lordosis. The shoulders are taped down to facilitate visualization of the caudal cervical segments. (**b**) Intraoperative photograph of the operating room setup with the microscope draped and ready on the side of the approach, the fluoroscope in position, and the image intensifier on the opposite side of the fluoroscope. (Used with permission from Barrow Neurological Institute, Phoenix, Arizona)

optimize the anesthetic parameters and ensure that there is no interference with monitoring.

In the patient with severe myelopathy, having the patient fully extend the neck for a period in the preoperative area offers a sense of whether a fiber-optic or GlideScope (Verathon, Inc.) intubation might be necessary. The presence of Lhermitte sign with either flexion or extension should prompt precautions to minimize either flexion or extension during intubation. Although hypotension should be avoided in all patients with induction of anesthesia, such precaution is especially necessary in patients with myelopathy, because an elevated pressure may be required to adequately perfuse the spinal cord [18]. An arterial line can be helpful for these myelopathic patients. Clear communications between the surgeon and the anesthesiologist regarding concerns about hypotension during induction allow for adequate preparation in the event that vasopressors are required for a period after induction. Transient hypotension is of less concern in otherwise healthy patients with cervical radiculopathy but no myelopathy, which makes an arterial line less helpful.

Positioning and Incision Planning

My preference is to plan an incision opposite the side with the patient's symptoms. For example, in a patient with a left C6 radiculopathy, the incision is planned on the right side of the cervical spine. Although the entire cervical segment may be exposed, the contralateral recess is in the direct line of sight, while the ipsilateral recess tends not to be. Other surgeons tend to favor either one side or the other. However, an adequate decompression may always be accomplished regardless of the side of the incision. Laterality of the incision is less important and should be left entirely to the preference of the surgeon.

Numerous reports have been published detailing the risk of recurrent laryngeal nerve palsy and the laterality of the incision; a left-sided approach may particularly be associated with a lower incidence [19]. The greatest risk in my experience has been with ACDFs at C7–T1 and previous recurrent laryngeal palsy after an ACDF. Evidence suggests that lowering the endotracheal cuff pressure may decrease the incidence of recurrent laryngeal nerve palsy [19, 20].

Whether a head holder or a donut gel pillow is used, the patient should be positioned to optimize the capacity to either preserve cervical lordosis or restore it. Although landmarks (i.e., carotid tubercle or thyroid cartilage) can be used to plan the incision, a preoperative fluoroscopic image taken after positioning the patient can precisely guide the incision and thereby minimize the extent of exposure and dissection. The added value of a preoperative fluoroscopic image is confirmation of the ideal positioning of the patient without rotation. The fluoroscopic image should demonstrate crisp end plates and clearly visible joint space, with the facets perfectly aligned at the operative segment.

For a single-level operation, the incision is planned immediately over the disc space. For a two-level operation, the incision is planned over the top of the intervening body (e.g., a C5–6, C6–7 ACDF will have the incision planned over the C6 vertebral body) (Fig. 22.7). For a three-level operation, the incision is centered over the middle disc space (e.g., a C4–5, C5–6, and C6–7 ACDF will have an incision centered over the C5–6 segment). Finally, for a four-level ACDF, a single transverse incision has potential challenges, and traditionally a carotid endarterectomy type of incision has been used, which is a viable option. However, it has become my preference to make two incisions, as described by Chin et al. [21], as if performing two distinct ACDFs. For example, a four-level C3–4, C4–5, C5–6, and C6–7 ACDF will have incisions centered over the top of the C4 vertebral body and over the C6 vertebral body (Fig. 22.8). If a natural neck crease is in the vicinity of the planned incision, the incision may be adjusted upward or downward to optimize the aesthetics.

The sternal notch of the patient is marked with a prominent "V" to become a visual reference for the midline, and the final incision is marked (Fig. 22.9). An electrocardiogram (ECG) lead may be placed on the nose of the patient to provide a palpable reference point for the midline.

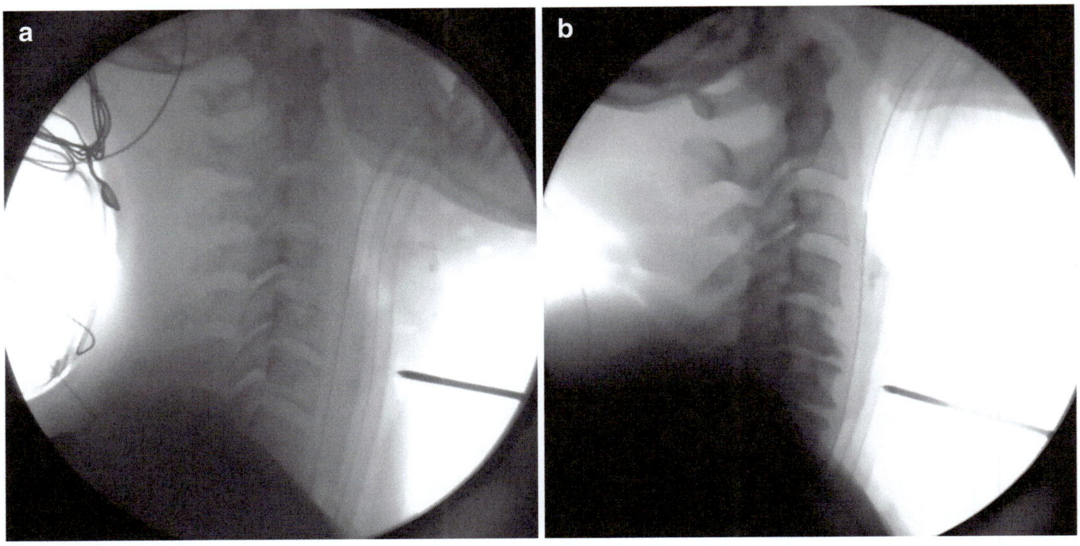

Fig. 22.7 Planning the incision. (**a**) A lateral fluoroscopic image with a Kirschner wire (with a protected tip) for planning an incision for a C5–6 anterior cervical discectomy and fusion (ACDF). The Kirschner wire points directly to the disc space. (**b**) Lateral fluoroscopic image for planning a two-level ACDF at C5–6 and C6–7. The incision will be centered over the top of the C6 vertebral body. (Used with permission from Barrow Neurological Institute, Phoenix, Arizona)

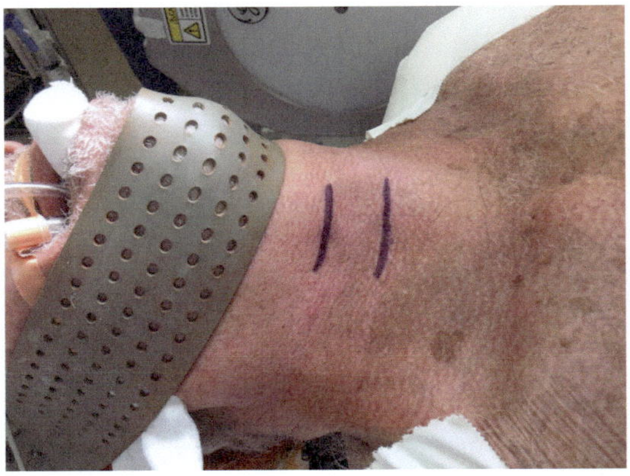

Fig. 22.8 Planning a four-level anterior cervical discectomy and fusion (ACDF). Intraoperative photograph of a planned skin incision for a four-level ACDF from C3–4 to C6–7. The rostral incision is planned over the C4 vertebral body, and the caudal incision is planned over the C6 vertebral body. Doing so overcomes the challenges of a single transverse incision for so many levels while avoiding the carotid endarterectomy type of incision, which is not as aesthetic as a transverse incision. (Used with permission from Barrow Neurological Institute, Phoenix, Arizona)

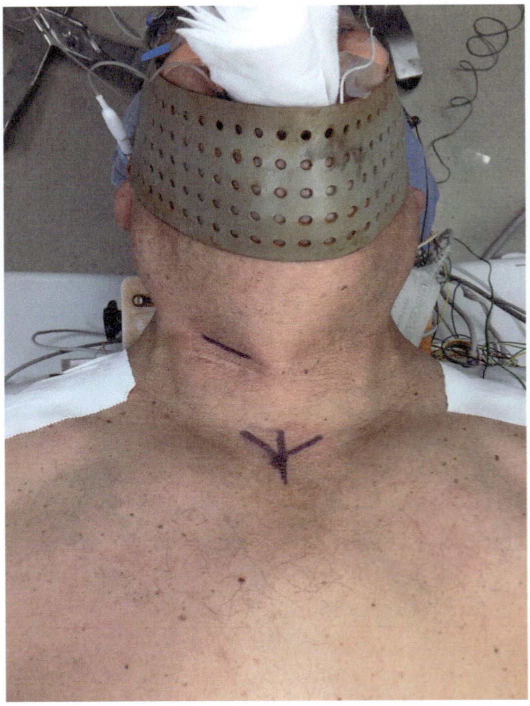

Fig. 22.9 Planning the incision. Intraoperative photograph of a patient positioned in a Caspar head holder with the sternal notch marked and the incision planned over the top of the cervical segment. (Used with permission from Barrow Neurological Institute, Phoenix, Arizona)

Because the midline is where the relevant surgical anatomy lies and also where the interbody and the anterior cervical plate should be positioned, the transverse incision will extend right up to the midline. The sternal notch is draped into the surgical field to provide added visualization of a midline reference point. The sternal notch along with the palpable ECG lead serves as the reference points for the eventual placement of an orthogonal midline cervical plate.

Surgical Technique

After the incision is made, the platysma is elevated with DeBakey forceps and sharply divided either with cautery or Metzenbaum scissors. An avascular plane is identified along the medial border of the sternocleidomastoid muscle, which guides a path onto the precervical fascia. A handheld Cloward retractor and Metzenbaum scissors that do nothing more than spread can be used to reliably cleave an avascular plane of dissection on the precervical fascia. At times, when the platysma is divided, large veins will be encountered, and every effort should be made to preserve them. Minimal dissection is typically necessary to adequately mobilize these veins before continuing along the avascular plane onto the precervical fascia of the spine. Blunt dissection with a Kittner dissector then exposes the precervical fascia. At times, engorged veins on the surface of the precervical fascia will be encountered. These veins should be cauterized before their inadvertent interruption obscures the operative field.

Confirmation of the level is accomplished by holding a Kittner dissector over the top of the presumptive level and obtaining a low-dose fluoroscopic image (Fig. 22.10). Using the Kittner dissector instead of a spinal needle avoids the risk of puncturing the annulus of the wrong level. Disrupting the annulus of a cervical disc in such a manner may begin a degenerative cascade for that particular cervical disc [16]. At this point in the operation, only blunt dissection has been used to expose the level to be operated on. For a single-level operation, only after the level is confirmed should cautery be used to expose only the inferior one-third of the vertebral body above the disc space and the superior one-third of the vertebral body below the disc space. For multiple-level operations, the entire intervening vertebral body is exposed in addition to the inferior and superior one-third of the levels above and below (e.g., for a C5–6 and C6–7 ACDF, the entire C6 vertebral body is exposed, along with the inferior one-third of C5 and the superior one-third of C7). The goal is to minimize dissection of the uninvolved segments to reduce the risk of adjacent segment degeneration. However, the entire exposure that will be needed for the operation, including cervical plating (if applicable), should be accomplished at the outset before the placement of any self-retaining retractors.

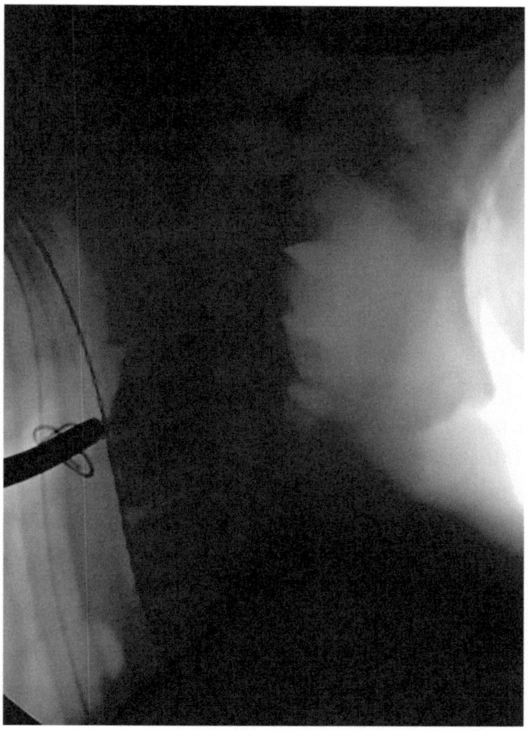

Fig. 22.10 Localization. Lateral fluoroscopic image demonstrating a Kittner dissector placed to confirm the operative segment of C4–5 in lieu of a spinal needle, which could inadvertently puncture the annulus of an uninvolved segment. (Used with permission from Barrow Neurological Institute, Phoenix, Arizona)

Fascial bands along the dissection plane of the sternocleidomastoid muscle have the capacity to limit exposure and may cause difficulty with exposing a segment or placing the cervical plate. These fascial bands should be identified and released. Individually, these fascial bands offer little resistance and are readily dealt with by nothing more than the spreading of the blades of the Metzenbaum scissors. However, altogether, the fascial bands can coalesce and restrict passage of a cervical plate or the rostral or caudal exposure in a multiple-level operation.

The longus colli muscles on either side of the segment are the next target for dissection. Cautery may be used to elevate the longus colli from over the top of the vertebral body and the disc space. Mobilizing the longus colli in this manner creates a cuff of muscle that will be able to engage the blade of the self-retaining retractor and to add stability to the retractor. Before the placement of retractors, all levels that will be operated on are exposed in a similar fashion. Ensuring approximately 22 mm of exposure for each segment (slightly more for larger patients and less for smaller) will enable the placement of the self-retaining retractors, optimize visualization for the decompression, and facilitate placement of the anterior cervical plate. Achieving the exposure at this phase in the operation is easier than struggling to expand an inadequate exposure later.

Upon completion of the entire exposure, self-retaining retractors are secured over the operative segment. Caspar posts are secured into the vertebral bodies above and below the disc to be operated on (Fig. 22.11). The goal is to place the Caspar posts perpendicular to the posterior wall of the vertebral body so that distraction will reverse any kyphosis of the segment. These steps optimize the capacity to restore and maintain cervical lordosis with discectomy and placement of an interbody.

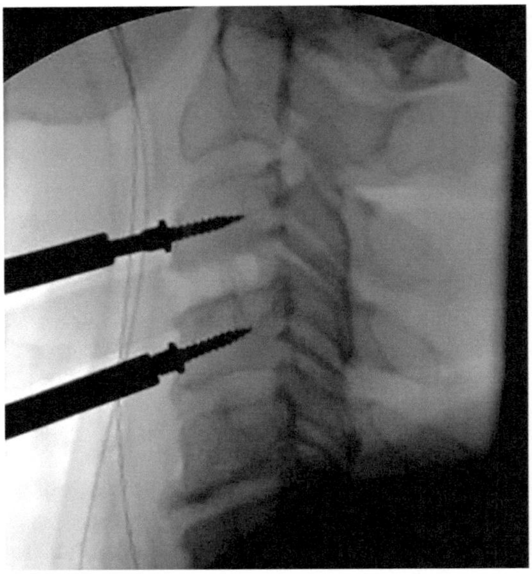

Fig. 22.11 Placement of the Caspar posts. Lateral fluoroscopic image demonstrating placement of the Caspar posts perpendicular to the posterior wall of the vertebral body. Placing the posts in this manner allows for correction of kyphosis and restoration of lordosis of the segment. (Used with permission from Barrow Neurological Institute, Phoenix, Arizona)

Discectomy, End Plate Preparation, and Osteophyte Removal

There are three goals for this phase of the operation: (1) to prepare the end plates for arthrodesis, (2) to decompress the neural elements, and (3) to restore segmental lordosis and disc height. The first step is to distract the disc space with the Caspar post distractor and to incise the disc space with a no. 11 blade. The disc material is removed with pituitary forceps, and the cartilaginous end plate is removed with straight curettes. If a scalloped end plate is present within the rostral vertebral body, the anterior and posterior aspects of the scallop are flattened with a drill. Removal of the scallop allows for clear visualization of the posterior aspect of the disc space. Visualization of the rise of each uncovertebral joint is critical for confirming the midline and ensuring adequate decompression of the spinal cord and nerve roots.

In patients with advanced spondylosis, disc space may be nearly absent, making distraction difficult. In these circumstances, the inferior and superior aspects of the disc space should be drilled to reach the canal. Despite advanced spondylosis, the uncovertebral joints tend to be well preserved and remain a reliable guide for the extent of decompression. Patients with advanced disc collapse and spondylosis will have lost lordosis at that particular segment. Drilling in a parallel manner on the inferior and superior aspects of the end plates with the disc space distracted will reliably restore the segmental lordosis, especially when a lordotic implant is secured into the disc space after decompression.

In patients with a posterior osteophyte, drilling the posterior end plate of the inferior aspect of the caudal segment and the posterior aspect of the superior aspect of the rostral end plate will reliably remove any osteophyte protruding into the canal and foramen. This drilling pattern creates a trumpet appearance to the posterior aspect of the disc space and ensures wide decompression (see Case 1).

Division and Resection of the Posterior Longitudinal Ligament

Upon completion of the bone work, the posterior longitudinal ligament (PLL) is identified and divided (Fig. 22.12). This ligament tends to be thickest in the middle but thinner in the lateral aspects of the canal. Typically, a nerve hook or microcurette can be used to cleave a plane beneath the PLL and provide a glimpse of the dura of the cervical spinal cord. A no. 1 or no. 2 Kerrison Rongeur can then be used to widely resect the PLL, incorporating the underside of the posterior vertebral body above and below. Resection extends out to where the uncovertebral joint was drilled bilaterally. A forward-angled microcurette can be used to readily palpate the pedicle of the caudal segment to confirm adequate decompression of the nerve root. Vigorous venous bleeding can indicate that the limit of the decompression has been reached. Such venous bleeding is readily controlled with thrombin-soaked or particle Gelfoam (FloSeal, Baxter Healthcare Corp.) and a half-by-half-inch cottonoid patty. A full 20–22 mm of decompression ensures adequate decompression of the spinal cord and nerve roots, because the vertebral arteries reside 25 mm apart [22].

Placement of Interbody Graft

The options for the interbody grafts that may be used for anterior cervical fusions are numerous. Harvested structural autograft, at one point the gold standard, has largely fallen out of favor because of the risk of infection from the second incision and perhaps most importantly because of the postoperative discomfort related to harvesting the graft. Donor-site discomfort may last years and is the main source of postoperative discomfort for patients. The donor-site pain, along with

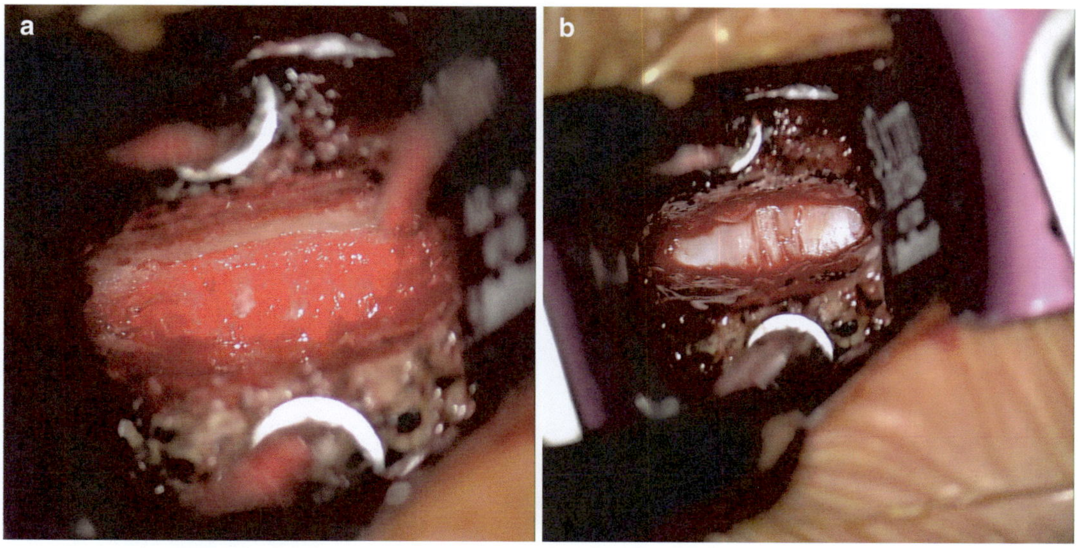

Fig. 22.12 Division of the posterior longitudinal ligament (PLL). (**a**) Intraoperative photograph demonstrating a C5–6 anterior cervical discectomy and fusion. The cortical end plates are prepared, and the posterior annulus and PLL are exposed. (**b**) The PLL is resected with the posterior osteophytes from the uncovertebral joint for wide decompression of the spinal cord and nerve roots. (Used with permission from Barrow Neurological Institute, Phoenix, Arizona)

the wide availability of allograft and biomechanical options, has in large part led to the use of structural autografts in many centers [23]. As a result, the use of structural allograft, cortical cancellous combinations, and metallic and polymer (i.e., polyether ether ketone [PEEK]) interbodies has become commonplace, with demonstrated clinical success. A shift from PEEK implants has begun to occur because of the unfavorable reactions that occur at the interface of the polymer and osteoblasts. Compared to titanium, PEEK has been shown to be less osteoconductive and bioactive [24]. In contrast, an irregular metallic surface seems to create an environment favorable for osseointegration of the implant [25]. As a result, interest has increased in metallic-coated PEEK implants and completely metallic implants.

Regardless of the type of interbody used, the goals remain the same—maintain the disc height achieved by the distraction, the bone work, and the decompression and restore lordosis while reliably achieving arthrodesis. Complete removal of the cartilaginous end plate is the essential first step, followed by adequate preparation of the cortical end plate and securing a tightly fitting interbody graft into the anterior aspect of the disc space. Abiding by those key principles is essential to achieving the aforementioned goals. Packing the interbody graft with local bone collected from drilling or with a demineralized bone matrix further adds to the capacity to achieve arthrodesis, but doing so will not overcome the challenges of an inadequately prepared end plate or an end plate still covered with cartilage.

The dimensions of the interbody can be determined first by reviewing the lateral fluoroscopic image and determining the distance from the tip of the Caspar post to the posterior aspect of the vertebral body. Knowledge that the post is either 12 mm or 14 mm provides insight as to how deep to place the interbody. A trial with the corresponding depth can be selected and tested to determine the appropriate height. A mallet is required to secure the ideal height for the interspace, and testing should be done with the Caspar post distractor released. A tight fit can be appreciated by toggling the handle of the trial with gentle upward traction. Any movement, especially if the trial can be withdrawn from the interspace

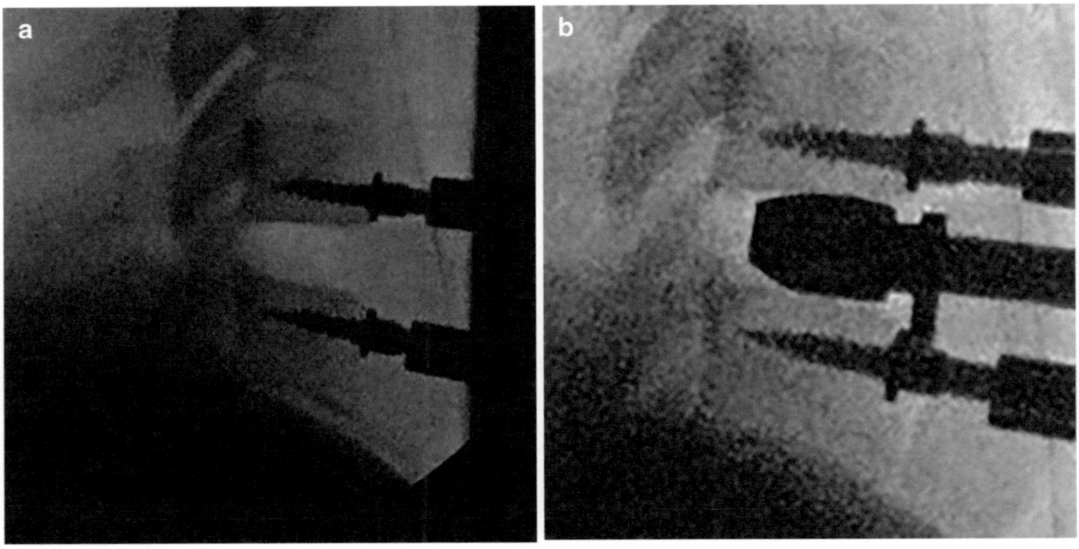

Fig. 22.13 Dimensions of the interbody spacer. (**a**) Lateral fluoroscopic image demonstrating 12-mm Caspar posts in position after completion of the decompression. Estimating the depth at 14 mm based on the lateral fluoroscopic image requires an interbody trial 14 mm wide and 11 mm deep, so that it can be recessed without encroaching upon the canal. (**b**) Lateral fluoroscopic image demonstrating the positioning of an interbody trial 7 mm tall by 14 mm wide by 11 mm deep. (Used with permission from Barrow Neurological Institute, Phoenix, Arizona)

without much force, should prompt a trial of the taller interbody. That sequence is repeated until the appropriate height for an interbody is identified (Fig. 22.13).

Anterior Instrumentation

The introduction of anterior cervical plating to stabilize a cervical segment decreases the incidence of pseudarthrosis and kyphosis [8, 10]. Methods to stabilize the segment have continued to evolve throughout the years, and research has led not only to lower-profile anterior cervical plates but also to anterior instrumentation through the interbody device itself [26]. These standalone instrumented interbodies have become popular, especially for an adjacent segment above or below a long construct, thereby preventing the need to remove the anterior cervical plate. Regardless of the type of fixation chosen, the segment must be adequately immobilized to create an ideal environment for arthrodesis.

When anterior cervical plates are used, the plate should be positioned midline orthogonally, with a minimum of 5 mm between the plate and the disc space above and below to mitigate the risk of adjacent segment degeneration [27, 28]. Therefore, the shortest plate that adequately covers the segment or segments should be used (Fig. 22.14).

A well-positioned interbody spacer typically has no coronal imbalance and resides in the geometric midline of the disc space. The key to securing the plate in the geometric midline is to use that interbody as an index for the midline. Most cervical plating systems have a window in the center of the cervical plate that allows the surgeon to see the interbody spacer. When a symmetrical view of the interbody spacer is maintained in the center of the window, the position of the plate should be midline orthogonal.

Regarding fixation of the plate, the geometry of the cervical screws and the way they will interface with the cervical plate should be considered, because the interface will affect the manner in which the forces act upon the interbody space. In particular, the concern for stress shielding the graft because of a fixed geometry of the screws into the cervical plate will prevent the optimiza-

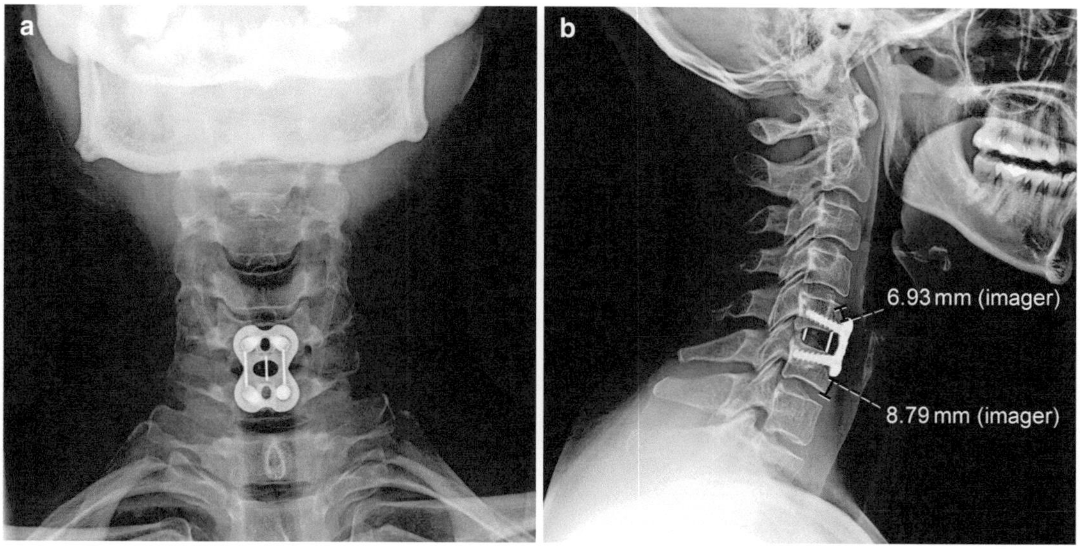

Fig. 22.14 Orthogonal midline cervical plate. (**a**) Anteroposterior radiograph of a C6–7 anterior cervical discectomy and fusion (ACDF) with the plate indexed off the interbody spacer. As a result, the plate was secured in the midline in an orthogonal position. (**b**) Lateral radiograph of a C5–6 ACDF where the plate-to-disc distance is greater than 5 mm from the segment above and below. (Used with permission from Barrow Neurological Institute, Phoenix, Arizona)

tion of Wolff's law. Over time, our growing understanding of the forces that act on the interbody led to modifications in how the screw interfaces with the plate. Cervical screws designed with a round geometry can still allow for variable angles when interfaced with the cervical plate, which prevents stress shielding of the interbody graft and creates an ideal environment for arthrodesis to occur. These variable-angled screws can be used in the entire construct, at the level of the most caudal segment or at the levels above the most caudal segment [29]. Commonly, a screw with a fixed head will have minimal settling after it interfaces with the plate, so it is typically placed at the caudal segment of the construct. Stand-alone constructs have fixed-angle screws that interface into the fixation housing that holds the interbody spacer. The same concern for stress shielding has led to an interbody spacer design with simultaneous stabilization within the segment and uncoupling of the forces of fixation of the housing unit from the spacer itself.

Closure

After completion of the anterior instrumentation, final AP and lateral fluoroscopic images are obtained, the retractors are removed, hemostasis is obtained, and the incision is closed. The decision to place a drain is made based on the number of levels and the degree of hemostasis achieved. My preference is to use a drain in three- or four-level ACDFs and revision ACDFs that involved explantation of a cervical plate. The platysma is reapproximated with interrupted Vicryl sutures (Ethicon US, Somerville, NJ), as is the subcutaneous layer, and the skin edges are joined by subcuticular sutures.

Postoperative Care and Concerns

All patients should be advised that some degree of dysphagia will occur after the operation. Typically, the extent of dysphagia is proportional to the number of levels. Postoperative dysphagia is self-limited and will gradually regress over the course of several weeks to months [30–33]. Patients should also be advised that some degree of posterior discomfort is to be expected after the operation and that it is related to the restoration of height of the disc space and correction of kyphosis. Similar to postoperative dysphagia, that degree of discomfort will be proportional to the number of levels addressed during surgery.

Difficulty with phonation after the operation may represent recurrent laryngeal nerve palsy. It is important to identify this complication and to educate the patient about the transiency of most of these palsies. Patients may also report having a normal voice but complain about the inability to project well. If no improvement occurs after a period of observation, then a referral to an ENT surgeon for evaluation may be appropriate.

Patients undergoing a C4–5 ACDF should be advised of the risk for C5 nerve root palsy, and immediate assessment should be made of deltoid function [33, 34]. These postoperative complications also tend to be self-limited and improve over time. In the event of C5 nerve root palsy, immediate imaging should be obtained to identify any need for additional decompression from a posterior approach.

The most concerning postoperative event is the potential for an expanding hematoma that can compromise the airway. Such complications are typically self-evident within the first hour after an operation. Observation in the postanesthesia care unit by nurses experienced in the management of cervical spine surgery is critical for all patients, whether they have same-day surgery or overnight observation.

Complication Management and Avoidance

Each phase of the operation—exposure, decompression, instrumentation, and closure—has the potential for its own unique set of complications. Thus, reducing the likelihood of such complications requires special focus at each phase.

Complication Avoidance with Exposure

During the exposure phase, recurrent laryngeal nerve palsy is perhaps the most common complication. Identifying the avascular plane medial to the sternocleidomastoid muscle and using Metzenbaum scissors to spread instead of cut will result in nearly bloodless dissection of the precervical fascia. The use of blunt dissection with a Kittner dissector is essential. No effort should be made to identify the recurrent laryngeal nerve, but if it is identified during dissection, ensuring that it is not tethered and can be safely mobilized without undue traction is advisable to mitigate the risk of injury.

Esophageal injury is also a risk of an anterior cervical exposure. However, most esophageal injuries occur as a result of hardware failure and present in a delayed fashion. A review of the neurosurgical literature indicates that few esophageal injuries occur at the time of exposure.

Complication Avoidance with Decompression

During the decompression phase, the main complications include vertebral artery injury, inadequate decompression and persistent radicular symptoms, and cerebrospinal fluid leak. The risk of vertebral artery injury can be mitigated with certain knowledge of the midline. Complete exposure of the uncovertebral joints on the left and right is essential to orient to the midline. Before beginning the operation, the surgeon should scroll through the axial MRIs to ensure that there is no tortuosity of the vertebral artery at the segment of surgery, which can increase the risk of a vertebral artery injury [22].

Decompression of the nerve root exiting the foramen may result in venous bleeding after bone removal. As vigorous as that bleeding may seem initially, the use of particle Gelfoam and a half-by-half-inch cottonoid patty will typically achieve hemostasis. This maneuver is always the first to use when encountering bleeding in the vicinity of the uncovertebral joint. If hemostasis is not achieved with Gelfoam, then an assessment for possible vertebral artery injury should be made. The midline should be reassessed and a determination should be made of whether a vertebral artery injury has occurred by being too far lateral.

In the unlikely event of a vertebral artery injury, proximal and distal control of the vertebral artery can be obtained by holding down a cottonoid patty with suction and then widening the exposure over the top of the foramen transversarium. Doing so will involve opening up the self-retaining retractor and exposing the lateral aspect of the vertebral body. Descending along the lateral aspect of the vertebral body leads directly to the foramen transversarium. Once the foramen transversarium has been adequately exposed, the use of temporary aneurysm clips above and below the vessel injury will allow determination of whether a primary repair is feasible. If the injury is to the left vertebral artery, careful consideration of primary repair is advisable because of the statistical probability of left vertebral artery dominance for the posterior circulation. If primary repair is untenable, the following actions should be taken: permanent clip ligation with aneurysm clips to stop the bleeding, completion of the operation, and immediate assessment of the posterior circulation with conventional angiography, CT angiography, or magnetic resonance angiography, including assessment of perfusion of the vertebrobasilar system. Fortunately, the incidence of vertebral artery injuries is low, and they are preventable with certain knowledge of the midline.

In the absence of an anatomical irregularity of the vertebral artery, 20 mm of decompression of the entire segment can be safely achieved after the midline has been firmly established. Ensuring such a wide exposure prevents the next potential complication, which is inadequate decompression that results in persistent radicular symptoms. As mentioned above, the nerve root may be completely decompressed by drilling out the uncovertebral joints and resecting any osteophyte within the foramen. The pedicle can be palpated with a microcurette or nerve hook to check for adequate decompression.

Finally, the risk of cerebrospinal fluid leak is heightened in the management of patients with OPLL. The key to avoiding this complication in these patients is to recognize the presence of OPLL at the outset and to determine whether a posterior approach can be used to accomplish all the goals of an anterior surgery. If not, and a dural defect occurs during the decompression, direct repair is typically untenable in an anterior approach. Instead, the cerebrospinal fluid leak can be adequately addressed by using a combination of a dural matrix and sealant (Tisseel, Baxter Healthcare Corp.) over the top of the defect, followed by placement of the interbody graft. The use of a lumbar drain to divert the cerebrospinal fluid away from the repair will optimize the environment for sealing the defect.

Complication Avoidance with Instrumentation

Complications from instrumentation tend to present in delayed fashion and result from a pseudarthrosis. Failure to achieve arthrodesis will ultimately lead to instrumentation failure (Fig. 22.15). Complete removal of the cartilaginous end plate and cortical bone bleeding are essential for arthrodesis. A well-sized, tight-fitting graft, regardless of the type of interbody, is also essential. Educating patients about the increased risk for pseudarthrosis with active tobacco use and encouraging smoking cessation are valuable components of preoperative counseling.

The management of pseudarthrosis may be performed with an anterior or a posterior revision. An anterior revision is advisable for a screw or plate backing out, which may contribute to swallowing issues and lead to esophageal irritation or injury [35]. In the absence of any migrating or symptomatic hardware, I prefer to manage pseudarthrosis, even with hardware failure, with posterior lateral mass fixation, which reliably achieves arthrodesis.

Case Presentations

Case Illustration 1: Cervical Spondylosis with Radiculopathy

Clinical History

A 46-year-old right-handed man presented with a 6-month history of increasing left radic-

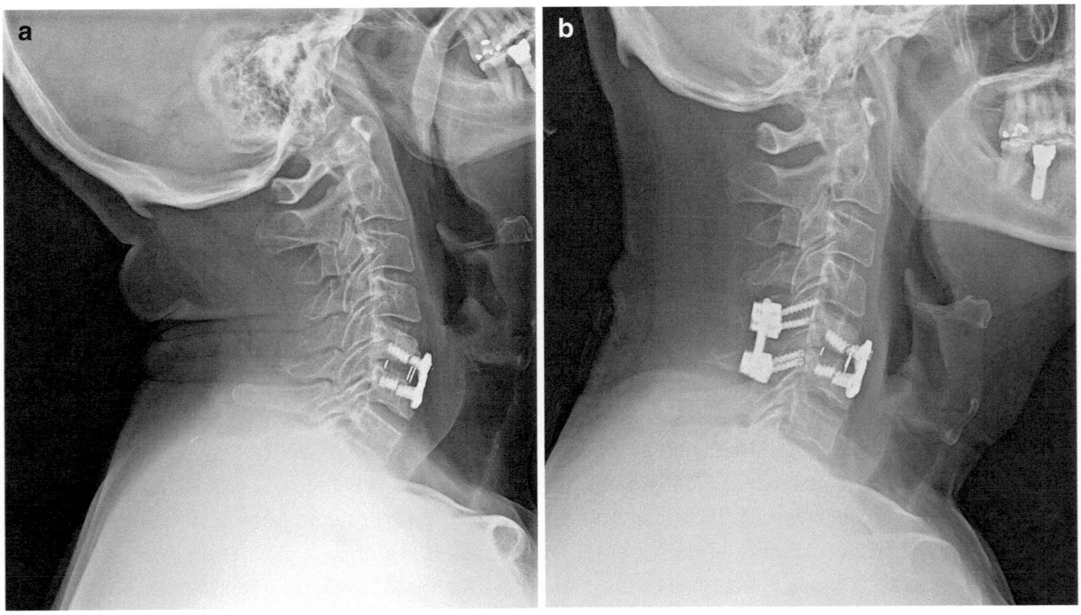

Fig. 22.15 Pseudarthrosis and instrumentation failure. (**a**) Lateral radiograph demonstrating a pseudarthrosis and fractured cervical screws that were identified in a patient 5 years after the initial surgery. The patient, an active smoker, returned with increasing neck pain but no radicular symptoms. (**b**) Lateral postoperative radiograph after lateral mass fixation for management of pseudarthrosis. (Used with permission from Barrow Neurological Institute, Phoenix, Arizona)

ular arm pain. The patient had undergone two cervical epidural injections, along with a regimen of physical therapy and cervical traction. Progressive weakness in the left arm interfered with his capacity to work, prompting a surgical evaluation.

Neurological Examination and Radiographic Studies

The neurological examination was notable for decreased sensation in the thumb, index finger, and middle finger. Motor examination by confrontation demonstrated 4/5 in the biceps and triceps on the left and 5/5 on the right. Reflexes were 1/4 bilaterally in the biceps, brachialis, and triceps and 2/4 bilaterally in the patellar and Achilles. A positive Spurling sign was elicited when the patient's head was tilted left. Plain radiographs demonstrated spondylosis at C5–6 and C6–7, with anterior osteophytes and loss of disc heights but no abnormal motion on flexion extension. MRIs demonstrated disc osteophyte complexes at C5–6 and C6–7, with flattening of the spinal cord at C5–6 and severe narrowing of the left C6 neural foramen and left C7 (Fig. 22.16).

Intervention

The patient was taken to the operating suite for a C5–6 and C6–7 ACDF. With the patient positioned supine, the head was stabilized in a Caspar head holder, and the shoulders were taped down to facilitate visualization of the C7 vertebral body. A transverse incision was made on the right side of the neck over the top of the C6 vertebral body. The platysma was sharply divided, and an avascular plane was identified medial to the sternocleidomastoid muscle. The esophagus and trachea were swept medially, and the carotid and the jugular venous complex were swept laterally. The entire exposure was completed from C5 to C7. After self-retaining retractors and Caspar posts were placed at C5–6, a complete discectomy was performed (Fig. 22.17).

The advanced collapse of the disc space, which did not correct with distraction of the Caspar posts, prompted drilling of the underside of C5 and the superior aspect of C6. The posterior aspects of the disc space at C5 and C6 were drilled obliquely to remove the posterior osteophytes in the canal and foramen. The PLL was identified, divided, and resected, and a titanium-coated PEEK implant containing demineralized bone matrix was positioned. The identical procedure was then performed at the C6–7 level. A cervical plate was affixed to the spine, with fixed screws placed into C7 and variable-angle screws placed at C5 and C6.

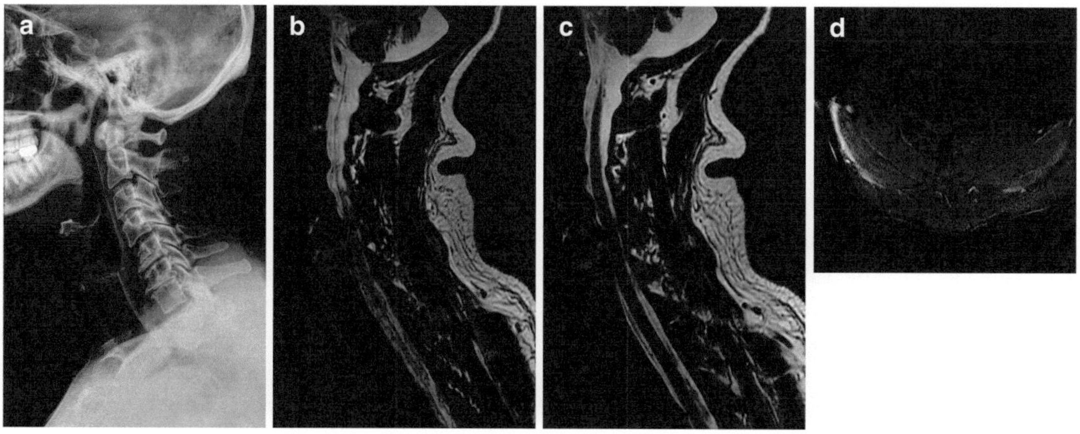

Fig. 22.16 Cervical spondylosis with radiculopathy. (**a**) Lateral radiograph demonstrating spondylosis at C5–6 and C6–7 with formation of an anterior osteophyte. (**b**, **c**) Sagittal T2-weighted magnetic resonance images (MRIs) demonstrating the disc osteophyte complex causing central stenosis, more so at C5–6 than at C6–7. (**d**) Axial T2-weighted MRI demonstrating central stenosis at C5–6, with flattening of the spinal cord and severe narrowing of the left C6 neural foramen. (Used with permission from Barrow Neurological Institute, Phoenix, Arizona)

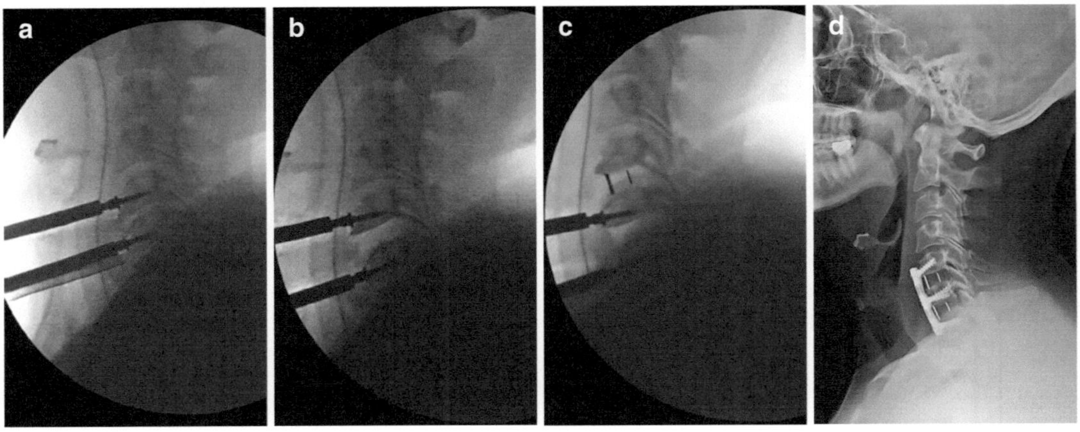

Fig. 22.17 C5–6 and C6–7 anterior cervical discectomy and fusion. (**a**) Lateral fluoroscopic image of Caspar posts in position at C5–6. Little restoration of height was accomplished with distraction of the posts. (**b**) After the discectomy, a drill was used to remove the underside of C5. Note the oblique cut removing the posterior osteophyte from the underside of C5 and C6. (**c**) Complete discectomy with decompression of C6–7. (**d**) Postoperative lateral radiograph demonstrating restoration of the disc height, removal of the anterior and posterior osteophytes, and the widely decompressed spinal canal. (Used with permission from Barrow Neurological Institute, Phoenix, Arizona)

Postoperative Course

The patient was discharged on the same day of surgery with resolution of his left radicular arm pain. He had mild dysphagia and minimal posterior cervical discomfort, both of which resolved by the second postoperative week. Thirty days after surgery, the patient was able to return to work as a maintenance engineer, with a 25-pound weight-carrying limit. By the third postoperative month, he had no restrictions or limitations.

Case Illustration 2: Adjacent Segment Degeneration with Myelopathy

Clinical History

A 67-year-old right-handed man with a surgical history significant for an uninstrumented C5–6 and C6–7 ACDF performed 22 years earlier presented with progressive gait imbalance and decreased manual dexterity. The patient could no longer dress himself with any clothing that required buttoning. He recently began using a cane to assist with ambulation because of his unsteady gait.

Neurological Examination and Radiographic Studies

On examination, the patient was incapable of a tandem walk. His Romberg test results were positive. Brisk patellar reflexes and three beats of clonus were present bilaterally. A positive Hoffman sign was present on the left but not on the right. Strength was remarkably preserved in the proximal muscle groups of the upper extremity (5/5 in the deltoid, biceps, and triceps). However, the patient had decreased strength in the intrinsic muscles of the hand, and he demonstrated difficulty holding a pen and performing tasks of fine motor dexterity.

Sagittal T2-weighted MRIs demonstrated severe cervical stenosis at C3–4 and moderate stenosis at C4–5 above the level of the uninstrumented fusion at C5–6 and C6–7 (Fig. 22.18). Lateral radiographs demonstrated robust fusion at C5–6 and C6–7.

Intervention

Preoperatively, the patient had undergone indirect laryngoscopy by an ENT surgeon who identified an incomplete recurrent laryngeal nerve palsy related to his initial surgery. The patient subsequently had a chronic cough but reported having normal swallowing function and was otherwise asymptomatic. An approach for a two-level ACDF through the same side as his previous surgery was performed at C3–4 and C4–5 with plate fixation. Because of the degree of stenosis at C3–4, a considerable amount of the inferior

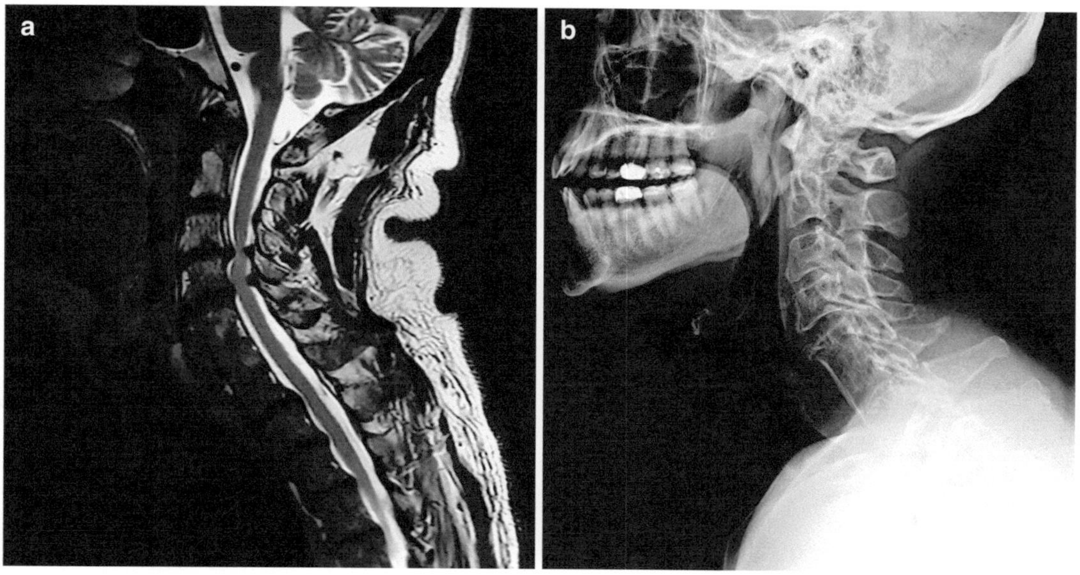

Fig. 22.18 Adjacent segment degeneration. (**a**) Sagittal T2-weighted magnetic resonance image demonstrating severe stenosis at C3–4 and moderate stenosis at C4–5. Myelomalacia was evident at C3–4. (**b**) Lateral radiograph of previous fusion at C5–6 and C6–7. Flexion extension studies (not shown) demonstrated mobility of the C4–5 segment. (Used with permission from Barrow Neurological Institute, Phoenix, Arizona)

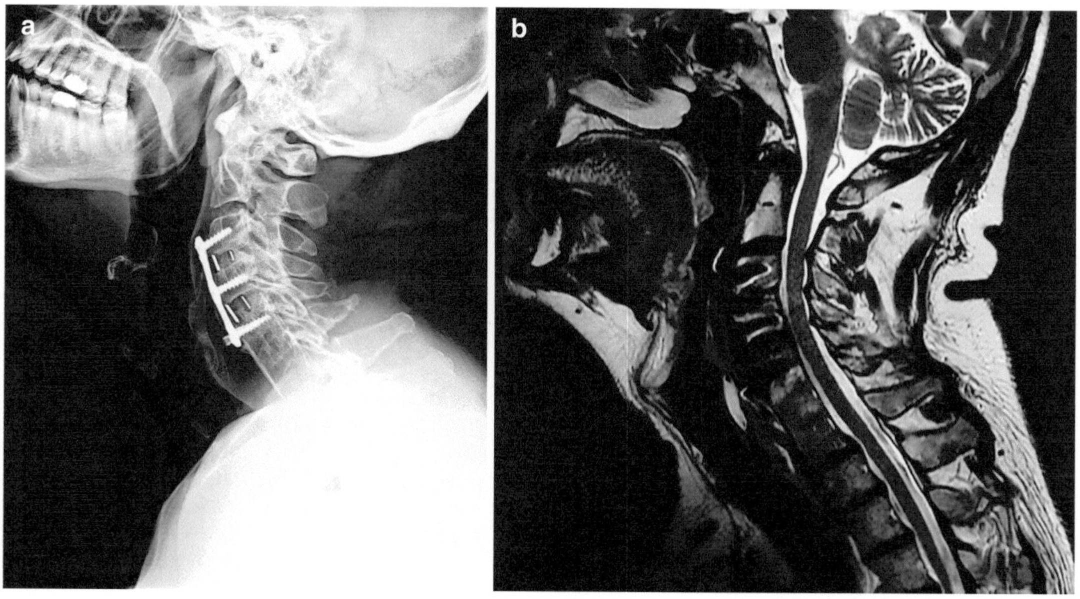

Fig. 22.19 Management of adjacent segment degeneration. (**a**) Lateral postoperative radiograph at 4-month follow-up demonstrating the anterior cervical discectomy and fusion performed at C3–4 and C4–5. A maturing arthrodesis is becoming evident within the interbody spacers. Note that one screw at C6 has begun to pull out past the locking mechanism; this pullout remained unchanged over the 4 months after surgery, and no further intervention was necessary. (**b**) Postoperative sagittal T2-weighted magnetic resonance image demonstrating decompression of the spinal cord at C3–4 and C4–5. (Used with permission from Barrow Neurological Institute, Phoenix, Arizona)

end plate was removed to adequately remove the disc osteophyte and completely decompress the spinal cord (Fig. 22.19).

Postoperative Course

The patient experienced a transient recurrent laryngeal nerve palsy, which returned to his preoperative baseline by the second postoperative month. Over the ensuing months, he experienced gradual improvement in gait and manual dexterity. By the third postoperative month, he was walking independently.

Conclusion

The ACDF is one of the most reliable and effective operations in spine surgery. The unique muscular and vascular anatomy of the cervical spine offers essentially bloodless dissection planes and almost painless exposures. Anterior approaches to the cervical vertebral bodies allow for wide decompressions, restoration of lordosis, and stabilization of segments. As a result, the ACDF is unparalleled in addressing the hallmarks of the degenerating cervical spine: kyphosis, compression, and instability. It is also through the ACDF experience that the foundation for cervical arthroplasty was laid. An essentially identical approach is used for placement of a motion preservation device, a topic covered in depth in the motion preservation section of this book.

The ACDF has undergone continuous refinement since its introduction, from the interbody grafts that are used to the anterior fixation that is applied to optimize arthrodesis. That refinement continues to this day with greater understanding of the mechanical aspects of fusion, biology of fusion at the surface of the interbody, and the emerging role of pharmacological neuroprotection before surgery. Today we have a greater appreciation of adjacent segment degeneration and the measures that can prevent it. From a socioeconomic standpoint, a transition has occurred from inpatient settings to outpatient settings, which continues to decrease the cost and increase the value of the procedure. In the years to come, an emerging understanding of osteoinduction at the interface of the interbody graft and the cortical end plate with various surfacing technologies promises to increase fusion rates even further. Three-dimensional printing will undoubtedly play a role in the manufacture of implants, which may become patient specific. The potential neuroprotection of riluzole promises to improve outcomes in cervical myelopathy. The safety, efficacy, and value of the ACDF will continue to increase in the years to come as we build on these experiences, expand the current knowledge base, and improve the technology.

Disclosures Dr. Tumialán is a consultant to Medtronic, plc. He is an investor in LessRay, which is owned by NuVasive.

References

1. Smith GW, Robinson RA. The treatment of certain cervical-spine disorders by anterior removal of the intervertebral disc and interbody fusion. J Bone Joint Surg Am. 1958;40-A(3):607–24.
2. Cloward RB. The anterior approach for removal of ruptured cervical disks. J Neurosurg. 1958;15(6):602–17. https://doi.org/10.3171/jns.1958.15.6.0602.
3. McGirt MJ, Godil SS, Asher AL, Parker SL, Devin CJ. Quality analysis of anterior cervical discectomy and fusion in the outpatient versus inpatient setting: analysis of 7288 patients from the NSQIP database. Neurosurg Focus. 2015;39(6):E9. https://doi.org/10.3171/2015.9.FOCUS15335.
4. Mansfield HE, Canar WJ, Gerard CS, O'Toole JE. Single-level anterior cervical discectomy and fusion versus minimally invasive posterior cervical foraminotomy for patients with cervical radiculopathy: a cost analysis. Neurosurg Focus. 2014;37(5):E9. https://doi.org/10.3171/2014.8.FOCUS14373.
5. Alvin MD, Lubelski D, Abdullah KG, Whitmore RG, Benzel EC, Mroz TE. Cost-utility analysis of anterior cervical discectomy and fusion with plating (ACDFP) versus posterior cervical foraminotomy (PCF) for patients with single-level cervical radiculopathy at 1-year follow-up. Clin Spine Surg. 2016;29(2):E67–72. https://doi.org/10.1097/BSD.0000000000000099.
6. Tumialán LM, Ponton RP, Gluf WM. Management of unilateral cervical radiculopathy in the military: the cost effectiveness of posterior cervical foraminotomy compared with anterior cervical discectomy and fusion. Neurosurg Focus. 2010;28(5):E17. https://doi.org/10.3171/2010.1.FOCUS09305.
7. Witiw CD, Tetreault LA, Smieliauskas F, Kopjar B, Massicotte EM, Fehlings MG. Surgery for degenerative cervical myelopathy: a patient-centered qual-

ity of life and health economic evaluation. Spine J. 2017;17(1):15–25. https://doi.org/10.1016/j.spinee.2016.10.015.

8. Matz PG, Ryken TC, Groff MW, Vresilovic EJ, Anderson PA, Heary RF, et al. Techniques for anterior cervical decompression for radiculopathy. J Neurosurg Spine. 2009;11(2):183–97. https://doi.org/10.3171/2009.2.SPINE08721.
9. Xie JC, Hurlbert RJ. Discectomy versus discectomy with fusion versus discectomy with fusion and instrumentation: a prospective randomized study. Neurosurgery. 2007;61(1):107–16; discussion 116–7. https://doi.org/10.1227/01.neu.0000279730.44016.da.
10. Jagannathan J, Shaffrey CI, Oskouian RJ, Dumont AS, Herrold C, Sansur CA, et al. Radiographic and clinical outcomes following single-level anterior cervical discectomy and allograft fusion without plate placement or cervical collar. J Neurosurg Spine. 2008;8(5):420–8. https://doi.org/10.3171/SPI/2008/8/5/420.
11. Smith JS, Lafage V, Ryan DJ, Shaffrey CI, Schwab FJ, Patel AA, et al. Association of myelopathy scores with cervical sagittal balance and normalized spinal cord volume: analysis of 56 preoperative cases from the AOSpine North America Myelopathy study. Spine (Phila Pa 1976). 2013;38(22 Suppl 1):S161–70. https://doi.org/10.1097/BRS.0b013e3182a7eb9e.
12. Scheer JK, Tang JA, Smith JS, Acosta FL Jr, Protopsaltis TS, Blondel B, et al. Cervical spine alignment, sagittal deformity, and clinical implications: a review. J Neurosurg Spine. 2013;19(2):141–59. https://doi.org/10.3171/2013.4.SPINE12838.
13. Odate S, Shikata J, Soeda T, Yamamura S, Kawaguchi S. Surgical results and complications of anterior decompression and fusion as a revision surgery after initial posterior surgery for cervical myelopathy due to ossification of the posterior longitudinal ligament. J Neurosurg Spine. 2017;26:1–8. https://doi.org/10.3171/2016.9.SPINE16430.
14. Iwasaki M, Okuda S, Miyauchi A, Sakaura H, Mukai Y, Yonenobu K, et al. Surgical strategy for cervical myelopathy due to ossification of the posterior longitudinal ligament: Part 2: advantages of anterior decompression and fusion over laminoplasty. Spine (Phila Pa 1976). 2007;32(6):654–60. https://doi.org/10.1097/01.brs.0000257566.91177.cb.
15. Iwasaki M, Okuda S, Miyauchi A, Sakaura H, Mukai Y, Yonenobu K, et al. Surgical strategy for cervical myelopathy due to ossification of the posterior longitudinal ligament: Part 1: clinical results and limitations of laminoplasty. Spine (Phila Pa 1976). 2007;32(6):647–53. https://doi.org/10.1097/01.brs.0000257560.91147.86.
16. Nassr A, Lee JY, Bashir RS, Rihn JA, Eck JC, Kang JD, et al. Does incorrect level needle localization during anterior cervical discectomy and fusion lead to accelerated disc degeneration? Spine (Phila Pa 1976). 2009;34(2):189–92. https://doi.org/10.1097/BRS.0b013e3181913872.
17. Smith PN, Balzer JR, Khan MH, Davis RA, Crammond D, Welch WC, et al. Intraoperative somatosensory evoked potential monitoring during anterior cervical discectomy and fusion in nonmyelopathic patients—a review of 1,039 cases. Spine J. 2007;7(1):83–7. https://doi.org/10.1016/j.spinee.2006.04.008.
18. Kalb S, Fakhran S, Dean B, Ross J, Porter RW, Kakarla UK, et al. Cervical spinal cord infarction after cervical spine decompressive surgery. World Neurosurg. 2014;81(5–6):810–7. https://doi.org/10.1016/j.wneu.2012.12.024.
19. Jung A, Schramm J. How to reduce recurrent laryngeal nerve palsy in anterior cervical spine surgery: a prospective observational study. Neurosurgery. 2010;67(1):10–5; discussion 15. https://doi.org/10.1227/01.NEU.0000370203.26164.24.
20. Apfelbaum RI, Kriskovich MD, Haller JR. On the incidence, cause, and prevention of recurrent laryngeal nerve palsies during anterior cervical spine surgery. Spine (Phila Pa 1976). 2000;25(22):2906–12.
21. Chin KR, Ricchetti ET, Yu WD, Riew KD. Less exposure surgery for multilevel anterior cervical fusion using 2 transverse incisions. J Neurosurg Spine. 2012;17(3):194–8. https://doi.org/10.3171/2012.5.SPINE111112.
22. Vaccaro AR, Ring D, Scuderi G, Garfin SR. Vertebral artery location in relation to the vertebral body as determined by two-dimensional computed tomography evaluation. Spine (Phila Pa 1976). 1994;19(23):2637–41.
23. Maharaj MM, Phan K, Mobbs RJ. Anterior cervical discectomy and fusion (ACDF) autograft versus graft substitutes: What do patients prefer? A clinical study. J Spine Surg. 2016;2(2):105–10. https://doi.org/10.21037/jss.2016.05.01.
24. Najeeb S, Bds ZK, Bds SZ, Bds MS. Bioactivity and osseointegration of PEEK are inferior to those of titanium: a systematic review. J Oral Implantol. 2016;42(6):512–6. https://doi.org/10.1563/aaid-joi-D-16-00072.
25. Gittens RA, Olivares-Navarrete R, Schwartz Z, Boyan BD. Implant osseointegration and the role of microroughness and nanostructures: lessons for spine implants. Acta Biomater. 2014;10(8):3363–71. https://doi.org/10.1016/j.actbio.2014.03.037.
26. Scholz M, Reyes PM, Schleicher P, Sawa AG, Baek S, Kandziora F, et al. A new stand-alone cervical anterior interbody fusion device: biomechanical comparison with established anterior cervical fixation devices. Spine (Phila Pa 1976). 2009;34(2):156–60. https://doi.org/10.1097/BRS.0b013e31818ff9c4.
27. Kim HJ, Kelly MP, Ely CG, Dettori JR, Riew KD. The risk of adjacent-level ossification development after surgery in the cervical spine: are there factors that affect the risk? A systematic review. Spine (Phila Pa 1976). 2012;37(22 Suppl):S65–74. https://doi.org/10.1097/BRS.0b013e31826cb8f5.
28. Lee DH, Lee JS, Yi JS, Cho W, Zebala LP, Riew KD. Anterior cervical plating technique to prevent adjacent-level ossification development. Spine J. 2013;13(7):823–9. https://doi.org/10.1016/j.spinee.2013.03.009.
29. Dipaola CP, Jacobson JA, Awad H, Conrad BP, Rechtine GR 2nd. Screw orientation and plate type

(variable- vs. fixed-angle) effect strength of fixation for in vitro biomechanical testing of the Synthes CSLP. Spine J. 2008;8(5):717–22. https://doi.org/10.1016/j.spinee.2007.06.016.
30. Olsson EC, Jobson M, Lim MR. Risk factors for persistent dysphagia after anterior cervical spine surgery. Orthopedics. 2015;38(4):e319–23. https://doi.org/10.3928/01477447-20150402-61.
31. Cho SK, Lu Y, Lee DH. Dysphagia following anterior cervical spinal surgery: a systematic review. Bone Joint J. 2013;95-B(7):868–73. https://doi.org/10.1302/0301-620X.95B7.31029.
32. Yue WM, Brodner W, Highland TR. Persistent swallowing and voice problems after anterior cervical discectomy and fusion with allograft and plating: a 5- to 11-year follow-up study. Eur Spine J. 2005;14(7):677–82. https://doi.org/10.1007/s00586-004-0849-3.
33. Nassr A, Eck JC, Ponnappan RK, Zanoun RR, Donaldson WF 3rd, Kang JD. The incidence of C5 palsy after multilevel cervical decompression procedures: a review of 750 consecutive cases. Spine (Phila Pa 1976). 2012;37(3):174–8. https://doi.org/10.1097/BRS.0b013e318219cfe9.
34. Sakaura H, Hosono N, Mukai Y, Ishii T, Yoshikawa H. C5 palsy after decompression surgery for cervical myelopathy: review of the literature. Spine (Phila Pa 1976). 2003;28(21):2447–51. https://doi.org/10.1097/01.BRS.0000090833.96168.3F.
35. Halani SH, Baum GR, Riley JP, Pradilla G, Refai D, Rodts GE Jr, et al. Esophageal perforation after anterior cervical spine surgery: a systematic review of the literature. J Neurosurg Spine. 2016;25(3):285–91. https://doi.org/10.3171/2016.1.SPINE15898.

Anterior Cervical Corpectomy

23

Anthony C. Lau and Allan D. Levi

Pearls and Pitfalls

- Being aware of the individual nuances and anatomic variants of each case is essential to reducing avoidable complications in an anterior cervical corpectomy.
- Know the advantages and disadvantages of techniques and implants available for the anterior cervical corpectomy.
- Consider posterior constructs when there is concern that an anterior approach alone may fail. This consideration applies especially to patients with CSM requiring three or more corpectomy levels, possessing severe pre-op kyphotic deformity (greater than 15°) or diagnosed with systemic diseases potentially compromising fusion.
- Extending construct level increases complication rates and should be considered only when absolutely necessary.

A. C. Lau · A. D. Levi
Department of Neurological Surgery, University of Miami Miller School of Medicine, Miami, FL, USA
e-mail: alevi@med.miami.edu

Introduction

The anterior approach to the cervical spine was initially described in the 1950s [9, 38] and has since become a fundamental part of the spine surgeon's armamentarium. Originally conceived to decompress the spinal cord and exiting nerve roots by removing disc material and posterior osteophytes, the development of the median corpectomy technique subsequently allowed surgeons to effectively access and treat most pathology ventral to the cervical spinal cord. As usage of corpectomies became more widespread, industry innovation followed with various graft and plating systems, leading to a wide variation in clinical practice and application. In this chapter, we will describe our approach to the anterior cervical corpectomy, as well as review the available evidence in the literature.

Our Approach

Preoperative Workup

A comprehensive preoperative workup should address both local and systemic factors that could affect the operation or its results. An exhaustive list of all factors to be considered prior to an anterior cervical corpectomy is well beyond the scope of this chapter, but we will provide a general overview in the next section.

M. G. Kaiser et al. (eds.), *Degenerative Cervical Myelopathy and Radiculopathy*,
https://doi.org/10.1007/978-3-319-97952-6_23

Aberrant anatomy, though relatively rare, is an important cause of complications and should be considered in every case. For example, an unidentified anomalous course of the vertebral artery can lead to profound unexpected blood loss and severe neurologic compromise. Similarly, an injury to the recurrent laryngeal nerve can lead to permanent unilateral vocal cord paralysis if unrecognized during the exposure. These anatomical anomalies will be discussed in further detail later in the chapter.

Any previous manipulation of the cervical spine must also be considered preoperatively. In general, surgical and/or radiation treatments to the neck will cause increased scarring and difficulty with dissection. For example, preoperative unilateral vocal paralysis would likely shift the surgeon's decision on operative approach to the ipsilateral side or opt for a posterior approach to minimize risk of complete bilateral vocal cord paralysis.

Osteoporosis and ankylosing spondylitis are examples of systemic diseases resulting in poor bone quality, the latter with highly vascular bone. Inadequate appreciation and/or treatment of these conditions can lead to graft subsidence and subsequent extrusion.

The prudent surgeon will adopt a treatment plan and operative approach based on the individual patient's unique clinical circumstances.

Preoperative Imaging

The standard imaging battery obtained in our institution prior to performing a corpectomy includes a plain MRI, a plain CT scan, upright neutral X-rays (A/P and lateral), and dynamic (flexion and extension) X-rays. The plain MRI is ideal to evaluate soft tissue and for visualizing neural compression. T2 flow voids can be traced to screen for anomalous major vessels. A shortfall of a plain MRI lies in the diagnosis of ossification of the posterior longitudinal ligament (OPLL), as a calcified PLL appears very similar to thickened ligament.

Routine CTs are best for evaluating bony anatomy and can help distinguish OPLL from ligamentous hypertrophy, which can significantly change the operative plan. The presence of osteophytes and calcified discs are also much easier to appreciate on the CT. Accurate length measurements for screws are also best determined on CT. Supplementing with intrathecal myelographic dye can enhance information obtained by CT in cases where MR is contraindicated or instrumentation artifact precludes adequate imaging of the nerve roots and spinal cord.

Upright neutral plain X-rays are useful to determine the degree of lordosis or kyphosis in addition to a number of other cervical parameters now being employed (T1 slope, neck tilt, etc.). Dynamic X-rays are ideal for determining presence of instability or the degree of rigidity or flexibility in deformity cases. Additionally, they afford the surgeon an idea of what visualization to expect with intraoperative X-rays.

Additional imaging is obtained as necessary including vascular imaging for aberrant vessels, contrast for suspected neoplasms or infections, and others.

Positioning and Room Setup

Patients are positioned supine in the middle of the room on an operating table, and the table is slid rostrally to allow easy manipulation and entry of the C-arm. The patient's head is placed in Gardner-Wells tongs to allow for manipulation of the head and the ability to distract if necessary. Ten pounds of weight is applied initially. A bolster is placed between the scapulae and, to prevent too much extension and head movement, a donut cushion is placed underneath the head. Rolled towels are placed beneath the neck for stability. Shoulders are taped gently caudally straight down, without flexion, extension, or rotation of the shoulder. The C-arm enters on the opposite side of the surgeon and is rolled rostrally between the surgical team and anesthesia when not in use. An initial radiograph is obtained to ensure adequate alignment of the cervical spine prior to incision. The microscope enters on the side of the surgeon. The C-arm screens are at the foot of the bed; the anesthesia team is at the head of the bed.

Neuromonitoring and Pre-op Anesthesia Medications

We routinely use neuromonitoring in our patients and thus must ensure that inhalational anesthetics and muscle paralytics are minimized after induction. The role of neuromonitoring varies based on the individual case but generally allows the identification of excessive shoulder traction and positioning palsies. Losses in somatosensory evoked potentials or motor-evoked potentials intraoperatively might suggest a spinal cord injury, necessitating elevation of mean arterial pressure above 85mmHg, administration of steroids, and/or cooling the patient [22]. Somatosensory evoked potentials are generally recorded in addition to motor-evoked potentials. Care should be taken to hold retractors in place during MEP runs to avoid dislodgment of the retraction system.

Our preoperative antibiotic prophylaxis regime includes cefazolin, which is replaced by levofloxacin in penicillin-allergic patients. Steroids are used judiciously, usually in the setting of neoplastic lesions with cord compression or in suspected intraoperative injuries.

Operative Technique

Incision

Classically, transverse and longitudinal incisions have been used for anterior cervical exposure. The transverse incision runs along a neck crease on the skin of the patient and is the most cosmetically acceptable approach. The longitudinal incision runs along the medial border of the sternocleidomastoid muscle and obviates the need for an extensive sub- or supra-platysmal dissection. In our experience, a properly placed transverse incision can be used in most circumstances which allows safe and adequate exposure up to four disc levels.

The laterality of exposure largely depends on surgeon preference in virgin cases. The advantage of the right is that there is no thoracic duct at the upper thoracic levels; the advantage of the left is that the recurrent laryngeal nerve has a more consistent route and longer route around the aorta before turning back rostrally into the tracheoesophageal groove. Clinical studies have shown no difference in rates of vocal cord paralysis based on laterality [4]. Thus, it is our practice to approach the cervical spine from the right in most cases, as it is also more ergonomic for the right-handed surgeon.

Special consideration should be given to extremely low-lying pathology requiring access to the low cervical and upper thoracic spine. In this case, we employ a midline incision over the top of the manubrium, slightly deviating to the side of preferred access along the medial border of the sternocleidomastoid. Occasionally, it is necessary to resect the upper portion of the manubrium to achieve adequate access. The subsequent exposure and identification of anatomical structures remain unchanged.

Platysmal Exposure

Depending on the incision used, there are various methods for manipulating the platysmal layer. The most common approach, and the one we employ, is sharply incising the playtsma along the skin incision used. If the longitudinal incision was employed, minimal undercutting of the playtsma is necessary, as the caudal/rostral extent of the exposure is already established with the platysmal incision. If a transverse incision was employed, the platysmal layer is undercut with sharp or blunt dissection as far rostral and caudal as possible. At this stage, the most commonly encountered large vessels are the external jugular and common facial veins. These vascular structures can both be safely transected if identified early.

An alternative to incising the platysma directly is a supra-platysmal dissection of the skin off the platysma in a rostral-caudal direction. Once the platysma layer is identified, blunt dissection can be used to open the platysma in a rostral-caudal direction along its fibers and natural planes.

Approach to the Spine

With blunt dissection following the medial border of the sternocleidomastoid, the carotid sheath should be identified. Care should be taken at every stage of the approach to extend the dissection as far caudally and rostrally as possible. This will allow easier mobilization of tissues, minimizing undue mechanical stretch on critical structures with the retraction system. The identity of the carotid sheath itself is confirmed by palpation and is retracted laterally. The omohyoid may be visualized at this time and can usually be mobilized rostrally or caudally sufficiently for the operation. If the omohyoid is too large and remains an obstacle to visualization, it is fully mobilized and sharply incised. The omohyoid is responsible for depression of the hyoid and can be divided with minimal consequence.

The dissection is continued medially until the prevertebral fascia is seen, which is then elevated with forceps to ensure no vascular or neural structures lie within. The prevertebral fascia is then incised sharply rostrally and caudally as necessary. A localizing X-ray is then taken, with a bayonetted spinal needle in the disc space. The disc space is marked by incising the annulus under direct visualization.

The longus colli muscle on each side is then identified, and its insertion is sharply dissected off the vertebral body with a monopolar cautery, taking care not to venture too laterally into the vertebral artery or too superficially in the sympathetic chain.

Placement of Retractors

Once the longus colli have been sufficiently dissected from vertebral body, a free-standing retraction system is placed in situ. It is our practice to place 3-pronged plates both medially and laterally to minimize movement of the retractors during MEP stimulation or during the procedure. Smooth retractors are placed in the caudal-rostral direction. It is imperative to deflate and reinflate the endotracheal tube at this time to minimize retraction and compression injury to the recurrent laryngeal nerve. The final pressure of the endotracheal tube cuff in our institution largely depends on the practice of the attending anesthetist. However, we recommend deflating the endotracheal tube cuff completely and reinflating to a pressure just enough to prevent an air leak around the cuff. Forced over-distraction at this stage is a common error which can lead to further soft-tissue injury. If retraction causes taut soft tissue around the exposure site, it is recommended that the retractors be removed and further soft-tissue dissection be attempted.

Corpectomy

As with most techniques in neurosurgery, there are a myriad of ways to perform the cervical corpectomy. We will outline the method by which this technique is performed in our institution, but with the understanding that this is highly variable. The width of the corpectomy is generally delineated by the uncovertebral joints on either side, often measuring 15 mm.

Discectomies are performed on the disc spaces adjacent to the proposed corpectomy site. The posterior longitudinal ligament is left intact. A Leksell rongeur is used to remove as much of the vertebral body as reasonably possible, using the discectomies as a general guide to depth. The removed bone is saved for autograft to be placed in the subsequent graft. The remaining vertebral body is cored out using a M8 matchstick head, again with the uncovertebral joints serving as a guideline for the lateral extent of the corpectomy. Absorbable gelatin or another hemostatic agent is used occasionally throughout the drilling process to minimize blood loss. When only a cortical shell remains, this bone is removed with a Kerrison punch. The PLL is then pierced and removed. When the PLL is calcified, we drill around the calcification laterally until soft tissue is seen in an attempt to isolate an island of centrally calcified PLL. This section of PLL is then carefully dissected from the dura using a blunt nerve hook and removed piecemeal. If it is believed that the floating piece of calcified PLL cannot be safely dissected from the dura, it is left in place.

Graft Selection

Of all the graft choices, autograft remains the gold standard, being osteogenic, osteoconductive, and osteoinductive. Accordingly, several studies have demonstrated better fusion rates with autograft versus allograft in multilevel fusions. Zdeblick and Ducker [46] reported non-union rates of 62% with iliac allograft compared to 17% with iliac autograft in multilevel fusions. Fernyhough et al. [13] similarly showed a pseudoarthrosis rate of 36% with fibular allograft compared to 25% with fibular autograft in anterior cervical corpectomies. However, autograft harvest sites have been known to cause significant donor site morbidity of up to 30% (MacDonald et al. 1997). Allograft has been shown to have similar fusion rates compared to autograft in one-level corpectomies [45].

Titanium mesh cages have been used since the 1980s with impressive reported fusion rates. An initial case series of one- to two-level corpectomies demonstrated fusion into the titanium cage in 94% of cases with available imaging (Narotam et al. 2003). Hee et al. [14] reported similar fusion rates of 95%, additionally noting failure with osteopenic patients which is likely due to the larger difference in the modulus of elasticity between titanium and osteopenic bone leading to increased subsidence and subsequent failure.

A newer subset of titanium cages has been recently adopted in cervical spine corpectomies. Expandable titanium cages were initially designed to facilitate cage implantation and provide precise distraction. A prospective case series from the Netherlands reported fusion rates of 93% with expandable cages, though this case series included spinal pathology from cervical, thoracic, and lumbar spine [3]. An initial case series of 22 patients with cervical corpectomies alone reported no hardware-related complications and 100% fusion rates with a mean follow-up of 22 months (Auguste et al. 2006). It should be noted, however, that 14/22 patients had a posterior fusion upfront in this series.

Although Kischner wires [36] or screws [1] and methyl methacrylate constructs have been used in the past, there have been significant criticisms with their use, as the fusion rates have not been ideal [23]. As such, these constructs can only be recommended for salvage operations where the life expectancy is short and fusion is not expected to occur.

The uses of many other materials (such as PEEK or carbon fiber) have been described, but regardless of the graft material selected, certain principles remain constant in technique. In general, we attempt to select a fibular allograft with the largest diameter possible without surpassing the prepared endplate area. The internal diameter of the allograft is enlarged to allow placement of autograft and bone morphogenic protein as necessary. The fibular allograft itself is then shaped using a high-speed drill to an appropriate length with slight lordotic angle. The specific graft length is determined by removing the weights off the Gardner-Wells tongs and approximating a length a couple of millimeters longer than the resultant space between the endplates. The weights are reapplied to distract the vertebral bodies and the graft is carefully inserted. The weight is then removed again, and the sizing of the graft is assessed by applying gentle ventrally directed force with a nerve hook to ensure no movement. Adequate endplate contact is assessed with a plain radiograph.

Bone Morphogenetic Protein

Bone morphogenetic protein 2 has been extensively studied as an adjunct for spinal fusions. Initial enthusiasm with BMP was tempered by reports of prevertebral swelling leading to dysphagia and/or airway obstruction in up to 27.5% of cases [40]. Subsequent reports described complications including local inflammation, sterile cyst formation, ectopic bone formation, and even possibly increased risk of malignancy [37]. However, recent publications suggest safety and efficacy of BMP in promoting bony fusion in anterior cervical procedures. To clarify the literature, a recent systematic review by Hofstetter et al. (2016) looked at the dose-dependent effect of BMP on bony fusion and adverse effects. Interestingly, they found minimal differences in fusion rates with arbitrarily assigned low-dose (0.2–0.6 mg per disc level) BMP and high-dose (0.7–2.1 mg per level) BMP. More importantly, they determined that the adverse effect rate was not significantly elevated with low-dose BMP compared to the non-BMP controls, while higher dosing leads to adverse effect rates of 8–10%. It was also noted that the effect of BMP on fusion rate was greater based on the number of levels fused. It should be noted that currently the use of BMP in anterior cervical spine surgery is considered off-label usage by the FDA. While this section on the use of bone morphogenic protein is included for completeness, it must be noted that the use of biologics in anterior cervical spine surgery remains highly controversial.

Plating

The options for plating following an anterior corpectomy includes long anterior plate (either fixed or dynamic), transitional (or buttress) plates, or no plate.

Overall, graft dislodgement has been reported in 5–50% of anterior corpectomies without plating. Fraser and Hartl (2007), in a systematic review, reported fusion rates of 92.9% and 95.9% for one-level corpectomies with or without plates, respectively. In two-level corpectomies, the fusion rates reported were 96.2% and 89.8% with or without anterior plates, respectively.

Prior to the development of anterior cervical plates, a medial corpectomy was supported by a fibular graft alone. To this end, various techniques have been devised to lodge the graft into the adjacent endplates through drilling notches or wedges. A more detailed overview of these techniques is outlined in Thongtrangan et al. (2003). Extensive drilling of the endplates, however, has been shown in cadaveric studies to increase the risk of subsidence and graft failure rates [20].

Long Anterior Plates: Fixed Versus Dynamic Plating

Long anterior cervical plates essentially come in two varieties: fixed or dynamic. Both have been studied extensively, and biomechanical studies have demonstrated higher pullout strength with dynamic plates compared to fixed-angle plates [10]. In addition, fusion rates appear higher, and hardware complications appear lower with dynamic plating [29, 41]. In our institution, fixed anterior plates are only used in the setting of trauma where there is a need to minimize loss of segmental lordosis subsequently. In our practice, the ideal plate length will span the entire area to be fused, but will not cover more than 1/3 of the most rostral vertebral body. The rationale for this practice is based on studies that have shown increased rates of radiographic adjacent segment disease when this threshold is surpassed [28].

Transitional or Buttress Plates

Since the most common mechanism of graft failure appears to be rostral settling with caudal "kicking out," buttressing the caudal portion of the construct may prevent kicking out while allowing settling and subsequent fusion rostrally. Buttressing plates may also avoid the theoretical distraction afforded by long anterior plates (especially those of the fixed variety) possibly hindering fusion.

An et al. [2] reported 11 cases of multilevel corpectomies with transitional plates and had a 0% failure rate. However, these constructs were all supplemented with posterior constructs. Riew et al. [31] showed similar results with buttress plates with 4/11 failures with anterior fixation alone: 1 graft extrusion and 3 pseudoarthroses. No failures were seen with posterior supplementation. An important observation made in this report was that failures of buttress plates are slightly different mechanistically, but with potentially devastating clinical consequences. Specifically, the rostral portion of the buttress plate projects anteriorly causing pretracheal compression and respiratory compromise.

In our practice, we generally use a fibular allograft strut with autograft harvested from osteophyte removal or the corpectomy itself. The endplates are left intact but are decorticated. A long anterior dynamic plate is used in most cases. BMP is used only in multilevel corpectomies.

Clinical Issues

Indications for Anterior Cervical Corpectomies

In general, the rationale for performing an anterior cervical corpectomy can be thought of as access, decompression of neural elements, correction of deformity, or a combination thereof.

The indications for treatment of CSM and OPLL with a corpectomy warrant special discussion, as the decision to treat these disorders from a posterior or anterior approach remains controversial. A recent systematic review by Lawrence et al. (2013) attempted to address the long-standing debate as to whether an anterior or posterior approach to spinal surgery was favored for multilevel CSM. Eight comparative studies were included in their analysis which encompassed a variety of anterior and posterior approaches. Overall, the authors concluded that there was insufficient evidence in the literature to make a statement favoring either an anterior or posterior surgical approach. However, they stressed that the important factors to consider when deciding on the optimal approach include: ventral vs. dorsal compression, sagittal alignment, focal vs. diffuse disease, presence or absence of axial pain or radiculopathy, age, comorbidities, and surgeon preference/familiarity. With respect to OPLL, Chen et al. [8] performed a meta-analysis comparing a laminoplasty to an anterior cervical corpectomy for multilevel OPLL. They included 10 nonrandomized controlled case studies (1 prospective nonrandomized trial and 9 retrospective studies) with a total of 819 patients. They concluded that corpectomies resulted in better neurologic outcomes as measured by JOA scores, but with significantly higher complication rates (25% vs. 19%) compared to laminoplasty. This effect was especially pronounced with OPLL patients with an occupying ratio greater or equal to 60% and OPLL patients with preoperative kyphotic deformities.

Increasing Corpectomy Levels and Associated Risks

The overall reported complication rate in a 31-patient retrospective study of four-level corpectomies was 38.7% [35]. While larger constructs are certainly possible, and may be necessary in rare circumstances, it is well documented that increasing the length of the corpectomy increases complication rates. In one of the largest series on complications following corpectomy to date, Boakye et al. [5] reviewed 1560 patients undergoing a cervical corpectomy in Veterans Affairs from 1997 to 2006. Overall, they determined that three or more corpectomy levels increased risk of postoperative complications over twofold (OR: 2.51). Additionally, they reported increased frequency of complications requiring reoperation in two-level (OR: 1.67) and three-level (OR: 3.15) corpectomies compared to one-level corpectomies. Biomechanical studies have also shown decreased immediate postoperative stability in three-level versus two-level corpectomies [30].

Increasing corpectomy levels similarly increases the chances of graft failure and migration. Vaccaro et al. [42] reported a failure rate of 9% with two-level corpectomies, compared to 50% with three-level corpectomies. Sasso et al. [34] reported a 6% failure rate with a two-level corpectomy compared to a 71% failure rate in a three-level corpectomy with a fixed plate. Wang et al. [43] showed graft migration rates increasing with increasing corpectomy levels using autograft without a plate, reporting 4%, 5%,10%, and 17% migration rates for one-, two-, three-, and four-level corpectomies, respectively.

Need for a Posterior Construct Upfront

There remains some controversy with regard to when a corpectomy should be supplemented with a posterior construct upfront. Not surprisingly, multiple cadaveric studies have shown that posterior construct supplementation provides a sturdier construct (Galler et al. 2007). McAfee et al. [24] reported a failure rate of essentially 0% when their anterior corpectomies were supplemented with a posterior construct, though the addition of a posterior construct upfront obviously increases surgical risk compared to anterior intervention alone. In addition, biomechanical cadaveric models have suggested that posterior supplementation may increase forces on adjacent levels compared to anterior corpectomies alone (Hussain et al. 2013), leading to increased rates of adjacent segment disease, though this has yet to be demonstrated in the clinical setting.

In our experience, supplementation of an anterior cervical corpectomy with posterior instrumentation is generally required in the following circumstances: three or more corpectomy levels, severe pre-op kyphotic deformity (greater than 15°), patients with systemic disease potentially compromising fusion (osteoporosis, ankylosing spondylitis, etc.), neoplastic processes, and/or circumferential pathology (fracture dislocations, etc.).

Complications and Complication Avoidance

Recurrent Laryngeal Nerve Injury

Among the most common injuries in an anterior cervical approach is injury to the recurrent laryngeal nerve. Cadaveric studies have shown that course of the RLN on the left is more redundant and allows for more stretch and thus may contribute to lower rates of vocal cord palsy [44]. Additionally, a nonrecurrent laryngeal nerve can occur on the right side, though this occurs in less than 1% [7]. A retrospective analysis of 16 cases of vocal cord paralysis due to anterior cervical spine approaches that showed all but 1 case was a right-sided paralysis [26]. Clinical studies, however, have not shown any difference in rates of RLN injury based on laterality of approach [4].

Estimates of permanent RLN injury range from 0.15% [6] to 2% (Cloward 1962). Apfelbaum et al. (2000) reported an incidence of 3% temporary RLN dysfunction and 0.33% permanent dysfunction. Practically, one method shown to reduce RLN injury rates is deflating and reinflating the endotracheal tube cuff after retractor placement, which reduces the incidence from 6% to 2% (Apfelbaum et al. 2000). Additionally, ensuring the retractors do not move during the operation (especially during MEPs), ensuring a generous dissection, and reducing surgical times have all been suggested to reduce RLN injury rates, though no definitive clinical studies exist.

Vertebral Artery Injury

Vertebral artery injuries can be devastating but fortunately rare. A recent survey of spine surgeons resulted in a reported incidence of 0.07% in all cervical spine surgeries [21], though this is likely an underrepresentation of the true incidence. Other estimates have the incidence of vertebral artery injury in anterior cervical approaches at 0.5% [39]. Boakye et al. [5] reported a 0.96% rate of vessel laceration with cervical corpectomies, but did not identify the vessel injured.

Given normal anatomy, utilizing the uncal vertebral joint as a border for the discectomy/corpectomy should reduce the chance of vertebral artery injury. However, as noted earlier, the possibility of aberrant anatomy must always be considered and must be looked for on the MRI or CT angiogram if available. The most important times to consider the vertebral artery are during the exposure of the anterior neck and during the corpectomy.

The vertebral artery enters the transverse foramen at C6 92–95% of the time, with entry at C4,

C5, and C7 at 1.8%, 5.6%, and 0.6%, respectively [12, 16]. If the vertebral artery enters the foramen more cephalad than normal, it runs just posterior and lateral to the longus colli without bony protection, lending itself to inadvertent injury during the dissection of the longus colli.

A recent study looking at 250 patients undergoing MRI scans for neck pain, radiculopathy or myelopathy showed midline migration of a vertebral artery in 7.6% of patients [12]. A medially deviated vertebral artery obviously represents significant risk if unrecognized during the corpectomy.

If injured, treatment of vertebral artery injuries include tamponade, exposure and electrocoagulation, open suture or clip placement, or endovascular sacrifice.

Sympathetic Chain Injury

Sympathetic chain injury is a fairly rare complication and thus no large studies have been done, though case reports exist. Poor exposure of the longus will result in injury of the sympathetic trunk, as the plexus lies superficial to this muscle. Movement of retractors during the case superficial to the longus may similarly cause sympathetic chain injury. Anatomical studies have shown that the sympathetic trunk is more medial in the lower cervical spine (C6 vs. C3) [11] and may be at higher risk with lower cervical approaches, though the clinical relevance is difficult to ascertain. These patients are usually identified by the development of a Horner's syndrome postoperatively. The management of these patients is generally expectant.

C5 Radiculopathy

C5 palsy is a complication of cervical decompressive techniques and appears to have similar incidences in anterior and posterior approaches to cervical spine decompression (Gandhoke et al. 2011). Studies have estimated rates of up to 10–20% in some series (Yonenobu et al. 1991; Saunders 1995). The vast majority of cases are unilateral, with only about 8% being bilateral [32].

The exact pathophysiologic mechanism behind this complication is not completely understood, though several theories have been put forward. One of the more prominent theories includes the spinal cord shift theory put forth by Yononenbu (1991). In this theory, mostly derived from posterior decompressions, it is theorized that the decompression of the spinal cord posteriorly causes stretching of the C5 nerve root. This is supported by Saunders et al. (1995) that showed limiting the corpectomy width to 15 mm reduced the incidence of C5 palsies from 14% to 2%.

The onset of C5 palsies can also be quite variable, ranging from immediately postoperatively to almost 2 months postoperatively [25]. However, several case studies reported subsequently showed much lower incidence of C5 palsy of 4.6% with wider decompressions guided by anatomy (uncovertebral joints) rather than an arbitrary width. Several preoperative factors have also been implicated in increased C5 palsies postoperatively: the presence of kyphotic deformity, the severity of cervical myelopathy, and age above 60. When presented with a postoperative C5 palsy, patients are started on a course of steroids with subsequent physiotherapy, with most resolving spontaneously over weeks to months. MR imaging is performed to rule out any structural lesions amenable to surgical reintervention.

CSF Leaks

Rates of CSF leaks are generally the same as a discectomy except in the case of OPLL. In this patient population, the ossified ligament can be firmly attached to the dura, or in some rare cases, the dura can be completely deficient. To avoid an unintentional durotomy, it may occasionally be necessary to leave an island of floating ossified ligament and decompress posteriorly if needed.

Oftentimes, a dural tear from an anterior approach will not be amenable to primary closure. In these cases, Gelfoam fibrin glue will be required. Fat and muscle grafts may be left in place behind the graft but with great care, as undue expansion will undo the decompression achieved. Lumbar drains can divert CSF for the first several days and allow healing of the dural defect.

Adjacent Segment Degeneration

Adjacent segment degeneration (ASD) is a problem that plagues spinal fusions. ASD requiring reoperation is estimated at 2.4% per year in a retrospective analysis of 1038 cases of cervical arthrodesis [18], whereas symptomatic ASD has been reported to be 2.9% [15]. In a small retrospective analysis of 44 patients looking specifically at corpectomies, radiographic ASD has been reported as high as 75% (Kulkarni et al. 2004).

ASD is believed to be a result of increased forces on joints adjacent to the construct causing compensatory hypermobility at these levels. Longer constructs result in higher forces exerted on the remaining joints, though a number of studies have shown that increasing the number of fusion levels actually decreases the rate of ASD ([15, 18], Kulkarni et al. 2004). Despite the added physical demands on the remaining segments with longer segments, it is believed that the inclusion of levels at high risk of ASD reduces this effect.

To reduce the incidence of ASD, we practice anterior plating over no more than 1/3 of the vertebral body at the rostral and caudal ends of the construct [28].

Graft Failure

Graft and plate displacement rates have been reported to be 5–50% in various case series. The most common mechanism of graft failure in corpectomies includes subsidence at the rostral end with anterior displacement of the caudal end of the graft. The mechanism is similar even with the application of long anterior cervical plates, likely attributable to increased screw loosening at the caudal end of the construct with repetitive motion as seen in biomechanical studies [27]. Efforts to minimize graft movement postoperatively have been described above and include anterior plating and endplate manipulation. In addition to the suggestions above, removing too much cortical bone with the osteophytes can increase screw pullout rates. Bicortical screws are an option when the risk of fusion failure is high but runs obvious risks to the underlying dura and spinal cord. Graft fractures can also occur but can be minimized by avoiding screw placement into the graft itself. Adequate sizing of the graft additionally minimizes overt subsidence and rates of graft fracture while promoting adequate fusion.

Management of graft failures depends on the severity of the clinical situation. Airway management is paramount and should be established immediately with strict spinal precautions. Surgical airways may be required. Once medically stable, an anterior approach is usually adopted to remove the failed graft and reestablish anterior column stability. Posterior construct support is generally recommended at the same time.

Non-union and Pseudoarthrosis

Pseudoarthrosis following corpectomies has been reported to be 7.6% at 1 year follow-up [17]. Though many technical considerations have already been mentioned to minimize non-union and pseudoarthrosis including appropriate graft sizing, BMP usage, and others, many controllable systemic risk factors also play a large role in successful fusions. For example, higher rates of pseudoarthrosis have been reported in smokers in a retrospective analysis of 132 patients compared to non-smokers (16% vs. 4%). Minimizing pseudoarthrosis risk often requires controlling systemic disease.

Plate Complications

In addition to plate migration, a poorly placed plate can result in dysphagia, throat irritation, or even erosion into the esophagus [19]. To minimize these complications, we ensure that the plate is flush against the vertebral bodies to minimize its profile. Removing anterior osteophytes is often necessary to accomplish this, though care should be taken to minimize cortical disruption which would reduce screw pullout strength.

Management of minor plate complications such as persistent esophageal irritation can include removal of the offending plate, assuming the underlying cervical spine has already fused. In esophageal perforations, consultation with ENT specialists is advised, as the esophagus may require primary repair of muscle flaps to adequately treat.

Postoperative Hematoma

One of the most feared complications following an anterior cervical approach to the spine is the development of an acute hematoma compromising the airway or impinging the spinal cord. Sarkar et al. [33] documented an incidence of 0.2% in a large single-institution series of 468 patients out of India, whereas a US Veterans Affairs experience reported a 1.47% postoperative hematoma complication rate [5]. Unfortunately, the severity and consequences of the latter study were not described and thus likely overestimate life-threatening postoperative hematomas. Regardless, it is our practice to leave a Jackson-Pratt drain following every corpectomy. Though more common following carotid endarterectomy surgery, acute hematomas compromising the airway in the recovery room requires immediate reopening of the surgical wound.

Postoperative Care

In our practice, plain X-rays are acquired immediately (1–2d postoperatively), in the acute phase (3 weeks) and the chronic phase (~6 months). Routine CT scans are performed only in the context of studies requiring documentation of fusion and performed at 1 year. Flexion and extension X-rays are taken once radiographic bony fusion is observed and external orthosis is removed to look specifically for pseudoarthrosis and adjacent segment disease. Additional and/or subsequent imaging (including MRI and CT scans) are only obtained if there are new symptoms or suspicious findings radiographically. Esophageal perforations are best diagnosed with barium swallow and/or gastrografin imaging, though CT/MRI alone may detect abscesses or fluid collections.

Compared to posterior approaches to the spine, anterior approaches tend to require less pharmacologic pain management. In our practice, we stress the use of non-pharmacologic pain management techniques (correct usage of orthotics, ice packs, physical/massage therapy, etc.) prior to using any medication. However, if needed, we employ the use of acetaminophen for mild pain, long-acting benzodiazepines for muscle spasm, and small doses of opioids for severe pain. NSAIDs are generally avoided to reduce the risk of non-union.

External Orthosis

Vaccaro et al. [42] demonstrated similar fusion rates in two- and three-level corpectomies with halo application compared to cervical collars. It is our practice to apply Miami J collars immediately postoperatively to be maintained generally for 10 weeks or earlier if radiographic evidence of fusion without pseudoarthrosis is seen on X-rays. However, it should be noted that the duration of collar use is highly variable and unique to the individual patient and surgeon.

Case Illustration

A 42-year-old female presented to clinic with increasing numbness in both upper extremities and difficulty walking. She also complained of persistent pain in her left arm with associated clumsiness that worsened with activity and was alleviated with rest. She did not complain of any bowel or bladder symptomology, and there was no history of trauma. The patient had already tried physiotherapy and injections, but these did not alleviate her symptoms to her satisfaction. She was taking gabapentin and naproxen at the time of clinic presentation and was otherwise systemically well. On examination, the patient demonstrated bilateral upgoing plantar reflexes and a positive left Hoffman's sign. She demonstrated a mildly ataxic gait and subtle weakness in hand intrinsic muscles, again worse on the left side. MR imaging demonstrated significant cervical stenosis at the level of C5/6 and C6/7, with indentation and displacement of the spinal cord on the left (Fig. 23.1a, b). Subsequent CT scans demonstrated calcification of the osteophytic-ligamentous complex dorsal to the vertebral body of C6 (Fig. 23.2a, b). An incidental note was made of a previously implanted odontoid screw. Preoperative plain films showed straightening of cervical lordosis, but no overt kyphosis.

The decision was made to offer the patient surgery based on the progressive nature of her clinical symptoms with radiologic evidence of

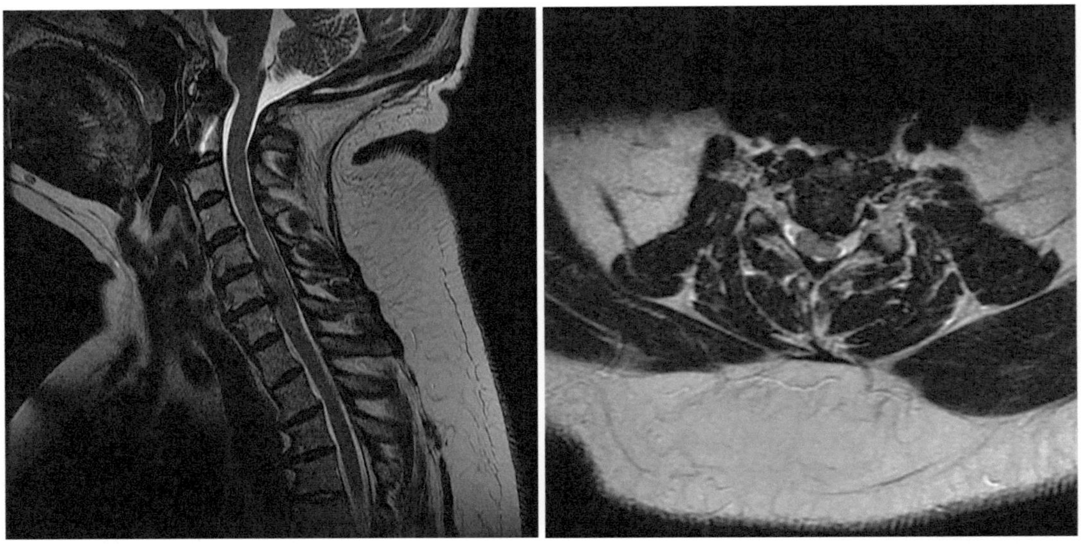

Fig. 23.1 (**a**) Sagittal T2-weighted magnetic resonance imaging demonstrating spinal cord compression posterior to the vertebral body of C6. (**b**): Axial T2-weighted magnetic resonance imaging at the midsection of the C6 vertebral body demonstrating spinal cord compression eccentric to the left

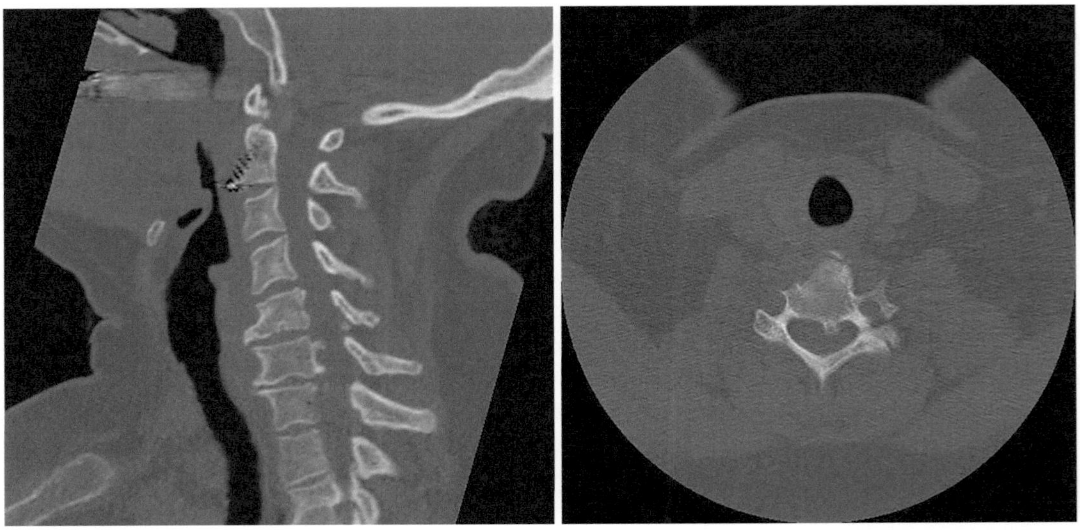

Fig. 23.2 (**a**) Sagittal CT scan confirming suspected calcification of the osteophyte-ligamentous complex behind the C6 vertebral body. (**b**): Axial CT scan showing calcification of the osteophyte-ligamentous complex behind the C6 vertebral body eccentric to the left

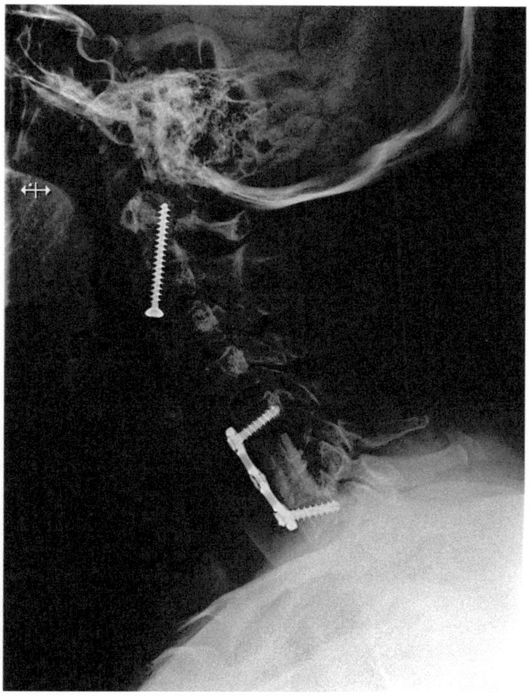

Fig. 23.3 Postoperative films. A full C6 corpectomy was performed with partial corpectomies at C5 and C7. The upright neutral plain film demonstrates good endplate contact with signs of early arthrodesis. No screw lucency or plate dislodgment is seen

spinal cord compression. Because of the primary location of compression behind the vertebral body, a C6 corpectomy was offered.

Intraoperatively, there were no complications, and the patient tolerated the procedure well. The patient was instructed to remain in a hard collar until reassessed in follow-up. At 9 weeks, the patient still had some residual numbness on the left upper extremity, but this was much improved. The patient's gait had also improved compared to her preoperative state but still had difficulty with tandem gait testing. Finally, plain films demonstrated early arthrodesis (Fig. 23.3) with no evidence of instability on dynamic films.

Conclusions

It is incumbent upon the surgeon to know the benefits and limitations of each procedure they perform. The anterior cervical corpectomy is no different, and the surgeon must weigh the benefit of increased exposure, decompression, or deformity correction with high rate of complications with increasing corpectomy levels. Moreover, adequate knowledge and extent of dissection of the anterior cervical soft tissues are paramount in facilitating the operation and reducing complication rates. Finally, while there exists a large variation in clinical practice, one should be aware of the advantages and disadvantages of each type of instrumentation or graft and apply them according to individual patient requirements.

References

1. Alleyne CH Jr, Rodts GE Jr, Haid RW. Corpectomy and stabilization with methylmethacrylate in patients with metastatic disease of the spine: a technical note. J Spinal Disord. 1995;8(6):439–43.
2. An HS, Gordin R, Renner K. Anatomic considerations for plate-screw fixation of the cervical spine. Spine (Phila Pa 1976). 1991;16(Suppl):S548–51.
3. Arts MP, Peul WC. Vertebral body replacement systems with expandable cages in the treatment of various spinal pathologies: a prospectively followed case series of 60 patients. Neurosurgery. 2008;63:537–44.
4. Beutler WJ, Sweeney CA, Connolly PJ. Recurrent laryngeal nerve injury with anterior cervical spine surgery risk with laterality of surgical approach. Spine (Phila Pa 1976). 2001;26(12):1337–42.
5. Boakye M, Patil CG, Ho C, Lad SP. Cervical corpectomy: complications and outcomes. Neurosurgery. 2008;63(Suppl 2):295–301.
6. Bulger RF, Rejowski JE, Beatty RA. Vocal cord paralysis associated with anterior cervical fusion: considerations for prevention and treatment. J Neurosurg. 1985;62(5):657–61.
7. Cannon RC. The anomaly of nonrecurrent laryngeal nerve: identification and management. Otolaryngol Head Neck Surg. 1999;120:769–71.
8. Chen Z, Liu B, Dong J, Feng F, Chen R, Xie P, Zhang L, Rong L. Comparison of anterior corpectomy and fusion versus laminoplasty for the treatment of cervical ossification of posterior longitudinal ligament: a meta-analysis. Neurosurg Focus. 2016;40(6):E8.
9. Cloward RB. The anterior approach for removal of ruptured cervical disks. J Neurosurg. 1958;15(6):602–17.
10. Dipaola CP, Jacobson JA, Awad H, et al. Screw orientation and plate type (variable- vs. fixed-angle) effect strength of fixation for in vitro biomechanical testing of the Synthes CSLP. Spine J. 2008;8:717–22.
11. Ebraheim NA, Lu J, Yang H, Heck BE, Yeasting RA. Vulnerability of the sympathetic trunk during the anterior approach to the lower cervical spine. Spine (Phila Pa 1976). 2000;25(13):1603–6.

12. Eskander MS, Drew JM, Aubin ME, Marvin J, Franklin PD, Eck JC, Patel N, Boyle K, Connolly PJ. Vertebral artery anatomy: a review of two hundred fifty magnetic resonance imaging scans. Spine (Phila Pa 1976). 2010;35(23):2035–40.
13. Fernyhough JC, White JI, LaRocca H. Fusion rates in multilevel cervical spondylosis comparing allograft fibula and autograft fibula in 126 patients. Spine (Phila Pa 1976). 1991;16(Suppl 10):561–4.
14. Hee HT, Majd ME, Holt RT, et al. Complications of multilevel cervical corpectomies and reconstruction with titanium cages and anterior plating. J Spinal Disord Tech. 2003;16:1–9.
15. Hilibrand AS, Carlson GD, Palumbo MA, Jones PK, Bohlman HH. Radiculopathy and myelopathy at segments adjacent to the site of a previous anterior cervical arthrodesis. J Bone Joint Surg Am. 1999;81(4):519–28.
16. Hong JT, Park DK, Lee MJ, et al. Anatomical variations of the vertebral artery segment in the lower cervical spine analysis by three-dimensional computed tomography angiography. Spine (Phila Pa 1976). 2008;33:2422–6.
17. Lau D, Chou D, Ziewacz JE, Mummaneni PV. The effects of smoking on perioperative outcomes and pseudarthrosis following anterior cervical corpectomy: clinical article. J Neurosurg Spine. 2014;21(4):547–58.
18. Lee JC, Lee SH, Peters C, Riew KD. Adjacent segment pathology requiring reoperation after anterior cervical arthrodesis: the influence of smoking, sex, and number of operated levels. Spine (Phila Pa 1976). 2015;40(10):E571–7.
19. Lee SH, Mesfin A, Riew KD. Delayed esophageal perforation after anterior cervical fusion and retropharyngeal steroid use: a report of two cases. Spine J. 2015;15(10):e75–80.
20. Lim TH, Kwon H, Jeon CH, et al. Effect of endplate conditions and bone mineral density on the compressive strength of the graft endplate interface in anterior cervical spine fusion. Spine (Phila Pa 1976). 2001;26:951–6.
21. Lunardini DJ, Eskander MS, Even JL, Dunlap JT, Chen AF, Lee JY, Ward TW, Kang JD, Donaldson WF. Vertebral artery injuries in cervical spine surgery. Spine J. 2014;14(8):1520–5.
22. Madhavan K, Benglis DM, Wang MY, Vanni S, Lebwohl N, Green BA, Levi AD. The use of modest systemic hypothermia after iatrogenic spinal cord injury during surgery. Ther Hypothermia Temp Manag. 2012;2(4):183–92.
23. McAfee PC, Bohlman HH, Ducker T, Eismont FJ. Failure of stabilization of the spine with methylmethacrylate. A retrospective analysis of twenty-four cases. J Bone Joint Surg Am. 1986;68(8):1145–57.
24. McAfee PC, Bohlman HH, Ducker TB, et al. One-stage anterior cervical decompression and posterior stabilization. A study of one hundred patients with a minimum of two years of followup. J Bone Joint Surg Am. 1995;77:1791–800.
25. Nassr A, Eck JC, Ponnappan RK, Zanoun RR, Donaldson WF III, Kang JD. The incidence of C5 palsy after multilevel cervical decompression procedures: a review of 750 consecutive cases. Spine (Phila Pa 1976). 2012;37(3):174–8.
26. Netterville JL, Koriwchak MJ, Winkle M, Courey MS, Ossoff RH. Vocal fold paralysis following the anterior approach to the cervical spine. Ann Otol Rhinol Laryngol. 1996;105:85–91.
27. Panjabi MM, Isomi T, Wang JL. Loosening at the screw-vertebra junction in multilevel anterior cervical plate constructs. Spine (Phila Pa 1976). 1999;24:2383–8.
28. Park JB, Cho YS, Riew KD. Development of adjacent-level ossification in patients with an anterior cervical plate. J Bone Joint Surg Am. 2005;87(3):558–63.
29. Pitzen TR, Chrobok J, Stulik J, et al. Implant complications, fusion, loss of lordosis, and outcome after anterior cervical plating with dynamic or rigid plates: two-year results of a multi-centric, randomized, controlled study. Spine (Phila Pa 1976). 2009;34:641–6.
30. Porter RW, Crawford NR, Chamberlain RH, Park SC, Detwiler PW, Apostolides PJ, et al. Biomechanical analysis of multilevel cervical corpectomy and plate constructs. J Neurosurg. 2003;99(1 Suppl):98–103.
31. Riew KD, Sethi N, Devney J, et al. Complications of buttress plate stabilization of cervical corpectomy. Spine (Phila Pa 1976). 1999;24:2404–10.
32. Sakaura H, Hosono N, Mukai Y, Ishii T, Yoshikawa H. C5 palsy after decompression surgery for cervical myelopathy: review of the literature. Spine (Phila Pa 1976). 2003;28:2447–51.
33. Sarkar S, Nair BR, Rajshekhar V. Complications following central corpectomy in 468 consecutive patients with degenerative cervical spine disease. Neurosurg Focus. 2016;40(6):E10.
34. Sasso RC, Ruggiero RA Jr, Reilly TM, et al. Early reconstruction failures after multilevel cervical corpectomy. Spine (Phila Pa 1976). 2003;28:140–2.
35. Saunders RL, Pikus HJ, Ball P. Four-level cervical corpectomy. Spine (Phila Pa 1976). 1998;23(22):2455–61.
36. Scoville WB, Palmer AH, Samra K, Chong G. The use of acrylic plastic for vertebral replacement or fixation in metastatic disease of the spine. Technical note. J Neurosurg. 1967;27(3):274–9.
37. Shields LB, Raque GH, Glassman SD, Campbell M, Vitaz T, Harpring J, et al. Adverse effects associated with high dose recombinant human bone morphogenetic protein-2 use in anterior cervical spine fusion. Spine (Phila Pa 1976). 2006;31:542–7.
38. Smith GW, Robinson RA. The treatment of certain cervical-spine disorders by anterior removal of the intervertebral disc and interbody fusion. J Bone Joint Surg Am. 1958;40-A(3):607–24.
39. Smith MD, Emery SE, Dudley A, et al. Vertebral artery injury during anterior decompression of the cervical spine. J Bone Joint Surg Br. 1993;75:410–5.
40. Smucker JD, Rhee JM, Singh K, Yoon ST, Heller JG. Increased swelling complications associated with

off-label usage of rhBMP-2 in the anterior cervical spine. Spine (Phila Pa 1976). 2006;31:2813–9.
41. Stulik J, Pitzen TR, Chrobok J, et al. Fusion and failure following anterior cervical plating with dynamic or rigid plates: 6-months results of a multicentric, prospective, randomized, controlled study. Eur Spine J. 2007;16:1689–94.
42. Vaccaro AR, Falatyn SP, Scuderi GJ, Eismont FJ, McGuire RA, Singh K, Garfin SR. Early failure of long segment anterior cervical plate fixation. J Spinal Disord. 1998;11(5):410–5.
43. Wang JC, Hart RA, Emery SE, Bohlman HH. Graft migration or displacement after multilevel cervical corpectomy and strut grafting. Spine (Phila Pa 1976). 2003;28:1016–21.
44. Weisberg NK, Spengler DM, Netterville JL. Stretch-induced nerve injury as a cause of paralysis secondary to the anterior cervical approach. Otolaryngol Head Neck Surg. 1997;116:317–26.
45. Young WF, Rosenwasser RH. An early comparative analysis of the use of fibular allograft versus autologous iliac crest graft for interbody fusion after anterior cervical discectomy. Spine (Phila Pa 1976). 1993;18:1123–4.
46. Zdeblick TA, Ducker TB. The use of freeze-dried allograft bone for anterior cervical fusions. Spine (Phila Pa 1976). 1991;16:726–9.

Multilevel ACDF Versus Corpectomy

24

Hani R. Malone and Michael G. Kaiser

Pearls

- The laterality of pathology should dictate the side of exposure – contralateral exposure offers the best line of sight, particularly with foraminal pathology.
- Evaluate patients for dynamic myelopathy preoperatively by determining if symptoms can be elicited with physiologic range of motion, including extension and flexion (Lhermitte's sign).
- Preoperative skin localization should be performed with fluoroscopy and slightly rostral to the intended level, as most surgeons follow a slightly caudal trajectory during exposure.
- Release retractors, and irrigate the wound every 15–20 min to mitigate the risk of retraction injury and swelling.
- Transect the omohyoid to decrease tension during retraction, particularly in multilevel operations involving the caudal cervical spine.
- Attaching a retractor system to a table-mounted articulating arm or utilization of a table-mounted retractor system will stabilize retractor blades and prevent blades from riding over the longus colli muscles.
- Maintain the integrity of the posterior longitudinal ligament if decompression is not required to accentuate lordosis during distraction.
- Maximize surface area contact between the graft interface and vertebral endplate.

Pitfalls

- Insufficient evaluation of preoperative imaging and failure to recognize anatomic anomalies, such as a medially displaced vertebral artery.
- Failure to utilize preoperative upright x-rays to assess cervical alignment.
- Neglecting the relative position of the mandible angle or sternum when attempting to access the rostral or caudal extremes of the cervical spine.
- Inadequate soft tissue exposure (especially superficial/sub-platysmal), compromising the assessment of midline and the width of decompression as well as increasing retraction force.

H. R. Malone · M. G. Kaiser (✉)
Department of Neurological Surgery, Columbia University Medical Center, New York, NY, USA
e-mail: mgk7@cumc.columbia.edu

M. G. Kaiser et al. (eds.), *Degenerative Cervical Myelopathy and Radiculopathy*, https://doi.org/10.1007/978-3-319-97952-6_24

- Asymmetric, and potentially insufficient, decompression resulting from the limited line of sight provided by inadequate exposure.
- Failure to resect prominent lateral/ventral osteophytes that obstruct proper retractor blade position under the longus colli muscles and placement of ventral cervical stabilization plate.
- Aggressive endplate decortication leading to graft subsidence.
- Overestimation of anterior cervical plate length leading to mechanical compromise of the adjacent disc space or potential screw violation of the adjacent disc space.

Introduction

Cervical spondylosis and the resulting neurological impairment are among the most common conditions treated by spine surgeons. Affected patients may present with an array of signs and symptoms, including axial neck pain, radicular arm pain, focal weakness or numbness, and myelopathy. When surgery is indicated, the most appropriate strategy depends on both established clinical principles, the experience of the operating surgeon, and the wants/desires of the patient. Effective management requires a comprehensive and individualized approach rooted in an evidence-based treatment algorithm.

Anterior approaches to the cervical spine are routinely used to treat degenerative cervical spondylosis, as well as traumatic, neoplastic, and infectious pathologies [1–3]. Improved clinical outcomes following the two most common procedures, anterior cervical discectomy and fusion (ACDF) and cervical corpectomy, are well established in the literature [4–8]. Both techniques can be effectively used to alleviate pain and improve function by decompressing the neural elements and restoring stability and alignment to the cervical spine. However, there are inherent advantages and disadvantages associated with each technique that may favor ACDF or corpectomy in a given case.

In this chapter, we will discuss anterior approaches to multilevel cervical pathology, including indications, surgical strategy, and technique. The advantages and disadvantages of cervical corpectomy will be compared and contrasted with multilevel ACDF. Special attention will be paid to a growing body of evidence that supports the use of a hybrid approach in select clinical scenarios, which incorporates both ACDF and corpectomy in a single construct.

ACDF and Corpectomy

Surgical strategy for anterior approaches to the cervical spine is contingent upon a myriad of factors, including but not limited to the extent, location, and nature of the compressive pathology, regional and global alignment, risk of pseudoarthrosis, and biomechanical stability. The extent of the pathology is a primary factor to consider when determining an appropriate surgical approach. When the pathology is confined to the disc space across one or two levels, discectomy is the straightforward choice (Figs. 24.1a and 24.2a). When the compressive pathology extends beyond two levels, the decision-making process regarding surgical approach becomes more complicated (Fig. 24.1b). Multilevel discectomies may be selected if compression is isolated to the intervertebral discs; however, an increased risk of swallowing complications has to be accepted with a multilevel ventral exposure [9]. Although definitive evidence is lacking, recent comparative studies indicate that in the presence of clinical equipoise, the ventral approach may provide improved outcomes [10].

Once the decision is made to undertake a ventral approach, the location and nature of the compressive pathology becomes an important consideration. If the offending ventral pathology is immobile calcified, and/or extends behind the vertebral body (Fig. 24.2b, c), corpectomy is often necessary for a safe and effective decompression. This is particularly true for patients

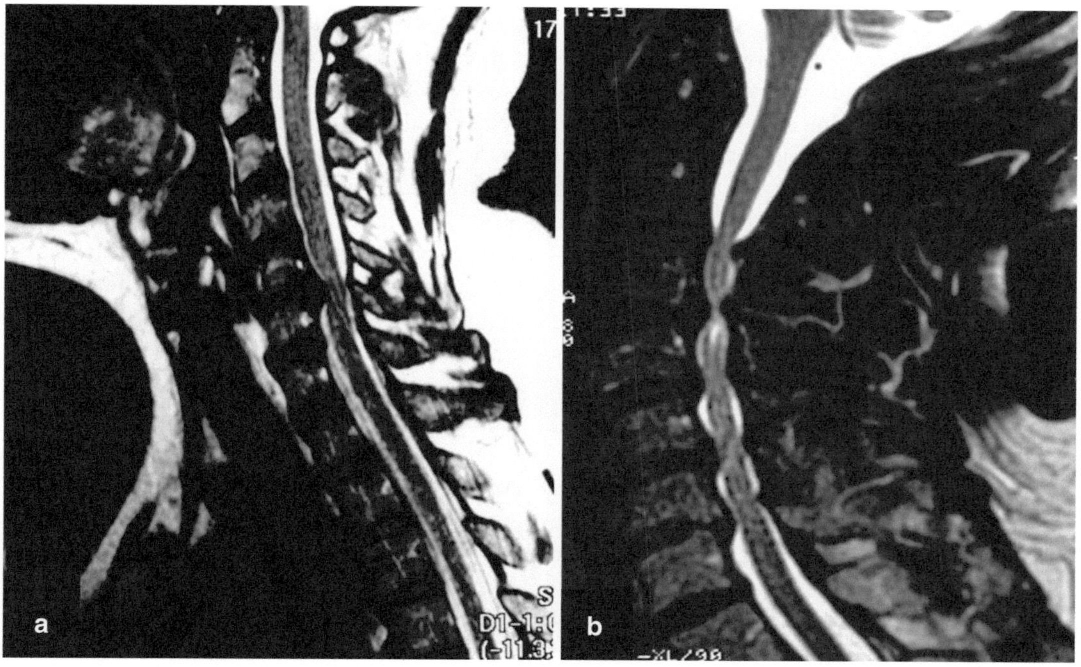

Fig. 24.1 Sagittal T2-weighted MRI sequences depicting cervical spondylosis. Cases that affect a single level (**a**) can generally be addressed with cervical discectomy. However, treatment paradigms for multilevel pathology (**b**) are often more complex

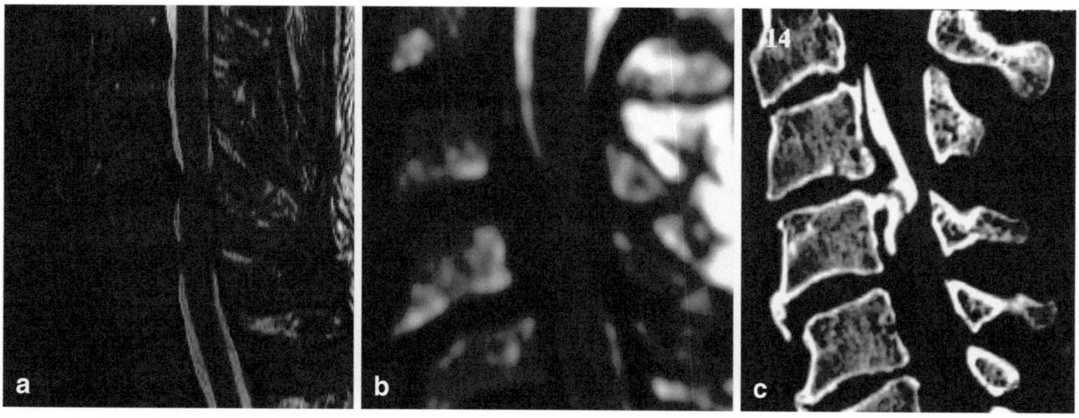

Fig. 24.2 When ventral pathology is confined primarily to the disc space (**a**), single- or multilevel discectomies are appropriate. However, when the offending pathology extends behind the vertebral body (**b**) or is calcified and immobile (**c**), corpectomy is required for safe decompression, regardless of the number of levels involved

with a kyphotic alignment due to the potential for "draping" of the spinal cord over persistent ventral pathology. Due to biomechanical limitations of corpectomies extending beyond two segments [11], consideration of either a supplemental posterior approach or a hybrid construct is required for pathology that extends beyond three levels.

The impact of sagittal alignment on clinical outcome has recently been recognized as a relevant factor for multilevel cervical reconstructions [12, 13]. The ability to restore or maintain appropriate sagittal balance is contingent on a careful preoperative assessment of upright lateral x-rays to determine the patient's baseline cervical posture. In general, multiple cervical discectomies are more effective at restoring cervical lordosis. The multiple release points allow for incremental reduction across each disc space, and the additional fixation points provide an opportunity to reduce the spine when applying the ventral cervical fixation plate [14]. The greater number of graft-endplate interfaces however comes with an increased risk of pseudoarthrosis [8, 15]. The development of dynamic cervical plates may partially mitigate this pseudoarthrosis risk by exposing the grafts to fusion-promoting forces, known as "load-sharing." [16] Although shorter fusion times have been associated with the use of dynamic plates, studies have failed to demonstrate an increased fusion rate due to this theoretical benefit [16–18]. Dynamic plates have also been associated with increased loss of lordosis and greater subsidence that may negatively impact adjacent segments over time (Fig. 24.3) [16–18]. A benefit of corpectomy is the reduced number of graft-endplate interfaces required for successful arthrodesis. Retrospective studies and a more recent meta-analysis comparing corpectomy with strut grafting to multilevel ACDF have consistently found lower pseudoarthrosis rates in the corpectomy group, although these studies are limited to one- and two-level corpectomies [8, 15, 19].

In addition to fewer fusion interfaces, a corpectomy allows for the harvesting of local autograft. Although autograft can be harvested from the iliac crest to augment fusion following multilevel discectomy, the morbidity associated with graft harvest is significant and often underestimated by the treating surgeon [20]. The evolution of synthetic interbody devices allows for the simultaneous use of local morselized autograft while providing structural support. For patients at increased risk of pseudoarthrosis, the use of bone morphogenetic protein (BMP) remains controversial. Complications, including dysphasia and respiratory issues, are dose-dependent and therefore more problematic when utilized during multilevel procedures [21]. These questions regarding appropriate dosing as well as the relative cost-effectiveness of BMP have to be carefully considered given the efficacy of traditional fusion alterantives [1, 6, 7, 21]. The use of BMP however remains an option under certain circumstances; however, a detailed discussion between patient and surgeon is advised, including the non-cleared FDA status of BMP for cervical surgery, so that there is complete understanding

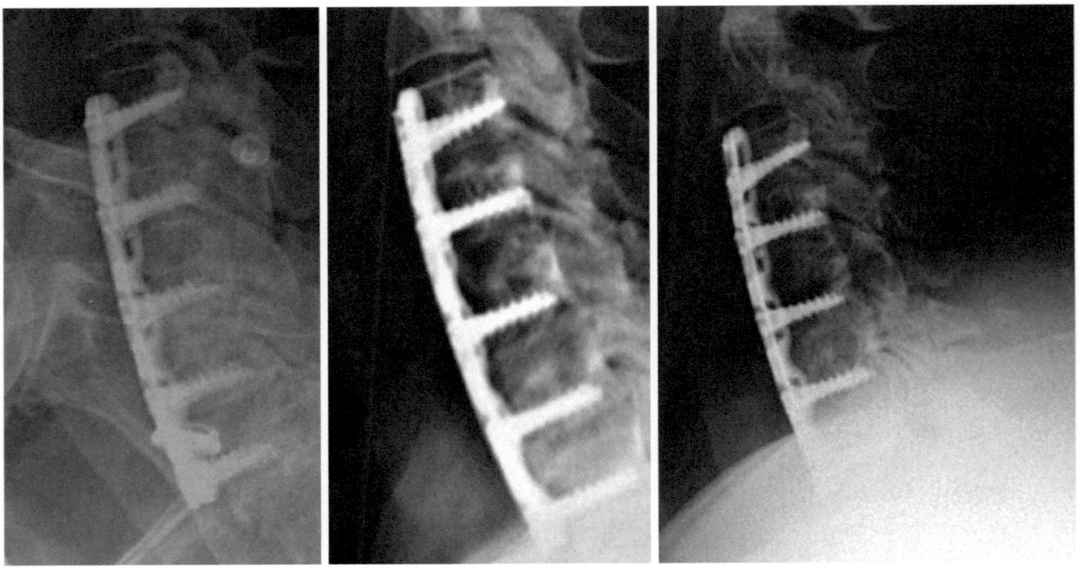

Fig. 24.3 The potential for excessive subsidence leading to plate impingement on adjacent segments can occur with dynamic plates across multiple levels. This sequence of postoperative x-rays demonstrates this phenomenon over time

regarding the risks and limitations associated with the application of BMP.

Despite the relative advantage of corpectomy in regard to fusion rate, data from retrospective clinical studies underscore several biomechanical limitations of the procedure, particularly with longer constructs. Sasso and colleagues found that corpectomies extending beyond two segments will generally fail [11]. At a mean follow-up of 21 months, after three-level corpectomy and reconstruction with iliac crest strut graft and a fixed cervical plate, the authors report 71% failure rate, while only 6% of two-level corpectomies failed at 31 months. The authors concluded that beyond two levels, corpectomy constructs should be supplemented by posterior instrumented fusion [11].

Biomechanically, the increased failure rate of longer corpectomy constructs is explained by the length of the lever arm and the resulting torque exerted on the sole fixation points at the terminal ends of the construct. The moment load transmitted at the intervertebral graft-endplate interface is directly proportional to the length of the graft. Likewise, longer cervical plates (without intervening screws) used across a multilevel corpectomy lead to increased stress and failure at the terminal ends of the construct. The application of an anterior plate also shifts the instantaneous axis of rotation (IAR) ventrally. This effectively reverses the loading pattern experienced in long strut grafts, with minimal loading in flexion and excessive compressive stress in extension. Clinically, this increases the likelihood of a "pistoning effect," a common failure pattern in which the cervical plate "kicks out" as the graft telescopes through the caudal vertebral body (Fig. 24.4). Augmenting a corpectomy construct with a posterior fusion shifts the IAR closer to its physiologic position toward the dorsal half of the vertebral body, protecting the graft from excessive loads in extension [22].

The segmental fixation points created across a multilevel discectomy significantly enhance rigidity with regard to flexion-extension and lateral bending, compared to the terminal fixation with a corpectomy [23, 24]. Segmental fixation truncates the acting lever arm and resulting moment loads that lead to early failure in longer corpectomy constructs. The importance of interval fixation was made salient in a retrospective study by Ashkenazi and colleagues in which patients underwent multiple corpectomies, but with an intervening vertebral body facilitating interval fixation. In this study, a 95% fusion rate with a stable or improved neurological exam was achieved at 29 months [25]. Cadaveric studies by Porter [24] and Singh [23] have also demonstrated that pullout and bending forces are more evenly distributed through multiple points of fixation. Interestingly, Porter and colleagues found that the addition of an intervening fixation point, by attaching the cervical plate to the midpoint of the strut graft, significantly improved the biomechanical stability of three-level (but not two-level) corpectomy constructs [24].

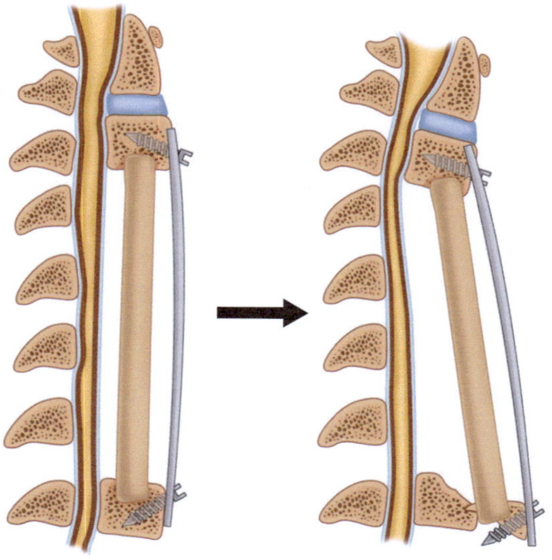

Fig. 24.4 Longer corpectomy constructs (beyond two levels) with a strut graft and cervical plate create significant lever arms that alter the IAR, stress the terminal ends of the construct, and often lead to distal failure with graft kick out. (From Benzel [36]; with permission)

Hybrid Constructs

There is growing evidence that hybrid constructs can be effectively used as an intermediate strategy that overcomes many of the limitations inherent to multilevel discectomy or corpectomy [26]. In a hybrid procedure, one or two corpectomies are performed in conjunction with one or more discectomies, and a single cervical plate is used to bridge the length of the construct (Fig. 24.5). The additional fixation point afforded by the intervening vertebral body improves biomechanical strength and provides an additional fulcrum for reduction and alignment correction. The corpectomy component of the hybrid construct allows access to pathology dorsal to the vertebral body, increases the line of sight for effective decompression, provides local autograft, and reduces the number of fusion interfaces and potentially the risk of pseudoarthrosis. The hybrid technique also offers the potential for enhanced deformity correction by "pulling" the spine to the plate through a lag effect and creating a three-point bending construct (Fig. 24.6), similar to what has been demonstrated across a multilevel discectomy.

In the aforementioned cadaveric study by Porter et al., hybrid constructs consisting of a two-level corpectomy and adjacent discectomy provided better immediate biomechanical stability than three-level corpectomy constructs of equal length [24]. Hussain and colleagues conducted a similar comparative analysis, attempting to quantify stress measurements at the graft-endplate and bone-screw interfaces following two-level corpectomy, three-level ACDF, and hybrid reconstructions. Instead of cadavers, a finite element computational model was used, again demonstrating the increased stability provided by interval fixation points in multilevel ACDF and hybrid constructs [27]. Importantly, the cadaveric and computational models above only estimate the short-term stability of these constructs and provide no information about implant fatigue and long-term stability.

There is retrospective clinical evidence supporting the durability of hybrid constructs. In the study by Ashkenazi et al., 24/25 (96%) CSM patients with hybrid constructs were fused at 29-month follow-up [25]. More recent data comes from Xu et al. who retrospectively analyzed 59 patients receiving either two-level corpectomy or a corpectomy/discectomy hybrid construct for CSM. In this study, 7 of the 39 (18%) patients treated with two-level corpectomy experienced graft/plate migrations or dislodgements, while there were no implant complications among 20 patients treated via the hybrid method [28]. Data from this study was recently pooled with four similar studies from China and Japan in a meta-analysis by Liu

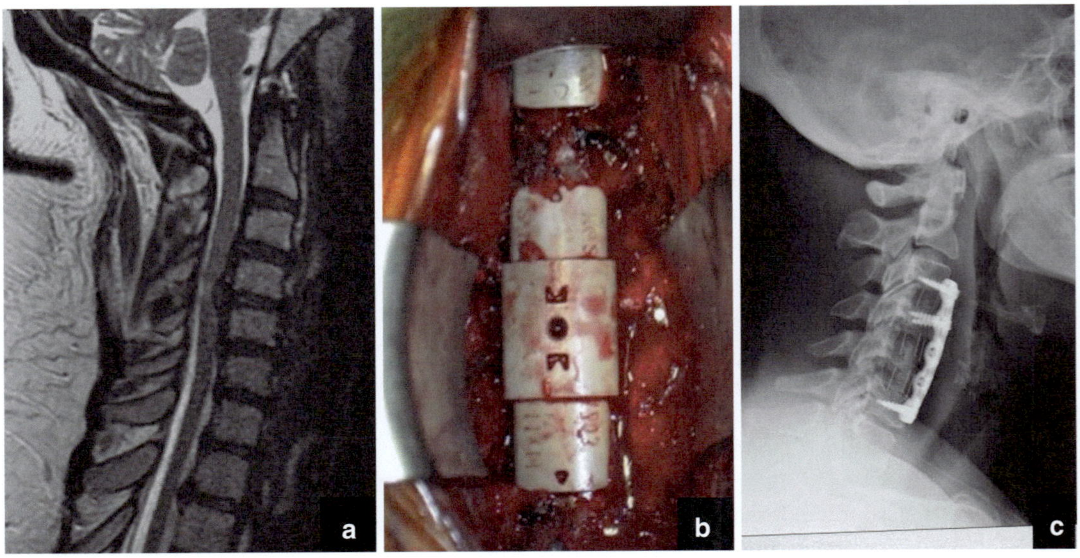

Fig. 24.5 Preoperative MRI (**a**), intraoperative image (**b**), and postoperative lateral x-ray (**c**) illustrating the combination of corpectomy and ACDF used in "hybrid" anterior cervical constructs

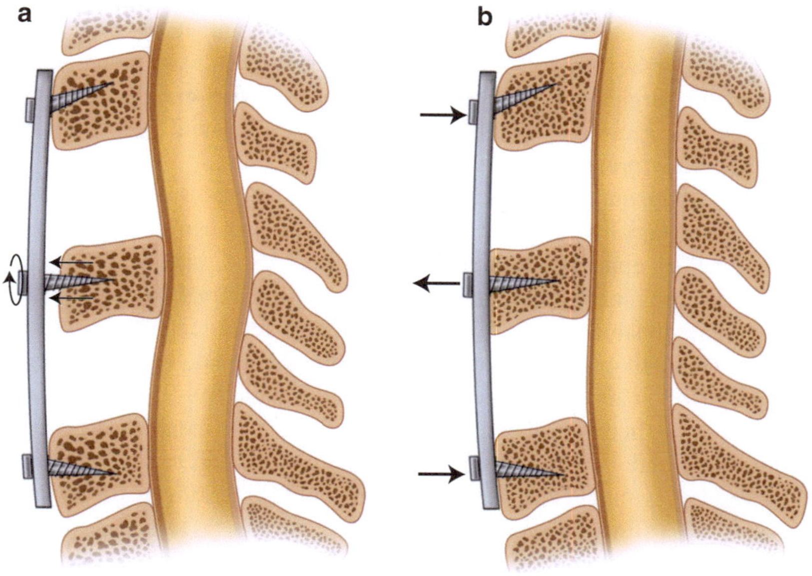

Fig. 24.6 There are significant biomechanical advantages to maintaining an intervening point of fixation when performing a multilevel ventral decompression. The intervening fixation points allow for "pulling" of the spine to the implant through a lag effect that enhances deformity reduction (**a**) and creates a three-point bending construct that increases resistance to translational stresses (**b**). (From Kaiser [3]; with permission)

et al., comparing clinical outcomes of the hybrid technique to corpectomy in the treatment of CSM. In total, 356 patients with 3–4-level CSM were studied (160 corpectomy, 196 hybrid). Hybrid constructs were associated with both higher rates of fusion and fewer complications, but no significant difference was found in clinical outcome measures (mJOA, NDI) [26].

Some have argued that the biomechanical advantages of hybrid constructs coupled with promising early clinical results obviate the need for staged circumferential procedures in the treatment of multilevel CSM [25]. But most agree that regardless of which anterior reconstruction strategy is utilized, the added durability of posterior stabilization should be considered whenever patients are at significantly increased risk of pseudoarthrosis or early implant failure [3, 22]. There is currently no prospective data available to compare and contrast the relative efficacy of multilevel ACDF, corpectomy, and hybrid constructs. The myriad of clinical factors that influence surgeons to favor a particular reconstruction strategy in a given clinical scenario makes treatment difficult to randomize. Nevertheless, retrospective data have demonstrated that, when used appropriately, multilevel ACDF, corpectomy, and hybrid constructs all represent effective treatment strategies for multilevel cervical pathology.

Indications/Contraindications

The most straightforward surgical indication remains the onset of significant or progressive neurologic deficits with a radiographic correlate. Surgery is also warranted for those patients with myelopathy or radicular pain that is unresponsive to conservative therapy and significantly compromises the patient's quality of life [6, 7]. Surgical treatment for purely axial neck pain without neurologic symptoms or significant spinal deformity remains controversial, as there is no definitive test to accurately identify the pain source.

Anterior Versus Posterior Approaches

When the decision to pursue surgery has been made, formulating the surgical plan starts by deciding on whether an anterior, posterior, or combined/circumferential procedure is most appropriate. Cervical alignment and the location/extent of pathology play equally important roles when determining which approach to pursue. When multilevel decompression is required, posterior approaches are reasonable in patients with lordotic alignment, which allows the spinal cord to migrate dorsally following decompression (Figs. 24.7a and 24.8a) [1]. In this scenario, laminectomy, laminoplasty, and laminectomy with fusion are all appropriate without clear superiority of one approach [1–3]. Although laminoplasty preserves the posterior ligamentous tension band, it is likely to be less advantageous in cases of kyphotic alignment [1, 29]. Conversely, multilevel laminectomy and fusion are viable options for patients with straight or kyphotic alignment, as long as postural reduction restores sagittal balance [2, 3].

However, most would advocate for an anterior approach for patients who lack cervical lordosis (Figs. 24.7b, c, and 24.8b) or with significant ventral pathology (Fig. 24.2c) [5]. A combined approach, featuring both anterior and posterior decompression and or stabilization, may be indicated for patients with a severe or fixed cervical deformity, poor bone quality, or other medical comorbidities that increase the risk of pseudoarthrosis [22]. Treatment paradigms outlining the order, timing, and reconstruction strategies involved with these staged procedures are

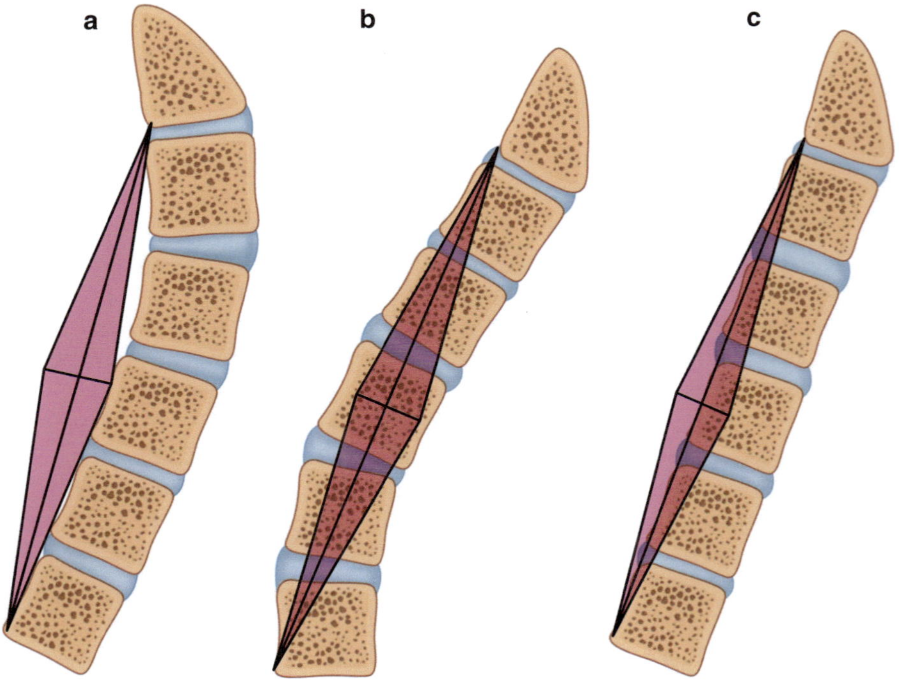

Fig. 24.7 A qualitative assessment of cervical sagittal alignment can be made by extending a line from the dorsocaudal aspect of C2 to the identical point on C7. Image (**a**) depicts lordosis with the vertebral bodies ventral to line between C2 and C7. Conversely, image (**b**) depicts kyphosis, where the line lies ventral to the subaxial vertebrae. Figure (**c**) depicts a straight spine, where the line runs parallel to the posterior aspect of the vertebrae. (From Benzel [36]; with permission)

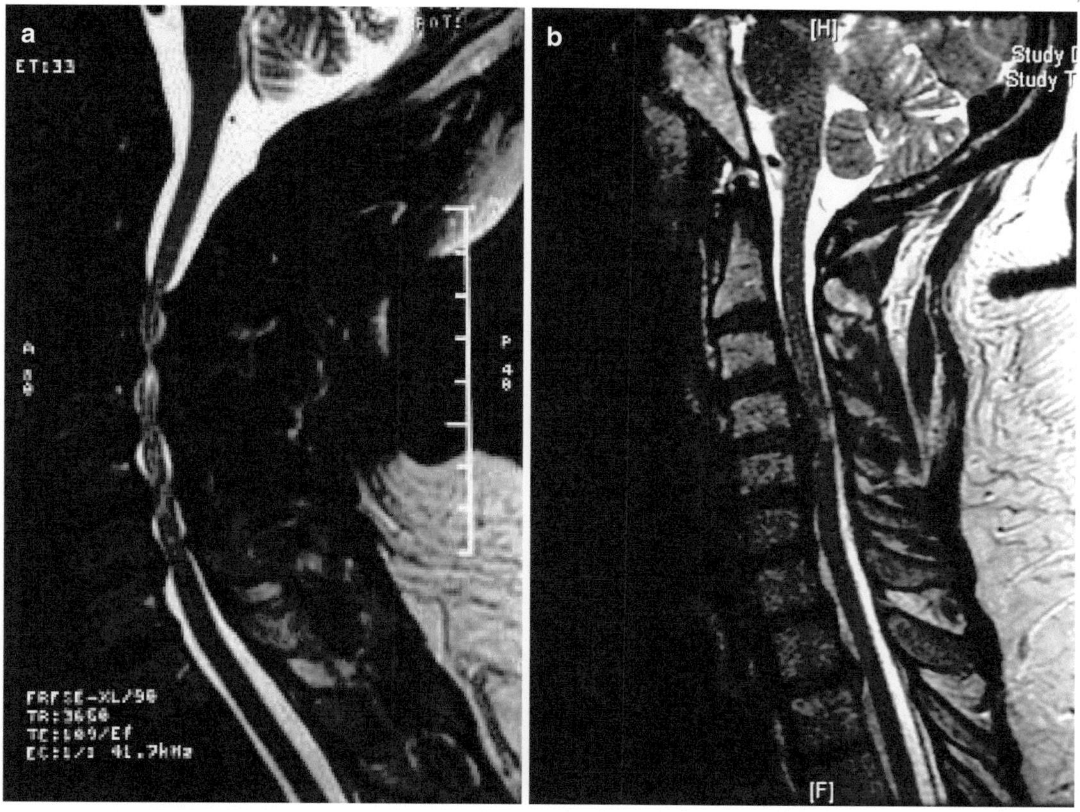

Fig. 24.8 T2-weighted sagittal MRI images contrasting patients who would be good candidates for posterior (**a**) versus anterior (**b**) surgical approaches to cervical spondylosis

multifactorial and highly dependent on surgeon preference/experience.

In general, patients should be involved in the decision-making process regarding the choice of surgical strategy. It is important, for example, that elderly patients are well-informed regarding the potential for dysphagia following multilevel ventral approaches. Likewise, previous anterior cervical surgery, radiation therapy, or the presence of a pre-existing recurrent laryngeal nerve (RLN) injury may lead the surgeon to favor a posterior approach for pathology that would be conventionally treated anteriorly. Accordingly, treatment algorithms cannot be broadly applied based on radiographic or clinical data alone. There remains no standard approach, and unique characteristics of each patient need to be considered to generate an optimal surgical strategy.

Preoperative Planning

Once the surgical plan has been formulated, detailed planning regarding instrumentation, patient positioning, and anesthetic considerations is critical to achieving an optimal outcome. Various preoperative assessments must be considered under certain circumstances. In reoperations, laryngoscopy can detect deficiencies of RLN function and resulting vocal cord paralysis that might dictate the side of approach [30]. Accordingly, anterior approaches contralateral to a pre-existing RLN injury should not be attempted given the potential for bilateral injury. Although not routinely performed, preoperative swallowing studies may also be helpful by alerting the surgeon to pre-existing subclinical pharyngeal dysfunction that increases the potential for significant postoperative dysphagia. Although most episodes of dysphagia are transient and resolve within 6 months, the complication remains underreported and poorly recognized by clinicians [30].

Imaging

Comprehensive assessment of preoperative radiographic studies is imperative. This should begin with upright cervical x-rays with dynamic flexion/extension views to appraise cervical alignment and stability. A qualitative assessment can be quickly made from upright lateral x-rays by drawing a midsagittal line from the dorsocaudal aspect of C2 vertebral body to the same point on C7. The cervical spine is considered to be in effective kyphosis if the dorsal aspect of any subaxial vertebral body crosses this line (Fig. 24.7). Upright x-rays should also be used to ensure that the relative position of the angle of mandible will not obstruct anterior access to the rostral cervical spine. Determining the level of the sternum, which may interfere with caudal access, may be difficult to assess with plain x-rays and often requires an analysis of either CT or MR imaging.

MR imaging is the primary modality for assessing the quality, location, and extent of pathology compressing the neural elements. Signal changes on T1- and T2-weighted sequences can identify acute disc herniation, presence of calcified tissue, acute or chronic spinal cord injury, and Modic changes in the vertebral endplates. CT myelogram remains advantageous in those patients who cannot undergo an MRI or who have had previous spinal instrumentation that would compromise the resolution of the MR image. Standard computed tomography remains the best method of assessing the quality of the bone and defining osteophytes or other calcified pathologies. Reformatted CT sequences in the sagittal and coronal planes are particularly useful in planning the appropriate length and trajectory of fixation points. Special attention should be given to the position of the foramen transversarium and potential anatomic aberrancies of the vertebral arteries, particularly if a corpectomy is planned.

Implants

There are numerous options to choose from when selecting an interbody graft. The joint guidelines from the AANS/CNS underscore available Class II evidence in support of the effectiveness of iliac crest autograft, cadaveric iliac or femur allograft, and titanium cages in promoting arthrodesis in one- or two-level ACDF [21]. Class III evidence is available for the use of polyetheretherketone (PEEK) and carbon fiber cages in the same clinical scenario. Although bone morphogenetic protein (*rhBMP-2*) may be a useful adjunct in patients at particularly high risk of pseudoarthrosis, it is associated with a complication rate of between 23% and 27%, and current evidence does not support its routine use [21].

A multitude of cervical plating systems with an array of different fixation and locking mechanisms are also available. There is retrospective evidence that the use of anterior cervical plating for 1–2-level ACDF significantly reduces the risk of pseudoarthrosis with minimal plate-associated complications [31]. Anterior cervical plates also serve to restore stability, maintain alignment, lower graft complications, and lessen the need for external orthosis [3]. When choosing a plate, the number of levels involved, availability of fixation points, bone quality, and risk of pseudoarthrosis should be considered. The best plates are strong, low profile, and easy to use. Dynamic plating systems are generally preferred for multilevel cervical spondylosis constructs, as they transmit fusion-enhancing forces to the graft according to Wolff's law [16]. For reasons previously discussed, appropriate plate sizing and positioning are important considerations for multilevel procedures.

Anesthesia, Preoperative Medications, and Neuromonitoring

When cervical cord compression or spinal instability causing myelopathy is present, an awake fiber-optic intubation may be considered to avoid unrestricted manipulation of the patient's neck leading to inadvertent cord compromise. Additional monitoring devices, including an esophageal thermometer or a nasogastric tube, may be avoided to minimize esophageal/laryngeal compression during operative retraction. Perioperative antibiotics with sufficient gram-positive coverage should be started within an hour prior to skin incision [32]. At our institution, weight-based dosing of cefazolin is routine, with vancomycin reserved for those patients allergic to penicillin. Pneumatic compression stockings are applied to mitigate the risk of lower extremity venous thrombosis.

The use of intraoperative neurophysiologic monitoring (IONM) for cervical surgery, even in the presence of cord compression, remains a controversial issue. The ability of IONM to *prevent* an injury has never been established. However, when reversible actions are considered, such as deformity correction or distraction, the use of IONM may be beneficial [33]. Baseline electrophysiological monitoring including somatosensory evoked potentials (SSEPs), motor evoked potentials (MEPs), and free-running electromyography are all modalities that can be utilized during ventral cervical surgery. The operating surgeon, the anesthesiologist, and the monitoring team must coordinate the anesthetic technique, with minimal use of paralytics, to allow for a recordable signal. Prepositioning baselines should be obtained in the context of cord compression/myelopathy or spinal instability so that changes can be detected during positioning and operative maneuvers.

Surgical Technique

Positioning

Patients' tolerance to cervical rotation, flexion, and extension should be assessed preoperatively while the patient is awake. This evaluation can disclose any dynamic aspect to the neurological dysfunction and provide information that can be incorporated during patient positioning. At our institution, patients are positioned for anterior cervical exposure with either a Jackson table (Mizuho OSI, Union City, CA) and flat board or a standard electric table with the Caspar head holder extension (Aesculap, Center Valley, PA). Using the Caspar head holder, the neck is placed in slight extension with the support bar high and angled caudally (Fig. 24.9). Additional extension and stabilization are then achieved with the chinstrap.

If the Jackson table or regular headrest is used, a shoulder roll can be placed to promote extension and head position maintained by placing tape across the forehead to the table. The Jackson table offers the ability to place patients in traction while supine, which may assist in any reduction maneuvers. Compression and stretch injury to exposed peripheral nerves is prevented by positioning extremities at angles less than 90° and padding all compression points. An added benefit of IONM is the ability to detect peripheral nerve irritation from inadequate positioning.

Planning the Incision

The laterality of pathology should dictate the side of approach. A contralateral approach offers the best line of sight. If pathology is midline or symmetric, some favor a left-sided approach because of the consistent course of RLN in the tracheoesophageal groove, as opposed to more variable course of the right RLN. Importantly, despite several cadaveric studies to the contrary, there is no definitive clinical data that suggests the right RLN is at greater risk during anterior cervical exposure [34].

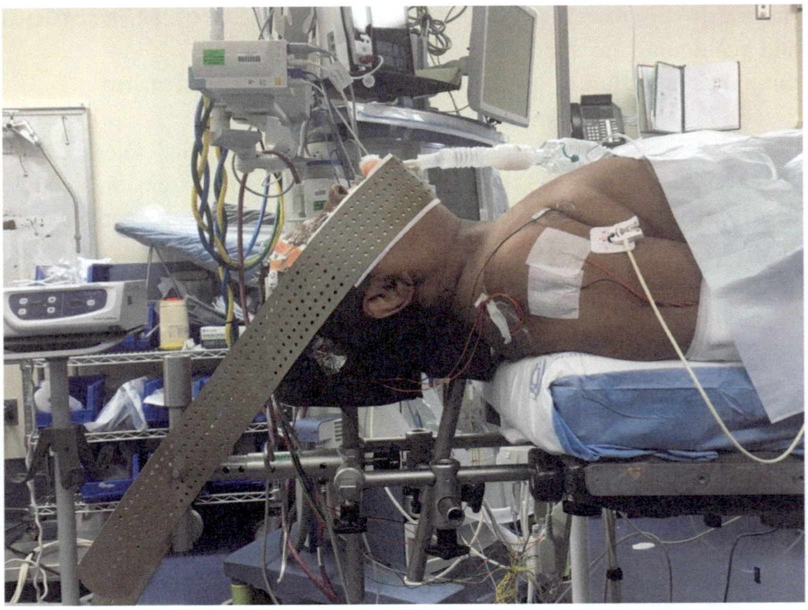

Fig. 24.9 Patient positioning for anterior cervical exposure using the Caspar head holder extension (Aesculap, Center Valley, PA). The neck is placed in slight extension with the neck bar high and angled caudally. Additional extension and stabilization are then achieved with the chinstrap, which is padded and placed firmly

As a result, some right-handed surgeons prefer the ergonomics of a right-sided approach if pathology does not dictate otherwise [30].

In most cases, we prefer a transverse skin incision, starting just lateral to the midline and extending to the medial border of the sternocleidomastoid. This incision generally measures 3–4 cm in length, but larger exposures require longer incisions. The incision should be planned in a skin crease when possible, to achieve the best cosmetic result. The hip should also be prepped if iliac crest autograft harvest is planned. Rostral-caudal localization can be achieved with lateral fluoroscopy. We generally bias the incision slightly rostral to the intended level to compensate for the caudal trajectory during the exposure. Prior to cutting the skin, local anesthetic (1% lidocaine with epinephrine) is injected subcutaneously along the incision, not only for analgesia but to limit bleeding and cautery near the skin edges.

Dissection and Exposure

The platysma is identified following the skin incision. Division of this muscle may be achieved both perpendicular and parallel to the muscle fiber orientation, depending on surgeon preference. A generous circumferential sub-platysmal dissection, achieved through a combination of blunt finger dissection and spreading with the Metzenbaum scissors, is critical. Failure to achieve an adequate sub-platysmal release will tether the soft tissue at its most superficial attachment and increase the pressure required for retraction. It is essential that all fascial attachments be released in a superficial to deep fashion to maximize exposure and decrease incidence of retraction injury.

The sternocleidomastoid (SCM) is a key anatomical landmark. Care should be taken to avoid entering the SCM fascia and muscle fibers. Instead, dissection should be carried out in the avascular plane of connective tissue just medial to the SCM. With this plane defined, the carotid artery is palpated. Dissection is continued just medial to the carotid sheath, retracting the tracheoesophageal bundle medially while bluntly dissecting toward the ventral cervical spine. Dissection may be limited by the omohyoid muscle, which intersects the field in an inferior-lateral to superior-medial direction usually at the level of C5/6. For multilevel procedures, we routinely transect the omohyoid to achieve wider release and improve line of sight. Bridging fascial attachments and/or vascular structures are identified and sharply divided. Larger venous channels may require a suture ligature prior to transection. Soft tissue dissection should be continued until the prevertebral fascia is encountered.

Once the ventral surface of the cervical spine is reached, recognizable landmarks include the elevated "peaks" representing the disc space/osteophytes and "valleys" representing the vertebral bodies and the paired bodies of the longus colli muscles. Localization is performed with intraoperative fluoroscopic imaging to confirm the appropriate levels. We utilize a bent spinal needle, placed into the exposed disc space to confirm localization, with the bend preventing the needle from being inadvertently inserted too deep. Once the appropriate level is localized, a localizing mark can be made with monopolar cautery without losing sight of the operative field and marked level.

Elevation of the anterior longitudinal ligament and longus colli muscles is then performed. A subperiosteal dissection can then be carried out using monopolar cautery along the ventral surface of the involved vertebral bodies and disc spaces. Dissection should extend rostrally and caudally to expose the proximal half of the vertebral bodies adjacent to the affected levels. The lateral dissection should free the longus colli from ventral surface of the spine. Dissection is initiated in the midline, where the ALL is clearly identified. Emphasis is placed on performing a symmetric dissection of the longus colli muscles, to the level of the uncinate processes, in order to maintain a midline orientation and provide exposure for a sufficient bilateral decompression. Care must be taken to avoid direct injury to the sympathetic chain, which runs along the ventral surface of the longus colli. Any remaining ventral or lateral osteophytes should be removed to further release the longus colli so that retracting blades can be securely placed under the muscle. Failure to resect lateral osteophytes will prevent proper seating of the retractor blades.

We prefer the Shadow-Line® (V. Mueller, Franklin Lakes, NJ) retractor system with a serrated blade directed laterally and a smooth blade deep to the medial longus colli muscle. It is essential that these retractors fit well and remain under the longus colli. "Riding up" of the retractors may rake the blades over the sympathetic chain or allow esophageal tissue to creep into the surgical field. Small (2 mm) medial, horizontal cuts in longus colli rostrally and caudally may aid in flush retractor placement. We advocate fixating the base of the Shadow-Line retractor to a rigid articulating arm attached to the bed in order to avoid unintended movement of the blades. A simple adaptor that attaches the Shadow-Line to the articulating arm of the MET-Rx® minimally invasive retractor system (Medtronic, Minneapolis, MN) is used at our institution. With retractor blades in place, distraction posts can be placed in the rostral and caudal vertebral bodies. It is important that these posts are placed as close to midline as possible, both for optimal purchase and to serve as a midline reference point for the ensuing decompression. Additional lordosis can be achieved upon distraction if the posts are placed with slightly convergent trajectories.

Structures at risk during anterior exposure of the cervical spine include the jugular vein, carotid artery, esophagus, recurrent laryngeal nerve, and sympathetic chain. Injury is often the result of insufficient soft tissue release leading to excessive compression and traction, as opposed to direct trauma [30]. Accordingly, the incidence of these complications can be greatly reduced by a thorough exposure with generous sub-platysmal dissection and release of all fascial attachments, as well as periodic retractor release. In regard to RLN injury, as previously discussed, there is no definitive evidence that the laterality of approach influences the incidence of RLN injury. However, Apfelbaum and colleagues found a reduction in the incidence of recurrent laryngeal nerve injury (from 6.4% to 1.69%) by monitoring endotracheal cuff pressure and intermittently releasing retractors. In regard to injury to the sympathetic chain, superficial dissection of the longus colli muscles off the midline can damage the sympathetic chain and produce a Horner syndrome. Wide release of the muscle and positioning the retractor blades deep to the muscle reduce the risk of this complication.

Discectomy

Once overhanging osteophytes are removed, the discectomy is initiated by sharply incising the annulus. Free disc fragments within the annulotomy can then be removed with a pituitary rongeurs. A combination of curettes and Kerrison rongeurs is used to perform the discectomy, progressing from superficial to deep and working laterally out to the uncinate processes in a stepwise fashion until the posterior longitudinal ligament (PLL) is encountered. Bilateral exposure of the uncinate processes will assist in determination of the midline. Decortication of the vertebral endplates is performed with either curettes or a drill. Excessive decortication can lead to graft subsidence and should be avoided.

Dorsal osteophytes are removed with either a drill or Kerrison rongeurs. A plane between the dorsal osteophyte and posterior ligamentous tissues is developed with a small upgoing curette and the osteophyte resected. If entry into the epidural space is intended, the fibers of the posterior ligamentous tissues can be separated with a small curette or nerve hook and the ligament resected with Kerrison rongeurs. If the Kerrison is in the appropriate epidural plane under the PLL, the footplate should slide easily, and the remainder of ligament can be removed.

Ligament that is adherent or calcified/incorporated into the dura, as can be the case with OPLL, may be left intact to avoid a spinal fluid leak. These areas of calcification typically exist in the midline, allowing for a circumferential release of surrounding attachments that will allow the ligament/dura complex to float freely and alleviate compression. If decompression is not necessary, the posterior longitudinal ligament should be preserved to act as a fulcrum accentuating lordosis during distraction. Foraminotomies are generally performed after the midline decompression as the epidural venous plexus around the nerve root can lead to bleeding. The base of the uncinate process is removed with either a drill, utilizing a matchstick burr, or Kerrison rongeurs. With severe foraminal stenosis however, insertion of the Kerrison footplate can lead to further nerve compression and possible injury, particularly for the C5 nerve root. Under these circumstances, drilling of the foramen is a better alternative. The foraminotomy should extend from the caudal pedicle to above the uncinate process to ensure adequate decompression. Free fragments of disc deep to the ligament in either the foramen or behind the vertebral body can be delivered with a nerve hook.

Corpectomy

If a corpectomy is to be performed, we will typically first perform discectomies adjacent to the vertebrae to be resected. With the vertebrae isolated, a Leksell rongeur can then be used to remove the bone and harvest autograft. Drilling of the bone is also possible; however, this makes harvesting more difficult. Vertebral resection should proceed until an “egg shell” of thin dorsal cortical bone remains. The posterior cortical wall can be drilled to the ligament, particularly in the midline where the PLL is thickest (Fig. 24.10). A plane beneath the remaining bone and the PLL can then be developed and the bone removed with a Kerrison rongeur. The PLL can then be resected in a fashion similar to discectomy, by making a small opening with a curette, establishing the epidural space, and then using the Kerrison punch to remove the ligament and decompress the dura.

Accurate identification of the midline is essential to carrying out a thorough and safe decompression. In most cases, an exposure width of 15–20 mm provides for an adequate decompression, but bilateral identification of the uncinate processes is a more reliable way to an appropriate decompression. This is particularly important because the line of sight provided by anterior exposure often limits visualization of the ipsilateral canal, creating a tendency to compromise the ipsilateral decompression (Fig. 24.11). The shape of a classic “Erlenmeyer” flask is often used as an example to guide the decompression. Extending

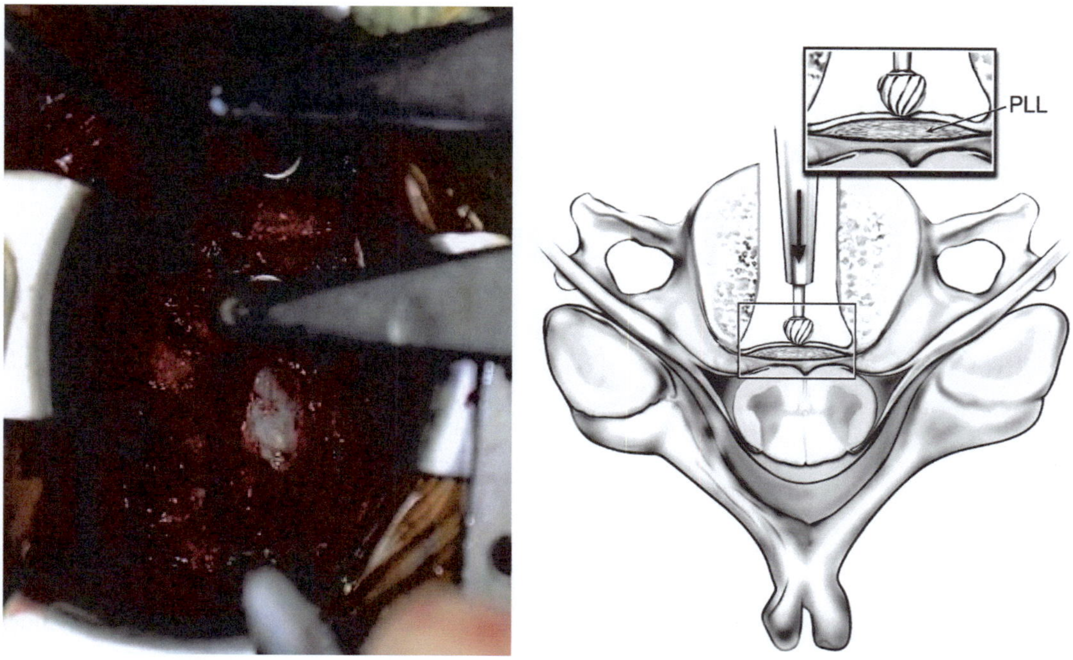

Fig. 24.10 Intraoperative image (left) and illustration (right) demonstrating the resection of posterior osteophytes by drilling to the level of the posterior longitudinal ligament (PLL) in the midline, where the ligament is thickest and provides maximal protection to the underlying dura. (From Kaiser [3]; with permission)

decompression beyond the uncinate processes however, which defines the lateral boundary of the vertebral body, puts the vertebral artery at risk. If resection of the lateral vertebral wall is intended, positioning a blunt dissector along the outside of the uncinate process can protect the artery. As previously mentioned, preoperative imaging always should be assessed for an aberrant course of the artery.

Interbody Grafting

Once the anterior decompression is complete, attention can be turned to the sizing and placement of interbody grafts. Final decortication of the endplates is performed prior to determining interbody graft size. A moderate amount of distraction during graft placement can help restore lordosis, but excessive distraction can lead to painful stretching of the facet capsule and increase postoperative pain. With this in mind, following discectomy, a series of metallic trials are inserted into the disc space to determine appropriate sizing. For discectomy procedures, we generally use prefabricated allograft bone, unless factors warrant harvesting iliac crest autograft. For a corpectomy, a sizing instrument is generally used to determine appropriate graft length, and we generally use synthetic interbody grafts, either titanium or PEEK, and fill the graft with local autograft, allograft, and/or demineralized bone matrix. For hybrid constructs, the amount of local autograft is generally sufficient for use in both the corpectomy and discectomy cages. In general, modest lordotic shaping of the graft enhances lordosis during impaction and optimizes the distribution of an axial load across the construct (Fig. 24.12a).

The potential for subsidence is inversely proportional to the cross-sectional area between the endplate and inserted graft. Accordingly, every

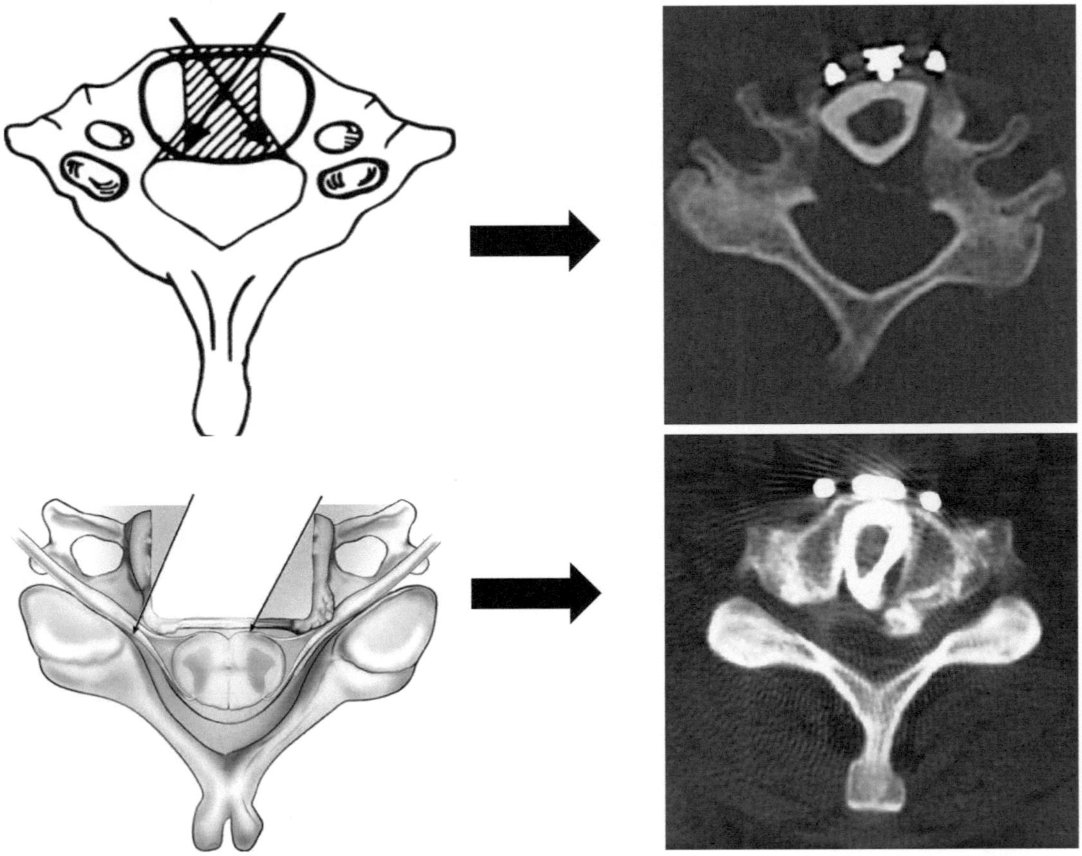

Fig. 24.11 Adequate soft tissue exposure is essential to accurate assessment of midline and achieving symmetric and wide decompression (shown above). Asymmetric and/or insufficient decompression may result from the limited line of sight provided by inadequate exposure (below). (From Kaiser [3]; with permission)

attempt should be made to maximize the contact surface area of the graft-endplate interface. Once the graft is positioned, distraction can be released, and a nerve hook can be used to probe the posterior to the graft, confirming appropriate fit and axial loading across the construct. Fluoroscopy can also be used to confirm placement prior to application of the anterior cervical plate.

Ventral Plate Stabilization

With the graft(s) in place, remaining ventral osteophytes should be removed allowing for flush application of the cervical plate (Fig. 24.12b, c). Ideally, the cervical plate will extend just beyond the rostral and caudal endplate, facilitating the placement of screws into dense subchondral bone. Screw trajectory should be medially oriented to allow for maximal pull-out resistance. With dynamic platting systems, we prefer fixed screws in the caudal vertebrae to act as a buttress, facilitating axial loading through the construct. An inappropriately long plate can impact motion at the levels above and below the construct, increasing the propensity for adjacent segment disease (Fig. 24.3). Long plates also increase the risk of placing a screw into the adjacent disc space. Plates should be flushed with the bone and low profile. A prominent plate has the potential to precipitate postoperative swallowing difficulty. Complications related to graft and plate placement are generally related to poor

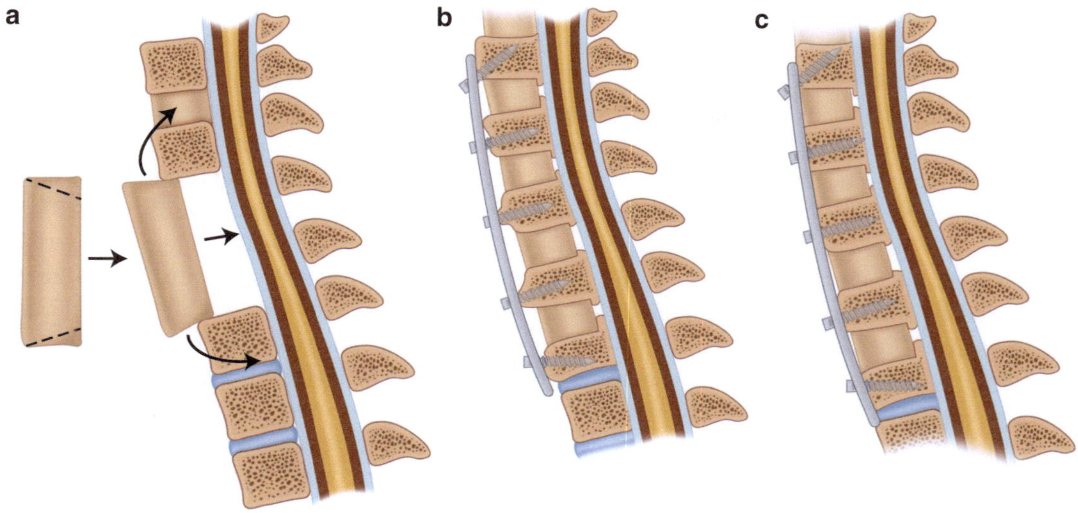

Fig. 24.12 Ideally, interbody strut grafts are shaped to promote lordosis during insertion (**a**). Anterior osteophyte resection ("gardening of the spine") allows for flush placement of the plate along the cervical vertebrae, distributing axial loads effectively between the construct and spine (**b**, **c**). (From Kaiser [3]; with permission)

visualization of the bony landmarks, inadequate removal of protruding osteophytes, or insufficient evaluation of preoperative imaging.

Closure

After obtaining meticulous hemostasis, the wound should be copiously irrigated with antibiotic irrigation. The trachea, esophagus, and carotid sheath should be inspected for potential injury. Use of a Hemovac drain is at the surgeon's discretion but is generally advised for multilevel procedures. The platysma and subcutaneous tissue should be reapproximated with interrupted 3-0 Vicryl sutures. The skin can then be closed with a running subcuticular 4-0 Biosyn stitch.

Postoperative Care and Concerns

Many of the standard postoperative concerns in spine surgery are present following anterior cervical approaches, including bleeding, infection, pseudoarthrosis, and hardware complications. More specific concerns are related to postoperative swallowing and respiratory function, as well as possible injury to the carotid artery, vertebral artery, esophagus, and recurrent laryngeal nerve. An analysis by the AANS/CNS Joint Committee identified age, duration of symptoms, and preoperative neurologic function as the primary predictors of outcome following surgery for cervical spondylotic myelopathy, and patients should be counseled accordingly [35]. Importantly, patients with multilevel cervical pathology treated from an anterior approach need to be well prepared for the possibility for postoperative dysphagia. This is particularly true in elder patients with rostral disease, who may require a gastrostomy tube in some cases.

Oral intake should be advanced slowly under close supervision. Postoperative upright x-rays provide valuable information regarding implant placement, alignment restoration, and soft tissue edema. In some cases, a postoperative CT scan may be indicated to better understand the construct in three dimensions. X-rays should be repeated periodically during the postoperative course to monitor for fusion maturation. For multilevel disease, we suggest a rigid cervical collar be worn for 6–12 weeks to minimize stress on the construct and augment arthrosis.

Case Presentation

The patient is a 45-year-old woman presenting with 4 weeks of diffuse right upper extremity pain, loss of fine motor control/weakness in both hands, and acute exacerbation of chronic neck pain (NDI of 54 at presentation). MR imaging reveals a multilevel ventral degenerative process extending from C3/C4 to C6/C7 with disc herniations causing spinal cord compression and T2 signal change (Fig. 24.13). Upright x-rays demonstrate a kyphotic cervical alignment (Fig. 24.14a). In this case, the ventral location of the offending pathology and the patient's kyphotic alignment both favored an anterior approach. A C6 corpectomy was performed to achieve adequate decompression of the disc herniations at C5/C6 and C6/7, both of which extended dorsal to the C6 vertebrae. Discectomies were then performed at C3/C4 and C4/C5. The corpectomy provided sufficient autograft to fill PEEK cages at C4–5 and C5–C7, and a structural allograft was inserted at C3/C4 (Fig. 24.14b, c). The patient made an excellent recovery, with full motor strength in all muscle groups and normal hand function at 1 year following the operation (NDI of 24 at 1 year).

Discussion

Like most of spine surgery, multilevel cervical disease can be successfully treated from many different approaches. The optimal approach for a given patient is generated by careful consideration of the three tenets of evidence-based medicine: best available medical evidence, surgeon expertise/experience, and patient characteristics and preferences. Failure to fully consider all of these factors can subvert an otherwise sound surgical plan.

The best available evidence confirms that multilevel cervical disease can be effectively treated from an anterior approach with either multilevel discectomy or corpectomy [1, 4–7]. Data from cadaveric, biomechanical, and limited clinical studies also support the potential benefit of using a hybrid construct when appropriate [24–28]. The ACDF versus corpectomy comparison has been thoroughly studied [4, 8, 15], but more data are needed to better understand how the long-term clinical and radiographic outcomes achieved via the hybrid approach holds up against these more traditional procedures.

Ultimately, the operating surgeon must be comfortable employing the techniques supported by the best available research in order to optimize

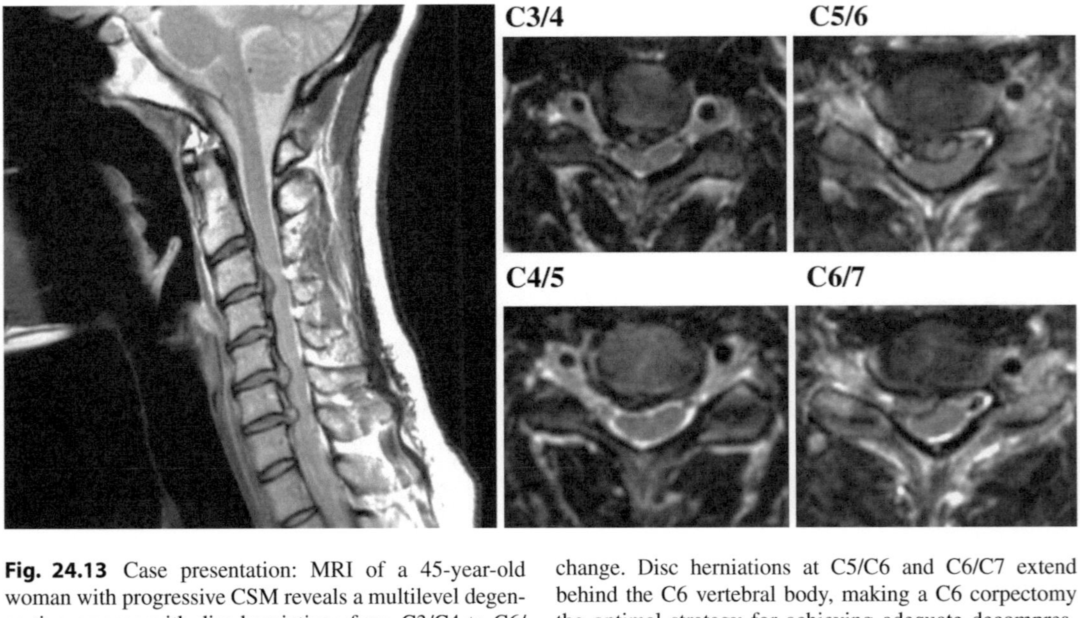

Fig. 24.13 Case presentation: MRI of a 45-year-old woman with progressive CSM reveals a multilevel degenerative process with disc herniations from C3/C4 to C6/C7 causing spinal cord compression with T2 signal change. Disc herniations at C5/C6 and C6/C7 extend behind the C6 vertebral body, making a C6 corpectomy the optimal strategy for achieving adequate decompression at these levels

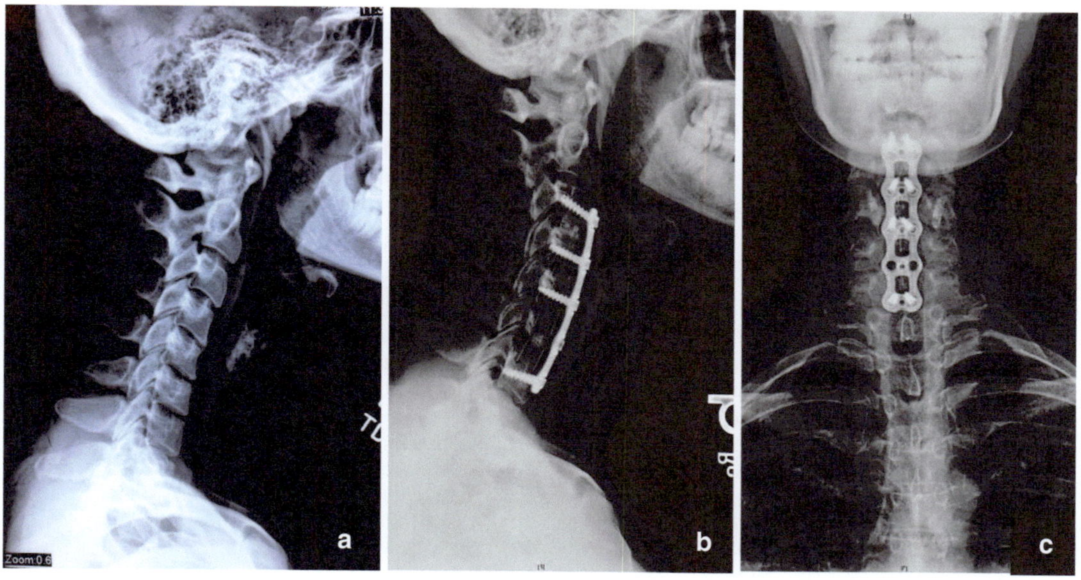

Fig. 24.14 Case presentation: upright cervical x-rays demonstrate a kyphotic cervical alignment (**a**), which, along with the ventral offending pathology in this case, favors an anterior approach. Cervical reconstruction was achieved with PEEK cages at C4/C5 and C5–C7, while a structural allograft was used at C3/C4, shown here on lateral (**b**) and AP (**c**) x-rays at 1-year follow-up

patient outcome. Due to the prevalence of cervical spondylosis and the efficacy of both ACDF and corpectomy, most spine surgeons have significant expertise performing these procedures. The incorporation of recent evidence into anterior cervical surgery is less about developing new surgical skills and more contingent on appropriate preoperative planning. As previously discussed, this planning must account for the patient's condition and preferences as well as the surgeon's experience.

Conclusion

Successful treatment strategies for multilevel cervical disease require a comprehensive and individualized approach. There is sufficient evidence demonstrating the comparative efficacy of both anterior cervical discectomy and corpectomy, particularly in cases of ventral pathology and/or kyphotic alignment. Although there is evidence that corpectomy reduces the risk of pseudoarthrosis, ACDF provides better short-term stability and restoration of alignment. In the appropriate clinical scenario, hybrid constructs may serve as an alternative, affording patients some of the benefits of each reconstruction strategy. However, long-term clinical data is needed to judge the comparative efficacy of hybrid constructs against corpectomy and multilevel ACDF. There is a multitude of factors that must be considered when planning anterior cervical surgery, and the potential for complications exists at each step. Success is contingent upon a treatment paradigm based on the best available research evidence and the operating surgeon's own experience, as well as an individualized approach to the patient.

References

1. Mummaneni PV, Kaiser MG, Matz PG, et al. Cervical surgical techniques for the treatment of cervical spondylotic myelopathy. J Neurosurg Spine. 2009;11(2):130–41.
2. Komotar RJ, Mocco J, Kaiser MG. Surgical management of cervical myelopathy: indications and techniques for laminectomy and fusion. Spine J. 2006;6(6 Suppl):252S–67S.

3. Kaiser MG. Multilevel cervical spondylosis. Neurosurg Clin N Am. 2006;17(3):263–275, vi.
4. Lau D, Chou D, Mummaneni PV. Two-level corpectomy versus three-level discectomy for cervical spondylotic myelopathy: a comparison of perioperative, radiographic, and clinical outcomes. J Neurosurg Spine. 2015;23(3):280–9.
5. Masaki Y, Yamazaki M, Okawa A, et al. An analysis of factors causing poor surgical outcome in patients with cervical myelopathy due to ossification of the posterior longitudinal ligament: anterior decompression with spinal fusion versus laminoplasty. J Spinal Disord Tech. 2007;20(1):7–13.
6. Matz PG, Holly LT, Groff MW, et al. Indications for anterior cervical decompression for the treatment of cervical degenerative radiculopathy. J Neurosurg Spine. 2009;11(2):174–82.
7. Matz PG, Holly LT, Mummaneni PV, et al. Anterior cervical surgery for the treatment of cervical degenerative myelopathy. J Neurosurg Spine. 2009;11(2):170–3.
8. Swank ML, Lowery GL, Bhat AL, McDonough RF. Anterior cervical allograft arthrodesis and instrumentation: multilevel interbody grafting or strut graft reconstruction. Eur Spine J. 1997;6(2):138–43.
9. Joaquim AF, Murar J, Savage JW, Patel AA. Dysphagia after anterior cervical spine surgery: a systematic review of potential preventative measures. Spine J. 2014;14(9):2246–60.
10. Ghogawala Z, Martin B, Benzel EC, et al. Comparative effectiveness of ventral vs dorsal surgery for cervical spondylotic myelopathy. Neurosurgery. 2011;68(3):622–30. discussion 630-621.
11. Sasso RC, Ruggiero RA Jr, Reilly TM, Hall PV. Early reconstruction failures after multilevel cervical corpectomy. Spine (Phila Pa 1976). 2003;28(2):140–2.
12. Etame AB, Wang AC, Than KD, La Marca F, Park P. Outcomes after surgery for cervical spine deformity: review of the literature. Neurosurg Focus. 2010;28(3):E14.
13. Grosso MJ, Hwang R, Mroz T, Benzel E, Steinmetz MP. Relationship between degree of focal kyphosis correction and neurological outcomes for patients undergoing cervical deformity correction surgery. J Neurosurg Spine. 2013;18(6):537–44.
14. Traynelis VC. Total subaxial reconstruction. J Neurosurg Spine. 2010;13(4):424–34.
15. Hilibrand AS, Fye MA, Emery SE, Palumbo MA, Bohlman HH. Increased rate of arthrodesis with strut grafting after multilevel anterior cervical decompression. Spine (Phila Pa 1976). 2002;27(2):146–51.
16. Pitzen TR, Chrobok J, Stulik J, et al. Implant complications, fusion, loss of lordosis, and outcome after anterior cervical plating with dynamic or rigid plates: two-year results of a multi-centric, randomized, controlled study. Spine (Phila Pa 1976). 2009;34(7):641–6.
17. Ghahreman A, Rao PJ, Ferch RD. Dynamic plates in anterior cervical fusion surgery: graft settling and cervical alignment. Spine (Phila Pa 1976). 2009;34(15):1567–71.
18. Kelly MP, Mok JM, Berven S. Dynamic constructs for spinal fusion: an evidence-based review. Orthop Clin North Am. 2010;41(2):203–15.
19. Fraser JF, Hartl R. Anterior approaches to fusion of the cervical spine: a metaanalysis of fusion rates. J Neurosurg Spine. 2007;6(4):298–303.
20. Heary RF, Schlenk RP, Sacchieri TA, Barone D, Brotea C. Persistent iliac crest donor site pain: independent outcome assessment. Neurosurgery. 2002;50(3):510–6. discussion 516-517.
21. Ryken TC, Heary RF, Matz PG, et al. Techniques for cervical interbody grafting. J Neurosurg Spine. 2009;11(2):203–20.
22. Singh K, Vaccaro AR, Kim J, Lorenz EP, Lim TH, An HS. Biomechanical comparison of cervical spine reconstructive techniques after a multilevel corpectomy of the cervical spine. Spine (Phila Pa 1976). 2003;28(20):2352–8. discussion 2358.
23. Singh K, Vaccaro AR, Kim J, Lorenz EP, Lim TH, An HS. Enhancement of stability following anterior cervical corpectomy: a biomechanical study. Spine (Phila Pa 1976). 2004;29(8):845–9.
24. Porter RW, Crawford NR, Chamberlain RH, et al. Biomechanical analysis of multilevel cervical corpectomy and plate constructs. J Neurosurg. 2003;99(1 Suppl):98–103.
25. Ashkenazi E, Smorgick Y, Rand N, Millgram MA, Mirovsky Y, Floman Y. Anterior decompression combined with corpectomies and discectomies in the management of multilevel cervical myelopathy: a hybrid decompression and fixation technique. J Neurosurg Spine. 2005;3(3):205–9.
26. Liu JM, Peng HW, Liu ZL, Long XH, Yu YQ, Huang SH. Hybrid decompression technique versus anterior cervical corpectomy and fusion for treating multilevel cervical spondylotic myelopathy: which one is better? World Neurosurg. 2015;84(6):2022–9.
27. Hussain M, Nassr A, Natarajan RN, An HS, Andersson GB. Corpectomy versus discectomy for the treatment of multilevel cervical spine pathology: a finite element model analysis. Spine J. 2012;12(5):401–8.
28. Wei-bing X, Wun-Jer S, Gang L, Yue Z, Ming-xi J, Lian-shun J. Reconstructive techniques study after anterior decompression of multilevel cervical spondylotic myelopathy. J Spinal Disord Tech. 2009;22(7):511–5.
29. Kaminsky SB, Clark CR, Traynelis VC. Operative treatment of cervical spondylotic myelopathy and radiculopathy. A comparison of laminectomy and laminoplasty at five year average follow-up. Iowa Orthop J. 2004;24:95–105.
30. Apfelbaum RI, Kriskovich MD, Haller JR. On the incidence, cause, and prevention of recurrent laryngeal nerve palsies during anterior cervical spine surgery. Spine (Phila Pa 1976). 2000;25(22):2906–12.
31. Kaiser MG, Haid RW Jr, Subach BR, Barnes B, Rodts GE Jr. Anterior cervical plating enhances arthrodesis after discectomy and fusion with cortical allograft.

Neurosurgery. 2002;50(2):229–36. discussion 236-228.
32. Shaffer WO, Baisden JL, Fernand R, Matz PG. North American Spine S. An evidence-based clinical guideline for antibiotic prophylaxis in spine surgery. Spine J. 2013;13(10):1387–92.
33. Kelleher MO, Tan G, Sarjeant R, Fehlings MG. Predictive value of intraoperative neurophysiological monitoring during cervical spine surgery: a prospective analysis of 1055 consecutive patients. J Neurosurg Spine. 2008;8(3):215–21.
34. Heeneman H. Vocal cord paralysis following approaches to the anterior cervical spine. Laryngoscope. 1973;83(1):17–21.
35. Holly LT, Matz PG, Anderson PA, et al. Clinical prognostic indicators of surgical outcome in cervical spondylotic myelopathy. J Neurosurg Spine. 2009;11(2):112–8.
36. Benzel EC. Complex Instrumentation Constructs and Force Application. In: Benzel EC, editor. Biomechanics of spine stabilization. Rolling Meadows: AANS Publications Committee; 2001.

Options for Interbody Grafting

25

Azam Basheer, Mohammed Macki, and Frank La Marca

Pitfalls/Pearls of Interbody Grafting

- The choice of interbody graft is based on the osteogenic potential to supply osteoprogenitor cells, osteoinductive signals to stimulate the differentiation of osteoprogenitor cells to osteoblasts, and an osteoconductive scaffold to support cellular architecture and neovascularization.
- Autografts allow for excellent bony arthrodesis across the interbody space; unfortunately, donor site morbidity limits the utility of autograft.
- Cages afford superior axial load-bearing of the cervical vertebral column and height restoration of the intervertebral space. While cages reduce stress on the adjacent vertebral bodies, the stimulus for bone remodeling necessary in fusion is also decreased.

A. Basheer
Department of Neurosurgery, Neuroscience Institute, Henry Ford Health System, Detroit, MI, USA

M. Macki
Department of Neurosurgery, Henry Ford Hospital, Detroit, MI, USA

F. La Marca (✉)
Department of Neurosurgery, Henry Ford Health System, Detroit, MI, USA
e-mail: flamarc1@hfhs.org

While it is generally agreed upon that the approach to address cervical degenerative pathology is based on individualized characteristics, there remains a wide variety of appropriate fusion constructs to address anterior cervical degenerative disease. Although the role of the cervical interbody grafting remains a time-honored tool in fusion operations, the surgical armamentarium for reconstruction of the anterior and middle column in the cervical spine has expanded to a myriad of materials and techniques. Cervical grafts/spacers alone have evolved exponentially over the decades as surgeons attempt to strike a perfect balance between the structural and biological roles of the interbody graft.

Background

A limitation of the posterior approach for cervical spondylosis is that a lamino-foraminotomy does afford easy access to ventral osteophytes compressing the nerve root in the intervertebral foramen; thus, the anterior cervical approach has become the mainstay for the surgical management of pathologies anterior to the posterior longitudinal ligament, such as degenerative disc disease. While authors have contested that discectomy alone results in spontaneous arthrodesis in 70–80% of cases [1], the procedure disrupts axial loading and normal cervical lordosis, especially since the disc traverses both the anterior

M. G. Kaiser et al. (eds.), *Degenerative Cervical Myelopathy and Radiculopathy*,
https://doi.org/10.1007/978-3-319-97952-6_25

column, responsible for 36% of cervical loading, and the middle column, responsible for 64% of cervical loading [2]. Thus, Robinson-Smith and [3] and RB Cloward [4] in the 1950s independently described the anterior cervical approach for interbody graft placement.

The principles of cervical interbody graft derive from Wolff's law, named after the German surgeon Julius Wolff in the nineteenth century [5]. In essence, he described remodeling of bone structure to adapt to the forces and loads applied. This response is achieved via mechanotransduction, wherein mechanical forces induce biochemical signals at the cellular level, resulting in the upregulation of certain growth factors that lead to bony remodeling [6]. This bony remodeling is what spine surgeons heavily rely on when implanting a graft between two vertebral bodies (interbody graft). Additionally, this remodeling is proportional to the amount of loading exerted on bone. Hence, larger grafts provide bigger surface area, friction, and more compressive forces on the endplates which can lead to changes in the trabeculae of bone and thickening of cortical endplates [6]. The inverse is true, where bony resorption and decreased bone density are seen when there is a lack of force.

Biomechanically speaking, the interbody spacer/graft (1) preserves disc height and angulation (distraction lever) necessary for the patency of the neuroforamen and the spinal canal, (2) maintains cervical alignment, (3) arrests the development of bone spurs, and (4) eliminates instability [7, 8]. A successful cervical interbody spacer/graft must account for the modulus of elasticity, characterized by a stress-strain curve which defines the resistance of elastic (nonpermanent) deformation to a certain force (stress):

$$\lambda = \frac{\text{Stress }(\text{Pascals})}{\text{Strain}}$$

Stiffer materials will have a larger modulus of elasticity. An ideal interbody graft will have an equivalent modulus of elasticity to the bone: 0.1–1.0 GPa for cancellous bone and 1.0–2.4 GPa for cortical bone. Otherwise, the substrate will have a tendency to subside into the adjacent endplate.

In addition to these structural mechanisms, cervical interbody grafts must also respect physiological principles that stimulate bone fusion across two vertebral bodies via hematoma formation, inflammation, neovascularization, and creeping substitution [1]. Three critical elements of the interbody graft affect new bone formation: the osteogenic potential to supply osteoprogenitor cells for the developing bone, osteoinductive signals to stimulate the differentiation of osteoprogenitor cells to osteoblasts, and an osteoconductive scaffold to support cellular architecture and neovascularization of bony ingrowth [9]. Classically only structural autografts provided all three features and thus are deemed the gold standard against which substitutes are measured.

Endplate Preparation

The discussion on interbody grafts/spacers must be couched in the surgical context of endplate preparation, a vital step in anterior cervical fusion. Endplate preparation refers to a surgical technique by which the entire rostral and caudal end of the intervertebral disc is removed. Next, scraping off a thin layer of the cortical endplate (e.g., with a Cobb elevator) exposes bone marrow osteoprogenitor cells from the cancellous bone into the intervertebral space. Overaggressive decortication of the endplate will not only induce excess bleeding but will also compromise endplate strength, as cancellous bone confers far less resistance compared to cortical bone. An interbody graft/spacer placed in these suboptimal conditions is more likely to undergo subsidence. A biomechanical study on regional biomechanical strength reported that the complete removal of the endplate decreased compressive strength by nearly 39% [10]. Interestingly, only a marginal decrease in endplate compressive strength was noted with the removal of only the anterior third of the endplate. This introduces the concept of "regional strength": a biomechanical concept, involving the removal of the weaker central endplate to increase vascularity while preserving the stronger peripheral cortex to increase stress resistance. Thus, in the geometric consideration of cages, the implant with a hollow center can accommodate the bleeding osteoprogenitor cells centrally and engage the cortical bone peripherally.

At the other end of the spectrum, inadequate removal of disc material and cartilaginous endplate increases the risk of pseudarthrosis. In a study on endplate preparation for Bagby and Kuslich (BAK) cage, complete discectomy, where disc material is removed and scraped off the bone till clean endplates are visualized, allows for 100% fusion rate, whereas partial reamed channel discectomy diminished the fusion rate to 16% [11]. The residual disc prevents cage access to the appropriate nutrient-rich environment and blood supply that comes from the endplates. Again, this emphasizes meticulous surgical technique to cultivate an optimal cross-sectional interface between the cage and the endplates.

Autograft

Traditionally harvested from the iliac crest, autografts spurred the initial interest in interbody fusions because of the ideal biological composition for in vivo bone formation and an equivalent modulus of elasticity to vertebral bodies. From a technical perspective, the graft height should measure at least 7 mm and a minimum of 2 mm higher than the original intervertebral space according to the operative description by Smith and Robinson [12]. The graft will then ideally countersink into the original disc space such that the ventral aspect is flush with or slightly deep to the anterior vertebral body cortical surface. With these appropriate techniques, a systematic review of the literature on cervical autografts published a mean arthrodesis rate of 77%, which ranges from 83% to 99% after single-level fusion, decreasing with higher number of interspaces [1].

Because autografts, specifically iliac crest, contain a cancellous bone core, in addition to the cortical bone covering, the biomechanical properties depend largely on the shape of the bone. The horseshoe shape in the Smith-Robinson graft upholds more resistance to compressive forces compared to other graft types: a dowel representative of the Cloward graft, an onlay strut in the Bailey-Badgley graft (the technique later evolved into anterior cervical corpectomy), and keystone in the Simmons-Bhalla graft [12, 13]. The Smith-Robinson graft provides more strength because the shorter square-shaped interbody graft can support a higher load compared to the other, longer grafts per elementary strength of material theory [13]. By that same token, the square interbody graft is more resistant to kyphotic deformity than the keystone graft, which does not maximize on the surface contact area with the rostral and caudal endplates.

Unfortunately, autografts require longer operative times, create donor site morbidity, and increased blood loss. Morbidity and mortality percentages are suggested to be overstated; be that as it may, prior studies have cited rates of 8.6% for major complications and 20.6% for minor complications following any-type autologous bone grafting [14]. Harvesting of iliac crest bone grafts, in particular, confers an upward of 20%–30% incidence of donor site infection, hematoma, fracture, pain, meralgia paresthetica, and abdominal herniation [9, 15]. Graft donor site pain, in particular, is underestimated by neurosurgeons according to a study that independently questioned the physicians and the patients [16]. The percentage of patients with iliac crest site discomfort was over four times higher than expected by the surgeons.

Furthermore, the length of autograft may limit long anterior fusion constructs, and there is a limited supply of autograft. To that end, revision operations become problematic because re-harvesting bone grafts from different locations and inserting additional grafts/spacers in the intervertebral space increase the risks of donor site morbidity. In order to circumvent these potential difficulties, different grafting substitutes marketed over the past few decades heralded a new generation in cervical interbody fusions.

Allograft

Allografts, by definition, derive from preserved cadaveric bone, the first engineered substitute to autograft. The specimen is harvested from iliac bone or fibula, the latter of which maintains disc height more effectively at the expense of decreased osteoconductivity, albeit these presumptions have not been corroborated in the literature. One prospective study comparing fibular versus iliac crest allograft did not find a statistically significant difference with non-union or collapse [17]. Regardless of the harvest site, mineralized allografts are hailed for their high osteoconduction with no osteogenic potential and, at best, mild osteoinduction, whereas demineralized allografts possess both osteoconductivity and variable osteoinduction [1]. Minimally manipulated and milled grafts now provide for more consistent graft design and modulus of elasticity as well as provide a varied selection of cortical and/or cancellous bone configurations.

Commensurate to rates cited in autograft constructs, allograft yields a mean arthrodesis rate of 74%, which ranges from 94% after single-level fusion, decreasing with more number of interspaces according to one institutional series of 170 patients [18]. The correlation of increasing spinal levels with pseudoarthrosis and collapse rates was more pronounced in allografts over autografts. One study reported that the 95% union rate after one-level fusion with autograft or allograft dropped precipitously among two-level fusions to 38% with allografts and 83% with autografts [19]. In fact, a meta-analysis of four studies on both one- and two-level ACDF concluded that allograft versus autograft exhibited inferior rates of radiographic fusion and higher rates of graft subsidence [20]. Comparatively speaking, allografts also fared worse with delayed union and kyphotic deformity [1]. Nevertheless, the principal advantage of the allograft over autograft points to the decreased postoperative pain scores and mean length of hospital stay as harvesting techniques have been completely circumvented [21].

The structural integrity of allografts depends on bone type and manufacture preparation. Cortical allografts maintain a stronger tensile strength as compared to corticocancellous allografts, whose larger surface area with the rostral and caudal endplates facilitates bone integration [22, 23]. Second, the allograft preservation process necessary to decrease the antigenicity of the bone transplant entails either freezing or lyophilization (freeze-drying). While the latter subdues immunogenicity, rehydration compromises mechanical strength by almost 50% [24].

Notwithstanding that allografts have been advertised for their favorable osteoconductive scaffold, certain preservation processes, in particular ethylene oxide or radiation, not only impair the osteoinductive factors but also abolish osteogenic cells in the interbody graft, whose aptitude for cervical arthrodesis has been subsequently questioned [9].

Failure to fuse could also be contributed by genetic incompatibility that causes immunological reactions ranging from localized soft tissue swelling around critical structures in the neck to systemic anaphylactic reactions [25]. To that end, while aseptic techniques conjure a theoretical risk of bacterial contamination, rigorous donor screening coupled with aggressive preservation has lowered the risk of HIV transmission, for example, to less than one per million transplants [26].

Ceramics

Ceramic interbody spacers incorporate a combination of various calcium phosphates, notably hydroxyapatite and/or beta-tricalcium phosphate (β-TCP). Ceramics have gained popularity in light of their nontoxic, biodegradable, and non-immunogenic properties [9]. The principle of ceramics relies on its favorable osteoconductive scaffold; however, these inert interbodies have no osteogenic or osteoinductive potential. Furthermore, the brittle nature and reduced shear strength/fracture resistance of ceramics predisposes the fusion construct to mechanical instability, especially in the immediate postoperative period when bone has not fused. Thus ceramics must be supplemented with autograft and/or allograft. Some studies have demonstrated that ceramics supplemented with rigid internal fixation provide a safe and efficacious alternative to bone replacement, but not ceramics alone [27]. β-TCP, for example, has gained most success in interbody cages. As the ceramic requires months to fuse, surgeons advocate for anterior plating to prevent migration of the unfused cage. In a randomized clinical controlled trial, successful fusion was noted in both the interbody cages containing β-TCP plus plating cohort versus the cage containing β-TCP without anterior plating cohort, but the non-plating group experienced higher rates of vertical cage migration [28]. Similar results are noted with hydroxyapatite ceramics-in-cage plus plating, in which complete fusion occurred in 98% of one-level and 100% of two-level fusions [29]. Although, unlike the previous studies with autograft and allograft, the current study is limited by a smaller study population size. Incidences of slight graft collapse (3%), deterioration (19%), and fracture (3%) did not affect clinical outcomes, defined as "good" or "excellent" in 91% of patients.

Polymethylmethacrylate (PMMA)

A synthetic polymer of methyl methacrylate, PMMA, is a soft compound that hardens upon polymerization in the interspace. Some surgeons advocate for tying at the endplates: using a drill, the rostral and caudal endplates are perforated to create a small burr hole to anchor the PMMA superiorly and inferiorly, respectively. After protecting the dura with a sponge, PMMA is injected into the intervertebral space. Two randomized clinical controlled trials found that PMMA did not improve rates of bony union compared to cervical discectomy alone [30] or cage-assisted fusion [8]. While the strength of PMMA is comparable to industrial grade resistance, the polymer interposition lacks osteogenesis, osteoinduction, and osteoconduction. In fact, the rigidity of the PMMA has been reported to necrose the adjacent vertebrae and even diminish ventral ossification [31]. Unsurprisingly then, appreciable bony arthrodesis requires approximately 2 years [31]. Spine surgeons have thus suggested the application of PMMA with a mixture of allograft cancellous bone into a cage with anterior plating [32]. The practice of mixing graft materials with rigid substrates introduced the concept of cages: synthetic prostheses intended to restore disc height and lordosis as well as to prevent graft collapse [33]. Advantages and disadvantages of cage types are discussed below.

Cages

A revolutionary addition in the surgeon's armamentarium for anterior cervical fusions, cages have been commercialized for their superior axial load-bearing of the cervical vertebral column and height restoration of the intervertebral space and neuroforamina. Cages must strike a mechanical balance between stress reduction and bone remodeling. According to Wolff's law, bone will adapt to stress loads such that increasing forces will encourage osteocytes to strengthen bone mineral density (BMD). Unfortunately, the reverse also holds true: a cage that reduces stress on the adjacent vertebral bodies will decrease the stimulus for bone remodeling necessary for fusion leading to osteopenia and possibly subsidence of the cage into the vertebral body. Additionally, the orthopedic literature emphasizes the causal relationship between force transference onto bony implants and subsequent pseudoarthrosis. This becomes particularly important when extremely rigid hardware with a very high modulus of elasticity actually promotes not only subsidence but shields the graft material from the compressive forces consistent with Wolff's law, a phenomenon known as stress shielding [34].

Aside from structural considerations, cages must also be discussed in the context of biological supplementation as traditional cages have no osteogenic, osteoinductive, or osteoconductive potential. Morselized local or harvested bone or iliac crest bone marrow aspirates represent two common autograft supplements, naturally rich in bone morphogenetic proteins, insulin growth factors, and fibroblast growth factors [34]. Systematic reviews comparing local autograft from the bony decompression versus harvesting autograft from the iliac crest found similar fusion rates of 89% and 79%, respectively [35]. In those patients without sufficient bone from local decompression or without interest in painful bone marrow aspirates, allograft powder, strips, and bone chips confer a cost-effective alternative to expensive synthetic proteins, albeit the aforementioned allogenic risks still apply. One particular allograft application, demineralized bone matrix (DBM), chemically isolates type I collagen and osteoinductive particles for placement into the fusion construct. Criticisms of DBM include an overabundance of marketed products with significant variability in the concentrations of osteoinductive properties, as seen in in vitro extraction of growth factors and in vivo animal fusion models. Without clinical or scientific evidence in humans to support its use, the efficacy can be unpredictable. Plus, in the absence of viable cells, the osteoinductive effects of DBM require an adjunctive biologic substrate, which again questions the utility of DBM all together.

Ceramics are another graft substrate that can be alternatively manufactured as a biologic supplement, including hydroxyapatite, tricalcium phosphate, calcium phosphate, collagen, and calcium sulfate. The large porosity (void) sizes allow for cell adhesion, proliferation, and differentiation into osteoblasts. Lastly, recombinant human bone morphogenetic protein-2 (rhBMP-2), despite its popularized success in fusion adjunctive therapy, should be considered with caution in the cervical spine because of prevertebral swelling/inflammation that may result in airway compromise, reintubation, and seroma-related compression. In addition, patients should be consoled that use of rhBMP-2 has not been approved by the FDA and there is an FDA warning regarding its use in anterior cervical surgery.

Polyetheretherketone (PEEK)

Inert semicrystalline polyaromatic linear polymers, PEEK cages, do not carry any osteogenic, osteoinductive, or osteoconductive potential. The implant is radiolucent with radiopaque markers to assist the surgeon for roentgenographic (X-ray) localization without significant artifact on magnetic resonance imaging (MRI). Furthermore, the radiolucent composition of these cages easily allows surgeons to monitor bone growth on serial X-rays in the long-term postoperative period. In the 1990s, polyetheretherketone (PEEK) cages were developed to facilitate the bone-cage-bone transition with a modulus of elasticity equal to 3 GPa, comparable to 1.0–2.4 GPa in cortical bone. Hence, the rate of arthrodesis with PEEK cages is comparable to autografts [36]. Extrapolation of evidence from the lumbar spine indicates that supplementation of PEEK with local autograft or demineralized allograft is necessary for fusion across these cervical constructs.

As compared to autograft, prospective clinical studies suggested equivalent results in terms of patient-reported outcomes [36]. In fact, obviating morbidity associated with donor site harvesting persuaded some authors to suggest PEEK cage over autografts. Surgical outcomes, on the other hand, unveiled surprisingly high rates of PEEK cage subsidence, ranging from 32% to 38% of operations [37, 38]. Causes for subsidence include over distraction, aggressive endplate preparation, or normal fusion processes.

The shape of the interbody graft also draws upon the modulus of elasticity, in which a larger surface area of the straining force decreases the stress on the adjacent endplate. This equates to a decreased modulus, closer to that of cortical bone. In a randomized prospective trial, a wider square-shaped PEEK cage, in comparison to a narrower circular cage, decreased subsidence and segmental kyphosis. Thus, while the height of the cage does impact lordosis, surgeons should not overlook the width of the interbody graft to optimize their fusion construct [39].

Surface-Coated Interbody Cages

The concept of surface-coated interbody cages arose from conflicting evidence in the literature on the efficacy of PEEK cages. While comparisons between allograft/autograft and PEEK cages indicated worse subsidence rates with the polymeric compound, comparisons with titanium cages demonstrated very different outcomes. In a randomized controlled trial comparing PEEK to titanium cages in the cervical spine, subsidence rates of 34.5% in the titanium cohort fell precipitously to 5.4% in the PEEK group [40]. Therefore, several studies ascertained that the polymeric insert preserved Cobb angles and intervertebral heights more effectively than metallic counterparts [41]. So despite near-perfect (100%) fusion success across PEEK and titanium groups, PEEK implants have consistently merited the final recommendations in the aforementioned studies [8, 40, 41]. Owing to lower elasticity compared to titanium, PEEK cages theoretically decrease the risk of subsidence. As different studies teetered between advantages and disadvantages of autograft/allograft, PEEK, and titanium, engineers designed surface-coated interbody cages to capture favorable properties of PEEK, metals, and biological supplements.

Surface-coated interbody cages increase bone-to-implant contact ratio and bioactivity. PEEK implants and other interbody models may be covered with a thin layer of various metals: hydroxyapatite, titanium, gold, titanium dioxide, diamond-like carbon, and *tert*-butoxides [42]. The most commonly used bioactive material is hydroxyapatite, the closest derivative of pure bone. Several studies have demonstrated the increased osteoconductivity of hydroxyapatite-coated PEEK cages, with some suggestion of osteoinduction [43]. Histologically speaking, these properties of surface-coated interbody cages speak to a phenomenon, known as osseointegration: the formation of bony tissue around the implant provides a direct anchor onto the bone endplate without fibrous tissue overgrowth at the bone-implant interface according to *Dorland's Illustrated Medical Dictionary* [44]. Clinically speaking, osseointegration is defined as "A process whereby clinically asymptomatic rigid fixation of alloplastic materials is achieved, and maintained, in bone during functional loading." [45] The surface-coated particles, thus, induct bony overgrowth and subsequent arthrodesis beginning at the cage-bone interface. For example, titanium and gold coating promotes osteoblast adhesion on the PEEK interbody graft [46]. Similar findings have been discovered with carbon fiber coatings. The rough nanometer terrain promotes bony fusion and precipitates calcium phosphate deposit and, thus, fusion at the cellular level [47]. Despite physiological optimism, surface-coated interbody cages have undergone intense scrutiny because, like titanium cages, their modulus of elasticity can range from 10 GPa to 100 GPa depending on the density of the coat (compared to 1.0–2.4 GPa in cortical bone).

Titanium-coated interbody cages have gained the most notoriety, however, for their load-bearing applications. The coating increases the shear strength between interbody and bone and thus reduces the risk of pseudoarthrosis; however, the benefits should be weighed with the risk of delamination – separation of the metallic layers. In a biomechanical study, repeated drop weight forces produced wear debris from titanium-coated PEEK [48]. Phagocytosis of the particulate matter promulgates a systemic inflammatory reaction, which may hinder arthrodesis.

Bioabsorbable Polymers

The inherent limitations of surface-coated interbody cages stimulated the development of the bioabsorbable polymers – a radiolucent implant on X-ray films. Composed of polylactic acid (PLA), the polymer exhibits slower degradation kinetics with higher crystallinity, molecular weight, and glass transition temperature (Tg) than other biodegradable implants. The interbody cage in vivo crystallizes after several months with final loss of polymer mass over several years. Clearance of these degradation products underscores the importance of neovascularization around the surgical bed. These products may also be responsible for local inflammation and osteolysis, which opposes propensity to fuse. Greater interbody thickness also expedites degradation often times before bony fusion, which may lead to pseudoarthrosis. Therefore, the bioabsorbable polymers are ill-suited for large distracting forces. Lastly, in general, bioresorbable materials confer less strength than metals or other nondegradable polymers, so the inserts should be reserved for single-level fusions. Clinical data on PLA implants have been largely limited to lumbar applications. In a study on single transforaminal lumbar interbody fusion, fusion rate reached 90% after a minimum of 3 years [49]. Two other studies reported arthrodesis rates up to 97% with biologic supplementation. One study on cervical fusion with bioresorbable cages reported no soft tissue swelling, dysphagia, or dysphonia [50]. Fusion rates reached 46.6%, 69.0%, and 74.1% after the 6-month, 12-month, and ultimate follow-up visits, respectively.

Addition of hydroxyapatite or tricalcium phosphate composites to the PLAs introduces an osteoconductive scaffold. However, decreasing the purity of the polymer with bone products must be tempered with the reduction of the PLA strength once hydrolysis begins [51]. A second technical pearl, endplate preparation, is of utmost importance because fibrous tissue from disc remnants more easily invades the graft than the bone from adjacent vertebral bodies.

Future Directions

Three-Dimensional Printed Interbody

Regardless of the interbody graft choice, a poorly selected interbody shape decreases the likelihood of fusion because of failure to restore normal loading patterns [52]. To engineer more ergonomic and organic shapes, the impetus on interbody technologies has shifted to three-dimensional (3D) printing, also known as additive manufacture. With a computer-aided design, the interbody cage is assembled with a layer-by-layer deposition of nanocomposite polymer. Degradable polyurethane renders an elastic scaffold that mimics the gelatinous nature of the native intervertebral discs. The polycarbonate base has a modulus of elasticity equal to 2.4 GPa, equivalent to that of the bone [53]. These fabricated scaffolds replicated elastic behavior similar to healthy intervertebral discs during compressive and shear testing, an important attribute in permitting fatigue resistance and preventing permanent deformation [54]. 3D printing also allows for seeding cells along the concentric lamellae of the polymer and allows for osteogenic and osteoconductive capacity, like the native disc. While the safety and efficacy of 3D printing clinical and biomechanical testing still require rigorous clinical and biomechanical testing, the prospect of custom design 3D printing bares a new horizon in interbody technology.

References

1. Chau AM, Mobbs RJ. Bone graft substitutes in anterior cervical discectomy and fusion. Eur Spine J. 2009;18(4):449–64.
2. Pal GP, Sherk HH. The vertical stability of the cervical spine. Spine. 1988;13(5):447–9.
3. Robinson RA. Anterolateral cervical disc removal and interbody fusion for cervical disc syndrome. Bull Johns Hopkins Hosp. 1955;96:223–4.
4. Cloward RB. The anterior approach for removal of ruptured cervical disks. J Neurosurg. 1958;15(6):602–17.
5. Frost HM. Wolff's law and bone's structural adaptations to mechanical usage: an overview for clinicians. Angle Orthod. 1994;64(3):175–88.
6. Ruff C, Holt B, Trinkaus E. Who's afraid of the big bad Wolff?: "Wolff's law" and bone functional adaptation. Am J Phys Anthropol. 2006;129(4):484–98.
7. An HS, Simpson JM, Glover JM, Stephany J. Comparison between allograft plus demineralized bone matrix versus autograft in anterior cervical fusion. A prospective multicenter study. Spine (Phila Pa 1976). 1995;20(20):2211–6.
8. Barlocher CB, Barth A, Krauss JK, Binggeli R, Seiler RW. Comparative evaluation of microdiscectomy only, autograft fusion, polymethylmethacrylate interposition, and threaded titanium cage fusion for treatment of single-level cervical disc disease: a prospective randomized study in 125 patients. Neurosurg Focus. 2002;12(1):E4.
9. Rothman RH, Simeone FA. The spine, vol. 2. Philadelphia: WB Saunders Company; 1982.
10. Lowe TG, Hashim S, Wilson LA, et al. A biomechanical study of regional endplate strength and cage morphology as it relates to structural interbody support. Spine (Phila Pa 1976). 2004;29(21):2389–94.
11. McAfee PC, Lee GA, Fedder IL, Cunningham BW. Anterior BAK instrumentation and fusion: complete versus partial discectomy. Clin Orthop Relat Res. 2002;394:55–63.
12. Song KJ, Choi BY. Current concepts of anterior cervical discectomy and fusion: a review of literature. Asian Spine J. 2014;8(4):531–9.

13. White AA 3rd, Hirsch C. An experimental study of the immediate load bearing capacity of some commonly used iliac bone grafts. Acta Orthop Scand. 1971;42(6):482–90.
14. Younger EM, Chapman MW. Morbidity at bone graft donor sites. J Orthop Trauma. 1989;3(3):192–5.
15. Silber JS, Anderson DG, Daffner SD, et al. Donor site morbidity after anterior iliac crest bone harvest for single-level anterior cervical discectomy and fusion. Spine (Phila Pa 1976). 2003;28(2):134–9.
16. Heary RF, Schlenk RP, Sacchieri TA, Barone D, Brotea C. Persistent iliac crest donor site pain: independent outcome assessment. Neurosurgery. 2002;50(3):510–6; discussion 516–7.
17. Tyerman SD, Terry BR, Findlay GP. Multiple conductances in the large K+ channel from Chara corallina shown by a transient analysis method. Biophys J. 1992;61(3):736–49.
18. Jagannathan J, Shaffrey CI, Oskouian RJ, et al. Radiographic and clinical outcomes following single-level anterior cervical discectomy and allograft fusion without plate placement or cervical collar. J Neurosurg Spine. 2008;8(5):420–8.
19. Zdeblick TA, Ducker TB. The use of freeze-dried allograft bone for anterior cervical fusions. Spine (Phila Pa 1976). 1991;16(7):726–9.
20. Floyd T, Ohnmeiss D. A meta-analysis of autograft versus allograft in anterior cervical fusion. Eur Spine J. 2000;9(5):398–403.
21. Young WF, Rosenwasser RH. An early comparative analysis of the use of fibular allograft versus autologous iliac crest graft for interbody fusion after anterior cervical discectomy. Spine (Phila Pa 1976). 1993;18(9):1123–4.
22. Stevenson S, Horowitz M. The response to bone allografts. J Bone Joint Surg Am. 1992;74(6):939–50.
23. Goulet JA, Senunas LE, DeSilva GL, Greenfield ML. Autogenous iliac crest bone graft. Complications and functional assessment. Clin Orthop Relat Res. 1997;339:76–81.
24. Hamer AJ, Strachan JR, Black MM, Ibbotson CJ, Stockley I, Elson RA. Biochemical properties of cortical allograft bone using a new method of bone strength measurement. A comparison of fresh, fresh-frozen and irradiated bone. J Bone Joint Surg Br. 1996;78(3):363–8.
25. Bauer TW, Muschler GF. Bone graft materials. An overview of the basic science. Clin Orthop Relat Res. 2000;371:10–27.
26. Asselmeier MA, Caspari RB, Bottenfield S. A review of allograft processing and sterilization techniques and their role in transmission of the human immunodeficiency virus. Am J Sports Med. 1993;21(2):170–5.
27. Thalgott JS, Fritts K, Giuffre JM, Timlin M. Anterior interbody fusion of the cervical spine with coralline hydroxyapatite. Spine (Phila Pa 1976). 1999;24(13):1295–9.
28. Dai LY, Jiang LS. Anterior cervical fusion with interbody cage containing beta-tricalcium phosphate augmented with plate fixation: a prospective randomized study with 2-year follow-up. Eur Spine J. 2008;17(5):698–705.
29. Bruneau M, Nisolle JF, Gilliard C, Gustin T. Anterior cervical interbody fusion with hydroxyapatite graft and plate system. Neurosurg Focus. 2001;10(4):E8.
30. van den Bent MJ, Oosting J, Wouda EJ, van Acker RE, Ansink BJ, Braakman R. Anterior cervical discectomy with or without fusion with acrylate. A randomized trial. Spine (Phila Pa 1976). 1996;21(7):834–9; discussion 840.
31. Boker DK, Schultheiss R, Probst EM. Radiologic long-term results after cervical vertebral interbody fusion with polymethyl methacrylate (PMMA). Neurosurg Rev. 1989;12(3):217–21.
32. Chen JF, Wu CT, Lee SC, Lee ST. Use of a polymethylmethacrylate cervical cage in the treatment of single-level cervical disc disease. J Neurosurg Spine. 2005;3(1):24–8.
33. Yoo M, Kim WH, Hyun SJ, Kim KJ, Jahng TA, Kim HJ. Comparison between two different cervical interbody fusion cages in one level stand-alone ACDF: carbon Fiber composite frame cage versus Polyetheretherketone cage. Korean J Spine. 2014;11(3):127–35.
34. Benzel EC. Spine surgery: techniques, complication avoidance, and management. New York: Churchill Livingstone; 2005.
35. Hsu WK, Nickoli MS, Wang JC, et al. Improving the clinical evidence of bone graft substitute technology in lumbar spine surgery. Global Spine J. 2012;2(4):239–48.
36. Lied B, Roenning PA, Sundseth J, Helseth E. Anterior cervical discectomy with fusion in patients with cervical disc degeneration: a prospective outcome study of 258 patients (181 fused with autologous bone graft and 77 fused with a PEEK cage). BMC Surg. 2010;10:10.
37. Konig SA, Spetzger U. Distractable titanium cages versus PEEK cages versus iliac crest bone grafts for the replacement of cervical vertebrae. Minim Invasive Ther Allied Technol. 2014;23(2):102–5.
38. Kao TH, Wu CH, Chou YC, Chen HT, Chen WH, Tsou HK. Risk factors for subsidence in anterior cervical fusion with stand-alone polyetheretherketone (PEEK) cages: a review of 82 cases and 182 levels. Arch Orthop Trauma Surg. 2014;134(10):1343–51.
39. Kast E, Derakhshani S, Bothmann M, Oberle J. Subsidence after anterior cervical inter-body fusion. A randomized prospective clinical trial. Neurosurg Rev. 2009;32(2):207–14; discussion 214.
40. Chen Y, Wang X, Lu X, et al. Comparison of titanium and polyetheretherketone (PEEK) cages in the surgical treatment of multilevel cervical spondylotic myelopathy: a prospective, randomized, control study with over 7-year follow-up. Eur Spine J. 2013;22(7):1539–46.
41. Niu CC, Liao JC, Chen WJ, Chen LH. Outcomes of interbody fusion cages used in 1 and 2-levels anterior cervical discectomy and fusion: titanium cages versus polyetheretherketone (PEEK) cages. J Spinal Disord Tech. 2010;23(5):310–6.

42. Ma R, Tang T. Current strategies to improve the bioactivity of PEEK. Int J Mol Sci. 2014;15(4):5426–45.
43. Lee JH, Jang HL, Lee KM, et al. In vitro and in vivo evaluation of the bioactivity of hydroxyapatite-coated polyetheretherketone biocomposites created by cold spray technology. Acta Biomater. 2013;9(4):6177–87.
44. Bucy PC. Dorland's illustrated medical dictionary. Surg Neurol. 1982;17(5):369.
45. Zarb G, Albrektsson T. Osseointegration: a requiem for the periodontal ligament. Int J Periodontics Restorative Dent. 1991;11(1):88–91.
46. Yao C, Storey D, Webster TJ. Nanostructured metal coatings on polymers increase osteoblast attachment. Int J Nanomedicine. 2007;2(3):487–92.
47. Devine DM, Hahn J, Richards RG, Gruner H, Wieling R, Pearce SG. Coating of carbon fiber-reinforced polyetheretherketone implants with titanium to improve bone apposition. J Biomed Mater Res B Appl Biomater. 2013;101(4):591–8.
48. Kienle A, Graf N, Wilke HJ. Does impaction of titanium-coated interbody fusion cages into the disc space cause wear debris or delamination? Spine J. 2016;16(2):235–42.
49. Lowe TG, Tahernia AD. Unilateral transforaminal posterior lumbar interbody fusion. Clin Orthop Relat Res. 2002;394:64–72.
50. Vaccaro AR, Sahni D, Pahl MA, et al. Long-term magnetic resonance imaging evaluation of bioresorbable anterior cervical plate resorption following fusion for degenerative and traumatic disk disruption. Spine (Phila Pa 1976). 2006;31(18):2091–4.
51. Wuisman PI, Smit TH. Bioresorbable polymers: heading for a new generation of spinal cages. Eur Spine J. 2006;15(2):133–48.
52. Palissery V, Mulholland RC, McNally DS. The implications of stress patterns in the vertebral body under axial support of an artificial implant. Med Eng Phys. 2009;31(7):833–7.
53. Serra T, Capelli C, Toumpaniari R, et al. Design and fabrication of 3D-printed anatomically shaped lumbar cage for intervertebral disc (IVD) degeneration treatment. Biofabrication. 2016;8(3):035001.
54. Whatley BR, Kuo J, Shuai C, Damon BJ, Wen X. Fabrication of a biomimetic elastic intervertebral disk scaffold using additive manufacturing. Biofabrication. 2011;3(1):015004.

26 Anterior Fixation Plating

Harel Deutsch and Mena G. Kerolus

Pitfalls/Pearls Outline

- Anterior cervical plating systems promise to provide internal fixation and stabilization for the cervical spine, promoting fusion and maintenance of alignment, and decrease the rate of pseudoarthrosis and graft extrusion.
- In one-level anterior cervical discectomy and fusion (ACDF) cases, benefits of cervical plating are difficult to prove. Anterior cervical plating is shown to increase fusion rates and is especially likely to help in more challenging fusion cases such as multilevel cases, ACDFs involving allograft, and in smokers.
- Failure due to high screw and plate fractures were seen with early rigid anterior cervical plates. New dynamic stabilization plates have reduced complications related to screw and plate fractures. All modern anterior cervical plates seem to be equally effective.
- When placing a cervical plate intraoperatively, the shortest plate should be used to avoid adjacent segment disease.
- Graft subsidence will occur over time which will result in the plate encroaching on the adjacent cranial and caudal disc space. The plate should cover less than half of the adjacent cranial and caudal vertebral body to avoid this complication.

Introduction

The anterior cervical discectomy and fusion (ACDF) is currently a favored treatment option for most degenerative cervical spine pathology. The ACDF has been shown to be a safe and effective treatment alternative for patients with cervical degenerative myelopathy and radiculopathy. The first anterior cervical procedure was performed in the early 1950s. The anterior cervical plate was developed to address problems with anterior interbody fusions such as graft extrusion, kyphotic deformity, and low fusion rates [1–3]. Initial rigid anterior cervical plating systems were found to have complications related to screw and plate fracture. As unrestricted and rigid constructs have been replaced by dynamic rotational and translation plating systems, the

H. Deutsch (✉)
Department of Neurologic Surgery, Rush University Medical Center, Chicago, IL, USA

M. G. Kerolus
Department of Neurosurgery, Rush University Medical Center, Chicago, IL, USA

M. G. Kaiser et al. (eds.), *Degenerative Cervical Myelopathy and Radiculopathy*,
https://doi.org/10.1007/978-3-319-97952-6_26

incidence of screw and plate fractures along with screw loosening have all decreased; however, there have been no reported significant clinical differences in outcomes with different plating systems [4].

The goals of anterior cervical spine surgery include stabilization of the cervical spine, maintenance of cervical alignment and decompression of the neural structures, all of which have improved with the use of an anterior cervical plate, especially in smokers [5, 6]. The adoption of an anterior cervical plate was rapidly adopted by surgeons despite lack of convincing evidence supporting the use of plating [7–9]. The widespread adoption was likely due to the less demanding technical step after discectomy and graft placement and compelling belief among surgeons that the plating would improve fusion rates and therefore results. Additionally, complications related to anterior cervical plating were rare. This chapter addresses the fundamental biomechanics and development of the anterior cervical plate, the surgical nuances of securing the anterior cervical plate, and the radiographic and clinical outcomes of anterior cervical plating in degenerative myelopathy and radiculopathy.

Main Ideas Supported by Relevant Literature and References

Anterior cervical discectomy and fusion was pioneered in the 1950s by Bailey, Badgley, and Cloward [1, 2]. In 1964, Bohler developed anterior internal fixation to address problems with kyphosis and pseudoarthrosis after uninstrumented fusion [3]. Anterior cervical plating was developed to prevent graft dislodgement and maintain cervical alignment by improving fusion rates and preventing subsidence [5]. Anterior cervical plating must abide by the principles of Wolff's law, that the mechanical force placed on the graft promotes bone remodeling, through a series of biochemical changes, a process of mechanotransduction. A rigid plate may result in stress shielding when some subsidence occurs. The load is carried by the plate-screw construct rather than by the graft. The result is resorption of the graft which increases the risk of nonunion, destabilization, and deformity of the cervical spine [10].

Anterior cervical plates are least helpful in flexion but promote stiffness and stability in extension and lateral bending [11]. Anterior plating after a prior posterior instrumentation enhances stability in longer constructs, but in surgical construct less than two levels, plating does not provide significantly improved rigidity [11–13].

Cervical plating can be broadly divided into two categories: unrestricted and restricted plating systems [14]. Unrestricted plating systems were the first plating systems developed in ACDF procedures. In the 1970s and early 1980s, unrestricted cervical plates were used for the first time. Orozco and Llovet first described the use of a unrestricted cervical plate in a patient with a history of trauma [15]. This was later followed by Caspar who reported a series of 60 patients with an anterior cervical plate in patients with cervical spine trauma [16]. The lack of a screw mechanism to prevent screw back out required a more technically demanding procedure with bicortical screw purchase. The rigid construct was at times complicated by screw and plate fractures which were reported as high as 22% [17, 18].

Restricted cervical plates can be broadly divided into constrained and semiconstrained constructs [14]. The first constrained plate was developed in Switzerland in the late 1980s by Morscher allowing unicortical screw placement and a decrease in screw pullout [19]. This plate was later brought to the United States in 1991 which was known as the Synthes CSLP (DePuy, [Raynham, MA]) [20]. The CSLP plate was rigid and had an increased rate of screw fractures [17]. The Orion plate (Medtronic Sofamor Danek [Memphis, TN]) was later developed with variable screw lengths, plate lengths, and built-in lordosis [14, 17].

Semiconstrained plating systems are considered dynamic plating systems and can be divided into rotational and translational semiconstrained systems. Semiconstrained plating systems allow screw plate motion while providing a locked screw [14]. The Codman plate (Depuy [Raynham,

MA]) was the first rotational plating system allowing both cranial and caudal variable angle screws providing rotational subsidence and decreasing the stress on the plate screw interface. Several case series have demonstrated fusion rates of 88–93% with screw failure rates of 8% [21, 22]. Several other rotational plating systems have been developed including the Atlantis plate (Medtronic Sofamor Danek [Memphis, TN]). The Atlantis plate allowed for mixing fixed and variable screws within the same construct [14]. Fusion rates are as high as 94% with a decreased screw failure rate of 3% [23, 24]. The first semi-constrained translational plate was developed by Acromed (DePuy, [Raynham, MA]), the DOC plate in which the screw interface slide along a rail on the plate. Several other plates including the ABC plate by Aesculap (Tuttlingen, Germany) and the Premier plate by Medtronic Sofamor Danek (Memphis, TN, USA) combine features of rotational and translational semiconstrained plates. Fusion rates with the ABC dynamic plate have been reported to range from 83% to 88% with 4.7% rate of implant-related complications [4, 25, 26]. In conclusion, the rigid screw-plate constructs generally had unacceptable instrumentation failure, but the newer plating systems with a variable screw-plate angle or dynamic plates all seem to have similar improvements over rigid plating systems [27, 28].

Currently, the majority of prospective data regarding the ACDF procedure is obtained during FDA IDE studies for artificial cervical disc procedures. Burkus et al. described a 7-year follow-up in the control for one-level cervical fusion cases and noted a 13.7% (29 of 265 patients) reoperation rate at the index level and an 11.9% reoperation for adjacent level problems (24 of 265 patients) [29].

Surgical Technique

Indications

The treatment of cervical spondylosis involves decompression of the neural structures and maintenance of cervical alignment and stabilization. The ACDF procedure is commonly used to treat patients with cervical spondylosis because it allows for ventral decompression with relatively minimal morbidity. The use of anterior cervical plating is standard in ACDF procedures and corpectomies for the treatment of degenerative cervical disease. Most surgeons routinely use cervical plating in all ACDF surgeries. An ACDF is done in patients to address ventral pathology including the disc space, vertebral body, and correction of cervical alignment. Patients with cervical disc herniation presenting with radiculopathy, cervical spondylosis, cervical stenosis, or cervical kyphosis may benefit from an ACDF with an anterior cervical plate. ACDFs are also effective for anterior osteophytes, fractures, and the majority of cervical degenerative conditions.

Contraindications

Contraindications to ACDF with an anterior cervical plate in patients with cervical spondylosis remain rare. Patients with underlying swallowing dysfunction may not be ideal candidates for an anterior cervical approach. A prior history of cervical radiation or radical neck dissection may limit the approach to the anterior cervical spine in these patients. Once an ACDF procedure is performed, the use of a cervical plate may be considered optional but has no strict contraindications.

Preoperative Planning

The ACDF is traditionally performed in hospital operating rooms although now one- and even two-level ACDFs are increasingly done in ambulatory surgical centers [30]. Patients undergo general anesthesia with general endotracheal intubation. In cases of myelopathy, fiberoptic asleep or fiberoptic awake intubation is considered to avoid hyperextending the cervical spine. The endotracheal tube is usually taped up over the head to allow a surgeon and an assistant to work on either side. The shoulders are taped caudally to allow better visualization of the lower cervical spine with fluoroscopy. The head is usually placed on a donut headrest. In situations when distraction is required, some surgeons use inline Gardner-Wells tongs. Intraoperative monitoring may be considered based on the clinical scenario and surgeon preference, but its role in preventing neurologic injury in ACDF has yet to be significant [31]. Preoperative imaging is closely reviewed and vertebral body depth is assessed. Additionally, anomalous vertebral anatomy can also be assessed.

Surgical Technique

A standard approach for an anterior cervical discectomy is performed. After the discectomy and graft placement, the Caspar pins or disc distractor is removed and the cervical plate is ready to be secured. Contouring of the plate and anterior cervical vertebral bodies is essential for appropriate placement of the cervical plate. Anterior osteophytes should be drilled to ensure that the anterior cervical plate is flush with the vertebral bodies. If anterior osteophytes are not appropriately removed and the vertebral bodies are not contoured appropriately, the cervical plate may be proud and may contribute to swallowing difficulty as well as place increase stress on screw-plate interface. The length of the cervical plate should be the shortest length while providing adequate screw purchase in the vertebral bodies. As subsidence of the surgical construct occurs, a plate that is too long will encroach on adjacent levels and accelerate degenerative changes at these levels as the plate "moves" closer to the adjacent disc. When using longer plates for longer surgical constructs, holding pins may be used to keep the plate aligned as there may be significant manipulation during screw placement.

Screws are typically placed subcortically and are typically 14 mm in length although the vertebral bodies can be measured preoperatively and screws up to 16 or even 20 mm can be placed. There is a higher risk of neurologic injury when bicortical purchase is desired. Additionally, more fluoroscopy would be necessary for bicortical screw placement. Screws are either self-tapping or self-drilling and can be placed angled away from the graft in the sagittal plane and medially. Screws are placed at an angle to promote bone purchase. In a variable screw plate construct, as settling occurs, diverging sagittal plane screws will become parallel over time. If screws are initially placed parallel in the sagittal plane, after subsidence, the screws will appear converging in a variable angle screw construct. Fluoroscopy can be used to confirm proper screw trajectory. Ideally the plate should be in line with the coronal plane in the center of the vertebral body. Once all the screws are placed, the locking mechanism of the cervical plate is engaged to prevent screw backup. The locking mechanisms do vary from plate to plate which may include a positive stop usually with turning of a cam to prevent screw back out. Other screw-plate systems allow for automatic engagement of the mechanism to prevent screw back out once the screw advances into the plate.

Patients with osteoporosis may benefit from anterior cervical plating, but poor bone mineral density and bone purchase may lead to screw loosening and subsequent complications [32, 33]. Bicortical screw purchase provides increased holding power and increases cyclic loading, but the differences between bicortical and subcortical screw placement are minimal [33–35].

Postoperative Care/Concerns

The patients are monitored in the postoperative period for any swelling at the surgical site that may indicate a hematoma that may result in airway problems. A postoperative lateral and anteroposterior cervical radiograph is obtained to establish baseline instrumentation placement. A drain is placed if there is bleeding at the operative site. The use of an anterior cervical plate is suggested as a reason to reduce the need for bracing in the postoperative period [36, 37]. Cervical radiographs are obtained at approximately 6 weeks, 3 months, 6 months, and a year out to assess instrumentation. A cervical CT scan may be considered at 1 year to assess for fusion.

Complication Management/ Avoidance

Complications related to anterior cervical plating remain rare [30, 38]. A misaligned plate rarely results in a complication; fluoroscopy and attention to detail can be used to confirm a midline placement of the plate. Extreme deviation of the plate could result in an inadvertently placed screw. If the screw-plate mechanism is not appropriately engaged, screw loosening can occur and back out of the vertebral body. A millimeter of screw back out may be followed closely with serial X-rays. If a screw backs out significantly, there is a concern the screw may erode into the esophagus, and therefore the screw is often revised. Additionally, if the anterior cervical plate is proud, the plate may result in swallowing difficulty as well.

Anterior cervical plates have the choice of built-in lordosis. Self-contouring of the plate has been reported to place stress on the plate and subsequently lead to fracture [39]. Plate/screw fractures were common when the plating system was rigid. With the use of a hybrid plate with variable screws or a dynamic plate, plate or screw fractures are rare. Incomplete discectomy or improperly placed grafts may lead to hardware loosening or fractures suggest pseudoarthrosis and should be evaluated with a CT scan. Complications of cervical plating include stress on adjacent segments, implant-related stress shielding on bone and graft, and late tissue injury.

Case Presentations

Case 1: Rigid Plate Construct

A 50-year-old female presented with a 6-month history of progressive, intermittent right scapular pain. One month prior to evaluation, she began experiencing right hand weakness and occasional left arm pain as well. She underwent physical therapy and steroid injections with no relief. On physical examination, she has full range of motion of her neck and grade 4/5 strength in her right wrist dorsiflexion and hypalgesia in her right C6 dermatome. Her reflexes were symmetric. Plain neutral lateral radiographs done revealed disc space collapse and osteophyte formation at C5/C6 (Fig. 26.1a). Magnetic resonance imaging (MRI) demonstrated central canal stenosis and right greater than left foraminal narrowing (Fig. 26.1b, c). Due to her symptomatic right C6 radiculopathy, she underwent a C5/C6 ACDF and plating (Fig. 26.1d) with bicortical screw fixation to form a rigid construct (Fig. 26.1e).

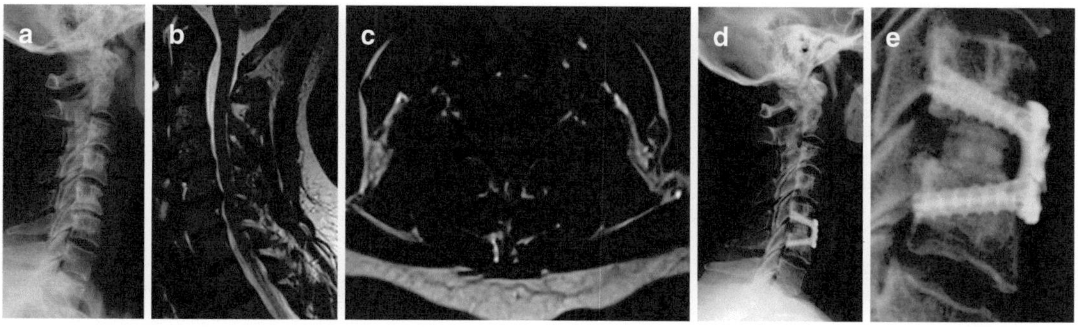

Fig. 26.1 Plain neutral lateral radiograph (**a**) demonstrating disc collapse at C5/C6, osteophyte formation, and loss of lordosis. T2-weighted sagittal (**b**) and axial (**c**) magnetic resonance imaging (MRI) of the cervical spine demonstrating severe cervical stenosis at C5/C6 and right greater than left foraminal narrowing. Postoperative lateral neutral radiographs (**d**) demonstrate correction of lordosis and successful placement of the graft and instrumentation. Note the length of the cervical plate (**e**) in relationship to the vertebral body. The plate covers less than half of the adjacent vertebral bodies. Screws are placed in a bicortical manner as to create a rigid construct

Case 2: Hybrid Cervical Plate

A 59-year-old female presented with a history of neck discomfort, progressive gait difficulty, and paresthesias in her bilateral hands. On physical examination, she did not have any weakness. She had bilateral Hoffman's, a positive Babinski sign, and hyperreflexia 3+ in both her patellar and Achilles reflexes. She also had unsteady gait with tandem heel to toe walk. Sagittal MRI revealed T2 hypertintensity in the cord behind the C4 vertebral body and some cervical stenosis at C3/C4 due to osteophyte formation (Fig. 26.2a). Plain neutral lateral radiographs demonstrated loss of lordosis, osteophyte formation at C3/C4, and multilevel degenerative changes (Fig. 26.2b). Thoracic MRI was normal. Due to failure of improvement in her symptoms, she underwent a C3/C4 and C4/C5 ACDF and plating (Fig. 26.2c). A hybrid construct was used with bicortical purchase at the caudal end of the construct and subcortical screw placement in the cranial vertebral body (Fig. 26.2d). The cervical plate was flush with the vertebral bodies. After 1 year, settling along the caudal graft is evident (arrow) with evidence of fusion (Fig. 26.2e).

Case 3: Swift Plate as Dynamic System

A 50-year-old female presented with 9-year history of neck pain and a 9-month history of right upper extremity and shoulder pain with occasional paresthesias along her right fifth digit. The pain was sharp and intermittent. She underwent conservative management including cervical epidural steroid injections and physical therapy. On physical examination, she had grade 4/5 strength in her deltoids, biceps, triceps, and hand flexors. Reflexes were normal. Plain neutral radiographs (Fig. 26.3a) demonstrated appropriate cervical alignment. Cervical MRI (Fig. 26.3b) demonstrated a large disc herniation at C4/C5 and severe cord compression with subtle white matter changes. There was less severe compression at C5/C6. Due to physical exam findings concerning for myelopathy and severe cord compression on MRI, she underwent a C4–C6 ACDF and plate fixation utilizing a dynamic translational plate (Fig. 26.3c). Lateral and AP X-rays immediately after surgery (Fig. 26.3d, e) and after 1 year demonstrate the dynamic translation within the plate as controlled settling occurs, leading to a solid arthrodesis (Fig. 26.3f, g).

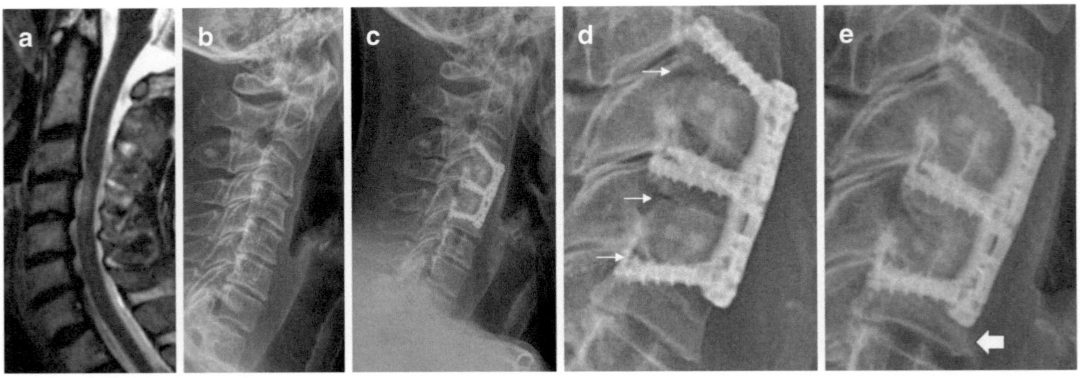

Fig. 26.2 Sagittal T2-weighted MRI (**a**) demonstrating severe cervical stenosis at C3/C4 and osteophyte formation. Plain neutral lateral radiograph (**b**) demonstrating loss of cervical lordosis and multiple levels of cervical degenerative disease and disc collapse. The patient underwent a C3–C5 ACDF (**c**) with plate fixation. Bicortical screw purchase was obtained in the caudal vertebral body and subcortical in the cranial end of the construct. The cervical plate is flush with the vertebral bodies and covers less than half of the superior and inferior adjacent vertebral bodies (**d**). Subsidence of the graft is apparent as the air gaps present on the prior film are gone. The inferior aspect of the cervical plate has subsided into the inferior vertebral body (**e**). Note that the adjacent inferior disc level is still several millimeters away from the inferior edge of the cervical plate (*arrow*)

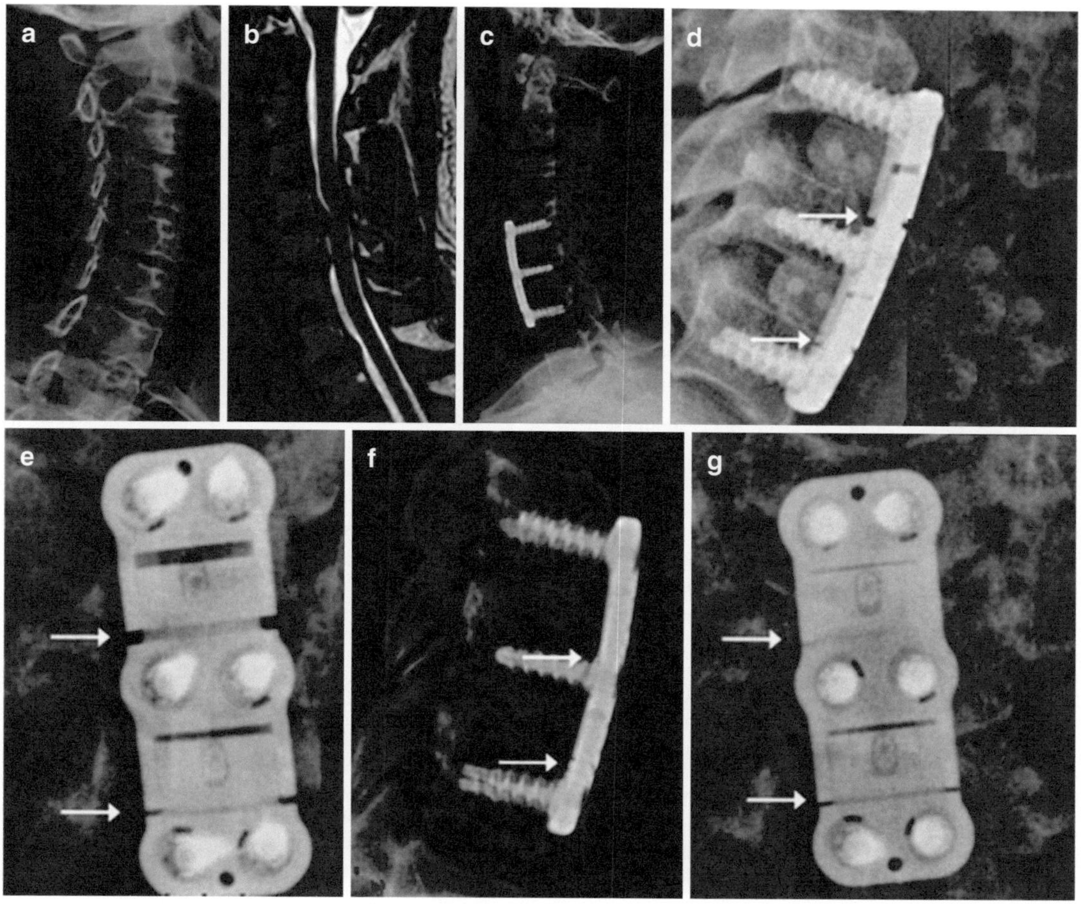

Fig. 26.3 Plain neutral oblique radiograph (**a**) demonstrating overall cervical lordosis. Sagittal T2-weighted MRI (**b**) demonstrating multiple levels of cervical stenosis, most prominent at C3/C4 with T2 cord signal change behind the C4 vertebral body. A C4–C6 ACDF was performed (**c**). A semiconstrained translational plate was used. Note the grooves on the lateral (**d**) and AP (**e**) radiographs indicating the "open" position of the plate. As subsidence of the graft takes place and fusion occurs, the plate collapses on itself, hence its translational construct. The 1-year lateral (**f**) and AP (**g**) radiographs demonstrate the dynamic changes of the plate

Discussion/Conclusions

ACDFs are the most common option for treating cervical spondylosis. Anterior cervical plating is typically applied with all ACDFs. Cervical plating is most frequently used in cases of degenerative cervical disease including anterior cervical corpectomies. Plate biomechanics have evolved to address different clinical scenarios and early plate's failures. The new systems have improved on the plate/screw fractures seen in rigid cervical plate systems. However, there is no strong evidence to support one particular cervical plate system over another. The surgical placement of anterior cervical plates is relatively straightforward and safe. It is important to pay close attention to the cervical plate's relationship to the adjacent cranial and caudal segments to establish the best outcome and avoid long-term complications.

References

1. Bailey RW, Badgley CE. Stabilization of the cervical spine by anterior fusion. J Bone Joint Surg Am. 1960;42-A:565–94.
2. Cloward RB. The anterior approach for removal of ruptured cervical disks. J Neurosurg. 1958;15(6):602–17. https://doi.org/10.3171/jns.1958.15.6.0602.
3. Böhler J, Gaudernak T. Anterior plate stabilization for fracture-dislocations of the lower cervical spine. J Trauma. 1980;20(3):203–5.
4. Pitzen TR, Chrobok J, Stulik J, et al. Implant complications, fusion, loss of lordosis, and outcome after anterior cervical plating with dynamic or rigid plates: two-year results of a multi-centric, randomized, controlled study. Spine. 2009;34(7):641–6. https://doi.org/10.1097/BRS.0b013e318198ce10.
5. Bose B. Anterior cervical instrumentation enhances fusion rates in multilevel reconstruction in smokers. J Spinal Disord. 2001;14(1):3–9.
6. Martin GJ, Haid RW, MacMillan M, Rodts GE, Berkman R. Anterior cervical discectomy with freeze-dried fibula allograft. Overview of 317 cases and literature review. Spine. 1999;24(9):852–8. discussion 858–9.
7. Wang JC, McDonough PW, Endow KK, Delamarter RB. Increased fusion rates with cervical plating for two-level anterior cervical discectomy and fusion. Spine. 2000;25(1):41–5.
8. Wang JC, McDonough PW, Kanim LE, Endow KK, Delamarter RB. Increased fusion rates with cervical plating for three-level anterior cervical discectomy and fusion. Spine. 2001;26(6):643–6. discussion 646–7.
9. Wang JC, McDonough PW, Endow K, Kanim LE, Delamarter RB. The effect of cervical plating on single-level anterior cervical discectomy and fusion. J Spinal Disord. 1999;12(6):467–71.
10. Hakało J, Wroński J, Ciupik L. Subsidence and its effect on the anterior plate stabilization in the course of cervical spondylodesis. Part I: definition and review of literature. Neurol Neurochir Pol. 2003;37(4):903–15.
11. Clausen JD, Ryken TC, Traynelis VC, Sawin PD, Dexter F, Goel VK. Biomechanical evaluation of Caspar and Cervical Spine Locking Plate systems in a cadaveric model. J Neurosurg. 1996;84(6):1039–45. https://doi.org/10.3171/jns.1996.84.6.1039.
12. Griffith SL, Zogbi SW, Guyer RD, Shelokov AP, Contiliano JH, Geiger JM. Biomechanical comparison of anterior instrumentation for the cervical spine. J Spinal Disord. 1995;8(6):429–38.
13. Singh K, Vaccaro AR, Kim J, Lorenz EP, Lim T-H, An HS. Biomechanical comparison of cervical spine reconstructive techniques after a multilevel corpectomy of the cervical spine. Spine. 2003;28(20):2352–8. discussion 2358. https://doi.org/10.1097/01.BRS.0000085344.22471.23.
14. Haid RW, Foley KT, Rodts GE, Barnes B. The cervical spine study group anterior cervical plate nomenclature. Neurosurg Focus. 2002;12(1):E15.
15. Omeis I, DeMattia JA, Hillard VH, Murali R, Das K. History of instrumentation for stabilization of the subaxial cervical spine. Neurosurg Focus. 2004;16(1):E10.
16. Caspar W, Barbier DD, Klara PM. Anterior cervical fusion and Caspar plate stabilization for cervical trauma. Neurosurgery. 1989;25(4):491–502.
17. Lowery GL, McDonough RF. The significance of hardware failure in anterior cervical plate fixation. Patients with 2- to 7-year follow-up. Spine. 1998;23(2):181–6. discussion 186–7.
18. Paramore CG, Dickman CA, Sonntag VK. Radiographic and clinical follow-up review of Caspar plates in 49 patients. J Neurosurg. 1996;84(6):957–61. https://doi.org/10.3171/jns.1996.84.6.0957.
19. Morscher E, Sutter F, Jenny H, Olerud S. Anterior plating of the cervical spine with the hollow screw-plate system of titanium. Chir Z Alle Geb Oper Medizen. 1986;57(11):702–7.
20. Grubb MR, Currier BL, Shih JS, Bonin V, Grabowski JJ, Chao EY. Biomechanical evaluation of anterior cervical spine stabilization. Spine. 1998;23(8):886–92.
21. Casha S, Fehlings MG. Clinical and radiological evaluation of the Codman semiconstrained load-sharing anterior cervical plate: prospective multicenter trial and independent blinded evaluation of outcome. J Neurosurg. 2003;99(3 Suppl):264–70.
22. Mayr MT, Subach BR, Comey CH, Rodts GE, Haid RW. Cervical spinal stenosis: outcome after anterior corpectomy, allograft reconstruction, and instrumentation. J Neurosurg. 2002;96(1 Suppl):10–6.
23. Barnes B, Haid RW, Rodts GE, Subach BR, Kaiser M. Early results using the Atlantis anterior cervical plate system. Neurosurg Focus. 2002;12(1):E13.
24. Kaiser MG, Haid RW, Subach BR, Barnes B, Rodts GE. Anterior cervical plating enhances arthrodesis after discectomy and fusion with cortical allograft. Neurosurgery. 2002;50(2):229–36. discussion 236–8.
25. Epstein NE. Anterior cervical dynamic ABC plating with single level corpectomy and fusion in forty-two patients. Spinal Cord. 2003;41(3):153–8. https://doi.org/10.1038/sj.sc.3101418.
26. Ragab AA, Hodges FS, Hill CP, McGuire RA, Tucci M. Dynamic anterior cervical plating for multi-level spondylosis: does it help? Evid Based Spine Care J. 2010;1(1):41–6. https://doi.org/10.1055/s-0028-1100892.
27. Yang S, Wang L-W. Biomechanical comparison of the stable efficacy of two anterior plating systems. Clin Biomech (Bristol Avon). 2003;18(6):S59–66.
28. Lehmann W, Briem D, Blauth M, Schmidt U. Biomechanical comparison of anterior cervical spine locked and unlocked plate-fixation systems. Eur Spine J. 2005;14(3):243–9. https://doi.org/10.1007/s00586-004-0746-9.

29. Burkus JK, Traynelis VC, Haid RW, Mummaneni PV. Clinical and radiographic analysis of an artificial cervical disc: 7-year follow-up from the prestige prospective randomized controlled clinical trial: clinical article. J Neurosurg Spine. 2014;21(4):516–28. https://doi.org/10.3171/2014.6.SPINE13996.
30. Adamson T, Godil SS, Mehrlich M, Mendenhall S, Asher AL, McGirt MJ. Anterior cervical discectomy and fusion in the outpatient ambulatory surgery setting compared with the inpatient hospital setting: analysis of 1000 consecutive cases. J Neurosurg Spine. 2016;24(6):878–84. https://doi.org/10.3171/2015.8.SPINE14284.
31. Ajiboye RM, Zoller SD, Sharma A, et al. Intraoperative neuromonitoring for anterior cervical spine surgery: what is the evidence? Spine. 2017;42(6):385–93. https://doi.org/10.1097/BRS.0000000000001767.
32. Ryken TC, Clausen JD, Traynelis VC, Goel VK. Biomechanical analysis of bone mineral density, insertion technique, screw torque, and holding strength of anterior cervical plate screws. J Neurosurg. 1995;83(2):324–9. https://doi.org/10.3171/jns.1995.83.2.0324.
33. Hitchon PW, Brenton MD, Coppes JK, From AM, Torner JC. Factors affecting the pullout strength of self-drilling and self-tapping anterior cervical screws. Spine. 2003;28(1):9–13. https://doi.org/10.1097/01.BRS.0000038185.73138.CB.
34. Spivak JM, Chen D, Kummer FJ. The effect of locking fixation screws on the stability of anterior cervical plating. Spine. 1999;24(4):334–8.
35. Chen IH. Biomechanical evaluation of subcortical versus bicortical screw purchase in anterior cervical plating. Acta Neurochir. 1996;138(2):167–73.
36. Aebi M, Zuber K, Marchesi D. Treatment of cervical spine injuries with anterior plating. Indications, techniques, and results. Spine. 1991;16(3 Suppl):S38–45.
37. Vaccaro AR, Balderston RA. Anterior plate instrumentation for disorders of the subaxial cervical spine. Clin Orthop. 1997;335:112–21.
38. Shapiro SA, Snyder W. Spinal instrumentation with a low complication rate. Surg Neurol. 1997;48(6):566–74.
39. Baldwin NG, Hartman GP, Weiser MW, Benzel EC. Failure of a titanium anterior cervical plate implant: microstructural analysis of failure. Case report. J Neurosurg. 1995;83(4):741–3. https://doi.org/10.3171/jns.1995.83.4.0741.

Cervical Laminectomy and Fusion

27

Jacob Januszewski and Juan S. Uribe

Pitfalls/Pearls

- Cervical laminectomy is a relatively simple technique with a moderate number of technical steps mainly used to treat degenerative cervical myelopathy (DCM).
- It is an effective method for efficient decompression of multilevel, extensive caudal-to-rostral compression.
- Laminectomy alone is a motion-sparing procedure good for elderly patients with osteoporosis or other morbid conditions.
- It may potentially destabilize the posterior tension band and cause progressive kyphosis over time, requiring revision surgery with stabilization and fusion.
- Patients with signs of dynamic instability, moderate to severe spondylosis, listhesis, or lack of lordosis require at least supplemental dorsal instrumentation and arthrodesis.
- Instrumentation and fusion is a complex and potentially more morbid surgery especially in the elderly and patients with osteoporosis.
- Detailed and careful technique must be utilized in laminectomy with fusion to avoid perioperative complications.
- Posterior decompression is not adequate to address mainly anterior compression or presence of anterior osteophytes and a limited number of stenotic segments (three or less). In such cases, either combination anterior/posterior or anterior only approach has to be utilized.

J. Januszewski (✉)
Department of Neurosurgery, Barrow Neurological Institute, Phoenix, AZ, USA

Department of Neurosurgery, The B.A.C.K Center, Melbourne, FL, USA
e-mail: Lionel.Metz@ucsf.edu

J. S. Uribe
Department of Neurosurgery, Barrow Neurological Institute, Phoenix, AZ, USA

Introduction

Degenerative cervical myelopathy (DCM), which includes cervical spondylotic myelopathy (CSM), OPLL, and other entities, is a result of combination of compressive, dynamic and biomolecular factors on the spinal cord (Table 27.1) [1, 2]. Compression arises from narrowing of the ventral/dorsal cervical canal, disc degeneration, spondylosis, and ossification of the posterior longitudinal ligament (PLL) and ligamentum flavum leading to direct pressure on the spinal cord. Dynamic forces arise from abnormal cervical spinal alignment or motion as in cases with

M. G. Kaiser et al. (eds.), *Degenerative Cervical Myelopathy and Radiculopathy*,
https://doi.org/10.1007/978-3-319-97952-6_27

Table 27.1 Overview of forces involved in cervical spinal pathology necessitating either laminectomy alone or laminectomy with fusion

Compressive forces	Dynamic forces	Biomolecular forces
Narrowing of the ventral/dorsal cervical canal, disc degeneration, spondylosis, ossification of the posterior longitudinal ligament (PLL) and ligamentum flavum	Abnormal cervical spinal alignment or motion (degenerative spondylosis/listhesis, subluxation, or kyphotic deformity) Physiological narrowing of cervical vertebral canal diameter with neck extension, causing strain/stretch forces on the spinal cord	Ischemic injury from chronic compression, subsequent release of inflammatory factors, glutamate-mediated excitotoxicity, and eventually neuronal apoptosis

degenerative spondylolisthesis, subluxation, or kyphotic deformity. Physiological narrowing of canal diameter with neck extension as well as strain/stretch forces placed on the spinal cord with physiological neck movements also contribute to dynamic pathophysiological stresses [1, 2]. Finally, ischemic injury from chronic compression, subsequent release of inflammatory factors, glutamate-mediated excitotoxicity, and eventually neuronal apoptosis contribute to CSM on a molecular and cellular level [1]. The goal of surgery, in turn, is first to decompress the neural structures and reduce the effect of static and biomolecular factors and, second, to stabilize the dynamic factors if such need exists.

Cervical laminectomy for degenerative cervical myelopathy from compressive forces is commonly performed in either minimally invasive (MIS) or open fashion. Addition of dorsal instrumentation and arthrodesis should be used when abnormal dynamic forces exist and result in instability. Additionally, attention must be paid to maintenance of cervical sagittal balance, correction of loss of lordosis, or cervical kyphosis that may result in symptomatic cervical deformity. This chapter discusses the importance of preoperative imaging and patient workup on successful surgical planning and clinical outcome. Meticulous surgical technique is also required to avoid potentially avoidable complications from technical errors. Surgical techniques for both open and MIS approaches are discussed in detailed, followed by surgical pearls for complication avoidance, management, and postoperative care.

Main Ideas

While DCM has been traditionally treated with mainly posterior approaches in the past, the national trend has dramatically changed over the last decade. A recent retrospective nationwide database analysis showed that combined anterior/posterior approaches have increased sixfold, while posterior-only approach increased threefold, and anterior-only approach doubled while at the same time increasing morbidity [3]. There is no clear indication as to why this trend is occurring, but the wide variability in patient selection, preoperative imaging and workup, and technique used undoubtedly plays a role. The role of anterior vs. posterior surgery or both is still not established and frequently debated. The main goal of surgery is decompression of the spinal cord and the exiting nerve roots. If stabilization is also required, successful arthrodesis becomes a secondary goal. True fusion rates for laminectomy with instrumentation and fusion are still not clearly defined and may depend on several factors such as adequate preparation of the bony articular surfaces and bone substitute material used. Autogenous corticocancellous bone may be used from the laminectomy performed or from a harvested dorsal iliac crest or a rib and is placed over the decorticated dorsal elements of the articular surfaces and lateral masses [4]. Biologic allograft use has recently become a popular option in fusion surgery but however has been on a decline since the 2008 FDA advisory and 2011 *The Spine Journal* warning regarding rhBMP use in cervical spine [5]. Prior to this, fusion rate with rhBMP has been shown to be 100% [6]. Use of mesenchymal cellular bone matrix in cervical spine also has fusion rates approaching that of rhBMP, and autograph at 12 months with good clinical outcomes and stem cell augmentation of spinal fusion is now considered the equivalent to the gold standard for iliac crest graft in fusion models [3, 7]. When combined with anterior surgery, however, pseudoarthrosis rates decrease depending on the type of instrumentation/plating and bone supplementation used for the anterior portion, though new randomized controlled studies on this topic are lacking [2].

Surgical Options

Patient Selection

Proper patient selection should be carefully approached keeping in mind the pathological process involved (Fig. 27.1). Patients with mild to moderate clinical DCM, without radiographic signs of myelomalacia, with good lordosis may be favorable candidates for laminectomy as their symptoms are likely mainly compressive in nature. Elderly patients requiring a multilevel decompression who may have poor bone quality (osteomalacia, osteopenia, osteoporosis) and severe subsystem disease would also be better candidates for laminectomy alone, as they have higher morbidity associated with more complex procedures. However, multilevel laminectomies may result in kyphotic deformity over time, and younger patients may benefit from instrumentation and fusion even with initially good cervical lordosis so as to minimize the likelihood of progression to degenerative kyphoscoliosis in the future. In patients with advanced DCM (T2 cord signal changes), while still debatable, it may also be beneficial to limit the dynamic component by dorsal instrumentation and arthrodesis. Finally, for patients who present with frank signs of instability (antero−/retrolisthesis, subluxation, dynamic instability on flexion/extension radiographs, significant loss of lordosis, or frank kyphoscoliosis), it is advised to stabilize the dynamic instability with dorsal instrumentation and arthrodesis [8].

Preoperative Workup and Imaging

Equally important is thorough preoperative workup and imaging, as it itself leads to proper

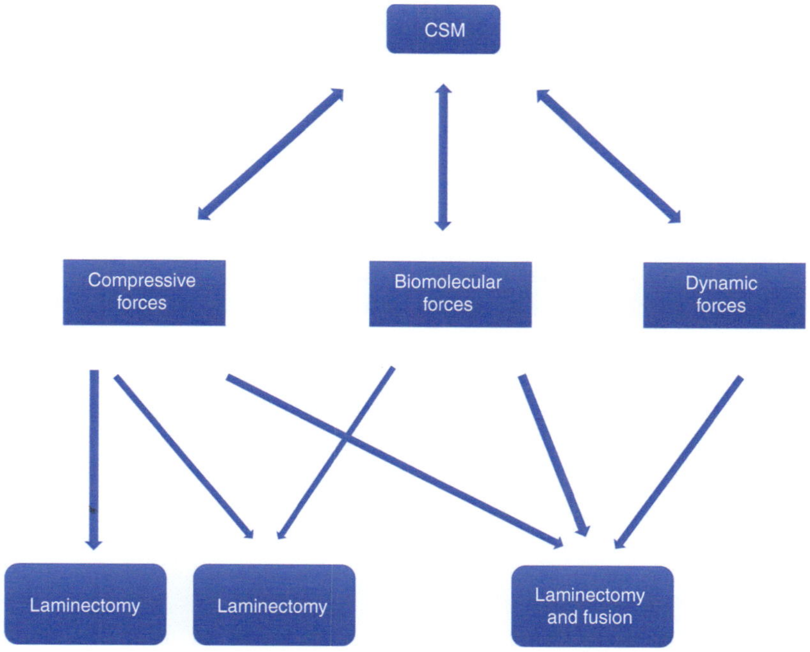

Fig. 27.1 Surgical decision-making flowchart based on pathology being addressed

patient selection and aids in surgical approach decision-making. Almost all patients who present with clinical signs of DCM will already have a non-contrast cervical MRI to evaluate compressive forces done prior to their surgical consultation. However, it is important not to rely solely on one imaging modality. Upright cervical AP/lateral and flexion/extension radiographs will provide substantial information that a cervical MRI performed in a supine position simply cannot. Patient presenting with good alignment on an MRI may actually show kyphosis or anterolisthesis on upright radiographs. Similarly, if instability is suspected based on the plain radiograph possibility leading to a laminectomy with fusion, a non-contrasted CT of cervical spine should also be obtained. A CT can better delineate anterior osteophytes, ossified ligament, lateral mass size, and location of aberrant vertebral artery in rare situations. However, having a full picture of the patient prior to surgical planning will aid in deciding on surgical approach and potentially decrease patient morbidity.

Occasionally, in patients with a confusing clinical picture or combination of myelopathy and radiculopathy, other tests such as electromyeographs (EMGs) and bone scans can be used to facilitate evaluation of the patient. For women who are over the age of 55 and men with risk factors for osteoporosis, evaluation of bone mineral density (BMD) with a DEXA scan could help to assess potential perioperative and long-term morbidity, especially if dorsal instrumentation and arthrodesis are planned. BMD has been strongly associated with higher complications and instrumentation failure rates [9–13]. Finally, the use of objective health-related quality of life measures (HRQOL) such as visual analog scale (VAS), SF-12, or SF-36 should be used both in preoperative and postoperative settings. These allow for better evaluation of postoperative clinical outcomes and can be used to trend the efficacy of the treatment provided over time.

Preoperative Assessment and Workup in Cervical Deformity

Cervical kyphosis, or ventral angulation of 5° or more, is a result of the same processes involved in degenerative cervical myelopathy: concurrent ligamentous laxity, loss of disc height, and bony remodeling. Spinal malalignment can, in turn, lead to neck pain, myelopathy, radiculopathy, or loss of mobility regardless of compressive radiographic findings on cervical spine MRI. A considerable variation in the amount of cervical lordosis is observed in general population. While the loss of cervical lordosis may be a normal part of aging, and not all patients with loss of lordosis have refractory neck pain, there certainly is a subset of patients with chronic neck pain secondary to loss of lordosis, cervical sagittal imbalance, and dorsal neck pain secondary to chronic muscle fatigue. Evaluation of cervical sagittal balance is, therefore, a crucial component of preoperative patient assessment.

Multitude of studies has been performed to normalize cervical lordosis (CL) measurements with a range from −10° to −39° reported [14–18]. There isn't, however, a normal cervical lordosis value yet agreed upon due to a variable range in the general population, increase of the CL with age as a compensatory mechanism for the increased thoracic kyphosis and reduced lumbar lordosis, and influence of posture on CL as demonstrated by an average increase of CL by 3.45° from standing to sitting [19, 20]. However, accepted range falls somewhere between −15 and 20 ± 15° measured as a Cobb angle between C1 or C2 and C7 [2]. This value is measured from standing upright lateral radiographs. For proper cervical deformity assessment, AP/lateral and flexion/extension radiographs are needed to provide information about the deformity levels involved, severity, dynamic instability, listhesis, or pseudoarthrosis and whether deformity appears reducible or fixed. Another useful measure in cervical deformity correction is the chin-brow vertical angle.

This angle should be as close to neutral as possible to facilitate the position of the eyes in line with the horizon. The goal of surgical realignment, however, should be to restore neutral sagittal balance rather than a specific value of cervical lordosis. The C2–C7 SVA (cSVA) plumb line should be maintained or corrected close to neutral. While there isn't a specific normal value for cSVA, symptomatic patients tend to have cSVA >40 mm with the surgical correction goal of under 20 mm [16, 21, 22]. Overall sagittal and coronal balance should be taken into consideration, and the head should be balanced over the sacrum. Recently, higher T-1 slope (T1S) has been associated with modic changes in the cervical spine, which may be contributory to the development of axial neck pain [23]. T1S slightly increase with each decade but range from 32 to 36° in men and 28 to 37° in women, respectively. T1S > 40° and T1S-CL > 20° have worse HRQOL scores and should be addressed with surgical deformity correction [20, 24]. Complete upright standing scoliosis films should be considered in every preoperative workup where cervical deformity is suspected. Cervical C2–C7 SVA, T-1 slope, cervical lordosis, and global sagittal alignment should all be evaluated as part of routine preoperative evaluation. Craniocervical angle (CCA), which combines the slope of McGregor's line and the inclination from C7 to the hard palate, and the C2-pelvic tilt (CPT), which combines C2 tilt and pelvic tilt, account for both cervical sagittal alignment and upper cervical compensation and can be utilized in assessment of complex cervical deformity patients [25].

Most deformities are reducible with positioning (flexion/extension) of the patient's neck and can be addressed with dorsal surgical reconstruction alone or ventrally if ventral compression is present on MRI. On average, ventral approaches can achieve segmental correction of 6° and overall cervical lordosis correction of 9 to 32° [26]. However, ventral approach alone without dorsal instrumentation for support allows for long-term loss of lordosis of approximately 2° [26]. Patients that do not reduce with neck extension deserve a trial of traction before surgery to determine "reducibility" of the spine. If successful, patient can then be fused dorsally in that position. If deformity is fixed and does not reduce with traction, ventral approach can be used for correction. If there is a presence of ankylosed facets, a dorsal osteotomy with combined dorsal-ventral approach may be indicated. Dorsal-only approaches can achieve approximately 6 to 54° of overall lordosis correction (23 to 54° with osteotomy) and chin-brow vertical angle correction of 35 to 52°. Combined ventral-dorsal approaches can achieve approximately 24 to 61° of correction of overall cervical lordosis [26, 27].

Relevant Anatomy

Nuchal Ligament

Nuchal ligament is an extension of the supraspinous ligament of the thoracolumbar spine and attaches from the spinous process of C7 to the external occipital protuberance. It serves as an attachment for the adjacent paraspinal muscles; however, it is surgically relevant as dissection along the middle of this ligament provides an avascular plane. Minimal to no blood loss occurs if dissection is carried out along this ligament followed by the subperiosteal plane along the spinous processes.

Superficial Nerves of the Posterior Neck

Cutaneous branches of the posterior primary rami are found adjacent to spinous process at every level below C2. The dorsal root ganglion is located just anterior to the superior articulating facet sandwiched between the facet and the vertebral artery. From here the nerves divide into anterior primary rami and dorsal primary rami. The anterior primary rami of C1 to C4 form the cervical plexus and from C5 to T1 for the brachial plexus. The dorsal rami send motor fibers to the deep paraspinal muscles and sensory fibers to the facet joint, deep muscles, and soft tissue. The largest branch of the dorsal primary ramus is the greater occipital nerve, and the lesser occipital nerve lies just lateral to it. However, these two nerves are located just below the suboccipital triangle and are rarely encountered during subaxial laminectomies and fusion. In an approach to the lateral area of the facet joint during a laminectomy, it is likely that trunks of the medial branches of the dorsal rami will be encountered and injured; however, this does not seem to negatively affect patient clinical outcome.

Surgical Techniques

Open Surgical Options

Midline Posterior Approach

Patient position for posterior open laminectomy is always prone with head placed either in Mayfield pins or on a flat top table with head in a facemask. However, placing the patient in pins facilitates intraoperative manipulation of cervical alignment if needed. Direct, open posterior approach involves a midline incision centered over the spinous process of the targeted levels. Tissue dissection should be performed in an avascular plane through the ligamentum nuchae, and muscle dissection is always performed in a subperiosteal fashion, as close to the midline as possible to avoid substantial blood loss and unnecessary injury that may lead to increased postoperative pain. Gentle subperiosteal elevation of muscles can be performed, rather than direct monopolar cautery, to avoid tissue damage. Dissection is taken to the lateral aspects of the facet joints. It is easier to start at the caudal end because the bleeding is less at the lower levels. To confirm the level, a small upgoing curette is inserted below the laminar edge, and lateral fluoroscopy is taken.

Bony decompression can be achieved with either a high-speed drill, thinning of the lamina, and a small 2 mm Kerrison rongeur. Ligamentum flavum is always left behind until the entire laminectomy is performed. The ligament is subsequently removed with a Kerrison rongeur to finish the decompression [28]. Alternately, a "lobster-tail" laminectomy can be performed in order to facilitate the operation and remove all of the laminas in one peace. This is accomplished by drilling out a small trough at the lateral edge of the lamina on both sides with a small 4 mm cutting burr or AM-8 drill bit. A small 2 mm Kerrison rongeur is then used to remove the ligamentum flavum from the troughs. Towel clamps are attached to the spinous process and can be used to facilitate the decompression with lamina elevation. Once both sides have been freed and the cephalad and caudal midline lamina has been drilled out, the entire laminectomy can be safely removed en bloc.

Lateral Mass Plating

Anatomical relationship of vertebral artery to lateral mass and lamina must be considered when placing lateral mass screws to avoid injury to the vertebral artery. The medial border of the facet is identified where the lamina joins the lateral mass and the vertebral artery and the exiting nerve root are just anterior to this point. Lateral mass screws must be lateral to this point, and the entry point of the screw is just lateral to it. The targeting angle is 25–30° lateral and 25–30° cephalad [28]. A good rule of thumb is to place the entry points prior to doing a laminectomy. The drill handle making contact with the spinous process forms approximately a 30 degree lateral angle, ideal for lateral mass screw placement.

Cervical Pedicle Screw Fixation

Pedicle screw fixation in cervical spine is mostly used at the cervicothoracic junction, as the lateral masses become thinner at the C7 level (approximately 9 mm and not enough for adequate purchase that generally requires 12–14 mm). The average pedicle size range from 3.5 to 6.5 mm, and the average height is 5–8 mm. The entry point of C7 transpedicular screw is located at the junction of (1) the vertical line passing through the middle of C6/C7 facet and (2) the horizontal line passing at the middle of C7 transverse process. The trajectory of the screw is 30–35° medial and 5° caudal [28].

MIS Surgical Options

Subaxial Laminectomy

Surgical level is identified and confirmed with intraoperative fluoroscopy. The incision is marked 1–1.5 cm off midline on the side of the target laminectomy and infiltrated with a local anesthetic. Incision is 2–2.5 cm in length. A longitudinal fasciotomy is the same length as the skin incision. A starting dilator is then placed and docked on a lamina-facet junction of interest under fluoroscopic guidance. Sequential intermuscular dilation is then followed until final 16–18 mm tubular retractor is inserted and secured to a mounted retractor arm. Retractor should be locked in a medial angulation toward the spinous process, with a lateral edge of the retractor at the medial edge of the lamina-facet junction. Once any residual muscle is removed with a combination of electrocautery and pituitary rongeur, a high-speed drill is used to remove the inferior part of the superior lamina, exposing the ligamentum flavum. Laminectomy is then continued to the superior part of the inferior lamina while preserving ligamentum flavum the entire time. Once the bony laminectomy is completed, ligamentum flavum is removed with a microscopic curette and Kerrison rongeur. Decompression of adjacent levels is then performed by angulating the tube retractor cephalad and caudal as needed. For three or more levels, an expandable retractor may be utilized. After completing the laminectomy, the contralateral side is decompressed in the same manner. Alternatively, the retractor can be angled medially to decompress the contralateral side from the same ipsilateral incision.

Subaxial Cervical Fusion

Surgical Exposure

Intraoperative lateral fluoroscopy is used to identify the surgical level(s) to be fused.

The surgical site is marked and infiltrated with a local anesthetic. For subaxial lateral mass screws in a single level fusion, a 2 cm longitudinal midline skin incision is made approximately two spinal segments below the level of fusion. This is done to match the trajectory of the tube with the facet joint. For a multilevel fusion, the incision is made one spinal segment above the most caudal level of fusion. For subaxial transfacet screws, a 1–2 cm longitudinal midline incision is placed one spinal segment cephalad to the level of fusion. For more horizontal facet orientation, incision is placed even more cephalad to accommodate screw trajectory.

Lateral Mass Screw-Rod Construct Detailed Procedure

A longitudinal fasciotomy is made approximately 1 cm lateral to the midline. Incision should be the same length as the skin incision. A dilator is passed under fluoroscopic guidance and docked on a lateral mass of interest. Tube trajectory should be parallel to the facet joint. Sequential intermuscular dilation is followed. A tubular or expandable retractor is then placed and locked into a retractor arm mounted to the operative table. Any remaining muscle is cleared with electrocautery and pituitary rongeur. Both facet joints and the medial and lateral edge of the lateral mass should be visualized (in a single-level fusion). For multilevel fusions, repositioning of the retractor either more caudal or cephalad can be achieved, or expandable retractor can be used that allows for visualization of all levels at once. Once the lateral mass is visualized, the screw trajectory is very similar to an open procedure and can be performed as either An, Anderson, Magerl, or Roy-Camille technique [29–31]. For rod placement, slight elevation of the retractor is necessary to accommodate the passage of the rod into each polyaxial screw head. At the end of the procedure, retractor is slowly withdrawn, and any active bleeding can be cauterized with bipolar cautery to achieve hemostasis. The procedure is then repeated with a new rod in the same fashion on the contralateral side.

Transfacet Screws Procedure

A small fascial incision is made overlying the targeted facet. More cephalad incision is required for more horizontal facets in order to address the more caudal trajectory needed. A cannulated drill guide is then docked on the dorsal surface of the middle of the superior lateral mass, and a pilot hole is made. A guidewire is advanced in a lateral trajectory until reaching the body of the inferior facet. The caudal direction should be perpendicular to the facet joint. At this point the smaller of the cannulated cancellous drills is used to drill the entire length. This is followed by a second drill equal to the major diameter of the screw that is advanced only through the superolateral mass. This allows lagging of the two segments when a screw is placed. A 7–10 mm cancellous screw is then inserted.

Postoperative Management and Expected Outcomes

Compared to traditional open approach, MIS outcomes are comparable short- and long-term alike with an advantage of smaller incision and less blood loss with the MIS approach [28, 32]. However, MIS cervical laminectomy has been noted to be less painful with shorter hospital stay and faster recovery [28, 33, 34]. MIS posterior cervical fusions are associated with low complication rate, reduced blood loss, and high fusion rates after 2 years [28, 35, 36]. Percutaneous transfacet screw placement may help reduce pseudoarthrosis rates due to the construct high pullout strength from penetration of four cortical bone surfaces [28, 37]. Surgeon preference and skill level should be used when deciding on surgical approach type. The rate of vertebral artery injury for C1–C2 lateral mass screw placement in MIS fashion is 0–2.5%; however, the overall incidence is closer to 0.14% [28, 38, 39]. Careful preoperative review of imaging should be instituted to note abnormal vertebral artery course and the dominant side of vertebral artery. Rod selection should be made appropriately to limit unnecessarily long constructs as they may cause compression of vertebral artery.

Complications and Complication Management

For MIS laminectomy and subaxial fusion, complications are similar to those of open procedures. Superficial wound infections resolve with oral antibiotics. For high-risk patients, intraincisional vancomycin powder can be considered. Incidental durotomy, if noted intraoperatively, can be covered with either muscle, fat, or gel foam followed by a fibrin glue or synthetic sealant. Large leaks not amenable for direct closure should be managed with a lumbar drain for CSF diversion for 2–3 days to prevent a wound leak.

Post-laminectomy kyphosis is an infrequent complication; however, some argue that laminectomy alone without stabilization is a significant risk factor for kyphotic deformity. Cervical deformity is more likely in patients who have evidence of preoperative kyphosis or preoperative instability [2, 40]. As mentioned in the previous sections, avoidance of postoperative kyphosis after laminectomy starts with proper patient selection and evaluation. Flexion/extension as well as AP/lateral radiographs should always be obtained preoperatively and evaluated for alignment and any presence of dynamic instability. Careful attention to minimal muscle dissection intraoperatively as well as prevention of extensive facet resection may also decrease postoperative iatrogenic cervical deformity after laminectomy.

Lastly, while C5 palsy rates are lower with posterior cervical decompression than with anterior approach, it may be attributed to 5.8% of the cases [41]. C4/C5 foraminal stenosis may be a risk factor, and some argue for prophylactic C4/C5 bilateral foraminotomy [42]. Surgeons doing so must remain cautious as doing a foraminotomy itself may irritate or injure the C5 nerve root and result in C5 palsy.

Conclusion

Cervical laminectomy with or without dorsal instrumentation and arthrodesis is a longstanding, commonly performed surgery for patients with cervical spondylotic myelopathy with or without radiculopathy. The main goal of surgery is spinal cord and nerve root decompression. Preoperative patient selection is crucial to identify patients who may also benefit from dorsal instrumentation and fusion. If the presence of deformity or dynamic instability is identified preoperatively, it is advisable to perform a laminectomy with fusion. Patients with good preoperative cervical lordosis and no instability are likely to benefit from laminectomy alone.

Case Presentation

A 72-year-old female presents with chronic mechanical neck pain with some left arm radiculopathy for 2 years. She has had three epidural steroid injections, two radio-frequency ablations, facet blocks, and at least 6 months of physical therapy without relief. Her neck pain is progressively getting worse especially when the patient is in the upright position and with exertion, which also causes her to have unrelenting occipital headaches. Pain improves with rest and recumbence.

On imaging patient has severe degenerative cervical spondylosis with retrolisthesis of C5/C6 with anterior and posterior spinal cord compression (Fig. 27.2a). There is severe loss of lordosis with mild swan neck deformity, CL +2°, and cSVA >40 mm. On flexion/extension radiographs, there is a fixed deformity with ankylosed facets. Patient underwent C5 and C6 corpectomy and C4–C7 laminectomy with facetectomies to deformity correction followed by C4–T1 lateral mass and pedicle screw instrumentation and fusion. Patient tolerated the procedure well and showed complete radiographic fusion on a 12-month follow-up (Fig. 27.2b).

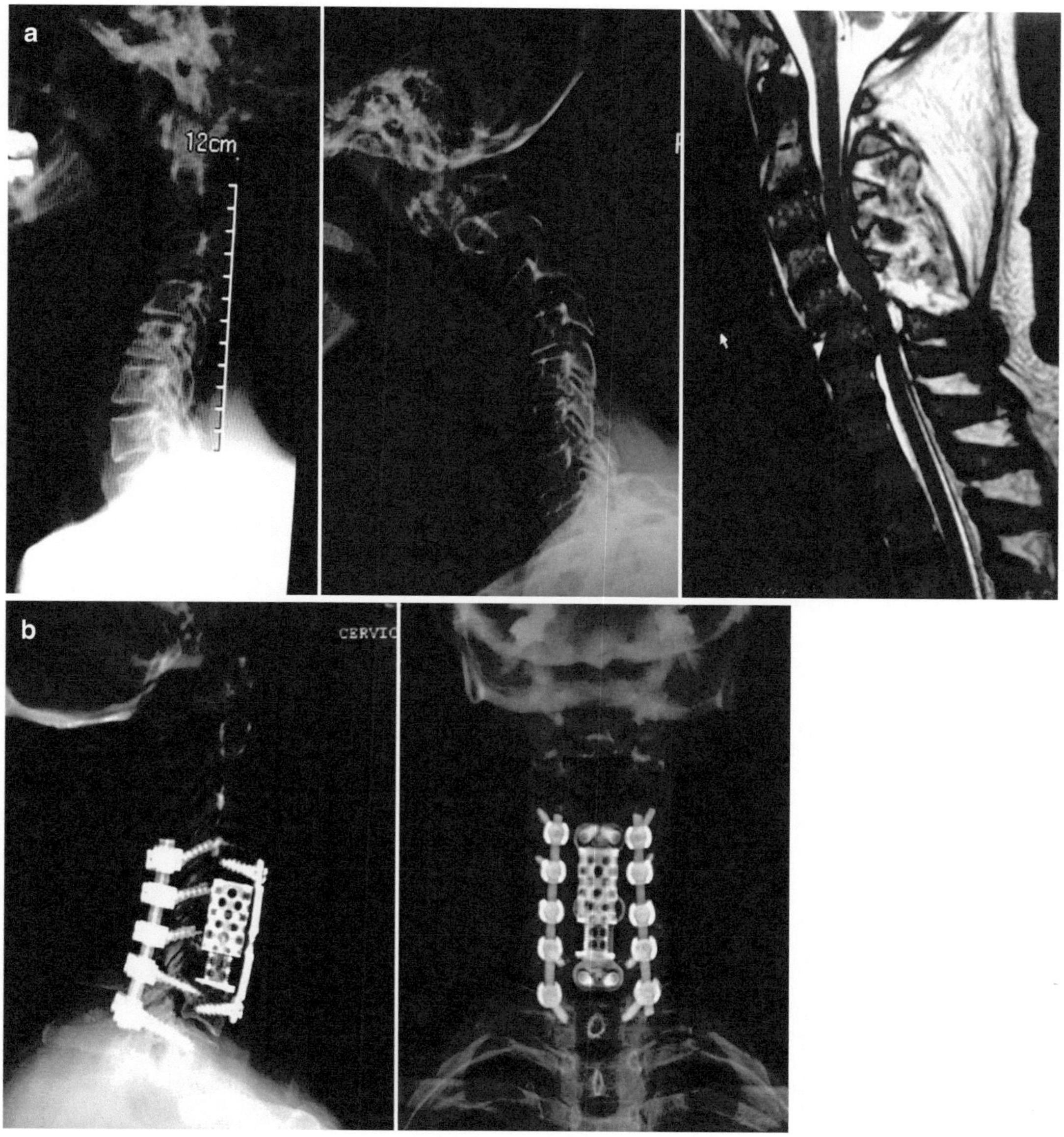

Fig. 27.2 (**a**) Patient has severe degenerative cervical spondylosis with retrolisthesis of C5/C6 with anterior and posterior spinal cord compression. (**b**) Patient underwent C5 and C6 corpectomy and C4–C7 laminectomy with facetectomies to deformity correction followed by C4–T1 lateral mass and pedicle screw instrumentation and fusion. Patient showed complete radiographic fusion on a 12-month follow-up

Key Recommendations

- Proper preoperative workup should be performed to analyze factors contributing to pathology being treated.
- Patient selection is key to correct surgical approach and improving clinical outcome and avoiding complications.
- MIS techniques result in similar clinical and radiographic outcomes, however may provide additional benefit of less blood loss, quicker recovery, decreased postoperative pain, and less complications compared to open surgery.
- MIS technique is associated with a steeper learning curve and should be used based on physician comfort level and preference.
- During laminectomy, more caudal levels should be addressed first to minimize bleeding in the surgical field.
- For adequate decompression, approximately 12 mm of lamina should be removed on each side.
- For lateral mass screws, if the trajectory is too low, it may violate the facet joint too; medial trajectory may cause vertebral artery injury.
- For lateral mass screws, pilot holes should be drilled first to maintain the anatomic relationships. If the pilot holes are too medial, screws will enter through the lamina and may cause spinal cord injury, too; lateral placement may cause a lateral breech and/or inability to accommodate a longer screw (Table 27.1).

Bibliography

1. Wilson JR, Tetreault LA, Kim J, et al. State of the art in degenerative cervical myelopathy: an update on current clinical evidence. Neurosurgery. 2017;80:S33–s45.
2. Steinmetz MP, Benzel EC. Benzel's spine surgery: techniques, complication avoidance, and management. 4th ed. Philadelphia: Elsevier; 2016.
3. Divi SN, Mikhael MM. Use of allogenic mesenchymal cellular bone matrix in anterior and posterior cervical spinal fusion: a case series of 21 patients. Asian Spine J. 2017;11:454–62.
4. Sawin PD, Traynelis VC, Menezes AH. A comparative analysis of fusion rates and donor-site morbidity for autogeneic rib and iliac crest bone grafts in posterior cervical fusions. J Neurosurg. 1998;88:255–65.
5. Guzman JZ, Merrill RK, Kim JS, et al. Bone morphogenetic protein use in spine surgery in the United States: how have we responded to the warnings? Spine J Off J North Am Spine Soc. 2017;17(9):1247–54.
6. Hamilton DK, Smith JS, Reames DL, et al. Safety, efficacy, and dosing of recombinant human bone morphogenetic protein-2 for posterior cervical and cervicothoracic instrumented fusion with a minimum 2-year follow-up. Neurosurgery. 2011;69:103–11; discussion 11.
7. Hansraj KK. Stem cells in spine surgery. Surg Technol Int. 2016;XXIX:348–58.
8. McAllister BD, Rebholz BJ, Wang JC. Is posterior fusion necessary with laminectomy in the cervical spine? Surg Neurol Int. 2012;3:S225–31.
9. Kim DK, Kim JY, Kim DY, et al. Risk factors of proximal junctional kyphosis after multilevel fusion surgery: more than 2 years follow-up data. J Korean Neurosurg Soc. 2017;60:174–80.
10. Liu FY, Wang T, Yang SD, et al. Incidence and risk factors for proximal junctional kyphosis: a meta-analysis. Eur Spine J Off Publ Eur Spine Soc Eur Spinal Deform Soc Eur Sect Cerv Spine Res Soc. 2016;25:2376–83.
11. Park SJ, Lee CS, Chung SS, et al. Different risk factors of proximal junctional kyphosis and proximal junctional failure following long instrumented fusion to the sacrum for adult spinal deformity: survivorship analysis of 160 patients. Neurosurgery. 2017;80:279–86.
12. Yagi M, King AB, Boachie-Adjei O. Incidence, risk factors, and natural course of proximal junctional kyphosis: surgical outcomes review of adult idiopathic scoliosis. Minimum 5 years of follow-up. Spine. 2012;37:1479–89.
13. Yagi M, Rahm M, Gaines R, et al. Characterization and surgical outcomes of proximal junctional failure in surgically treated patients with adult spinal deformity. Spine. 2014;39:E607–14.
14. Gore DR, Sepic SB, Gardner GM. Roentgenographic findings of the cervical spine in asymptomatic people. Spine. 1986;11:521–4.
15. Hardacker JW, Shuford RF, Capicotto PN, et al. Radiographic standing cervical segmental alignment in adult volunteers without neck symptoms. Spine. 1997;22:1472–80; discussion 80.
16. Iyer S, Lenke LG, Nemani VM, et al. Variations in occipitocervical and cervicothoracic alignment parameters based on age: a prospective study of asymptomatic volunteers using full-body radiographs. Spine. 2016;41:1837–44.
17. Janusz P, Tyrakowski M, Yu H, et al. Reliability of cervical lordosis measurement techniques on

long-cassette radiographs. Eur Spine J Off Publ Eur Spine Soc Eur Spinal Deform Soc Eur Sect Cerv Spine Res Soc. 2016;25:3596–601.

18. Lee SH, Kim KT, Seo EM, et al. The influence of thoracic inlet alignment on the craniocervical sagittal balance in asymptomatic adults. J Spinal Disord Tech. 2012;25:E41–7.
19. Hey HWD, Teo AQA, Tan KA, et al. How the spine differs in standing and in sitting-important considerations for correction of spinal deformity. Spine J Off J North Am Spine Soc. 2017;17:799–806.
20. Tan LA, Riew KD, Traynelis VC. Cervical spine deformity-part 1: biomechanics, radiographic parameters, and classification. Neurosurgery. 2017;81:197–203.
21. Tang JA, Scheer JK, Smith JS, et al. The impact of standing regional cervical sagittal alignment on outcomes in posterior cervical fusion surgery. Neurosurgery. 2012;71:662–9; discussion 9.
22. Tang JA, Scheer JK, Smith JS, et al. The impact of standing regional cervical sagittal alignment on outcomes in posterior cervical fusion surgery. Neurosurgery. 2015;76(Suppl 1):S14–21; discussion S.
23. Li J, Qin S, Li Y, et al. Modic changes of the cervical spine: T1 slope and its impact on axial neck pain. J Pain Res. 2017;10:2041–5.
24. Oe S, Togawa D, Nakai K, et al. The influence of age and sex on cervical spinal alignment among volunteers aged over 50. Spine. 2015;40:1487–94.
25. Protopsaltis TS, Lafage R, Vira S, et al. Novel angular measures of cervical deformity account for upper cervical compensation and sagittal alignment. Clin Spine Surg. 2017;30:E959–e67.
26. Cabraja M, Abbushi A, Koeppen D, et al. Comparison between anterior and posterior decompression with instrumentation for cervical spondylotic myelopathy: sagittal alignment and clinical outcome. Neurosurg Focus. 2010;28:E15.
27. Hann S, Chalouhi N, Madineni R, et al. An algorithmic strategy for selecting a surgical approach in cervical deformity correction. Neurosurg Focus. 2014;36:E5.
28. Kim DH, Vaccaro AR, Dickman CA, Cho D, Lee S, Kim I. Surgical anatomy and techniques to the spine. 2nd ed. Philadelphia: Saunders Elsevier; 2006.
29. Singh K, Vaccaro AR. Minimally invasive spine surgery: advanced surgical techniques. 1st ed. New Delhi: Jaypee Brothers; 2016.
30. Stemper BD, Marawar SV, Yoganandan N, et al. Quantitative anatomy of subaxial cervical lateral mass: an analysis of safe screw lengths for Roy-Camille and magerl techniques. Spine. 2008;33:893–7.
31. Xu R, Haman SP, Ebraheim NA, et al. The anatomic relation of lateral mass screws to the spinal nerves. A comparison of the Magerl, Anderson, and An techniques. Spine. 1999;24:2057–61.
32. Joseffer SS, Post N, Cooper PR, et al. Minimally invasive atlantoaxial fixation with a polyaxial screw-rod construct: technical case report. Neurosurgery. 2006;58:ONS-E375; discussion ONS-E.
33. Winder MJ, Thomas KC. Minimally invasive versus open approach for cervical laminoforaminotomy. Can J Neurol Sci. 2011;38:262–7.
34. Yabuki S, Kikuchi S. Endoscopic partial laminectomy for cervical myelopathy. J Neurosurg Spine. 2005;2:170–4.
35. Mikhael MM, Celestre PC, Wolf CF, et al. Minimally invasive cervical spine foraminotomy and lateral mass screw placement. Spine. 2012;37:E318–22.
36. Wang MY, Levi AD. Minimally invasive lateral mass screw fixation in the cervical spine: initial clinical experience with long-term follow-up. Neurosurgery. 2006;58:907–12; discussion −12.
37. Ahmad F, Sherman JD, Wang MY. Percutaneous trans-facet screws for supplemental posterior cervical fixation. World Neurosurg. 2012;78:716. e1–4.
38. Terterov S, Taghva A, Khalessi AA, et al. Symptomatic vertebral artery compression by the rod of a C1-C2 posterior fusion construct: case report and review of the literature. Spine. 2011;36:E678–81.
39. Neo M, Fujibayashi S, Miyata M, et al. Vertebral artery injury during cervical spine surgery: a survey of more than 5600 operations. Spine. 2008;33:779–85.
40. Albert TJ, Vacarro A. Postlaminectomy kyphosis. Spine. 1998;23:2738–45.
41. Gu Y, Cao P, Gao R, et al. Incidence and risk factors of C5 palsy following posterior cervical decompression: a systematic review. PLoS One. 2014;9:e101933.
42. Katsumi K, Yamazaki A, Watanabe K, et al. Analysis of C5 palsy after cervical open-door laminoplasty: relationship between C5 palsy and foraminal stenosis. J Spinal Disord Tech. 2013;26:177–82.

Biological Enhancers of Fusion

28

Matthew F. Gary and Scott D. Boden

Pitfalls/Pearls

- The goal of cervical stabilization procedures is ultimately arthrodesis. The surgeon must not lose sight of that fact.
- The most carefully placed instrumentation will serve little function if fusion across segments does not occur. To this end, the operator must be hyperaware of bone biology and the factors impacting arthrodesis.
- At the end of the operation, when all the hardware has been meticulously scrutinized and nerves methodically decompressed, we then hastily decorticate and lay down some substrate. This can have dire consequences for our patients as pseudoarthrosis leads to increased pain and disability and ultimately further surgeries.
- Spine surgery is frequently a three-staged operation: Decompression, instrumentation, and arthrodesis. The failure of one of these components will make the entire operation a failure. As such, we must have at least a basic understanding of bone biology and the processes involved in arthrodesis.
- There are frequently gaps in evidence for much of what we do in the spinal field, and the evidence for biological enhancers is no exception. It is just as important to understand these gaps so that we can better inform our patients preoperatively.

The goal of this chapter is to review the basic tenants of bone biology and examine the evidence for currently used enhancers of fusion.

Introduction

There are over 400,000 spinal fusions performed annually in the United States alone [1]. The reported incidence of nonunion following spinal fusion operations varies widely (5–45%) [2] and is dependent on multiple factors. For instance, Wang et al. found that the number of levels operated on for anterior cervical fusions greatly affected fusion rates (pseudoarthrosis was approximately 10% for single-level and 30% for three level fusions) [3]. Given the large number of fusion operations performed each year, even a

M. F. Gary · S. D. Boden (✉)
Department of Orthopaedic Surgery, Emory University School of Medicine, Atlanta, GA, USA
e-mail: scott_boden@emory.org

M. G. Kaiser et al. (eds.), *Degenerative Cervical Myelopathy and Radiculopathy*,
https://doi.org/10.1007/978-3-319-97952-6_28

low rate of pseudoarthrosis can have profound effects on outcomes and overall costs. A lack of understanding with regard to the basic biology involved with arthrodesis certainly contributes. There are three general properties that are needed in grafting materials: oseoinductive, osteogenic, and osteoconductive. Osteoinduction is the process by which immature cells are recruited to the fusion site and stimulated to differentiate into osteoblasts. Osteogenesis refers to the formation of the bone by implantation of a bone graft with live osteoblasts. Osteoconduction refers to substrates that serve as a scaffold for this new bone formation.

Autologous bone graft, particularly autologous iliac crest (AIC), has its own limitations. For cervical operations it requires a separate incision distant from the operative site. This brings added risks associated with longer operations, infection at a second operative site, and morbidity associated with high rates of chronic pain at the donor site [4–6]. In fact, a multicenter prospective study demonstrated that 31% of patients had significant donor site pain 24 months after surgery [6]. Given this limitation, bone graft substitutes which match the efficacy of AIC are needed.

Fracture healing and bone biology in general are complex topics and the subject of significant basic science research even today. Though we have a basic understanding of the processes involved in fracture healing, we are continually discovering new observations in this complex system. Fracture healing is a distinct entity from the fusion process that takes place following bone grafting in spine surgery; however there are many correlates. The three main phases of bone repair following fracture are (1) inflammation, (2) proliferation, and (3) remodeling [7–11]. The inflammatory phase occurs immediately following the fracture. A hematoma is caused as a result of the bleeding bone and periosteal vessels. Several proinflammatory mediators are released from the hematoma (interleukin-1 (IL-1), IL-6, IL-11, IL-18, and tumor necrosis factor (TNF)). These proinflammatory proteins serve as cytokines, attracting a multitude of inflammatory cells. The macrophages attracted to the fracture site phagocytize the necrotic tissue and release the growth factors that eventually promote the proliferative phase (bone morphogenetic proteins (BMPs), transforming growth factor (TGF), platelet-derived growth factor (PDGF), and insulin-like growth factor (IGF)). These growth factors are responsible for the migration, recruitment, and proliferation of mesenchymal stem cells (MSC). The MSC are now available for differentiation into angioblasts, chondroblasts, fibroblasts, and osteoblasts. These cells fill the fracture gap with granulation tissue thereby providing mild stabilization and preparing the site for the fusion process. The inflammatory phase usually occurs within the first week. The second phase of fracture healing is the proliferative phase. This phase is characterized by the formation of a callus with vascular ingrowth and the presence of collagen fibers. The chondrocytes turn the central fracture area into a cartilaginous zone and mechanically stabilizes it with a soft callus. Woven bone gradually replaces the cartilage by endochondral ossification resulting in a hard callus thereby increasing the stability of the fracture site. The third and final phase of fracture healing is the remodeling phase during which the immature woven bone callus is converted into mature lamellar bone. During this phase, osteoclasts reabsorb the woven bone callus, and osteoblasts replace it with lamellar bone. This final phase restores the mechanical strength at the fractured site [7–11]. As outlined briefly above, bone healing is a complex process involving a multitude of enzymes, cells, and matrixes. A bone graft enhancer focuses on complimenting one or more of these steps in the setting of autologous bone graft. On the other hand, a bone graft substitute is a material used in place of autologous bone graft with the goal of achieving equivalent or better fusion rates.

The process of spinal fusion has many similar properties as fracture healing but is a very distinct entity. In order to understand the properties of autologous bone graft that make it ideal for spinal fusion surgery, we must look to animal studies. Of the many animal models, the intertransverse process arthrodesis model has helped to heighten our understanding of basic biological processes and factors negatively impacting them [2]. For instance, these animal models have shown that the primary vascular supply to the fusion mass is from the decorticated bone and not the surrounding muscle, thus supporting the importance of thorough decortication during fusion operations. Also, histologic analysis demonstrated peripheral to central healing of the fusion mass whereby the area closest to the decorticated bone matured first followed by the central regions away from the decorticated bone. Nonunion usually occurred in these central regions where the levels of certain BMPs were much lower. In addition, it was shown that there are a number of factors that negatively impacted the fusion process including excessive spine motion, nicotine, and nonsteroidal anti-inflammatory drugs (NSAIDs) [2]. While these models tested posterior lumbar fusion, the mechanisms for posterior cervical fusion are assumed to be similar. Also, anterior interbody fusions have greater surface area and compressive forces that theoretically would make fusion more successful.

In addition to these external factors affecting bone healing, there are many internal factors detrimental to proper fusion, such as osteoporosis, renal osteodystrophy, primary bone tumors, metastases, and others. Understanding these processes is much more difficult given the lack of corresponding animal models and the inability to study them histologically in vivo. Nevertheless, we can apply the principles of bone biology learned in other settings to better treat these patients.

Autologous Bone Grafts

For posterior cervical fusion procedures, there is frequently ample local autograft. Morselized spinous processes and lamina for posterior fusions are in general sufficient for posterolateral and interfacet grafting. The benefits of autologous bone graft, compared to bone graft substitutes, is that it has all the necessary components for osteogenesis (MSCs and osteoblasts) and osteoconduction (extracellular matrix). When posterior fusion operations are performed without laminectomy (i.e., C1–C2 or occipital cervical fusions), then there is not ample local autograft. The same holds true for anterior cervical discectomy and fusion (ACDF) where there is not sufficient local autograft to fill the discectomy. In these instances one must harvest autologous iliac crest (AIC) or use a bone graft substitute. As with local autologous bone graft, AIC has all of the prerequisites for good fusion: osteoinductive, osteogenic, and osteoconductive. However, if harvested as a tricortical block, it also has the added benefit of providing structural support for use as an interbody. Most surgeons have gone away from using AIC in favor of bone graft substitutes due to longer operations, infection at a second operative site, and morbidity associated with chronic pain at the donor site.

Bone Graft Substitutes

There have been a number of bone graft substitutes developed, each of which has their own pros and cons. When evaluating each of these, it is important to keep in mind the osteoinductive, conductive, and genic properties of each. It is also important to find a substitute that provides structural support when needed for anterior reconstruction.

Allograft is an obvious first choice for bone substitutes. It can provide a weight-bearing strut and serves as a lattice for osteoconduction. Cancellous bone allograft is completely replaced over time by a process called creeping substitution, while cortical bone graft will remain a mixture of viable tissue at the ends and acellular matrix in the center [12]. For instance, the cortical fibular strut allograft in cervical corpectomies will eventually “spot weld” at the two ends where it comes in contact with the endplates. Unfortunately, allograft use alone is defined by high pseudoarthrosis rates because it is only osteoconductive [12]. In order to increase the rate of fusion, these grafts are hollowed out in the center and packed with local autograft or other agents described below to provide osteoinductive and osteogenic properties.

Demineralized bone matrix (DBM) was first described by Urist in the 1960s as an osteoinductive bone extender [13]. DBM is produced by an acid extraction processing of allograft bone resulting in the loss of mineralized elements with the remaining material consisting of collagen, non-collagenous proteins, and growth factors [14]. It is both osteoinductive and conductive but lacks structural integrity. Animal studies support the osteoinductive nature of DBM in both rabbit and primate models [15, 16]. Clinical data on the use of DBM is limited, and current studies mainly focus on its use as an extender for autograft (with the goal of limiting the amount of iliac crest that must be harvested) [17–19]. These studies by Vaccaro et al., Schizas et al., and Cammisa et al. compared the use of AIC alone versus DBM with AIC or DBM with iliac bone aspirate (IBA). There were no differences found. Recently, Zadegan et al. performed a systematic review of the literature looking at the effectiveness of DBM in ACDFs [20]. They were able to find 12 articles, 3 of which were randomized controlled trials. The authors concluded that the studies reported non-inferior results for DBM compared to other grafting material; however, the available evidence is limited.

Calcium phosphate salts are a class of graft extenders that provide a lattice framework for ingrowth of new bone. Examples include beta-tricalcium phosphate (TCP), hydroxyapatite (HA), and coral-based materials. Dai and Jiang performed a randomized controlled trial comparing TCP with local autograft versus AIC with local autograft in posterolateral lumbar fusion [21]. They had 100% fusion rates in both groups, and thus there was no difference in the two groups. The authors concluded that TCP and local autograft is an adequate substitute for AIC. Though this was a well-designed study, one limitation was the use of plain radiographs in determining fusion. Korovessis et al. also conducted a randomized controlled trial comparing AIC and coralline hydroxyapatite (CH) with local bone and BMA for lumbar posterolateral fusion [22]. They did not find a difference between the two groups; however, there are animal studies showing that CH and BMA is not efficacious. Thus, the authors concluded that CH with local autograft and BMA is a substitute for AIC. A number of other nonrandomized studies have been performed for calcium phosphate salts showing efficacy as an extender in lumbar fusion [23–25].

Bone Morphogenetic Proteins

Bone morphogenetic proteins (BMPs) are found in low quantities within demineralized bone matrix. These proteins are a part of the transforming growth factor-Beta (TGF-Beta) family and, despite the name, serve a multitude of functions throughout all organisms. In the spine world, however, they are best known for their osteoinductive properties. These proteins are found in very low doses within demineralized bone matrix. Early studies looking at the doses of recombinant BMPs needed for bone formation in vitro required nanomolar doses, and efficacy in rabbit studies required significantly higher doses and in humans even higher doses still, thus partly explaining why DBM is not a very strong osteoinductive substrate in its own right. In 2002, the FDA approved the use of recombinant human(rh)-BMP-2 for single-level ALIF procedures from L4 to S1 utilizing the LT-CAGE Lumbar Tapered Fusion Device [26]. rhBMP-7 was subsequently approved under a humanitarian device exemption for revision of posterolateral lumbar fusion. However, the application of rhBMP has extended beyond these applications with approximately 85% of primary spine procedures utilizing BMP off label (physician-directed applications) [26, 27].

There are a number of randomized controlled trials (RCT) evaluating the use of rh-BMP in the lumbar spine. Unfortunately, most studies to date looking at the role of BMPs for cervical pathology are not RCT. Reviewing the merits and flaws of these studies in detail is beyond the scope of this chapter; however a brief overview of the lumbar and cervical literature is important. Burkus et al. showed clinical equipoise in a RCT comparing rhBMP-2 as a substitute for AIC in single-level ALIFs [28, 29]. Haid et al. performed a RCT using rhBMP-2 as a substitute for AIC in posterior lumbar interbody fusions and found no statistically significant differences in outcomes; however, there was a significantly higher rate of heterotopic bone formation posterior to the grafts in the rhBMP-2 group [30]. Dimar et al., Dawson et al., and Glassman et al. performed three separate RCT comparing rhBMP-2 combined with a collagen matrix versus AIC for posterolateral instrumented fusions in the lumbar spine [31–33]. In all three studies, the rhBMP-2 group demonstrated a statistically significant higher fusion rate while the AIC group had a high rate of donor site pain. There were no significant differences in overall clinical outcomes between the two groups. Thus, the authors concluded that rhBMP-2 with collagen matrix was a suitable substitute to AIC. In the cervical literature, Baskin et al. published a pilot RCT for rhBMP-2 as a substitute to AIC in an allograft ring for anterior cervical interbody fusions [34]. There were a total of 33 patients enrolled in the study, and at 24 months, the investigational group had significant improvement in neck disability and arm pain scores compared to the control group. This study was not powered sufficiently to draw any worthwhile conclusions. A number of subsequent observational studies have demonstrated a higher rate of dysphagia and ectopic bone formation when rhBMP-2 is used in the anterior cervical spine. The application of lower doses of rhBMP-2 to mitigate these complications has shown promise. If rhBMP-2 is going to be used for anterior cervical interbody fusions, 0.5 mg/ml per level is what the author uses, but, again, there are no RCTs to evaluate the optimal dosage.

Over the last few years, there have been a number of articles expressing concern with regard to the risks associated with BMPs. In 2008, the Food and Drug Administration (FDA) issued a warning due to multiple reports of rhBMP-2 in anterior cervical fusion contributing to marked dysphagia, hematoma, seroma, and swelling [35]. Other concerns raised include possible increased risks of retrograde ejaculation, antibody formation, radiculitis, postoperative nerve root injury, ectopic bone formation, vertebral osteolysis/edema, interbody graft lucency, and wound healing complications [36]. Given that BMPs are a cytokine and induce an inflammatory response, those increased risks associated with inflammation are not surprising. Even the initial osteolysis can be explained by this profound inflammatory response which increases osteoclast bone reabsorption. As described earlier, inflammation is an important early step in bone induction. Unfortunately, the doses of rhBMP-2 required in humans for efficacy are an order of magnitude higher than in animal models. Since rhBMP-2 is not tightly bound to its collagen carrier (half-life of 3.5 days), very large local doses are released at once likely leading to some of the observed complications. It is important that the practitioner weigh these risks versus the risk of pseudoarthrosis and donor site pain when discussing fusion operations with patients. Finally, there have also been reported concerns about the theoretical carcinogenic risk associated with rhBMP-2. According to Cahill et al., analysis of three large healthcare data sets, as well as the initial clinical trial data for rhBMP-2, shows that there is no conclusive evidence linking rhBMP-2 to the formation of cancer locally or at a distant site [37].

Electrical and Electromagnetic Stimulation

One potential enhancer of bone healing is the use of electrical or electromagnetic bone stimulation. The effects of electrical stimulation on bone healing is a well-established concept in long bone healing [26]. The three forms of electrical stimulation used clinically are direct current stimulation (DCS), pulsed electromagnetic field stimulation (PEMFS), and capacitive coupled electrical stimulation (CCES). DCS requires the implantation of cathodes attached to an implanted battery, while PEMFS and CCES rely on external devices to provide electromagnetic energy to the fusion. There have been a number of studies looking at these techniques over the last few years. For instance, Simmons et al. looked at the use of PEMFS for the nonoperative treatment of pseudoarthrosis in a case series of 100 patients [38]. Fusion success rate was reported at 67%

with this nonoperative method. Kucharzyk et al. and Rogozinski et al. in retrospective reviews found that DCS improved fusion rates. However, Andersen et al. did not find significant improvement with DCS in a randomized controlled trial of patients over 60 undergoing noninstrumented fusion. Kaiser et al. reviewed the current literature in detail for evidence supporting these techniques in lumbar spinal fusion [26]. They found that the available literature to date was severely flawed limiting the ability to make any definitive recommendations. DCS may have a positive impact on fusion rates in patients younger than 60 years undergoing a lumbar fusion; however, it did not impact clinical outcomes. The strongest study design only looked at patients over 60 years of age for noninstrumented fusions and did not show efficacy. Finally, one could argue that though Simmons et al. study is flawed given the lack of a control group, the use of PEMFS is relatively benign carrying little risk other than added cost if it turns out to be ineffective. Unfortunately, the data supporting these therapies is even sparser for cervical fusion operations. In theory they should be helpful in high-risk populations, but there is limited clinical evidence to date.

Mesenchymal Stem Cells

Hypothetically, having pluripotent stem cells as part of a bone graft substitute would enable the graft to readily create new osteoblasts and release osteoinductive signals. Thus, products (such as Osteocel and Trinity Elite) have been developed which maintain cell viability during processing. These allograft products attempt to match AIC by maintaining viable stem cells along with osteoinductive BMPs [39, 40]. Eastlack et al. published a prospective nonrandomized study of Osteocel in a total of 182 patients [41]. They found patients had high fusion rates with low complications. However, this is a nonrandomized study making any generalizations very limited. Skovrlj B et al. recently searched the current literature for cellular bone matrices (CBMs) and found a wide variation in product composition (i.e., cellular concentration, age of donors, shelf life, and cell viability after defrosting) [42]. They also found that all current studies are industry funded with no independent studies under way. In addition, most of these CBMs are developed with proprietary techniques making it difficult to make direct comparison of products. While CBMs may be a promising spine bone graft substitute in the future, as of today, there is insufficient evidence to support them and their added expense.

Platelet-Rich Plasma

Autologous platelet-rich plasma (PRP) has been popularized as a treatment for various degenerative processes throughout the body and as a potential osteoinductive agent. When tissue is injured, platelets aggregate and release a number of cytokines and growth factors such as transforming growth factor-beta, insulin-like growth factor, platelet-derived growth factor (PDGF), vascular endothelial growth factors (VEGF), and others [43]. Since all of these factors play a role in the healing process, it was theorized that they would also assist in osteoinduction. Unfortunately, there are conflicting animal studies with PRP. Some of these studies demonstrate that PRP is actually inhibitory for osteoinduction, such as Ranly DM et al., who found that PRP inhibited DBM-induced bone formation in nude mice [44]. They theorized that it was the PDGF which contributed to this inhibitory effect. Scholz M et al. found no osteoinductive effect of PRP added to a mineralized collagen in a sheep spine fusion model [45]. Recently, Roffi A et al. performed a systematic review of the literature for studies on PRP from 2000 to 2012 [46]. They found 83 papers that fulfilled their inclusion criteria, the majority of which were for oral/maxillofacial surgery applications (only 4 for orthopedic applications). They found that the majority of the current studies were of low quality and preliminary in nature. "Among the RCT and comparative papers, 16 reported favorable results, 18 no significant difference with or without PRP and 6 underlined a doubtful role of PRP." [46]. Thus, there is insufficient data on the use of PRP as a bone graft substitute, especially given the fact that there are some studies showing an inhibitor effect.

Conclusion

Though bone substitutes and extenders are widely used in place of AIC for cervical fusions, there is still no consensus on best practices. The use of DBM, rhBMPs, allograft, calcium phosphate salts, and collagen sponges all have the goal of replicating the osteoinductive, osteoconductive, and osteogenic capabilities of AIC. Precursor cells, which make AIC so powerful, are the main component that these substitutes are lacking. The use of mesenchymal stem cells to provide the osteogenic precursor cells is the next step in achieving the ultimate goal of replacing AIC with products of equal efficacy and lower risk.

Key Recommendations

The gold standard for cervical spinal fusion continues to be autologous iliac crest. If the risks associated with donor site harvesting are not acceptable to the surgeon and patient, there are a multitude of possible substitutions each with their own merits and disadvantages. When deciding on a substitute, the goal is to achieve osteoinductive, osteoconductive, and osteogenic properties.

References

1. Rajaee SS, Bae HW, Kanim LEA, Delamarter RB. Spinal fusion in the United States: analysis of trends from 1998 to 2008. Spine. 2012;37:67–76.
2. Boden SD. Overview of the biology of lumbar spine fusion and principles for selecting a bone graft substitute. Spine. 2002;27:S26–31.
3. Wang JC, McDonough PW, Kanim LE, Endow KK, Delamarter RB. Increased fusion rates with cervical plating for three-level anterior cervical discectomy and fusion. Spine. 2001;26:643–6; discussion 646–647.
4. Delawi D, Dhert WJA, Castelein RM, Verbout AJ, Oner FC. The incidence of donor site pain after bone graft harvesting from the posterior iliac crest may be overestimated: a study on spine fracture patients. Spine. 2007;32:1865–8.
5. Fernyhough JC, Schimandle JJ, Weigel MC, Edwards CC, Levine AM. Chronic donor site pain complicating bone graft harvesting from the posterior iliac crest for spinal fusion. Spine. 1992;17:1474–80.
6. Sasso RC, LeHuec JC, Shaffrey C, Spine Interbody Research Group. Iliac crest bone graft donor site pain after anterior lumbar interbody fusion: a prospective patient satisfaction outcome assessment. J Spinal Disord Tech. 2005;18(Suppl):S77–81.
7. Oryan A, Monazzah S, Bigham-Sadegh A. Bone injury and fracture healing biology. Biomed Environ Sci BES. 2015;28:57–71.
8. Cottrell JA, Turner JC, Arinzeh TL, O'Connor JP. The biology of bone and ligament healing. Foot Ankle Clin. 2016;21:739–61.
9. Geris L, Gerisch A, Sloten JV, Weiner R, Oosterwyck HV. Angiogenesis in bone fracture healing: a bioregulatory model. J Theor Biol. 2008;251:137–58.
10. LaStayo PC, Winters KM, Hardy M. Fracture healing: bone healing, fracture management, and current concepts related to the hand. J Hand Ther Off J Am Soc Hand Ther. 2003;16:81–93.
11. Pilitsis JG, Lucas DR, Rengachary SS. Bone healing and spinal fusion. Neurosurg Focus. 2002;13:e1.
12. Goldberg VM, Stevenson S. Natural history of autografts and allografts. Clin Orthop. 1987;225:7–16.
13. Urist MR. Bone: formation by autoinduction. Science. 1965;150:893–9.
14. Gupta A, et al. Bone graft substitutes for spine fusion: a brief review. World J Orthop. 2015;6:449–56.
15. Choi Y, Oldenburg FP, Sage L, Johnstone B, Yoo JU. A bridging demineralized bone implant facilitates posterolateral lumbar fusion in New Zealand white rabbits. Spine. 2007;32:36–41.
16. Louis-Ugbo J, Murakami H, Kim H-S, Minamide A, Boden SD. Evidence of osteoinduction by Grafton demineralized bone matrix in nonhuman primate spinal fusion. Spine. 2004;29:360–6; discussion Z1.
17. Vaccaro AR, Stubbs HA, Block JE. Demineralized bone matrix composite grafting for posterolateral spinal fusion. Orthopedics. 2007;30:567–70.
18. Cammisa FP, et al. Two-year fusion rate equivalency between Grafton DBM gel and autograft in posterolateral spine fusion: a prospective controlled trial employing a side-by-side comparison in the same patient. Spine. 2004;29:660–6.
19. Schizas C, Triantafyllopoulos D, Kosmopoulos V, Tzinieris N, Stafylas K. Posterolateral lumbar spine fusion using a novel demineralized bone matrix: a controlled case pilot study. Arch Orthop Trauma Surg. 2008;128:621–5.
20. Zadegan SA, Abedi A, Jazayeri SB, Vaccaro AR, Rahimi-Movaghar V. Demineralized bone matrix in anterior cervical discectomy and fusion: a

systematic review. Eur Spine J Off Publ Eur Spine Soc Eur Spinal Deform Soc Eur Sect Cerv Spine Res Soc. 2016;26:958. https://doi.org/10.1007/s00586-016-4858-9.
21. Dai L-Y, Jiang L-S. Single-level instrumented posterolateral fusion of lumbar spine with beta-tricalcium phosphate versus autograft: a prospective, randomized study with 3-year follow-up. Spine. 2008;33:1299–304.
22. Korovessis P, Koureas G, Zacharatos S, Papazisis Z, Lambiris E. Correlative radiological, self-assessment and clinical analysis of evolution in instrumented dorsal and lateral fusion for degenerative lumbar spine disease. Autograft versus coralline hydroxyapatite. Eur Spine J Off Publ Eur Spine Soc Eur Spinal Deform Soc Eur Sect Cerv Spine Res Soc. 2005;14:630–8.
23. Lee JH, et al. A prospective consecutive study of instrumented posterolateral lumbar fusion using synthetic hydroxyapatite (Bongros-HA) as a bone graft extender. J Biomed Mater Res A. 2009;90:804–10.
24. Chang C-H, Lin M-Z, Chen Y-J, Hsu H-C, Chen H-T. Local autogenous bone mixed with bone expander: an optimal option of bone graft in single-segment posterolateral lumbar fusion. Surg Neurol. 2008;70 Suppl 1:S1:47–9; discussion S1:49.
25. Acharya NK, Kumar RJ, Varma HK, Menon VK. Hydroxyapatite-bioactive glass ceramic composite as stand-alone graft substitute for posterolateral fusion of lumbar spine: a prospective, matched, and controlled study. J Spinal Disord Tech. 2008;21:106–11.
26. Kaiser MG, et al. Guideline update for the performance of fusion procedures for degenerative disease of the lumbar spine. Part 17: bone growth stimulators as an adjunct for lumbar fusion. J Neurosurg Spine. 2014;21:133–9.
27. Ong KL, et al. Off-label use of bone morphogenetic proteins in the United States using administrative data. Spine. 2010;35:1794–800.
28. Burkus JK, Gornet MF, Dickman CA, Zdeblick TA. Anterior lumbar interbody fusion using rhBMP-2 with tapered interbody cages. J Spinal Disord Tech. 2002;15:337–49.
29. Burkus JK, Dorchak JD, Sanders DL. Radiographic assessment of interbody fusion using recombinant human bone morphogenetic protein type 2. Spine. 2003;28:372–7.
30. Haid RW, Branch CL, Alexander JT, Burkus JK. Posterior lumbar interbody fusion using recombinant human bone morphogenetic protein type 2 with cylindrical interbody cages. Spine J Off J North Am Spine Soc. 2004;4:527–38; discussion 538–539.
31. Dimar JR, Glassman SD, Burkus KJ, Carreon LY. Clinical outcomes and fusion success at 2 years of single-level instrumented posterolateral fusions with recombinant human bone morphogenetic protein-2/compression resistant matrix versus iliac crest bone graft. Spine. 2006;31:2534–9; discussion 2540.
32. Dawson E, Bae HW, Burkus JK, Stambough JL, Glassman SD. Recombinant human bone morphogenetic protein-2 on an absorbable collagen sponge with an osteoconductive bulking agent in posterolateral arthrodesis with instrumentation. A prospective randomized trial. J Bone Joint Surg Am. 2009;91:1604–13.
33. Glassman SD, et al. RhBMP-2 versus iliac crest bone graft for lumbar spine fusion: a randomized, controlled trial in patients over sixty years of age. Spine. 2008;33:2843–9.
34. Baskin DS, Ryan P, Sonntag V, Westmark R, Widmayer MA. A prospective, randomized, controlled cervical fusion study using recombinant human bone morphogenetic protein-2 with the CORNERSTONE-SR allograft ring and the ATLANTIS anterior cervical plate. Spine. 2003;28:1219–24; discussion 1225.
35. Health, C. for D. and R. Public health notifications (medical devices) – FDA public health notification: life-threatening complications associated with recombinant human bone morphogenetic protein in cervical spine fusion. Available at: http://www.fda.gov/MedicalDevices/Safety/AlertsandNotices/PublicHealthNotifications/ucm062000.htm. Accessed 18 Jan 2017.
36. Singh K, et al. Complications of spinal fusion with utilization of bone morphogenetic protein: a systematic review of the literature. Spine. 2014;39:91–101.
37. Cahill KS, McCormick PC, Levi AD. A comprehensive assessment of the risk of bone morphogenetic protein use in spinal fusion surgery and postoperative cancer diagnosis. J Neurosurg Spine. 2015;23:86–93.
38. Simmons JW. Treatment of failed posterior lumbar interbody fusion (PLIF) of the spine with pulsing electromagnetic fields. Clin Orthop. 1985;193:127–32.
39. Buser Z, Acosta FL Jr. Stem cells and spinal fusion—are we there yet? Spine J. 2016;16:400–1.
40. Eltorai AEM, Susai CJ, Daniels AH. Mesenchymal stromal cells in spinal fusion: current and future applications. J Orthop. 2017;14:1–3.
41. Eastlack RK, Garfin SR, Brown CR, Meyer SC. Osteocel plus cellular allograft in anterior cervical discectomy and fusion: evaluation of clinical and radiographic outcomes from a prospective multicenter study. Spine. 2014;39:E1331–7.
42. Skovrlj B, et al. Cellular bone matrices: viable stem cell-containing bone graft substitutes. Spine J Off J North Am Spine Soc. 2014;14:2763–72.
43. Civinini R, Macera A, Nistri L, Redl B, Innocenti M. The use of autologous blood-derived growth factors in bone regeneration. Clin Cases Miner Bone Metab. 2011;8:25–31.
44. Ranly DM, Lohmann CH, Andreacchio D, Boyan BD, Schwartz Z. Platelet-rich plasma inhibits demineralized bone matrix-induced bone formation in nude mice. J Bone Joint Surg Am. 2007;89:139–47.
45. Scholz M, et al. Cages augmented with mineralized collagen and platelet-rich plasma as an osteoconductive/inductive combination for interbody fusion. Spine. 2010;35:740–6.
46. Roffi A, Filardo G, Kon E, Marcacci M. Does PRP enhance bone integration with grafts, graft substitutes, or implants? A systematic review. BMC Musculoskelet Disord. 2013;14:330.

Part VI

Challenges of Cervical Fixation

Occipitocervical Stabilization 29

Robert F. Heary and Nitin Agarwal

Pitfalls and Pearls

- Flexion and extension of the head and neck are heavily dependent upon the interface of the cranium and upper cervical spine, and as such, indications must be carefully scrutinized prior to occipitocervical stabilization surgeries.
- Allograft and bone substitutes should be avoided in favor of autograft to promote bony arthrodesis and long-term stability.
- Given occiput is held still relative to cervical spine to allow for bony stabilization, achieving optimal sagittal alignment is paramount.

Introduction

The occipitocervical junction, also known as the craniocervical or craniovertebral junction (CVJ), consists of the two joints (the atlanto-occipital and atlantoaxial), the spinal cord, and several neurovascular elements supplying the head and neck [1]. Proper alignment of the occipitocervical junction relies upon several osseous and ligamentous complexes contributing to the aforementioned joints [2]. Key osseous structures include the occiput, atlas (C1), and axis (C2), while important ligamentous structures include the accessory atlanto-occipital, alar, apical, Barkow, nuchal, transverse, lateral atlanto-occipital, transverse occipital, anterior atlanto-occipital membrane, posterior atlanto-occipital membrane, and the tectorial membrane [1, 3]. The interplay of these elements affords stability for this complex anatomical location that functionally allows rotation, flexion, and extension of the cranium in relation to the cervical spine. The great majority of rotation occurs at the C1-C2 level. Historically, in the early 1900s, disruption of the aforementioned structural components, leading to CVJ instability, was not considered amenable to surgical intervention. Over time, treatment strategies have evolved with initial interventions involving only decompression and subsequent strategies also incorporating fusions with stabilization. However, since the first description of an occipitocervical fusion (OCF), by Forrester in 1927, multiple methods of CVJ fixation have been described enabling deformity correction to maintain proper spinal alignment [4]. Without intervention, spinal instability as a consequence of CVJ pathology may lead to severe neurological morbidity and/or mortality

R. F. Heary (✉)
Department of Neurological Surgery, Rutgers New Jersey Medical School, Newark, NJ, USA
e-mail: heary@njms.rutgers.edu

N. Agarwal
Department of Neurological Surgery, University of Pittsburgh Medical Center, Pittsburgh, PA, USA
e-mail: agarwaln@upmc.edu

M. G. Kaiser et al. (eds.), *Degenerative Cervical Myelopathy and Radiculopathy*,
https://doi.org/10.1007/978-3-319-97952-6_29

[2, 5]. While OCF is certainly an effective method to address pathology of the occipitocervical junction, given its important role in mobility, posterior fixation must ensure proper sagittal alignment. As such, this chapter discusses the relevant perioperative considerations to attempt to achieve the ideal posture following fixation.

Indications

Instability of the CVJ affecting the brainstem and cervical spinal cord can lead to pain, cranial nerve palsies, respiratory distress, paralysis, or death [6]. As such, the usual treatment of CVJ pathology should be for dorsal decompression with the objective of preventing and/or improving neurological injury. In addition, stabilization of a pain-inducing segment is another common reason for consideration of OCF at this level. A myriad of potential pathologies including traumatic, degenerative, congenital, neoplastic, inflammatory, and infectious can be responsible for alterations in the CVJ alignment [4, 6].

Fractures resulting from trauma comprise a substantial percentage of the CVJ pathologies requiring OCF. Examples include unstable Jefferson (C1, atlas) and dens (C2, axis) fractures. As most C1 Jefferson fractures are decompressive injuries, this rarely requires surgical intervention. Dens fractures require surgical intervention far more frequently as the fractured component can retropulse into the spinal canal and cause problematic compression of the upper cervical spinal cord. Pain from degenerative spondylosis can be another indication for OCF although the great majority of these surgeries are performed in the subaxial cervical spine. Congenital conditions including os odontoideum, Chiari malformation, osteogenesis imperfecta, basilar invagination, mucopolysaccharidosis, and Klippel-Feil syndrome may require OCF in some situations. Metastatic disease and primary tumors such as chordoma and myeloma can lead to CVJ instability as well. Lastly, inflammatory conditions for which OCF may be performed include ankylosing spondylitis and rheumatoid arthritis [6].

Alternatives to OCF to address the aforementioned CVJ pathologies include the application of a rigid collar or a halo-vest apparatus. These devices may also be utilized as postoperative adjuncts in scenarios where an OCF is performed. Rigid collars may augment good bony stabilization, but as a general rule, soft collars should be avoided as these provide comfort only but not adequate structural support. Halo-vests have received criticism for a variety of reasons; however, they are most effective in the upper cervical spine where they can immobilize the occiput to C2 region quite well. Furthermore, halo-vests allow for wounds to be left open without any external pressure on the healing site which can be beneficial to more rapid wound healing. In the lower cervical spine, halo-vests may be suboptimal due to the phenomenon of "snaking" – flexion at a given level with compensatory extension at adjacent levels which allows considerable individual-level motion with little total excursion of the entire cervical spine [7]. Some of the additional complications with halo-vests include pin loosening, cranial fractures, pin site infection, and skin breakdown [8].

Contraindications

While OCF is an effective method to address CVJ pathology, several structural and vascular conditions may preclude OCF or necessitate anterior support to ensure biomechanical stability. Patient characteristics, vasculature, and structural abnormalities are all important considerations.

Clinical

Patient characteristics may limit the ability to proceed with surgical intervention. Medical comorbidities may preclude safely placing a patient under general anesthesia. Furthermore, fusion of the CVJ typically requires the patient to be positioned in the prone position. Pre-existing cardiopulmonary conditions or morbid obesity may impact the ability to carefully conduct a major spine surgery in the prone position. Lastly, osteoporosis may increase the risk of fusion failure.

Vascular

A detailed preoperative understanding of a patient's vascular anatomy is of utmost importance to the surgeon. Prior to instrumentation of the CVJ, recognition of an aberrant vertebral artery (VA) on either side is essential. For example, Paramore et al. estimated 18–23% of patients may not be appropriate candidates for posterior C1–C2 transarticular screw placement given the anatomic variability of the foramen transversarium at this level [9]. In situations where the VA location prevents placement of either a C2 pedicle or pars screw, crossed laminar screws, as initially described by Wright et al., can be utilized if there is not a need to decompress the dorsal bony arch at the C2 level [10]. In a retrospective review of magnetic resonance angiography images obtained from 2739 patients, Uchino et al. described three types of VA variations with a prevalence of 5 percent and a female predominance within the CVJ: persistent first intersegmental artery, VA fenestration, and the posterior inferior cerebellar artery (PICA) origination from C1 to C2 level [11].

Structural

Structural abnormalities may prohibit fixation to the occiput or require support. An example includes absence or hypoplasia of the occipital bone. Another is body destruction of the anterior and middle columns of the spine resulting in loss of ventral support. In this case, compromise of cervicothoracic spinal stability may mean that posterior fixation alone will not be adequate. An anterior approach to provide additional fixation may also be necessary.

Preoperative Planning

Preoperative anteroposterior (AP) and lateral plain films and a computed tomography (CT) scan are obtained. In addition, a magnetic resonance imaging (MRI) without contrast as well as a CT angiogram may be obtained to evaluate for any aberrant vascular anatomy. Planned screw-rod constructs need to be biomechanically sound and improve or at a minimum preserve sagittal balance. In a retrospective review of 752 patients with spinal deformity, Glassman et al. demonstrated severity of symptoms increased in a linear fashion with progressive sagittal imbalance [12]. In keeping with studies focused on the thoracolumbar spine, Tang et al. noted the severity of disability increases with positive cervical sagittal malalignment [13, 14]. Another parameter to consider was described by Matsunaga et al., noting among 38 patients with rheumatoid arthritis who underwent OCF an association between subaxial subluxation and an occipitoaxial angle (measured between McGregor's line and the inferior surface of the axis) outside the normal range [15].

Surgical Technique

Patients are placed under general anesthesia in the prone position with the head secured with a three-pronged Mayfield skull clamp. Fluoroscopic guidance is utilized throughout the procedure. While it is not our practice (20-year experience without neurological morbidity) to utilize neurophysiological motoring, some surgeons will employ intraoperative somatosensory-evoked potentials and/or motor-evoked potentials, especially during operative positioning, placement of instrumentation, and deformity correction maneuvers.

A midline incision is made from the inion down to the appropriate cervical level based on a preoperative review of surgical pathology. This is followed by dissection and reflection of soft tissues with subsequent identification of osseous landmarks for instrumentation. Our typical approach will involve placement of all stabilizing screws first followed by performing any bony decompression that may be indicated as part of the procedure. We utilize a posterior screw-rod-plate system with midline screws placed through the plate into the thickest part of the occiput (referred to as the "keel"). Screws placed rostral to the superior nuchal line increase the risk for violation of the transverse sinus, and as such, a careful review of the location of the torcular Herophili is needed to determine its location. As a general rule, we avoid placing screws into the occiput more than 44 mm above the foramen magnum. The midline occipital screws are flat at the bottom and usually are between 10 and 12 mm in length. A ball-tipped probe is utilized to confirm the depth of the prepared hole prior to screw placement into the occipital keel. Screws placed into the cervical spine are dependent on the numbers of levels required for the construct. At the C2 level, we most often utilize C2 pars screws of 20 mm length. A careful review of the preoperative CT scan is needed to assure that the pars can accommodate this length of screw. If a pars screw is not possible, then either a C2 pedicle screw or crossed C2 laminar screws may be considered at the C2 level. From the C3 to C6 levels, lateral mass screws of 14 mm length are frequently utilized. While Abumi et al. have described the use of pedicle screws in the subaxial cervical spine with great success, we have avoided these out of concern for the neural structures medial to and the vascular structures lateral to the pedicle [16]. In the relatively rare OCF case that extends more distally than the mid-cervical spine, we favor the use of pedicle screws at the C7 level (usually 24–26 mm) and the T1 level (usually 25–30 mm). We have routinely avoided including the C1 level in OCF constructs. The rationale for this is that the amount of fixation strength gained is minimal and the need for a hyperacute bend of the rods develops a potential stress riser which could lead to delayed rod fracture.

Once the screws have been situated, any necessary neural decompression is performed. This is predicated on the preoperative neurological assessment and the review of the advanced neuroimaging studies. After sufficient decompression is achieved, the corrective maneuvers are performed whereby the head is maneuvered. We typically perform the initial portion of the surgery with head maintained in a relatively neutral position with respect to the cervical spine. After the bony decompression is completed, the Mayfield head holder is released, and the head is dorsally translated and extended, relative to the cervical spine, and the head holder is resecured. This maneuver is performed by one member of the team who breaks sterility, while the other team member directly observes the neural elements to assure that excessive kinking does not occur during the extension. The purpose of this maneuver is to improve the sagittal alignment and attempt to optimize horizontal gaze [17]. A lateral fluoroscopic view is obtained before and after the corrective procedure is performed. Once again, we do not use neuromonitoring on these cases and have not seen neurological deterioration as a result of this deformity correction procedure in over 20 years. The chin-brow vertical angle (CBVA) is utilized to ensure an optimal position has been achieved. The CBVA is defined as the angle subtended by a vertical reference line and a line drawn parallel to the chin and brow with the neck in a neutral position with the knees and hips extended. Overall, the CBVA allows for an objective measurement of the consequences of a flexion deformity of the spine on the horizontal gaze [17]. The CVJ is then locked into place. Autologous bone graft is utilized to promote fusion. The autograft can be a large structural graft, morselized graft, or a combination of these two forms. In our practice, no allograft, cement, or bone graft substitutes are employed in dorsal OCF surgeries. The overall objective with regard to corrective maneuvers is to hold the occiput still, in good sagittal alignment, relative to the cervical spine to allow for a bony arthrodesis to take place.

Postoperative Care

The instrumentation is assessed postoperatively with AP and lateral plain films and a CT scan on the day of surgery. Further follow-up consists of wound check and staple removal 10–14 days after surgery. Subsequent clinical visits are scheduled 6 weeks, 12 weeks, 6 months, 1 year, and 2 years postoperatively. At each postoperative visit, plain films are routinely obtained to assess the fusion and instrumentation. If any clinical or radiographical concerns exist, more frequent visits may be scheduled, and an advanced neuroimaging study may be obtained as well.

Complication Avoidance

Fusion Failure

Given the difficulty with achieving solid radiographic bony arthrodesis from the occiput to the cervical spine, whenever possible, we avoid fusing to the occiput. Screw loosening has been observed in 4–7% of cases [18]. Another study noted pseudarthrosis rates in 6% of cases [19, 20]. In our view, the method of assessment will directly affect the fusion failure rates. If CT scans are performed at times remote from the index surgery, substantially higher pseudarthrosis rates will be observed than if only clinical or plain film determinations are performed. It is our belief that the published literature markedly underreports the true incidence of fusion failures at the OC junction (when the presence of bridging trabecular bone with the absence of motion on flexion-extension views and no instrumentation issues are criteria of a successful fusion). As a solid bony arthrodesis occurring between the occiput and the cervical spine is most likely the most difficult area of the spine to fuse, we attempt to avoid this technique unless it is absolutely necessary.

Infection

Wound infection rates have been estimated to occur in up to 3% of cases [21]. Wound care is a priority if a rigid collar is utilized postoperatively. One 10-year review noted that the postoperative use of a rigid collar was a significant risk factor for surgical site infections with a relative risk of 15.30 [22]. One of the few advantages of halo-vest immobilization is wound care. When a halo-vest is utilized, the wound is often able to be left uncovered and open to air by the second postoperative day. Having no pressure on the wound seems to aid in wound healing speed and efficacy. Also in cases of OCF performed in the setting of rheumatoid arthritis, one should be aware of the potentially increased risk for wound complications with rheumatoid medications as well as the frequently fragile skin of rheumatoid arthritis patients.

Cerebrospinal Fluid Leak

The incidence of dural tears is estimated to occur up to 4% of cases with drilling of the occiput and screw placement. Violation of the dura with may occur in upward of 25% of cases utilizing wire-based fixation [4, 20]. Management of dural tears includes direct suture repair of the defect, dural grafting, intraoperative use of a fibrin sealant, and, in some cases, the use of cerebrospinal fluid (CSF) diversion with a lumbar subarachnoid drain. Valsalva maneuvers can be employed intraoperatively to confirm the presence or absence of an ongoing CSF leak.

Fusion Adjuncts

We only utilize autograft. No allograft or other bone substitutes are used. Of note, the Food and Drug Administration (FDA) sent out an advisory in 2008 alerting against the use of recombinant human bone morphogenetic protein-2 (rhBMP-2) in the cervical spine. Complications of rhBMP include, but are not limited to, wound seroma, hematoma formation, and increased inflammation at times clinically manifesting as a radiculopathy. While rhBMP-2 would likely increase the ultimate fusion rates, the excessive complication rates preclude its usage in the cervical spine. Fineberg et al. demonstrated among 20,334 posterior cervical fusions, those with rhBMP-2 had increased length of stay and associated costs [23].

Case Presentations

Case 1

A 68-year-old male with long history of neck pain and stiffness presented with signs and symptoms of progressive cervical myelopathy including difficulty with hand dexterity and poor balance. He was diagnosed 10 years prior with diffuse idiopathic skeletal hyperostosis (DISH) and opacification of the posterior longitudinal ligament (OPLL). On physical examination, he was diffusely hyperreflexic with a (+) Babinski sign, 5–8 beat clonus bilaterally, and (+) Hoffman's sign bilaterally. Plain films demonstrated autofusion ventrally of all vertebrae below C2 (Fig. 29.1). A large senile pannus was noted on MRI at C1 compressing the spinal cord (Fig. 29.1b). The patient underwent a C1 laminectomy with occiput to C4 fusion using a structural autologous iliac crest bone graft. Stabilization was achieved with occipital plating (two screws), bilateral C2 pars screws, and lateral mass screws bilaterally at C3 and C4 (Fig. 29.1c, d). Postoperatively he had excellent improvement over the first 2 years with dramatic changes in balance and hand function.

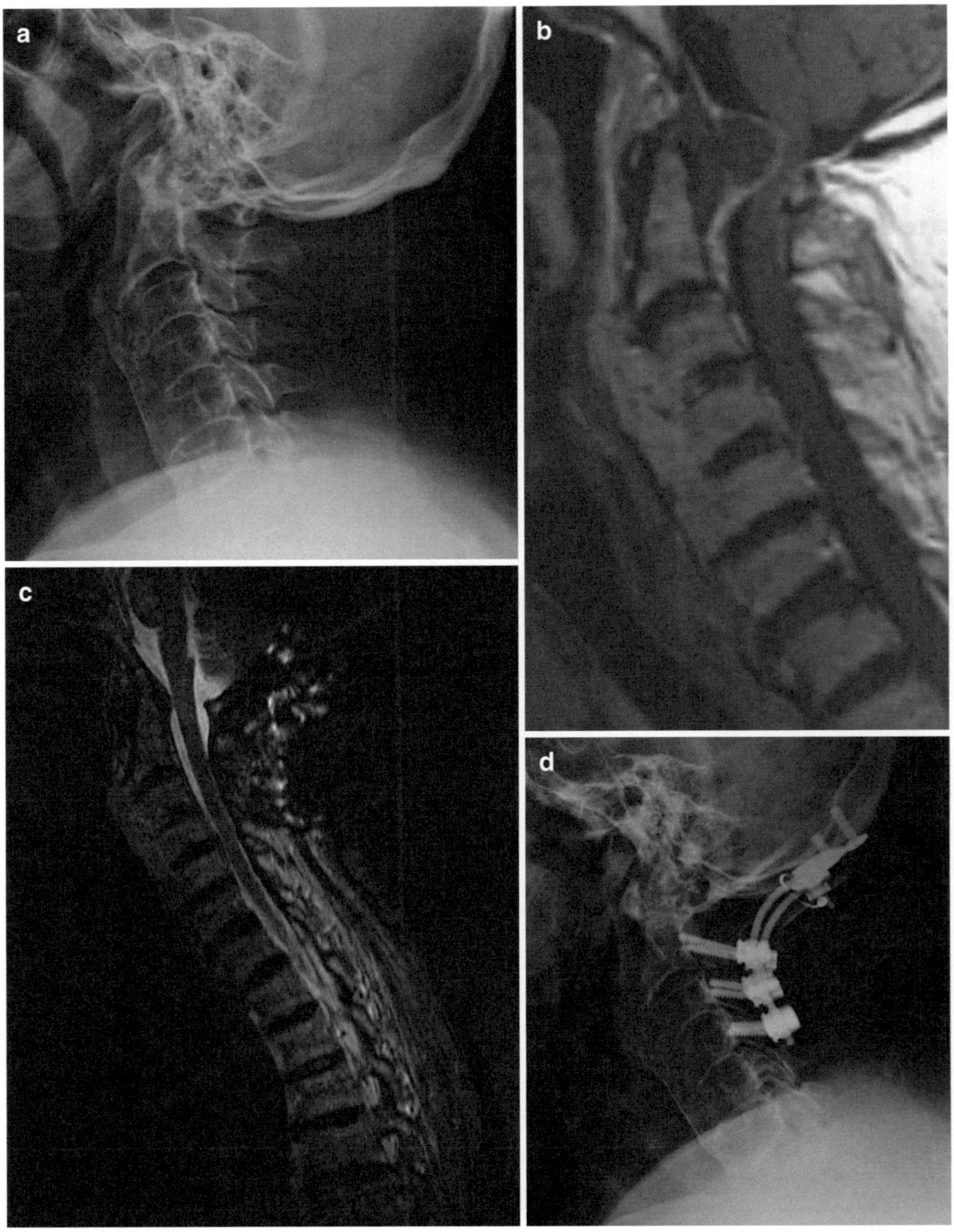

Fig. 29.1 (**a**) Lateral plain film demonstrating autofusion ventrally of all vertebrae below C2. (**b**) Sagittal T1-weighted MRI with large senile pannus at C1 compressing spinal cord. (**c**) Sagittal T2-weighted MRI demonstrating marked resolution of pannus at C1 following posterior stabilization only from occiput to C4. (**d**) Plain films obtain 6 months postoperatively with good alignment demonstrating a dorsal structural graft in place between occiput and C2 spinous process

Case 2

A 65-year-old female with a 15-year history of rheumatoid arthritis (RA) was recently diagnosed with basilar invagination, C2/3 klippel-feil deformity, and progressive myelopathy (Fig. 29.2a). Balance difficulties required her to use a 4-point walker. She also noted worsening hand function and was frequently dropping objects. Her hand difficulties were further complicated due to RA issues. She therefore underwent a suboccipital craniectomy with C1 laminectomy as well as an occiput to C5 fusion using a structural autologous iliac crest bone graft (Fig. 29.2b, c). Stabilization was achieved with an occipital plate (two screws), crossed laminar screws at C2 (Fig. 29.2d), and lateral mass screws bilaterally at C3 and C4. A Songer cable was utilized to hold the structural graft in place. Postoperative MRI obtained 1 year postoperatively demonstrated the CVJ was well

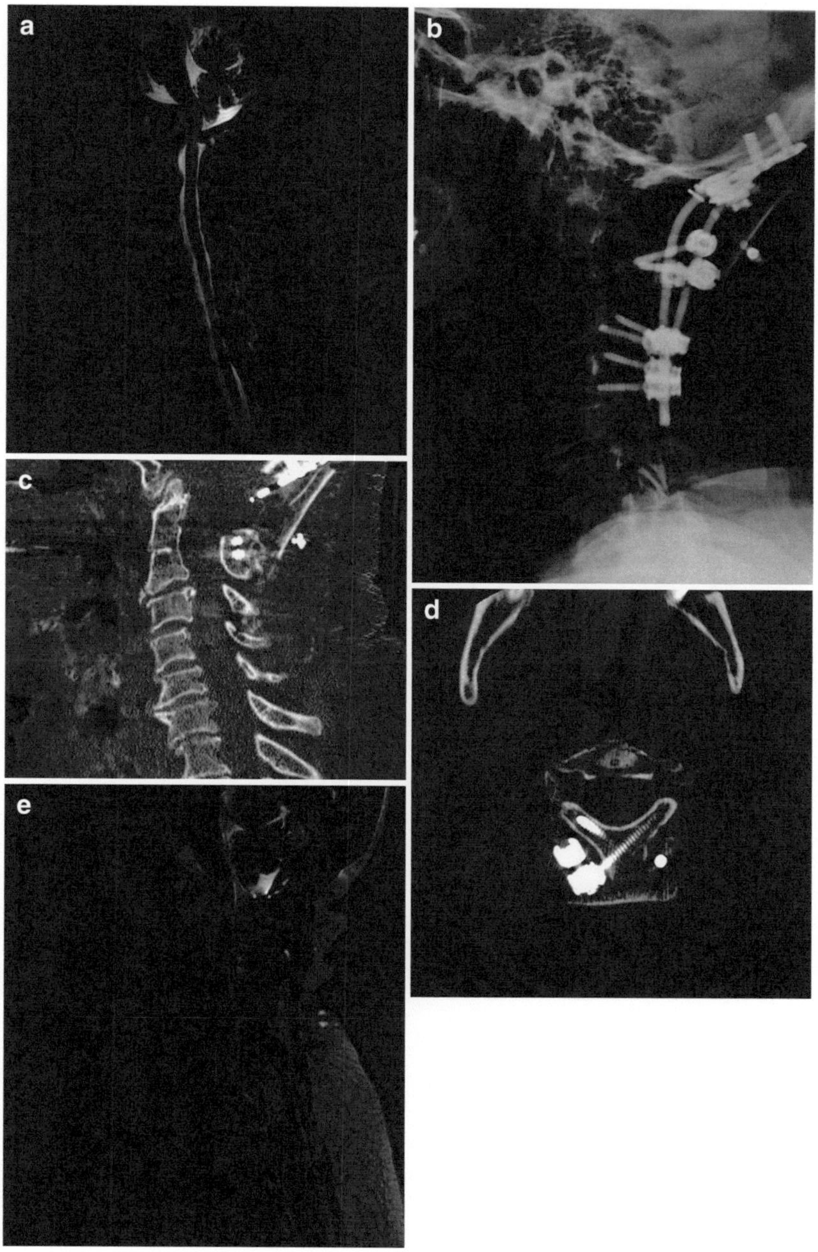

Fig. 29.2 (**a**) Sagittal T2-weighted MRI with basilar invagination secondary to a large rheumatoid pannus compressing the brain stem with increased T2 signal at level of foramen magnum. (**b**) Lateral plain film shows appropriate alignment in postoperative period with large iliac block bone graft extending between occiput and C2 spinous process. (**c**) Sagittal CT scan demonstrates the CVJ has been well decompressed with construct consisted of crossed laminar screws in C2 and a large structural graft from occiput to C2 held in place with a Songer cable. (**d**) Axial CT scan showing a large structural block iliac bone graft compressed against the C2 spinous process and crossed laminar screws placed at C2. (**e**) Sagittal T2-weighted MRI obtained 1 year postoperatively demonstrating a well-decompressed CVJ with resolution of rheumatoid pannus and an area of abnormal T2 signal in parenchyma of spinal cord in area where maximum compression had been present

decompressed with resolution of rheumatoid pannus and area of abnormal T2 signal in parenchyma of spinal cord in area where maximum compression had been present (Fig. 29.2e). The patient experienced modest improvements with independence. Her progressive symptoms related to RA complicated clinical picture, and she remained dependent on the use of a walker.

Case 3

A 70-year-old man with neck pain with a recent diagnosis of metastatic renal cell carcinoma was referred for evaluation. The patient was neurologically intact; however, imaging depicted a lytic lesion of the body of C2 with potential for neurological catastrophe (Fig. 29.3a) and a Spinal

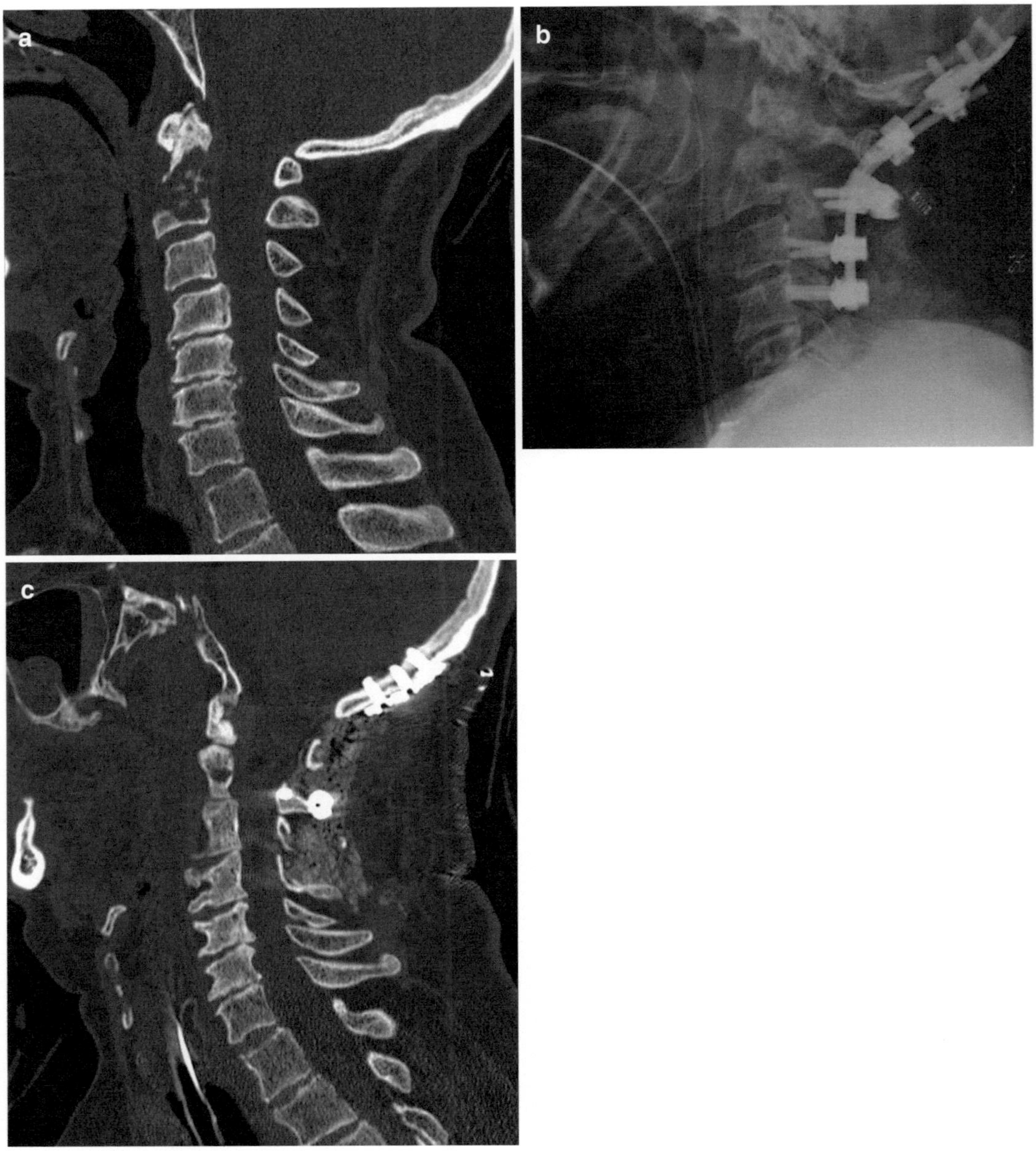

Fig. 29.3 (**a**) Sagittal preoperative CT scan with marked erosion of C2 vertebral body leading to impending neurological catastrophe. (**b**) Lateral postoperative plain film demonstrating occiput to C4 construct, sublaminar Songer cables at C1 that help align/stabilize C1 posterior arch, three screws fixated into occiput, and morselized autologous bone from occiput to C4. (**c**) Sagittal CT scan demonstrated anchor plate with three occipital screws and a generous quantity of autologous bone from occiput to C4 level

Instability Neoplastic Score (SINS) demonstrating an indication for surgical evaluation [24]. The patient underwent an occiput to C4 fusion using morselized autologous iliac crest bone graft. Stabilization was achieved with an occipital plate and three screws, sublaminar Songer cables at C1 which were attached to eyelet clamps attached to rods bilaterally, crossed C2 laminar screws, and lateral mass screws bilaterally at C3 and C4 (Fig. 29.3b, c). Postoperatively, the patient remained neurologically intact with marked improvement in neck pain. The plan was to hold off any radiation for a minimum of 4 weeks, if possible. This patient then moved to an outside state to be with his family. His local oncology team stated that no radiation was given for 3 months, while he fully fused. As needed, he could receive radiation therapy in the future, but it had not been given at last report as he remains symptom-free.

Conclusions

Posterior fixation of the occipitocervical junction is an effective method to address surgical pathology in this area. Failure to promptly address pathology affecting this complex area can lead to neurological morbidity and, possibly, mortality. The unique biomechanical and anatomical characteristics of the CVJ enable a large degree of motion and in particular flexion, extension, and rotation of the head relative to the spine without compromise of stability. As such, any surgical instrumentation of this complex area requires proper attention to sagittal alignment to optimize clinical and radiographic outcomes.

References

1. Tubbs RS, Hallock JD, Radcliff V, et al. Ligaments of the craniocervical junction. J Neurosurg Spine. 2011;14(6):697–709.
2. Martinez-Del-Campo E, Turner JD, Kalb S, et al. Occipitocervical fixation: a single surgeon's experience with 120 patients. Neurosurgery. 2016;79(4):549–60.
3. Lopez AJ, Scheer JK, Leibl KE, Smith ZA, Dlouhy BJ, Dahdaleh NS. Anatomy and biomechanics of the craniovertebral junction. Neurosurg Focus. 2015;38(4):E2.
4. Vender JR, Rekito AJ, Harrison SJ, McDonnell DE. The evolution of posterior cervical and occipitocervical fusion and instrumentation. Neurosurg Focus. 2004;16(1):E9.
5. Theodore N, Aarabi B, Dhall SS, et al. The diagnosis and management of traumatic atlanto-occipital dislocation injuries. Neurosurgery. 2013;72 Suppl 2(suppl_3):114–26.
6. Winegar CD, Lawrence JP, Friel BC, et al. A systematic review of occipital cervical fusion: techniques and outcomes. J Neurosurg Spine. 2010;13(1):5–16.
7. Glaser JA, Whitehill R, Stamp WG, Jane JA. Complications associated with the halo-vest. A review of 245 cases. J Neurosurg. 1986;65(6):762–9.
8. Lall R, Patel NJ, Resnick DK. A review of complications associated with craniocervical fusion surgery. Neurosurgery. 2010;67(5):1396–403.
9. Paramore CG, Dickman CA, Sonntag VKH. The anatomical suitability of the C1–2 complex for transarticular screw fixation. J Neurosurg. 1996;85(2):221–4.
10. Wright NM. Posterior C2 fixation using bilateral, crossing C2 laminar screws: case series and technical note. J Spinal Disord Tech. 2004;17(2):158–62.
11. Uchino A, Saito N, Watadani T, et al. Vertebral artery variations at the C1-2 level diagnosed by magnetic resonance angiography. Neuroradiology. 2012;54(1):19–23.
12. Glassman SD, Bridwell K, Dimar JR, Horton W, Berven S, Schwab F. The impact of positive sagittal balance in adult spinal deformity. Spine. 2005;30(18):2024–9.
13. Tang JA, Scheer JK, Smith JS, et al. The impact of standing regional cervical sagittal alignment on outcomes in posterior cervical fusion surgery. Neurosurgery. 2012;71(3):662–9; discussion 669.
14. Scheer JK, Tang JA, Smith JS, et al. Cervical spine alignment, sagittal deformity, and clinical implications. J Neurosurg Spine. 2013;19(2):141–59.
15. Matsunaga S, Onishi T, Sakou T. Significance of occipitoaxial angle in subaxial lesion after occipitocervical fusion. Spine. 2001;26(2):161–5.
16. Abumi K, Ito M, Sudo H. Reconstruction of the subaxial cervical spine using pedicle screw instrumentation. Spine. 2012;37(5):E349–56.
17. Kuntz C, Levin LS, Ondra SL, Shaffrey CI, Morgan CJ. Neutral upright sagittal spinal alignment from the occiput to the pelvis in asymptomatic adults: a review and resynthesis of the literature. J Neurosurg Spine. 2007;6(2):104–12.
18. Fehlings MG, Errico T, Cooper P, Benjamin V, DiBartolo T. Occipitocervical fusion with a five-millimeter malleable rod and segmental fixation. Neurosurgery. 1993;32(2):198–207; discussion 207–198.
19. Deutsch H, Haid RW Jr, Rodts GE Jr, Mummaneni PV. Occipitocervical fixation: long-term results. Spine. 2005;30(5):530–5.

20. Cheung JP, Luk KD. Complications of anterior and posterior cervical spine surgery. Asian Spine J. 2016;10(2):385–400.
21. He B, Yan L, Xu Z, Chang Z, Hao D. The causes and treatment strategies for the postoperative complications of occipitocervical fusion: a 316 cases retrospective analysis. Eur Spine J. 2014;23(8):1720–4.
22. Barnes M, Liew S. The incidence of infection after posterior cervical spine surgery: a 10 year review. Global Spine J. 2012;2(1):3–6.
23. Fineberg SJ, Ahmadinia K, Oglesby M, Patel AA, Singh K. Hospital outcomes and complications of anterior and posterior cervical fusion with bone morphogenetic protein. Spine. 2013;38(15):1304–9.
24. Fisher CG, DiPaola CP, Ryken TC, et al. A novel classification system for spinal instability in neoplastic disease: an evidence-based approach and expert consensus from the Spine Oncology Study Group. Spine. 2010;35(22):E1221–9.

Alternative Means of Posterior Cervical Stabilization

30

Hsuan-Kan Chang, David McCarthy, and Michael Y. Wang

Pitfalls/Pearls Outline

- Cervical pedicle screws, translaminar screws, and transfacet screws are viable alternatives to lateral mass screws (LMS) for posterior fixation when the lateral mass structure is compromised.
- Biomechanically, cervical pedicle screws provide stronger pullout strength, lower screw loosening rate at the bone-screw interface, and higher strengths in fatigue tests compared to LMS.
- There are anatomical limitations and significant neurovascular risks to insertion of the cervical pedicle screws.
- Spinal navigation (such as O-arm) demonstrated promising results in terms of accuracy and safety for a cervical pedicle screw but requires further investigation.
- The insertion of the translaminar screw is relatively straightforward and carries a low risk of neurovascular injury.
- The biomechanical feature of the translaminar screw is similar to LMS. Although the lamina is often undersized for translaminar screw placement, except in C2, C7, and upper thoracic segments, which are the more common locations.
- A transfacet screw is often used as a means of posterior fixation for substitution of LMS or cervical pedicle screw when the lamina is absent or as a supplement to multilevel anterior cervical fusion.
- Percutaneous insertion of the transfacet screw is feasible since no rod connection is necessary and the biomechanical stability still remains equivalent to LMS plus rod fixation.
- Screw length and trajectory are key factors for transfacet screws in order to avoid penetration of the anterior lateral mass wall and subsequent neurovascular injury.

H.-K. Chang · D. McCarthy · M. Y. Wang (✉)
Department of Neurological Surgery and Rehabilitation Medicine, University of Miami Miller School of Medicine, Miami, FL, USA
e-mail: mwang2@med.miami.edu

M. G. Kaiser et al. (eds.), *Degenerative Cervical Myelopathy and Radiculopathy*,
https://doi.org/10.1007/978-3-319-97952-6_30

Introduction

The posterior approach is commonly performed in the treatment of multilevel degenerative cervical myelopathy (DCM) with spinal cord compression. Both posterior laminoplasty and laminectomy with fusion can achieve adequate decompression of the spinal cord and obtain satisfactory neurologic outcomes. Lateral mass screw (LMS) fixation is the prevalent fixation technique for the posterior cervical approach. LMS fixation achieves a high fusion rate and is associated with a low complication profile. Neurologic injury, vascular injury, and hardware failure rarely occur in LMS cases [1]. LMS has become the standard technique for posterior fixation in the subaxial cervical spine for various pathologies. Nevertheless, LMS fixation has its own limitations and isn't indicated under certain circumstances. In such circumstances, alternative techniques including cervical pedicle screw, translaminar screw, and transfacet screw can be very useful for posterior cervical fixation instead of LMS. In this chapter, we will give a comprehensive explanation of these common alternatives for posterior cervical fixation.

Cervical Pedicle Screws

Indications/Contraindications

Although LMS fixation is the most common technique used for posterior cervical fusion, the cervical pedicle screw technique has its unique advantages. It is indicated in patients with primary and metastatic tumor, trauma with instability, spondylosis/spondylolisthesis, infectious discitis/osteomyelitis, and deformity correction. It is particularly beneficial in cases when the lateral mass is not available for screw placement, for example, if the lateral mass is incompetent due to tumor, erosion, infection, fracture, severe osteoporosis, small anatomical size, etc. Biomechanically compared to LMS, cervical pedicle screws provide stronger pullout strength, lower screw loosening rate at the bone-screw interface, and higher strength in the fatigue test [2]. These benefits allow the cervical pedicle screw technique to achieve satisfactory results in the posterior fixation for translational instability and kyphosis correction. Despite the advantages, cervical pedicle screws remain unpopular for posterior fusion because it is a technically challenging technique. The anatomical variations and limitations result in a high rate of pedicle breach complications. Due to the proximity of vital structures and the risk of a dural tear or CSF leak, a neurologic and vascular injury is the major concern for most spine surgeons performing cervical pedicle screw placement.

Contraindications for the cervical pedicle screw technique include (1) narrow or absent pedicle, (2) major vertebral artery anomaly located at the target level, (3) compression fracture at the targeted vertebral body, and (4) unfavorable conditions for a posterior approach, like infection, etc. Detailed inspection of preoperative images, including MRI and CT angiography, provides essential information for proper planning in cervical pedicle screw placement. Prior to a cervical pedicle screw operation, we recommend performing 1–2 mm thin-cut CT angiography as a routine evaluation. Thin-cut CT angiography allows surgeons to evaluate the pedicle diameter, the course of the vertebral artery, and the patency of bilateral vessels. If the pedicle width is less than 4 mm, the pedicle diameter is likely to be smaller than the screw diameter, making it difficult to create a proper tract for placement. Caution must be taken in patients with unilateral vertebral artery obstruction or hypoplasia because injury to the contralateral dominant artery can cause complete blockage of arterial flow to the brain stem, resulting in a devastating cerebrovascular event. In such cases, LMS or an alternative method, performed at the ipsilateral side of the dominant artery, can serve as a substitute for the pedicle screw. Occasionally the course of the vertebral artery varies and invades into the vertebral body. Placing a pedicle screw at a level with this vascular anomaly carries a high risk of damaging the ipsilateral vertebral artery. Thus, a cervical pedicle screw on the ipsilateral side should be avoided or skipped. If this is not possible, an

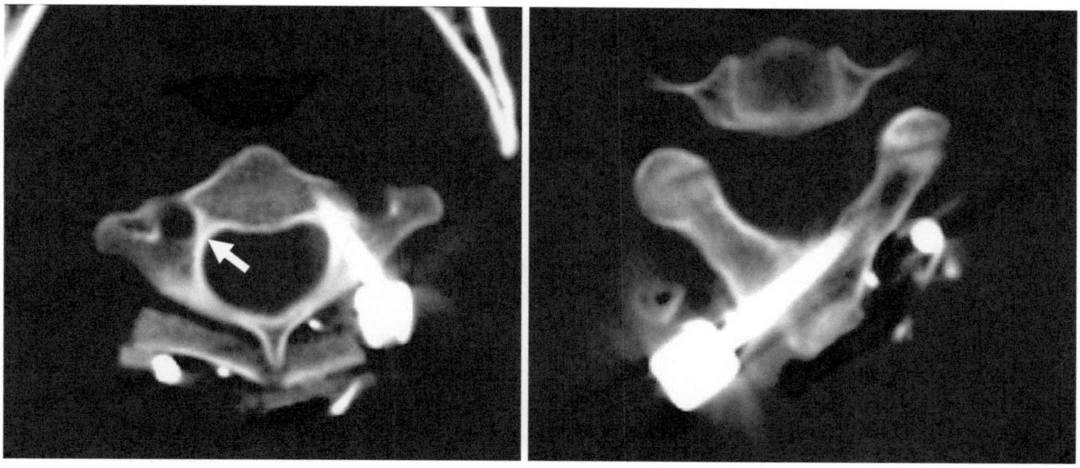

Fig. 30.1 A case example of the alternative techniques. A cervical pedicle screw (*left*) and a translaminar screw (*right*) at the same segment. Right pedicle screw is not feasible due to extremely narrow pedicle diameter and high risk of vertebral artery violation (*white arrow*)

alternative fixation method such as the translaminar screw, LMS, or transfacet screw techniques should be considered (Fig. 30.1).

Surgical Technique

The operative setting is similar to a routine posterior cervical spine approach. Following general anesthesia, the patient is positioned prone with the head fixed with a three- or four-point fixation device, like a Mayfield skull clamp. The neck is then placed parallel to the floor with a slightly lordotic curve. In a cautious fashion, avoiding injury to the shoulder joint or brachial plexus, the patient's shoulders are often taped and pulled caudally in order to allow clear visualization of the lower cervical spine. Neurological monitoring with somatosensory evoked potential (SSEP) or motor evoked potential (MEP) can be helpful for posterior cervical pedicle screw placement. A routine midline skin incision is made for the posterior approach, and an extensive muscular dissection is mandatory in order to explore the lateral edge of the lateral mass structure for pedicle screw insertion.

Abumi's technique has been adopted for cervical pedicle screw placement [3]. He describes a screw entry point slightly lateral to the midline of the lateral mass and just caudally bordering the superior articular facet at C3–C6. The lateral vertebral notch is approximately at the same level of, or slightly above, the pedicle, making it a useful landmark. Two to four millimeters (mm) medial to the lateral vertebral notch serves as another ideal entry point for the cervical pedicle screw (Fig. 30.2a). After determining the screw entry point at each level, a small pilot hole can be made in the cortical bone with a match head or small-diameter diamond burr. The optimal pathway for subsequent screw insertion is forged into the pedicle by inserting a small curved pedicle probe into the lateral mass. The sagittal trajectory of the pedicle probe should pass between the pedicle's cranial and caudal margin and remain parallel to the upper endplate of the vertebral body (Fig. 30.2b). The whole procedure should be performed under lateral fluoroscopic guidance. The oblique angle of the pedicle on the axial plane has high variation and can be estimated on a preoperative CT scan. Generally speaking, the angle ranges from 30° to 60°, in relation to the midline, with gradually larger angles at the more caudal levels (Fig. 30.3). By maintaining a medial probe angle, it decreases the likelihood of vertebral foramen and artery injury, but it increases the chance of a medial wall breach and violation the spinal canal. Structurally, the medial wall of the

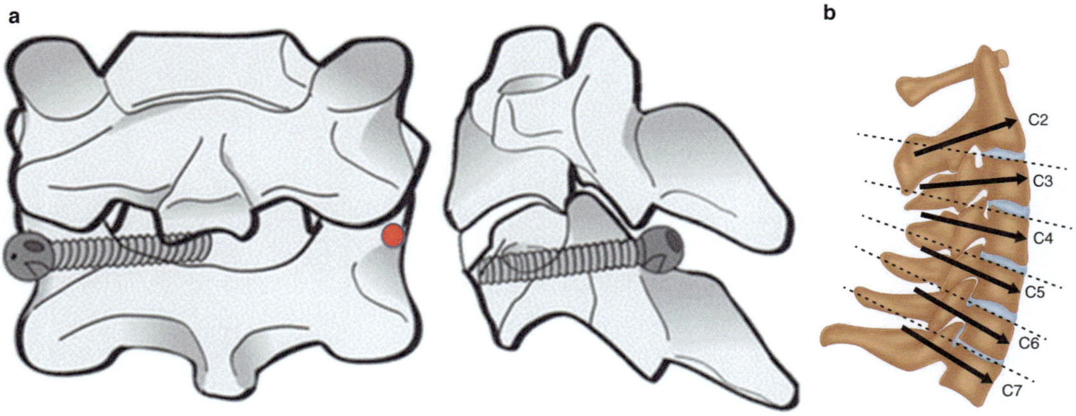

Fig. 30.2 (**a**) Ideal entry point for cervical pedicle screw (red dot); (**b**) screw trajectory in the sagittal plane. (Adapted from Abumi [23])

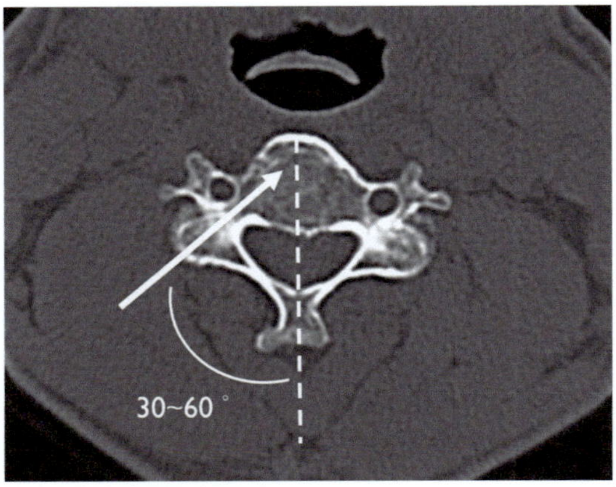

Fig. 30.3 Trajectory of cervical pedicle screw in the axial plane ranges from 30° to 60° at different level of subaxial spine

pedicle is thicker than the lateral wall and is not breached by the pedicle probe as easily. The medial wall can be palpated with a Penfield No. 4, serving as guidance for maneuvering the probe through the pedicle isthmus. During large-angle insertion of cervical pedicle screws, the aforementioned extensive soft tissue dissection is necessary to avoid blocking the pedicle probing and screw insertion. The depth of the pedicle probing can be monitored on lateral fluoroscopy.

A ball-tipped probe is helpful for ensuring pedicle probe tract accuracy and for screw length estimation. Ball-tipped probe palpation provides important feedback about the possible misplacement of screws. If the depth of probe tip is shorter than expected and there is soft tissue feedback, the probe has likely violated the vertebral foramen. Excessive bleeding from the pilot hole indicates that the pedicle probe has possibly penetrated the venous plexus around the vertebral artery. Under this circumstance, abandoning the pedicle screw technique and converting to alternative methods such as LMS are advised.

After the palpation with the ball-tipped probe, the tract is tapped, and then the screw is inserted. The screw length is estimated through measurements obtained by either the preoperative CT scan or the ball-tipped probe depth. The screw diameter, which is usually 3.5 or 4.0 mm, and the screw length, which usually ranges from 20 to 30 mm, are determined based on measuring the pedicle width and trajectory length on preoperative CT scan.

Fluoroscopic anteroposterior (AP) imaging is valuable in evaluating screw malposition intraoperatively. The screw tip should approximate to the midline or the spinal process on AP image. If any screws are not in the adequate position, they should be removed and a new tract re-explored, or the level with misplaced screws may have to be skipped. Postoperative AP and lateral X-rays should be obtained to confirm appropriate screw position (Fig. 30.4).

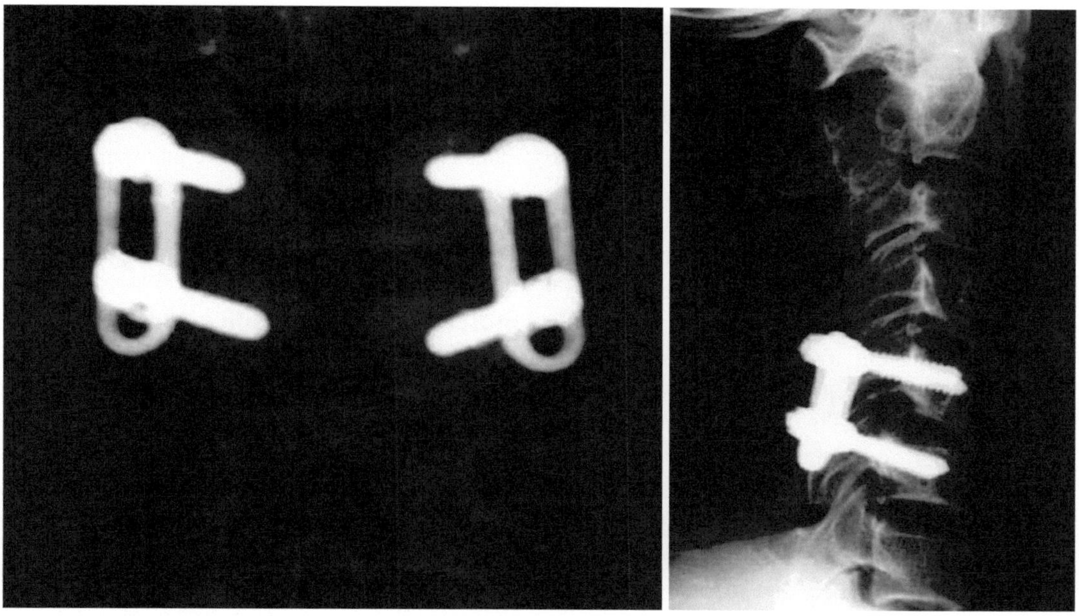

Fig. 30.4 Postoperative X-ray of cervical pedicle screw. (Adapted from Abumi et al. [3])

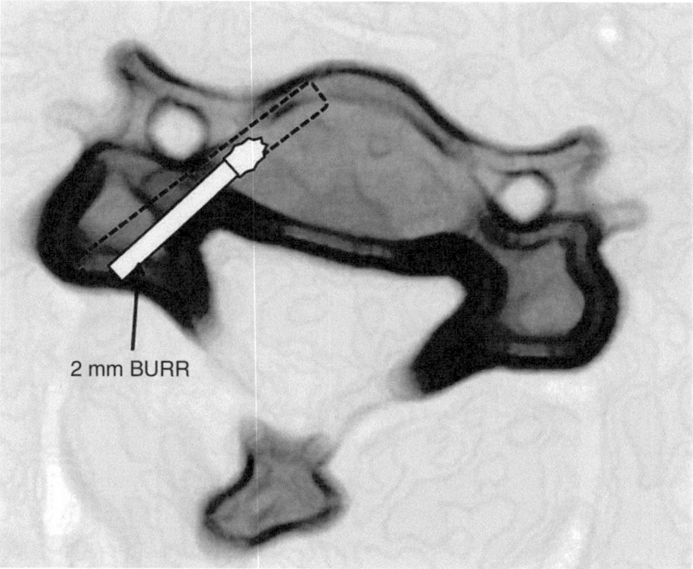

Fig. 30.5 The technique of medial cortical pedicle screws (MCPS). The dotted rectangle line represents the classic technique and trajectory of Abumi's. The 2 mm diamond-tipped burr demonstrates the entry point and trajectory of MCPS. (Adapted from Mahesh et al. [4])

Complication Management/ Avoidance

The major concerns involving cervical pedicle screw placement are possible nerve and vertebral artery injury. Vertebral artery injury is caused by lateral screw misplacement. This can be avoided by obtaining the optimal angle for screw tract purchase through extensive muscular dissection. Mahesh et al. described a medial cortical pedicle screw (MCPS) technique by partial drilling of the medial cortex and shifting the trajectory of pedicle screw along the medial cortex [4] (Fig. 30.5). He demonstrated that lateral perforation of the vertebral foramen is remarkably reduced by using this technique. A nerve root injury can result from cranially or caudally misplaced screws. In addition, medially misplaced screws may lead to dura injury, CSF leak, or even spinal cord injury in the worst-case scenario.

Spine surgeons must be aware of the aforementioned complications directly related to pedicle screw misplacement. Careful and thorough evaluation of the feasibility of the cervical pedicle screws, pedicle morphology, and vascular course from tomographic images are essential before surgery. Recently, it has become more popular to perform the cervical pedicle screws with the aid of navigation. Due to the pitfalls of the freehand technique, spinal navigation has become more utilized in posterior cervical fixation, improving accuracy and reducing the complication rate associated with pedicle screws [2, 5, 6]. O-arm and Stealth navigations are novel technologies based on intraoperative CT scans and three-dimensional guiding systems. Studies compared the outcome of O-arm navigation with the freehand method for cervical pedicle screw placement showing improvement in screw accuracy with O-arm assistance. A few studies demonstrated that O-arm-guided cervical pedicle screw placement can be performed with a remarkable decline in neurovascular injury [2, 5, 6]. O-arm navigation seems to be a promising tool for improving precision when compared to freehand technique, although the strength of evidence is weak since almost all existing studies are retrospective. In addition, O-arm assistance is under scrutiny because of its increased radiation exposure, hospital cost, personnel required, and operation time. The benefits of O-arm navigation for cervical pedicle screw placement require further investigation before they become established.

Originally documented by Heller et al. studying complications of LMS and posterior cervical plating, a few papers make note of iatrogenic foraminal stenosis following cervical pedicle screw placement at the C7–T1 levels. Several papers report a C8 radiculopathy following a cervical pedicle screw procedure for deformity correction [2, 5, 7, 8]. Though the mechanism of iatrogenic foraminal stenosis is not fully understood, it is thought to come from the reduction of the translation deformity and the resulting foraminal stenosis at cervicothoracic junction.

Translaminar Screws

Indications/Contraindications

A variety of fixation methods are available for a posterior cervical approach. Among them, the cervical LMS and pedicle screw techniques are widely studied and utilized in the subaxial spine. Although less popular than the LMS or pedicle screw, the translaminar screw is considered a practical alternative for subaxial spine fixation. The translaminar screw was first described by Wright et al. in 2004 using crossing screws through the C2 lamina in conditions for which C2 laminectomy is not required [9]. Traditionally, the translaminar screws are more frequently applied to the C2, C7, and cervicothoracic region.

A C2 pedicle screw provides stronger biomechanical stability and assists reliable fusion compared to a C2 pars screw. Unfortunately, the C2 pedicle screw is not always possible because of small pedicle diameters, high-riding vertebral grooves, and its high technical demand. Serious neurovascular complications may develop following a C2 pedicle screw misplacement, rendering a spine surgeon to seek substitute methods. C2 translaminar screws are a common substitution for the pedicle screw. Recently a number of publications have shown the clinical efficacy and safety of the C2 translaminar screw in place of the pedicle screw [10–12]. A biomechanical study demonstrated similar fixation strength between the C2 translaminar screw and the pedicle screw [13]. The clinical applications of the translaminar screw have been well established at C2 level.

At a lower level of the cervical spine, particular C7, the lateral mass structure can be very small and problematic for LMS insertion. Screw loosening and pullouts have been reported in C7

LMS placement. The pedicle screw is the most common method performed at C7 and biomechanically provides the most rigid fixation; however, it poses a risk of vascular injury and is also technically challenging due to anatomical variation and restrictive pedicle morphology. Translaminar screws have often replaced pedicle screws for posterior cervicothoracic fixation in the C7 and upper thoracic region. The indications for C7 and upper thoracic translaminar screws include trauma, neoplasm, degeneration, and pediatric patients requiring cervicothoracic region fixation.

For the subaxial spine (C3–6), applications for translaminar screws remain limited to select cases. In the last few years, morphology studies using radiographic images or computer simulation for translaminar screw insertion claim that translaminar screw is feasible in the subaxial spine [14]. Although, clinical studies reporting the outcomes and fusion rates are surprisingly rare.

Translaminar screws have their own advantages. First, the screw insertion technique is quite straightforward by only involving the posterior column of the cervical spine, therefore minimizes the risk of vertebral artery injury. Second, since the translaminar screw can be safely performed under direct visualization, there is almost no need for fluoroscopic monitoring during screw placement, remarkably reducing the radiation exposure. Additionally, the biomechanical strength was shown to be equivalent to a pedicle screw in terms of pullout force [15].

The indications for subaxial translaminar screws include degenerative conditions, traumas, tumors, and when LMS and pedicle screw techniques are impractical. This may occur in cases lacking substantial lateral mass structure, previous LMS and pedicle screw failed attempts, too much risk for neurovascular injury, narrow pedicles, abnormal vascular course, etc. Translaminar screw placement requires an intact lamina at the level intended to treat. Deficits or an absence of intact lamina may be caused by conditions like trauma, tumor, or post-laminectomy for decompression. In such cases, a translaminar screw placement is not feasible. There is a lack of literature showing translaminar screws as instrumentation for cervical deformity correction. It is unknown if the translaminar screw alone is sufficient for deformity correction with or without anterior column support.

Surgical Technique

According to a CT and cadaveric analysis from Cho et al., the typical screw size is 3.0 or 3.5 mm in diameter and about 23–26 mm in length [16]. However, a preoperative CT scan should be obtained to evaluate screw diameter, length, and projected insertion angle in advance. The operative setting is similar to the routine posterior cervical spine approach. Following general anesthesia, the patient is positioned prone with the head fixed with a three- or four-point fixation device like a Mayfield skull clamp. The neck is placed parallel to the floor with a slight lordotic curve in order to restore cervical lordosis after fixation. After a standard midline incision and muscular dissection, the bony structure of the posterior cervical lamina is prepared for screw placement. The placement of translaminar screw is under direct visualization of the involved bony structure and usually does not require fluoroscopy guidance. The entry point is usually at the junction between the spinous process and the contralateral lamina (Fig. 30.6, *right*). A pilot hole is made by a high-speed burr at the entry point. Either a hand drill or small-diameter high-speed diamond burr can be used to create the preoperatively measured trajectory which aims along the lamina. The tract is checked with a ball-tipped probe to ensure that it remains inside the cancellous bone and that the spinal canal is not violated. The screw is then placed and secured along the tract. If bilateral translaminar screws are to be executed at the same level, the entry points at the junction must stagger in order to avoid decussating tracts (Fig. 30.6). Rods are contoured and cut to the appropriate length and secured to the remaining screw heads or the concomitant cervical pedicle screws/lateral mass screws if in conjunction with them.

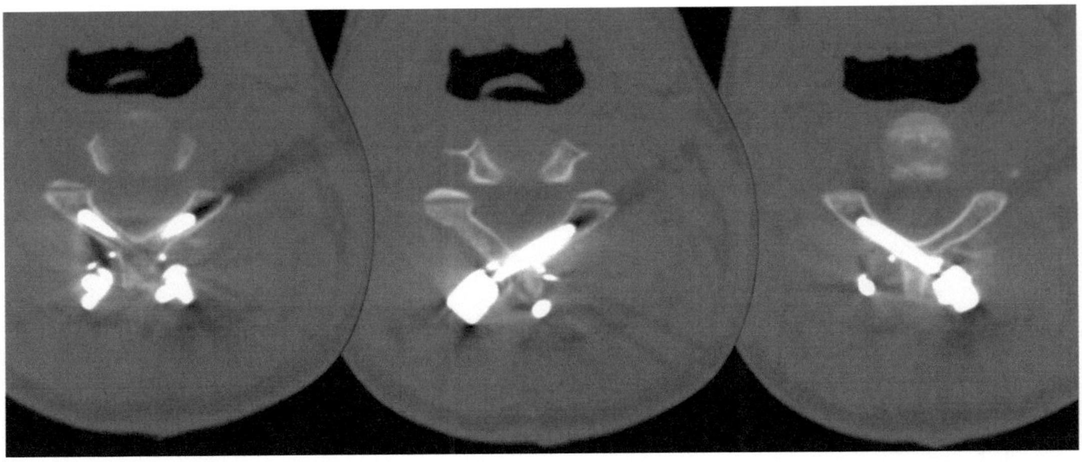

Fig. 30.6 Postoperative CT scan of translaminar screw at C2. The entry point of a translaminar screw is usually at the junction between the spinous process and the contralateral lamina *(right)*

Complication Management/ Avoidance

There are two major intraoperative complications associated with a translaminar screw. The breach to the inner cortical bone of the lamina and the subsequent risk of CSF leak/spinal cord injury are the most undesirable complications. These complications can be avoided by carefully following the trajectory of the lamina while drilling and detecting the spinal canal violation with dissectors. Ball-tipped probe is particularly useful in exploring screw tract and depth (usually between 20 and 30 mm), making sure that the laminar cortical bone is not violated. The second complication is a breach of the outer cortex of the lamina which may occur if the trajectory is directed dorsally. There may not be any serious consequence following an outer cortex breach, but theoretically the biomechanical stability can be compromised if the length of screw engagement is shorter than needed.

One disadvantage of the translaminar screw technique is that the lamina may be undersized for placement. The diameter and lengths of the lamina are the smallest in the subaxial spine and vary widely from individual to individual. This often raises doubt about the feasibility of translaminar screws. Alvin et al. measured the spatial anatomical environment for subaxial translaminar screws with CT scan to determine the applicability of translaminar screw placement at C3–C7. They found that C7 showed a universally high acceptance rate for 3.5 mm screw both unilaterally and bilaterally. C3–C6 only had an approximate 50–60% acceptance rate for a unilateral 3.5 mm screw. The acceptance rate for a bilateral screw at C3–C6 is extremely low [17]. The study concluded that bilateral translaminar screw placement is practical at C7, but not at C3–C6. Therefore, the standard use of a translaminar screw for posterior cervical fixation may be doubtful. Moreover, the study implicated that careful reviewing of the CT scan is warranted in order to measure the size of the lamina and to estimate the screw length prior to surgery.

Transfacet Screws

Indications/Contraindications

Many posterior cervical fixation techniques have been investigated for their outcome and biomechanical features. LMS remains the most popular method of posterior cervical fixation with low complication rates. Where LMS is limited, several other techniques are considered as salvage methods. Pedicle screws provide the strongest biomechanical rigidity but are technically demanding and highly risky. A translaminar screw is more practical at the C2, C7, and upper thoracic spine levels than the subaxial spine due to the limitation of lamina thickness. Recently, the transfacet screw has been a proposed alternative option for the subaxial spine.

Although uncommonly used, transfacet screw fixation can be an isolated fixation technique for segmental stabilization without rod connection. Transfacet screws are, for the most part, applied in adjunct with additional posterior screw fixation devices like an LMS and pedicle screws or as supplemental fixation in combination to a multilevel anterior cervical fusion. If transfacet screws are applied in conjunction with LMS or cervical pedicle screw, it is necessary to be coupled to the rod. Although the clinical reporting is scant for transfacet screws as an isolated posterior fixation system, the reported fusion rate is quite favorable [18]. Well-designed, long-term studies are required in order to validate the effectiveness of the transfacet screw. In contrast to a translaminar screw, the transfacet screw can be used in the absence of a lamina when decompression is necessary. Transfacet screw contraindications include conditions in which the facet joint and lateral mass are unavailable. Such conditions may arise due to fracture, trauma, infection, tumor, when foraminotomy or facetectomy is needed, etc. Transfacet screw placement is not indicated for deformity correction because it only provides motion restriction to the facet joint and does not involve rod connection and realignment of the spinal curvature. A biomechanical study discerned that the stability of transfacet screws (without rods) was equivalent to LMS with rod fixation [19]. The pullout strength of the transfacet screw is demonstrated to be superior to LMS since transfacet screws penetrate four cortical layers during purchase rather than the two seen in LMS.

Surgical Technique

The patient is placed in a prone position for transfacet screw placement. Cervical spine should be fixed in the neutral position with a slight lordosis to maintain the natural curvature. A three-point head fixation device, such as Mayfield skull clamp, is helpful in adjusting the relative position between head and neck. We recommend slightly flexing the skull so that the occiput does not interfere with the screw trajectory, particularly in procedures involving the upper cervical spine. There are different methods in terms of the entry point. Dal Canto suggested an entry point 2 mm below the center of the lateral mass, while Takayasu entered at a point rostral to Dal Canto, between the superior and median third of the vertical medial line (Fig. 30.7) [20]. The screw trajectory of Takayasu is 60–70° caudally and points toward the midline of ipsilateral lateral mass, which is often the location of the vertebral artery. We place our entry point at the center of the superior facet and aim for the body of the inferior facet. The trajectory is slightly lateral in an attempt to avoid the vertebral artery in front of lateral mass. The screw will purchase through the facet joint between the superior and inferior facet and then engage within the body of inferior facet (Fig. 30.8). The entry point and screw purchase in sagittal plane can be assessed with the assistance of a lateral fluoroscopic image. The placement of transfacet screw does not require rods to immobilize the spine, generating the potential for spine surgeons to perform the procedure in a minimally invasive fashion. Percutaneous screw placement could reduce the neck pain caused by extensive muscular dissection. In addition, when used for supplemental fixation to long anterior cervical fusion, percutaneous technique avoids a

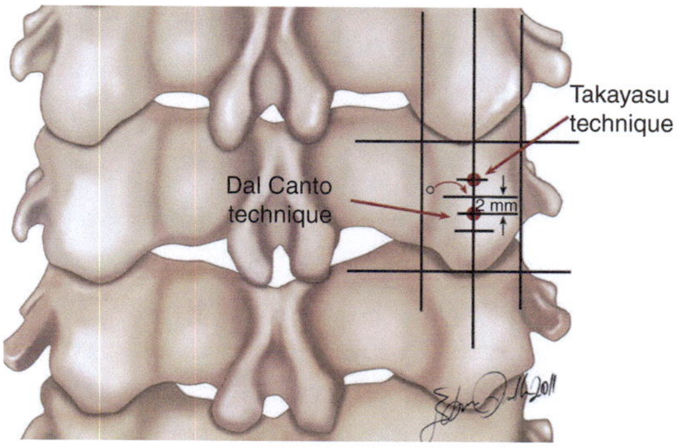

Fig. 30.7 The illustration of entry point for Takayasu's and Dal Canto's technique of transfacet screw. (Adapted from Aydogan et al. [20])

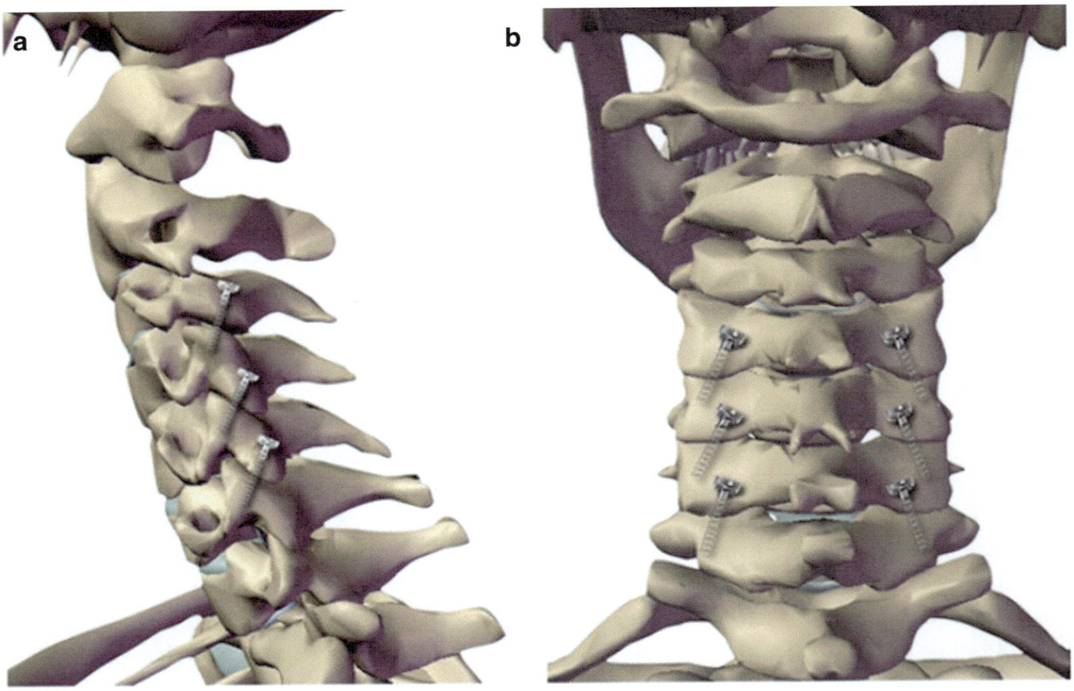

Fig. 30.8 The illustration of our starting point and screw trajectory in anteroposterior and lateral view. (Adapted from Ahmad et al. [24])

lengthy second incision. If percutaneous transfacet screws are primarily executed to supplement long anterior cervical fusion surgeries, the use of osteobiologic agents, like rhBMP-2, may improve the reliability of fusion simply through drilling and exposure of the facet joint. The use of rhBMP-2 in this setting however has not been cleared by the FDA and would be considered an off-label application of BMP.

Complication Management/Avoidance

The intraoperative complications of the transfacet screw include nerve root injury, vascular injury, and facet fracture. Since the cervical nerve root and vertebral artery are located directly anterior to the lateral mass, nerve root injury and vascular injury may occur if the ventral border of the inferior facet is penetrated. The screw length should be carefully determined because unnecessarily long screws may penetrate the lateral mass, compromising the vertebral artery and the nerve root. Compared to Takayasu's technique, we intend to slightly lateralize the screw trajectory in order to avoid impinging the vertebral artery. Liu et al. studied 20 cadaveric cervical spines and recommended a starting point 1 mm medial to the midline of the lateral mass. The drilling angle in their study is 37° inferiorly and 16° laterally. The ideal screw size in their study was 3.5 mm in diameter and 18 mm in length. No arterial or neurological violation is in their report [21]. Transfacet screws have been associated with lateral mass or facet fracture in the literature. The facet fracture may be related to the entry point and the angle of trajectory. Dal Canto's technique involves a lower entry point and a more oblique trajectory (about 40°), which may result in a larger risk of facet fracture than Takayasu's [20, 22].

Another potential drawback of the transfacet screw is the anatomical limitations. According to anatomic studies, upper levels are able to accommodate longer screws than the lower levels because of their longer transfacet lengths. The transfacet length decreases in the lower subaxial spine and in female patients, theoretically weakening the biomechanical strength. Although the upper levels could technically accommodate longer screws, the transfacet screw placement at C2–3 and C3–4 are challenging due to the interference from the occipital bone. Moreover, the trajectory at lower cervical spine is more desirable than at C2–3 and C3–4. Therefore, it is a great advantage to flex the head in an attempt to prevent the impediment from occiput [22].

Conclusions

Cervical pedicle screw placement at the subaxial spine is a viable alternative to LMS under certain circumstances. The biomechanical superiority allows the cervical pedicle screw to achieve excellent outcomes in cervical spine reduction and deformity correction from a posterior approach. Despite the technical challenges with the freehand approach, modern navigation may offer improvements in screw accuracy leading to reductions in neurologic and vascular complications. Careful preoperative planning on tomographic images is necessary to help select the proper surgical candidate and to avoid potential adverse events.

Translaminar and transfacet screws serve more as a conjunctional fixation technique with lateral mass and cervical pedicle screws. Translaminar screws carry a low risk of neurovascular injury but are more common at C2, C7, and upper thoracic segment due to the anatomical limitation. Transfacet screws can be used in the absence of a lamina when laminectomy is required. Percutaneous insertion of transfacet screws is feasible, and rod connection is not necessary for isolated transfacet screw fixation.

References

1. Coe JD, Vaccaro AR, Dailey AT, et al. Lateral mass screw fixation in the cervical spine: a systematic literature review. J Bone Joint Surg Am. 2013;95(23):2136–43.
2. Theologis AA, Burch S. Safety and efficacy of reconstruction of complex cervical spine pathology using pedicle screws inserted with stealth navigation and 3D image-guided (O-arm) technology. Spine (Phila Pa 1976). 2015;40(18):1397–406.
3. Abumi K, Ito M, Sudo H. Reconstruction of the subaxial cervical spine using pedicle screw instrumentation. Spine (Phila Pa 1976). 2012;37(5):E349–56.
4. Mahesh B, Upendra B, Vijay S, Arun K, Srinivasa R. Perforations and angulations of 324 cervical medial cortical pedicle screws: a possible guide to avoid lateral perforations with use of pedicle screws in lower cervical spine. Spine J. 2016;17(3):457–65.
5. Ishikawa Y, Kanemura T, Yoshida G, et al. Intraoperative, full-rotation, three-dimensional image (O-arm)-based navigation system for cervical pedicle screw insertion. J Neurosurg Spine. 2011;15(5):472–8.
6. Luther N, Iorgulescu JB, Geannette C, et al. Comparison of navigated versus non-navigated pedicle screw placement in 260 patients and 1434 screws: screw accuracy, screw size, and the complexity of surgery. J Spinal Disord Tech. 2015;28(5):E298–303.
7. Heller JG, Silcox DH 3rd, Sutterlin CE 3rd. Complications of posterior cervical plating. Spine (Phila Pa 1976). 1995;20(22):2442–8.
8. Abumi K, Shono Y, Ito M, Taneichi H, Kotani Y, Kaneda K. Complications of pedicle screw fixation in reconstructive surgery of the cervical spine. Spine (Phila Pa 1976). 2000;25(8):962–9.
9. Wright NM. Posterior C2 fixation using bilateral, crossing C2 laminar screws: case series and technical note. J Spinal Disord Tech. 2004;17(2):158–62.
10. Ma W, Feng L, Xu R, et al. Clinical application of C2 laminar screw technique. Eur Spine J. 2010;19(8):1312–7.
11. Hong JT, Sung JH, Son BC, Lee SW, Park CK. Significance of laminar screw fixation in the subaxial cervical spine. Spine (Phila Pa 1976). 2008;33(16):1739–43.
12. Dorward IG, Wright NM. Seven years of experience with C2 translaminar screw fixation: clinical series and review of the literature. Neurosurgery. 2011;68(6):1491–9; discussion 1499.
13. Reddy C, Ingalhalikar AV, Channon S, Lim TH, Torner J, Hitchon PW. In vitro biomechanical comparison of transpedicular versus translaminar C-2 screw fixation in C2-3 instrumentation. J Neurosurg Spine. 2007;7(4):414–8.
14. Shin SI, Yeom JS, Kim HJ, Chang BS, Lee CK, Riew KD. The feasibility of laminar screw placement in the subaxial spine: analysis using 215 three-dimensional computed tomography scans and simulation software. Spine J. 2012;12(7):577–84.
15. Cardoso MJ, Dmitriev AE, Helgeson MD, et al. Using lamina screws as a salvage technique at C-7: computed tomography and biomechanical analysis using cadaveric vertebrae. Laboratory investigation. J Neurosurg Spine. 2009;11(1):28–33.
16. Cho W, Le JT, Shimer AL, Werner BC, Glaser JA, Shen FH. Anatomy of lamina in the subaxial cervical spine with the special reference to translaminar screws: CT and cadaveric analysis with screw trajectory simulation. Clin Spine Surg. 2017;30(5):E535–9.

17. Alvin MD, Abdullah KG, Steinmetz MP, et al. Translaminar screw fixation in the subaxial cervical spine: quantitative laminar analysis and feasibility of unilateral and bilateral translaminar virtual screw placement. Spine (Phila Pa 1976). 2012;37(12):E745–51.
18. Takayasu M, Hara M, Yamauchi K, Yoshida M, Yoshida J. Transarticular screw fixation in the middle and lower cervical spine. Technical note. J Neurosurg. 2003;99(1 Suppl):132–6.
19. Miyanji F, Mahar A, Oka R, Newton P. Biomechanical differences between transfacet and lateral mass screw-rod constructs for multilevel posterior cervical spine stabilization. Spine (Phila Pa 1976). 2008;33(23):E865–9.
20. Aydogan M, Enercan M, Hamzaoglu A, Alanay A. Reconstruction of the subaxial cervical spine using lateral mass and facet screw instrumentation. Spine (Phila Pa 1976). 2012;37(5):E335–41.
21. Liu G, Xu R, Ma W, Sun S, Feng J. Anatomical considerations for the placement of cervical transarticular screws. J Neurosurg Spine. 2011;14(1):114–21.
22. Milchteim C, Yu WD, Ho A, O'Brien JR. Anatomical parameters of subaxial percutaneous transfacet screw fixation based on the analysis of 50 computed tomography scans: clinical article. J Neurosurg Spine. 2012;16(6):573–8.
23. Abumi K. Cervical spondylotic myelopathy: posterior decompression and pedicle screw fixation. Eur Spine J. 2015;24(Suppl 2):186–96.
24. Ahmad F, Sherman JD, Wang MY. Percutaneous trans-facet screws for supplemental posterior cervical fixation. World Neurosurg. 2012;78(6):716.e711–714.

Atlantoaxial Stabilization

31

Avery L. Buchholz, John C. Quinn,
Christopher I. Shaffrey, and Justin S. Smith

Pitfalls/Pearls Outline

C1 (atlas) and C2 (axis) surgery can be challenging given the complex anatomy. This chapter will detail a variety of atlanto-axial stabilization techniques providing a description of how to perform the surgery and when it is indicated. At the end, the reader should have a thorough understanding of C1 and C2 fixation options.

Introduction

Over the last few decades, atlantoaxial stabilization has evolved from simple posterior wiring techniques to a multitude of screw fixation points, trajectories, and constructs. Some of the earliest reports of C1 and C2 stabilization date back to 1910 when Mixter and Osgood described using heavy silk thread to tie the spinous processes together [1]. Gallie reported on his use of C1–C2 fixation using wire in 1939 [2]. This was followed by further modifications described by Brooks and Jenkins in 1978 and Dickman and Sonntag in 1991 [3, 4]. Interlaminar clamps were introduced in the 1980s along with C1 and C2 screw fixation techniques [5, 6]. These techniques have continued to evolve and will be discussed, along with the indications and variety of instrumentation options throughout this chapter.

The need for C1–C2 stabilization most commonly results from trauma. A variety of fracture patterns can cause instability at these segments. Some are amenable to a cervical collar, while others may warrant surgical fixation. Additional causes of instability include congenital malformations of C2 (e.g., odontoid agenesis and os odontoideum), tumors, infections, inflammatory disease, and degenerative disease. Specifically, rheumatoid arthritis can result in atlantoaxial subluxation or superior migration of the odontoid into the foramen magnum. This can cause compression of the brainstem and upper cervical spinal cord requiring decompression and fusion. Instability may be related to postsurgical changes such as C1 and C2 laminectomies. In addition, some patients may have ligamentous laxity and resultant C1–C2 instability.

The atlantoaxial junction is a highly specialized area of the spine. The anatomy is complex and as a result requires special attention. Throughout this chapter, we will discuss common

A. L. Buchholz
Department of Neurological Surgery, Medical University of South Carolina, Charleston, SC, USA

J. C. Quinn
Department of Neurosurgery, University of Virginia Health System, Charlottesville, VA, USA

C. I. Shaffrey (✉) · J. S. Smith
Departments of Orthopaedic and Neurological Surgery, Duke University Health System, Durham, NC, USA
e-mail: CIS8Z@hscmail.mcc.virginia.edu

M. G. Kaiser et al. (eds.), *Degenerative Cervical Myelopathy and Radiculopathy*,
https://doi.org/10.1007/978-3-319-97952-6_31

types of C1 and C2 pathology with treatment options. On completion of this text, the reader should have a good understanding of the variety of stabilization techniques for the atlas and axis segments.

Wiring/Clamps/Cement

Posterior wiring was one of the earliest techniques for C1–C2 fixation. Gallie was first to describe this method, which simply involved placement of a notched bone graft on the posterior arch of C1 and the spinous process and medial laminar arch of C2 [2]. The graft was originally secured by sublaminar wire passed beneath C1 and C2 [2]. More recent applications of this technique use a C2 spinous process wire made popular by the Sonntag wiring technique discussed below (Fig. 31.1a). Although easy to perform, the single midline fixation point is susceptible to rotational forces and very high non-union rates (25%) [7]. The Brooks type of fusion was a modification designed to overcome these rotational deficiencies by incorporating bilateral interlaminar bone grafts. This technique uses two separate bone grafts placed between the lamina of C1 and C2, each secured with sublaminar wiring (Fig. 31.1b). Often notches are placed in the bone to secure their position. Compression can be applied by tightening the wire [3]. Some surgeons have improved outcomes with this technique by using oversized iliac crest bone grafts and double strands of wire for each graft [8]. In each of these techniques, the placement of sublaminar wires increases the risk of neural injury during passage, although the evolution of braided cables has made the passage of these wires somewhat safer due to decreased rigidity [9]. Over time, the cables may cause encroachment of the spinal canal [10]. This is particularly troublesome with anterior translation of the atlas and an already decreased canal diameter.

To help reduce the risk of neural injury, a further modification was described by Sonntag, which eliminated the C2 sublaminar wiring and replaced it with wiring of the C2 spinous process. Autograft or allograft strut is fashioned similar to the Gallie technique. Notches may be placed to secure the wire. The inferior surface of C2 is also notched, and a looped wire passed sublaminar at C1 and over the C2 spinous process into the created notch. This secures the bone graft. The free ends of the wire are brought over the C2 spinous process and secured by crimping or twisting [4] (Fig. 31.1c).

In each of these wiring techniques, autograft or allograft strut may be used. The Iliac crest and rib are the most common harvest sites for these procedures. The last variation of wiring techniques is the Locksley intersegmental tie-bar technique [11]. With this method, bone grafts are secured with sublaminar wires twisted in a figure eight fashion. This method also incorporates a posterior stabilization plate, which is secured by wires to the C1 and C2

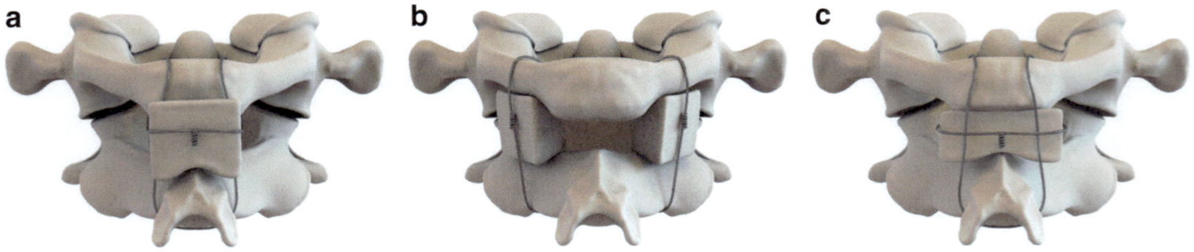

Fig. 31.1 (**a**) Gallie wiring technique with sublaminar wire at C1 and wire looped around the C2 spinous process. The original technique called for sublaminar wiring at C1 and C2. Spinous process wiring has been a more commonly used option. The graft is resting on posterior arch of C1 and C2 spinous process/medial lamina. (**b**) Brooks-Jenkins wiring technique with two interlaminar grafts and sublaminar wiring at C1 and C2. Some surgeons use double wiring at each graft for added security. (**c**) Sonntag wiring technique with an interlaminar graft wedged between the posterior arch of C1 and C2 spinous process/lamina. C1 sublaminar wire with wire under the C2 spinous process. The wire is tightened to wedge graft in place. Notches may be used in the bone with any of these techniques

spinous process. The Locksley method has the benefit of increased rigidity with three-point fixation. The rib graft offers a natural contoured fit for this technique [11]. All wiring techniques require an intact C1 and C2 posterior. They also are unable to provide sufficient stabilization alone, and external immobilization may be necessary. With newer fixation options, wiring techniques are more commonly used to enhance fusion and serve to augment these other techniques.

Clamp fixation has also been used successfully for C1–C2 immobilization but similar to wire options require an intact C1 and C2 posterior arch. The Halifax clamp was initially described in 1975 and has the benefit of immediate fixation without the risks of sublaminar wires. Bone grafts are again placed in the interlaminar space bilaterally using clamps to secure them in place. Early use saw screw loosening and clamp dislodgement, but newer devices have seen decreases in failure rates [10]. The clamps provide excellent biomechanical stabilization with flexion and extension and however are less effective with rotational maneuvers. The rounded C1 posterior arch creates a suboptimal interface between the arch and the clamp at this level. In addition, the large C2 spinous process creates angulation of the clamp from C1 to C2 lamina in the sagittal plane. This further decreases the clamp C1 surface area contact and increases susceptibility to loosening during rotation. Hanimoglu et al. have reported on the application of a C1–C2 claw system using a transverse connector to secure the two clamps reinforcing the stability of the construct in rotation [12].

Less common methods of atlantoaxial stabilization include the use of acrylic resins, cement, and Kirschner wires. These resins and cement may provide immediate stability to the C1–C2 interspace, but they do not promote fusion and do not bond directly to bone. As a result, they must be "anchored" to the bone by pins or wire. Pins are generally placed obliquely in the long arch of C1 and the articular pillar of C2 with heads protruding at least 4 mm. The acrylic is applied to appropriately cover the pins and resist the rotational forces. Kirschner wire may also be used as scaffolding between the pins but must be contained completely within the cement. In cases where this technique is employed, care must be taken to keep the area free of blood and CSF, while the acrylic hardens. The exothermic reaction that takes place while the acrylic hardens must also be managed so the spinal cord and nerve roots are not compromised [13].

Transarticular Screws

The first reported use of the transarticular screw was by Jeanneret and Magerl who had used the technique since 1979. In their description, bilateral screws are placed across the atlantoaxial joint to immobilize C1 and C2 [14] (Fig. 31.2). This technique has been used to treat atlantoaxial

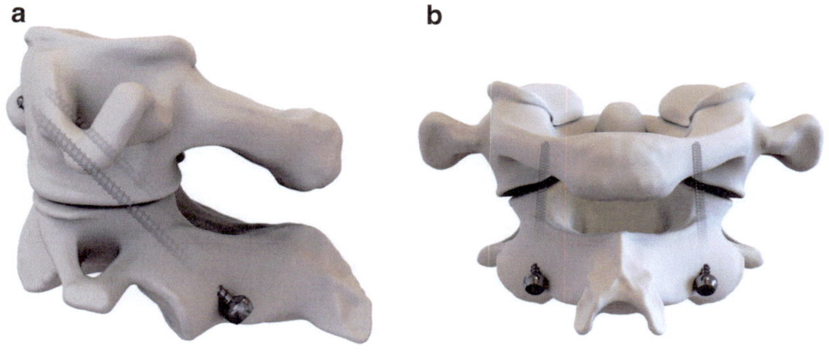

Fig. 31.2 Transarticular screw placement. (**a**) Lateral view of C1–C2 showing screw across the joint to anterior arch of C1. (**b**) Posterior view of C1–C2 with C2 entry point, 3 mm lateral and 3 mm cephalad from the inferior medial angle of the C2–C3 facet joint, the drill is directed toward the anterior arch of the atlas in the sagittal plane and 0–10° medially

trauma, instability, arthropathy, neuralgia, and inflammatory disease among other pathologies. It has the benefit of complete obliteration of rotational motion at the atlantoaxial joint but is a technically challenging operation with potential risk to the spinal cord, hypoglossal nerve, and vertebral artery [15–17].

To help avoid these complications, we recommend evaluation with CT imaging to look for an anomalous vertebral artery course and appropriate size of the C2 pars and ensure good bone quality at the intended fixation site. In addition, we use an MRI to assess the degree of neural compression and integrity of the transverse atlantoaxial ligament prior to performing this procedure. We consider this procedure only when the CT confirms appropriate anatomy and position of the vertebral artery. In the case of suspected vertebral artery injury, the screw should be placed on that side only to tamponade the bleeding. No attempt should be made to place the contralateral screw, and the patient should be taken for angiography to assess the injury and treat as needed.

To perform the atlantoaxial transarticular screw, the patient is positioned prone with a Mayfield head holder (OMI, Inc., Cincinnati, Ohio). The neck is kept neutral while the chin is tucked creating posterior translation and reduction of the C1–C2 complex. In the setting of a fracture, fluoroscopy can be used to verify adequate reduction and alignment. The chin tuck also improves access to the desired C1–C2 trajectory. Fluoroscopy can be used to determine the planned skin entry site for this trajectory. There are typically two separate incisions. One incision is for access to the C1–C2 posterior elements, and the other is for the planned screw trajectory, which is usually in the paramidline area near T1 spinous process.

The posterior anatomy of C1 and C2 should be clearly dissected and identified including the bony limits of the C2 lateral mass and superior and medial aspect of the C2 pars. A Penfield 4 can be useful to assess the C2 pars and determine the appropriate angle for the screw. Similarly, the Penfield may be used to inspect the C1–C2 joint and ensure proper alignment. In cases of subluxation, additional reduction can be achieved by manipulating the Mayfield head holder or by careful posterior traction on the C1 arch. There is often a significant epidural venous plexus in the area of the C1–C2 joint space, which may be managed with bipolar cautery. The second incision is determined using intraoperative fluoroscopic guidance or navigation with the instrument held outside the incision adjacent to the neck. The trajectory should cross the C1–C2 facet joint and enter the anterior arch of the atlas. A percutaneous entry site for the drill is usually made approximately 2 cm lateral to the T1 spinous process. A guide tube is then placed through the stab incision docking on the C2 entry point. Using a C2 entry point, 3 mm lateral and 3 mm cephalad from the inferior medial angle of the C2–C3 facet joint, the drill is directed toward the anterior arch of the atlas in the sagittal plane and 0–10° medially. The cortical bone is pierced with the drill, and a K-wire is advanced to a point 3–4 mm posterior to the anterior C1 tubercle being careful not to penetrate into the retropharyngeal area. After the K-wire is placed, a cannulated drill bit is passed over the K-wire drilling to the same target. It is important not to advance the K-wire as it is being drilled. The hole is then tapped over the K-wire followed by placement of a fully threaded 3.5 or 4 mm cortical screw, again taking care to ensure that the K-wire does not advance. Screw length can be measured from the drill or K-wire insertion but is usually 1–3 mm shorter than the measured length due to compression that occurs over the C1–C2 joint. Typical screw lengths are 34–44 mm [15]. This is performed on both sides assuming no vertebral artery injury. Instrumentation may be supplemented with one of the wiring techniques discussed for fusion. In cases where posterior elements are not intact, a direct atlantoaxial joint fusion may be required. Some authors have also suggested the use of graft and clamps to aid fusion while others have shown good results with no additional internal fixation [14, 15, 17]. Patients are generally also treated in a hard cervical collar for 6–12 weeks.

Atlantoaxial transarticular screw fixation can provide excellent stability, with high-published fusion rates and reports of successful outcomes in a variety of pathologies. At one point, this technique was considered the "gold standard" for atlantoaxial fixation partly because it could be used without the posterior elements being intact [18]. However, this technique does require reduction of C1–C2 and can be challenging to perform in patients with thoracic kyphosis due to an inability to achieve the proper screw trajectory. Anatomic studies have indicated bilateral transarticular screws would not be possible in 20% of patients due to anatomic variations [15, 19]. A meta-analysis has also shown a 3.1% incidence of vertebral artery injury and 7.1% incidence of a clinically significant malpositioned screws [17]. The relatively high complication rate, along with the success of less challenging techniques, has resulted in transarticular screws currently being used less often.

C1–C2 Segmental Fixation

The first C1–C2 screw construct was described by Goel and Laheri in 1994 and was based on a screw-plate system [20]. This study was the first to describe the C1 lateral mass technique. One of the benefits of this technique highlighted by Goel was that it provides immediate rigid immobilization without the need for anatomic alignment of the C1–C2 complex prior to fixation. It could also be utilized in patients with an aberrant vertebral artery anatomy, which can be problematic for transarticular screws. The plate acted as a tension band with good biomechanical stabilization in flexion, extension, and rotational movements, thereby obviating the need for additional midline procedures such as Gallie or Brooks wiring [20]. This surgery did require sacrifice of the C2 ganglion for hemostasis, placement of instrumentation, exposure of the atlantoaxial joint, and facet arthrodesis. Postoperative scalp numbness was noted in some, but reports indicate it was not a concern to patients [6]. More recently this technique has been modified to use polyaxial screws and rods as described by Harms and Melcher in 2001 [21] (Fig. 31.3).

In order to safely achieve screw placement, C1 and C2 anatomy must be thoroughly understood. There are a few anatomic considerations, which should be highlighted. Of critical importance when placing C1 lateral mass screws is the course of the vertebral artery. The vertebral artery and C1 nerve run along the superior lateral groove termed the sulcus arteriosus. In close to 15% of the population, this groove has a bony roof forming a foramen called the arcuate foramen. There is also variability in the extent of the sulcus arteriosus covering which may leave the distal portion of the vertebral artery exposed. The difference between the C2 pars and pedicle must also be understood. The C2 pars is defined as the portion of the C2 vertebra connecting the superior and inferior articular surfaces. The C2 pedicle is the portion of the C2 vertebra that connects its posterior elements to the vertebral body. The difference between entry point and screw position will be discussed.

This surgery again requires the patient to be in the prone position and typically fixed in a Mayfield head holder with the neck kept neutral and head in a military tuck position. The arms are tucked at

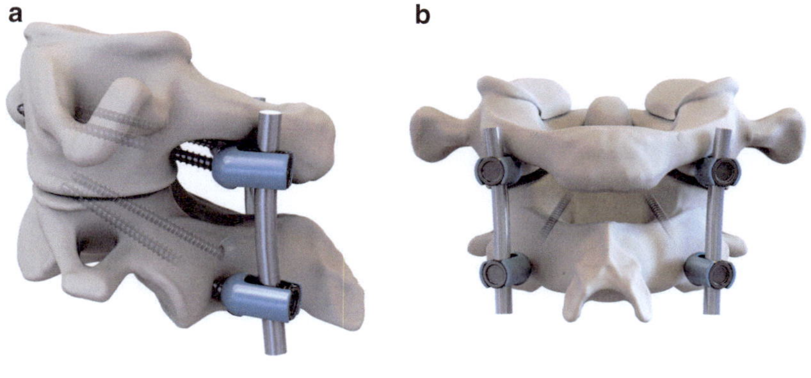

Fig. 31.3 C1–C2 Segmental fixation. (**a**) Lateral view of C1–C2 with lateral mass screw placed below the posterior arch of C1 and C2 pars screw. (**b**) Posterior view of C1–C2 with C1 lateral mass screws and C2 pars screws

the sides, and shoulders may be retracted using tape. The midline incision is carried through the nuchal ligament to minimize blood loss and muscle disruption exposing from the suboccipital area to the spinous process of C3. The dorsal arch of C1 and the lateral mass inferior to the arch are exposed laterally. The C2 nerve root is identified and may be sacrificed or mobilized inferiorly. There often is a large venous plexus surrounding the C2 nerve root, which must be controlled with bipolar cautery and hemostatic agents. The medial wall of the C1 lateral mass should be identified and palpated to appreciate the medial limit and angulation of screw placement. The medial aspect of the C1 and C2 transverse foramen can also be identified to serve as a lateral limit for screw placement (Fig. 31.4).

The entry point for C1 screws is identified at the center of the lateral mass in both the medial/lateral and superior/inferior quadrants. A pilot hole can be made with a 3 mm drill bit. The hole is drilled with an angle of approximately 10–15° medial and aiming toward the anterior cortex of C1. Use of fluoroscopy or navigation may be helpful to achieve an appropriate trajectory. The drill should just penetrate the ventral cortex of the lateral mass midway between the superior and inferior C1 facet. After tapping the hole, the C1 lateral mass screw is placed (usually 30–36 m in length) [15]. Importantly, approximately 10 mm of the screw shaft is left proud of the bone in order to facilitate connection to the C2 screw head.

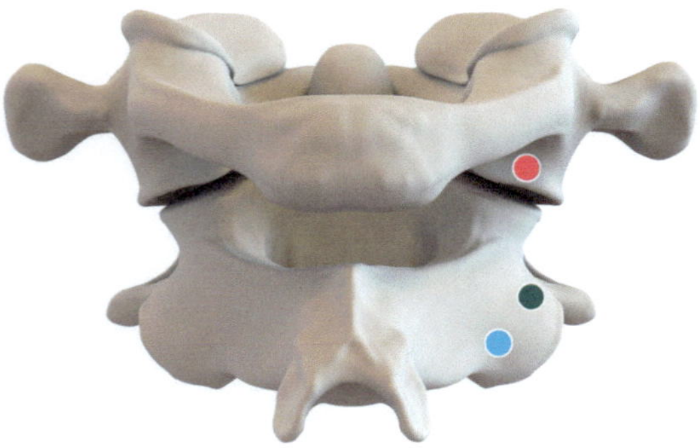

Fig. 31.4 Starting locations for C1 and C2 screws. Red – C1 lateral mass screw. Green – C2 pedicle screw. Blue – C2 pars screw. Note the differentiation between C2 pars and pedicle screws. Using a blunt dissection instrument to palpate the medial pedicle wall will help guide trajectory

The C2 screw can be placed in either the pars or the pedicle. The C2 pars is the portion of the C2 vertebra between the superior and inferior articular surfaces (Fig. 31.4). C2 pars screws are placed in a trajectory similar to a C1–C2 transarticular screws but shorter. The entry point is approximately 3 mm rostral and 3 mm lateral to the inferior medial aspect of the C2 inferior articulating surface. The screw should follow a steep trajectory, 45–60°, with 10–15 degrees of medial angulation. Typical screw length is 16–20 mm but should stop short of the transverse foramen. This length can be measured preoperatively on a CT scan. Because of the steep trajectory, a limited dissection or large-body habitus may make this screw difficult to place. Rarely, a separate stab incision may be needed to get proper angulation similar to the transarticular screw. The C2 pedicle, in contrast, is the portion of the C2 vertebra connecting the dorsal elements with the vertebral body and is anterior to the pars. The entry point for this screw is in the pars of C2, lateral to the superior margin of the C2 lamina. This is usually 2 mm lateral and 2 mm superior to the C2 pars screw entry point (Fig. 31.4). The pedicle screw requires a medial angulation of 15–25° with 20° upward trajectory. The thick medial wall of C2 can help reduce the risk of medial wall breach, but for patients with very narrow C2 pedicles, the risk of breach into the neural canal or transverse foramen is high, and CT scans should be evaluated preoperatively [15]. Bony anatomy should be carefully assessed prior to surgery for either C2 pars or pedicle screws, as anatomy may be more favorable for one of the techniques and in some cases may not be favorable for either technique. For the latter situation, unilateral or bilateral translaminar screws (discussed below) may be considered, although the rotational stability of these screws in providing rigid fixation and fusion may be less than for the pars and pedicle techniques [22–25].

Essential to the technique of Goel et al. was the routine bilateral sectioning of the C2 ganglion. Harms and Melcher did not sacrifice the C2 nerve root and instead used a C2 screw with a smooth unthreaded portion left proud of the bony surface to minimize irritation of the C2 nerve.

In their series of 37 patients, they were able to achieve 100% fusion rates with no vascular or neurologic complications, including C2 neuralgia [21]. However, increased use of this technique and subsequent studies have demonstrated an increasing number of reports citing postoperative onset of C2 neuralgia. This is likely from direct irritation caused by the abutting screw or mobilization of the C2 nerve root [26–28]. In some cases, this neuralgia resolves spontaneously [26], some improve with screw removal [28], and others are intractable [27].

C2 neuralgia typically causes pain in the back of the head or base of the skull. These symptoms may also frequently accompany atlantoaxial instability due to mechanical compression or injury to the C2 nerve root. Treatments for occipital neuralgia include percutaneous nerve blocks, rhizolysis, ganglionectomy, and C1 and C2 decompression. When placing C1 lateral mass screws, there are several advantages to a C2 neurectomy. It provides improved access to the atlantoaxial joint which aids in decortication, arthrodesis, and screw placement. In addition, improved access gives better hemostasis control and allows treatment of any preoperative C2 symptoms. Routine C2 neurectomy does however remain controversial due to the limited number of studies that have specifically assessed patient outcomes.

In one assessment, Hamilton et al. looked at 30 patients who underwent C1–C2 fixation with C2 neurectomy. In this report no patients reported allodynia. The authors noted that they were careful to perform a C2 ganglionectomy, since simple section of the nerve or ganglion may be more likely to produce postoperative neuralgia. Numbness in the C2 distribution was detected in 17 patients with only two patients self-reporting numbness. Neither of these patients was bothered or affected by this per report. While this study does not necessarily demonstrate the superiority of performing a C2 neurectomy, it does demonstrate that doing so does not appear to produce morbidity or negatively affect outcomes [29].

In an effort to avoid the C2 ganglion altogether, additional options for C1 instrumentation have been developed. The C1 posterior arch screw, first reported by Resnick and Benzel in 2002, involves a lateral mass screw inserted through a starting point in the posterior arch [30]. This screw provides increased pullout strength over standard lateral mass fixation, avoids bleeding risk from the venous plexus, and minimizes C2 nerve root irritation. The limitation of this technique is the variability in the sulcus arteriosus and narrow window for screw insertion [30]. Variability in anatomy may make this technique unfeasible in 8–53.8% of patients [19].

Some authors have also modified the C1 entry site to include the midpoint of the C1 lateral mass and the inferior aspect of the posterior arch. A 2–3 mm notch is drilled in the posterior arch at this entry site. This allows the screw to be placed farther from the C2 ganglion in an effort to reduce irritation. This is again a variation of the C1 posterior arch screw, and some authors have reported successfully avoiding postoperative C2 nerve dysfunction [31].

In 2008, Kelly et al. introduced a novel screw-plate system for C1–C2 fixation, which involved a posterior C1 locking plate combined with C2 translaminar screws [32]. It was devised to reduce surgical risk, and biomechanical testing showed similar stability compared to the Harms screw-rod system [32]. However, there have been no reported clinical applications of this method thus far. Other methods of C1–C2 fixation include C1 posterior arch screws, which involves crossing screws in the posterior arch of C1. Biomechanical testing has also shown this technique to provide rigid stabilization, but the clinical application of this remains to be seen, and the risk of vascular injury may be high.

Hooks may also be used in combination with C1 and C2 screw systems. Currently there are three systems that have been popularized: C1 hook with C2 screw, C1 hook with C1–C2 transarticular screw, and C1–C2 hook [19]. Usually these techniques are alternatives for atlantoaxial stabilization when screw-rod constructs are not feasible [19]. A fourth technique has also been described which involves a C1 lateral mass screw with a C2 claw formed by two opposing laminar hooks. In biomechanical testing, this fixation technique has shown results similar to the Harms screw-rod system [33]. Again, clinical applications of these techniques have not been reported.

Translaminar Screw

One of the limitations of the Magerl technique can be the dimension of a patient's C2 pedicle. Some reports have shown a diameter below 3.5 mm in 20% of the cadavers investigated. In other cases, a C2 pars/pedicle screw may fail, and a rescue screw is needed. Wright was the first to describe the use of the C2 translaminar screw technique (2004), but since then multiple reports have shown the anatomic and clinical application of this screw in both stand-alone constructs and as a rescue method [25] (Fig. 31.5).

For screw placement, a small cortical window at the junction of the C2 spinous process and rostral end of lamina is made with a high-speed drill. A hand drill is then used to drill the contralateral lamina to a depth of approximately 30 mm. The trajectory is kept visually aligned along the angle of the exposed lamina surface making it slightly less than the downslope of the lamina to help ensure any cortical breech would occur dorsally as opposed to near the spinal canal. Once no cortical breakthrough has been verified, a polyaxial screw can be carefully inserted along the same trajectory. In the final position, the screw head remains at the junction of the spinous process and lamina. When bilateral laminar screws are used, the method is repeated with the cortical window being made on the contralateral side at the caudal aspect of the lamina. These screws are then connected via rods to C1 lateral mass screws with bone graft packed onto remaining decorticated surfaces [25].

This method provides another option for rigid fixation of the atlas and axis. To date, there have been no reports of vascular or neural injury with translaminar screws, although the risk does remain while placing C1 lateral mass screws. In the case of failure of initial pars/pedicle screws, translaminar screws can be used as a salvage technique because the entry point is not yet violated. It can also be used as an initial screw trajectory with biomechanical studies showing it to be superior to the pars screw in both pullout strength and inspectional torque [23]. Gorek et al. and others have shown comparable biomechanical stability when compared to pedicle screws in flexion/extension, lateral bending, and rotation [22, 24]. In one clinical assessment, translaminar screws were found to have a lower cortical breach rate compared to C2 pedicle screws but with no clinical significance. These authors did however find a significantly higher pseudoarthrosis rate in patients with translaminar screw constructs compared to those with C2 pedicle screw [34]. Regardless, excellent clinical outcomes of this technique have been reported in several studies, and this technique may be utilized to address insufficient C2 pedicles, an aberrant vertebral artery course and for salvage.

Stand-Alone C2 Fixation

A bilateral C2 pars interarticularis or pedicle fracture, otherwise known as Hangman's fracture, is another reason for atlantoaxial stabilization.

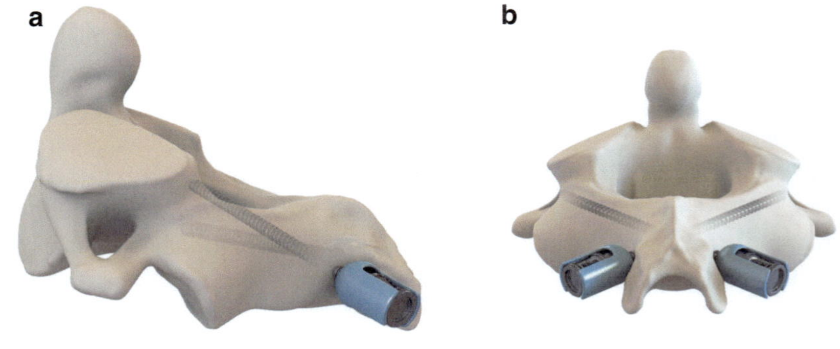

Fig. 31.5 C2 translaminar screws. (**a**) Lateral view of C2 with translaminar screw. (**b**) Posterior view of C2 showing bilateral translaminar screws. Starting points may need to be staggered to avoid screws hitting one another

Depending on the type of Hangman's fracture and degree of instability, these fractures may be treated either nonoperatively or may require surgical fixation. Common surgical options include C2–C3 and C1–C3 posterior instrumentation. An additional method of a stand-alone pars/pedicle screw fixation has also been described with good results in the treatment of Hangman's type II and III fractures.

With this technique, the patient is again prone with the head in a Mayfield head holder. Using intraoperative fluoroscopy, the fracture is reduced and the headframe locked in position. A posterior neck dissection is performed exposing C2 lamina and lateral mass. An exposure of the upper and lower cervical vertebrae may be useful for orientation. The pars and pedicle are both exposed as described previously. The fracture site will often be identified, and if reduction has not been properly achieved, it is done now using forceps to pull the C2 spinous process upward toward the occipital bone. A suitable entry point for C2 pars or pedicle screw is selected, and the trajectory drilled with two different diameter bits. The first has a diameter of 2.8 mm and is drilled to a depth of 30 mm, which crosses the fracture site and into the body of C2. The second drill bit has a diameter of 4 mm and is drilled only to the depth of the fracture. A 3.5 mm × 30 mm screw is then placed and tightened which will compress the fragments and secure the reduction [35].

Borne et al. have reported on their experience with this technique in 17 patients and found good results with no complications and no pseudoarthrosis. Functional results of the patients were also noted to be excellent. The proposed benefit of this technique is that it preserves range of motion at the atlantoaxial segment. Modifications of this technique have also been demonstrated to be successful with the use of lag screws and with drilling a single diameter on both sides of the fracture. Buchholz et al. reported on a series of five patients in whom screws were placed percutaneously with all patients having no breach, solid fusion, and good surgical outcomes [36].

Jefferson Fracture C1 Lateral Mass Screw

Jefferson fractures are in most cases treated successfully with immobilization in a hard collar. It is controversial whether an unstable fracture involving the transverse atlantal ligament should be treated nonoperatively or requires surgery. Some reports of nonsurgical management have been conferred to high rates of nonunions and cranial settling. Hence, C1–C2 or occiput to C2 fixation has been an increasingly popular option for treatment of unstable Jefferson fractures. Unfortunately, this sacrifices normal motion at these segments, which can also be debilitating. An additional more motion-preserving treatment option is a C1 lateral mass screw construct.

With this technique, C1 lateral mass screws are placed in the normal fashion with bicortical purchase. A rod is then used to connect the C1 screws across the midline. Compression of this construct facilitates reduction of the C1 burst fracture. After the fracture has been reduced, the construct is locked into place [37].

Anterior Options

Anterior C1 and C2 fixation is rarely used anymore in part due to decreased use of transoral surgery. Goel et al. were the first to describe it in 1994 for treatment of an unstable craniovertebral junction [38]. Harms and colleagues later described its use with transoral surgery for rotary dislocations, tumors, infections, and inflammatory disease. The advantage was the patient could avoid a subsequent posterior neck dissection and instrumentation.

For historical purposes, the technique is performed with the use of a "T-plate" (DePuy Spine, Raynham, MA). The horizontal portion of the plate is placed over C1 with screws securing the plate to bilateral C1 lateral mass with bicortical purchase. The vertical portion of the plate rests on the body of C2. Two vertebral body screws are placed just superior and parallel to the C2–C3 disc space. The high profile of the "T-plate" was prone to difficulty with wound healing and dysphagia. Again, this procedure is rarely used today [15].

Fusion

The ultimate goal of any atlantoaxial stabilization technique is to achieve immobilization so bone fusion can take place. Regardless of what instrumentation is used, a key component to this is the bone graft. Although multiple bone graft options are now available, autograft remains the preferred material. The most common sites for autograft harvest are the iliac crest and rib. Both sites are considered safe for harvest with excellent fusion outcomes although the reported graft morbidity rate has been higher in iliac crest harvest. Sawin et al. reviewed this in 600 patients (300 iliac crest and 300 rib harvests). Among patients undergoing posterior cervical fixation with rib (300) and iliac crest (52), fusion rates were 98.8% and 94.2%, respectively. Donor site morbidity was 3.7% for rib harvest and 25.3% for iliac crest [39].

Iliac crest and rib autografts are excellent bone graft sources because they have both osteoinductive and osteoconductive properties. In order to decrease the morbidity associated with harvesting, some surgeons have modified their techniques to incorporate iliac crest allograft in combination with recombinant human bone morphogenetic protein (rhBMP), which also supports osteoinduction and osteoconduction. Hood et al. looked specifically at the use of rhBMP in atlantoaxial fusion (C1 lateral mass and C2 pedicle) and reported a 100% fusion rate using corticocancellous allograft and rhBMP-2 [40]. A C2 neurectomy was performed in all cases. Hamilton et al. looked specifically at dosing and safety of rhBMP-2 and in their series of 23 patients found no complications with an average dose of 2.38 mg per level [41]. They also had a 100% fusion rate. Although off-label, we find rhBMP-2 to be a safe and effective alternative to the use autograft in the posterior cervical spine.

Discussion

Great advancements in posterior atlantoaxial fixation have been made in the last few decades. Many of these techniques are rarely used today, as superior options exist. We have utilized most of the methods discussed in this text over the years. The C1–C2 transarticular screw may remain the choice for atlantoaxial fusion for some surgeons; however, C1–C2 screw-rod constructs have become the most popular techniques. A transarticular screw combined with Sonntag-type interlaminar wiring has been shown to have excellent biomechanical stability and results in rigid fixation. While not superior to transarticular screws, C1 lateral mass and C2 pars/pedicle screws have also demonstrated biomechanical stability and excellent fusion rates and are technically easier to place [15, 19, 30]. They are also advantageous due to their lower risk of vertebral artery injury and the lack of need for complete realignment of the C1–C2 joints. We currently favor C1–C2 screw-rod fixation for almost all atlantoaxial stabilization procedures. Having a good understanding of the anatomy and the variety of stabilization techniques available is essential for the spine surgeon to address C1 and C2 pathology.

References

1. Mixter SJ, Osgood RB. IV. Traumatic lesions of the atlas and axis. Ann Surg. 1910;51(2):193–207.
2. Gallie WE. Fractures and dislocations of cervical spine. Am J Surg. 1939;46:495–9.
3. Brooks AL, Jenkins EB. Atlanto-axial arthrodesis by the wedge compression method. J Bone Joint Surg. 1978;60(3):279–84.
4. Dickman CA, Sonntag VK, Papadopoulos SM, Hadley MN. The interspinous method of posterior atlantoaxial arthrodesis. J Neurosurg. 1991;74(2):190–8.
5. Holness RO, Huestis WS, Howes WJ, Langille RA. Posterior stabilization with an interlaminar clamp in cervical injuries: technical note and review of the long term experience with the method. Neurosurgery. 1984;14(3):318–22.
6. Goel A, Desai KI, Muzumdar DP. Atlantoaxial fixation using plate and screw method: a report of 160 treated patients. Neurosurgery. 2002;51(6):1351–6; discussion 1356-1357.

7. Coyne TJ, Fehlings MG, Wallace MC, Bernstein M, Tator CH. C1-C2 posterior cervical fusion: long-term evaluation of results and efficacy. Neurosurgery. 1995;37(4):688–92; discussion 692-683.
8. McDonnell DEHS. Posterior atlantoaxial fusion: indications and techniques. In: Traynelis VCRS, editor. Techniques in spinal fusion and Stabialization. New York: Thiem; 1995. p. 92–106.
9. Huhn SL, Wolf AL, Ecklund J. Posterior spinal osteosynthesis for cervical fracture/dislocation using a flexible multistrand cable system: technical note. Neurosurgery. 1991;29(6):943–6.
10. Vender JR, Rekito AJ, Harrison SJ, McDonnell DE. The evolution of posterior cervical and occipitocervical fusion and instrumentation. Neurosurg Focus. 2004;16(1):E9.
11. Vender JR, Houle PJ, Harrison S, McDonnell DE. Occipital-cervical fusion using the Locksley intersegmental tie bar technique: long-term experience with 19 patients. Spine J. 2002;2(2):134–41.
12. Hanimoglu H, Hanci L, Kaynar MY, Hanci M. Bilateral C1-C2 claw for atlantoaxial instability. Turk Neurosurg. 2009;19(4):345–8.
13. Duff TA, Khan A, Corbett JE. Surgical stabilization of cervical spinal fractures using methyl methacrylate. Technical considerations and long-term results in 52 patients. J Neurosurg. 1992;76(3):440–3.
14. Jeanneret B, Magerl F. Primary posterior fusion C1/2 in odontoid fractures: indications, technique, and results of transarticular screw fixation. J Spinal Disord. 1992;5(4):464–75.
15. Mummaneni PV, Haid RW. Atlantoaxial fixation: overview of all techniques. Neurol India. 2005;53(4):408–15.
16. Claybrooks R, Kayanja M, Milks R, Benzel E. Atlantoaxial fusion: a biomechanical analysis of two C1-C2 fusion techniques. Spine J. 2007;7(6):682–8.
17. Elliott RE, Tanweer O, Boah A, et al. Atlantoaxial fusion with transarticular screws: meta-analysis and review of the literature. World Neurosurg. 2013;80(5):627–41.
18. Ni B, Zhou F, Guo Q, Li S, Guo X, Xie N. Modified technique for C1-2 screw-rod fixation and fusion using autogenous bicortical iliac crest graft. Eur Spine J. 2012;21(1):156–64.
19. Huang DG, Hao DJ, He BR, et al. Posterior atlantoaxial fixation: a review of all techniques. Spine J. 2015;15(10):2271–81.
20. Goel A, Laheri V. Plate and screw fixation for atlanto-axial subluxation. Acta Neurochir. 1994;129(1–2):47–53.
21. Harms J, Melcher RP. Posterior C1-C2 fusion with polyaxial screw and rod fixation. Spine. 2001;26(22):2467–71.
22. Gorek J, Acaroglu E, Berven S, Yousef A, Puttlitz CM. Constructs incorporating intralaminar C2 screws provide rigid stability for atlantoaxial fixation. Spine. 2005;30(13):1513–8.
23. Lehman RA Jr, Dmitriev AE, Helgeson MD, Sasso RC, Kuklo TR, Riew KD. Salvage of C2 pedicle and pars screws using the intralaminar technique: a biomechanical analysis. Spine. 2008;33(9):960–5.
24. Meyer D, Meyer F, Kretschmer T, Borm W. Translaminar screws of the axis--an alternative technique for rigid screw fixation in upper cervical spine instability. Neurosurg Rev. 2012;35(2):255–61; discussion 261.
25. Wright NM. Posterior C2 fixation using bilateral, crossing C2 laminar screws: case series and technical note. J Spinal Disord Tech. 2004;17(2):158–62.
26. Sciubba DM, Noggle JC, Vellimana AK, et al. Radiographic and clinical evaluation of free-hand placement of C-2 pedicle screws. Clinical article. J Neurosurg Spine. 2009;11(1):15–22.
27. Lee SH, Kim ES, Sung JK, Park YM, Eoh W. Clinical and radiological comparison of treatment of atlantoaxial instability by posterior C1-C2 transarticular screw fixation or C1 lateral mass-C2 pedicle screw fixation. J Clin Neurosci. 2010;17(7):886–92.
28. Liu G, Buchowski JM, Shen H, Yeom JS, Riew KD. The feasibility of microscope-assisted "free-hand" C1 lateral mass screw insertion without fluoroscopy. Spine. 2008;33(9):1042–9.
29. Hamilton DK, Smith JS, Sansur CA, Dumont AS, Shaffrey CI. C-2 neurectomy during atlantoaxial instrumented fusion in the elderly: patient satisfaction and surgical outcome. J Neurosurg Spine. 2011;15(1):3–8.
30. Resnick DK, Benzel EC. C1-C2 pedicle screw fixation with rigid cantilever beam construct: case report and technical note. Neurosurgery. 2002;50(2):426–8.
31. Lee SH, Kim ES, Eoh W. Modified C1 lateral mass screw insertion using a high entry point to avoid postoperative occipital neuralgia. J Clin Neurosci. 2013;20(1):162–7.
32. Kelly BP, Glaser JA, DiAngelo DJ. Biomechanical comparison of a novel C1 posterior locking plate with the harms technique in a C1-C2 fixation model. Spine. 2008;33(24):E920–5.
33. Reis MT, Nottmeier EW, Reyes PM, Baek S, Crawford NR. Biomechanical analysis of a novel hook-screw technique for C1-2 stabilization. J Neurosurg Spine. 2012;17(3):220–6.
34. Parker SL, McGirt MJ, Garces-Ambrossi GL, et al. Translaminar versus pedicle screw fixation of C2: comparison of surgical morbidity and accuracy of 313 consecutive screws. Neurosurgery. 2009;64(5 Suppl 2):343–348; discussion 348-349.
35. Borne GM, Bedou GL, Pinaudeau M. Treatment of pedicular fractures of the axis. A clinical study and screw fixation technique. J Neurosurg. 1984;60(1):88–93.
36. Buchholz AL, Morgan SL, Robinson LC, Frankel BM. Minimally invasive percutaneous screw fixation of traumatic spondylolisthesis of the axis. J Neurosurg Spine. 2015;22(5):459–65.

37. Jo KW, Park IS, Hong JT. Motion-preserving reduction and fixation of C1 Jefferson fracture using a C1 lateral mass screw construct. J Clin Neurosci. 2011;18(5):695–8.
38. Goel A, Karapurkar AP. Transoral plate and screw fixation of the craniovertebral region--a preliminary report. Br J Neurosurg. 1994;8(6):743–5.
39. Sawin PD, Traynelis VC, Menezes AH. A comparative analysis of fusion rates and donor-site morbidity for autogeneic rib and iliac crest bone grafts in posterior cervical fusions. J Neurosurg. 1998;88(2):255–65.
40. Hood B, Hamilton DK, Smith JS, Dididze M, Shaffrey C, Levi AD. The use of allograft and recombinant human bone morphogenetic protein for instrumented atlantoaxial fusions. World Neurosurg. 2014;82(6):1369–73.
41. Hamilton DK, Smith JS, Reames DL, Williams BJ, Shaffrey CI. Use of recombinant human bone morphogenetic protein-2 as an adjunct for instrumented posterior arthrodesis in the occipital cervical region: an analysis of safety, efficacy, and dosing. J Craniovertebr Junction Spine. 2010;1(2):107–12.

Reconstructive Procedures in the Osteoporotic Patient

32

Jacob Januszewski and Juan S. Uribe

Pitfalls/Pearls

- Bone mineral density (BMD) is increasingly thought of as one of the most important risk factors predicting failure of instrumentation and fusion, development of idiopathic spinal deformity, cage subsidence, and proximal junctional failure (PJF).
- The strict WHO definition of osteoporosis is not representative of the high frequency of failure with reconstructive spine procedures in the osteoporotic patient, as many patients with T scores above the 2.5 standard deviations below the average BMD present with complications related to failure of fusion.
- Patients with WHO definition of osteopenia are already at a high risk of fusion failure after reconstructive procedures.
- When reconstructive procedures of the spine are necessary in a patient with osteoporosis, attempt should be made to improve BMD prior to surgery.
- Preoperatively, perioperatively, and postoperatively, osteoclast inhibitors (denosumab/Prolia, zoledronic acid) or osteoblast activators (teriparatide/Forteo) should be used to improve bone density and promote fusion followed by bisphosphonate therapy for proper bone density maintenance.
- Spinal deformity correction, realignment, and maintenance of spinal balance are even more important in patients with osteoporosis to reduce abnormal excessive forces on fusion construct and prevent complications.
- Surgical techniques should be used to maximize cortical purchase of instrumentation such as the use of intraoperative fluoroscopy to facilitate bicortical anterior cervical screw purchase and neuronavigation for placement of cervical pedicle screws for more rigid dorsal instrumentation.
- Along with bicortical purchase, increased number of fixation points, use of cross-links and triangulation, use of hooks and wires instead of screws, cement augmentation of pedicle screws,

J. Januszewski · J. S. Uribe (✉)
Department of Neurosurgery and Brain Repair, University of South Florida, Tampa, FL, USA

M. G. Kaiser et al. (eds.), *Degenerative Cervical Myelopathy and Radiculopathy*,
https://doi.org/10.1007/978-3-319-97952-6_32

and use of expandable technology designed for an osteoporotic patient are all techniques previously tried and may be beneficial.

- Biologic allograft options such as allogenic mesenchymal cellular bone matrix, osteoprogenitor, and stem cells should be used to improve chances of arthrodesis.

Introduction and Main Ideas

Osteoporosis and osteopenia as defined by the WHO are based on bone mineral density (BMD) as measured by the dual-energy x-ray absorptiometry (DEXA) of the hip and spine. A T score below 2.5 standard deviations from the average BMD for a healthy young white female is defined as osteoporosis. This threshold was chosen on the basis of fracture risk in postmenopausal Caucasian women; however, several studies have shown that these values are similar in age-adjusted males and females [1, 2]. While indeed fragility fractures are highest in this group of patients, more than 80% of postmenopausal women with fractures have T scores better than −2.5 [3].

Current guidelines recommend pharmacologic treatment should be started in patients with a T score −2.5 or those who have experienced fragility fractures [4]. Patients who do not meet the DEXA criteria for osteoporosis and are over 50 years of age with a FRAX score greater than 3% 10-year risk of a hip fracture or 20% 10-year risk of a major osteoporotic fracture are also candidates for pharmacologic treatment [5]. While this may be sufficient to treat general osteoporosis and prevent fragility fractures, increasingly more studies show failure of this approach in an osteoporotic or osteopenic patient undergoing reconstructive spine surgery who may not necessarily meet the WHO criteria for pharmacologic treatment [6–10]. Kim et al. and a recent meta-analysis study reported that a pre-existing low BMD is a significant risk factor for patients in developing proximal junctional failure (PJF) after reconstructive spine surgery with an odds ratio of 2.37 [6, 7]. These reports strongly suggest an association between low bone density (osteoporosis/osteopenia) and increased complication rate after reconstructive surgery.

In this chapter we discuss options to improve cortical bone instrumentation purchase in reconstructive surgery of the cervical spine and promote arthrodesis in an osteoporotic patient. However, all current evidence begins to point toward avoidance of operating on an osteoporotic patient until bone mineral density is improved enough to better accommodate instrumentation without the risk of failure, non-union, or pseudoarthrosis. A short guideline for preoperative workup and management of an osteoporotic patient is suggested. This is followed by a short discussion of reconstructive techniques available for patients with osteoporosis as well as their postoperative care.

Indications and Preoperative Workup and Management

Patient Selection

Surgery for degenerative disease may be complicated by a diagnosis of osteoporosis. Many patients who require cervical spine reconstructive surgery are asymptomatic from their osteoporosis. Their clinical manifestation is the same as for patients who do not have osteoporosis and are affected by symptoms of degenerative spondylosis whether from degenerative disc disease, dynamic instability, or kyphosis and deformity. Indications for surgery for these patients have not changed in national guidelines and remain the same as those for patients without osteoporosis. However, in lieu of recent evidence, consideration should be given to screening postmenopausal women and men over the age of 70 for osteoporosis prior to undergoing a major reconstructive spine surgery requiring instrumentation and fusion.

Screening

A fracture risk assessment tool (FRAX) incorporates multiple risk factors into a 10-year probability of either a hip fracture or a major osteoporotic fragility fracture. Risk factors include low body mass index, history of a previous fracture or parental hip fracture, smoking, long-term use of glucocorticoids (more than 3 months), rheumatoid arthritis, and excessive daily alcohol consumption [1]. A calculation of a 10-year risk greater than 3% for hip fracture or 20% for a fragility fracture is generally enough to permit pharmacologic treatment in patients over 50 years of age even if the DEXA T score does not meet criteria for the WHO definition of osteoporosis. Also, patients with a T score in a range of osteopenia (−1.9 or lower) with radiographic evidence of a fragility or compression fracture are also candidates for pharmacological treatment of osteoporosis.

DEXA scan is considered a gold standard for measuring bone mineral density (BMD) and can be used as an initial screening test in patients described above as well as patients with secondary causes of osteoporosis such as hypogonadism, inflammatory bowel disease, prolonged immobility, type 1 diabetes, renal disease, thyroid disorders, and organ transplantation. DEXA has shown to be very precise with acceptable accuracy and good reproducibility so long as the same machine and technician are used on subsequent evaluations on the same patient [11–13]. Because there is no current agreement, or even scientific knowledge, on what should be a standard T score value below which a reconstructive spinal surgery would be postponed, clinical judgment and surgeon preference should be used. In our practice we consider a T score value −1.9 or lower at either the femoral neck or any vertebral body to be the threshold at which we would not perform a major reconstructive procedure requiring a multilevel instrumentation and arthrodesis.

Preoperative Pharmacological Management for Risk Reduction

As previously mentioned, there is strong new evidence associating low bone density with increased complication rate after reconstructive spine surgery. Most surgical techniques developed to combat the issue of instrumentation failure and non-fusion in spinal reconstruction in an osteoporotic patient are more than a decade old, with only a few developed within this past decade. There are also no long-term comparative studies that evaluate clinical outcomes of such techniques. It is very likely that risk reduction for fusion failure prior to reconstructive surgery may be a better workaround solution.

Pharmacologic therapy for osteoporosis centers around the antiresorptive and anabolic mechanisms. Antiresorptive drugs, such as bisphosphonates and a new class of human monoclonal antibody to osteoclast-activating receptor RANK (denosumab/Prolia), have been shown to reduce vertebral and nonvertebral fragility fractures by 50–68% [14–17]. However, both bisphosphonates and denosumab required 3–6 years of treatment prior to seeing any benefit in fracture rates.

Recently, a prospective, randomized, placebo-controlled, and triple-blinded study by Chen et al. evaluated 79 osteoporotic patients with single-level degenerative spondylolisthesis for effects of zoledronic acid on postoperative bone density, fusion rates, and adjacent-level vertebral body fractures. No patients in the zoledronic acid group developed adjacent-level fracture at 12 months, whereas 17% of control group patients did. Zoledronic acid also prevented a natural BMD decrease that occurred in the control group and even slightly improved it. While fusion rate between the groups was not different at 1 year, zoledronic acid allowed for faster bone formation on postoperative CTs and radiographs at 3, 6, and 9 months [18].

The biggest benefit of recombinant human parathyroid hormone (teriparatide/Forteo) is its ability to not only slow down bone resorption but to also stimulate bone formation by activating osteoblasts more than osteoclasts. It has been shown to increase bone mass by at least 10% and decrease fracture rate by 50% [19]. Its clinical response rate is also much faster than the other classes of drugs likely due to its anabolic activity rather than just antiresorptive properties. The maximum recommended duration of treatment, therefore, is 2 years, and observational studies suggest lasting benefit for at least 18 months after discontinuation [20]. Teriparatide, however, can significantly decrease DEXA T scores and promote significant new bone formation within only 6 months from the start of therapy [21–23]. Its perioperative use has also been shown to be more effective than bisphosphonates in preventing complications and maintaining fusion rates in osteoporotic patients [24–26].

There are currently no guidelines in regard to perioperative management of osteoporotic patients with pharmacologic therapy to reduce complication rates in reconstructive surgery. In many centers such management is still dictated in part by the insurance companies with decisions based on old or misinformed data. There are, however, many new recent studies in favor of perioperative pharmacotherapy for osteoporosis, which may soon change the direction of current management in patients requiring a high-risk reconstructive surgery. In our practice we screen all postmenopausal women and men over the age of 70 who require a multilevel deformity correction with a DEXA scan. If patients are below our T score threshold of −1.9, we then initiate treatment with teriparatide for 6 months (Fig. 32.1). We have noticed a significant improvement in DEXA T scores on repeat testing, allowing these patients to better tolerate the surgery and minimizing the risk of perioperative complications related to low BMD from osteoporosis.

Surgical Options in the Osteoporotic Patient

Decrease in bone mineral density that occurs in osteoporosis weakens the pullout strength of the spinal implants in bone. This in turn increases the rate of instrumentation failure, pseudoarthrosis, non-union, adjacent segment vertebral body fractures, proximal junctional failure, and idiopathic cervical kyphosis requiring revision surgery and poorer patient outcomes. Patients with osteoporosis, however, have fewer options when it comes to revision surgery, and prophylactic strategies for complication prevention are continuously sought after to minimize this issue in this patient population [27]. In rare cases, however, cervical kyphotic deformity in an osteoporotic patient may result in acute onset of symptoms from spinal cord compression, and surgical treatment on more urgent bases may be needed. There are several surgical techniques designed for patients with osteoporosis described in the literature, but most of the literature on these is one to two decades old without any new comparative analysis of clinical outcomes.

Increased Number of Fixation Points and Bicortical Purchase

In patients with osteoporosis, extension of fusion beyond the levels normally considered for instrumentation in a non-osteoporotic patient may be necessary. This way there are more rigid points of fixation distributed over a larger moment arm, allowing increased stiffness of the construct and reducing the chance of instrumentation failure [28]. There are case reports on the use of bicortical purchase of anterior cervical screws and placement of cervical pedicle screws with a use of intraoperative navigation to achieve increased pullout strength in an osteoporotic bone [29]. Distraction with Caspar screws or compression of the pedicle screws to improve cervical lordosis should be avoided due to increased risk of screw pullout or pedicle breach during such maneuvers on an osteoporotic bone.

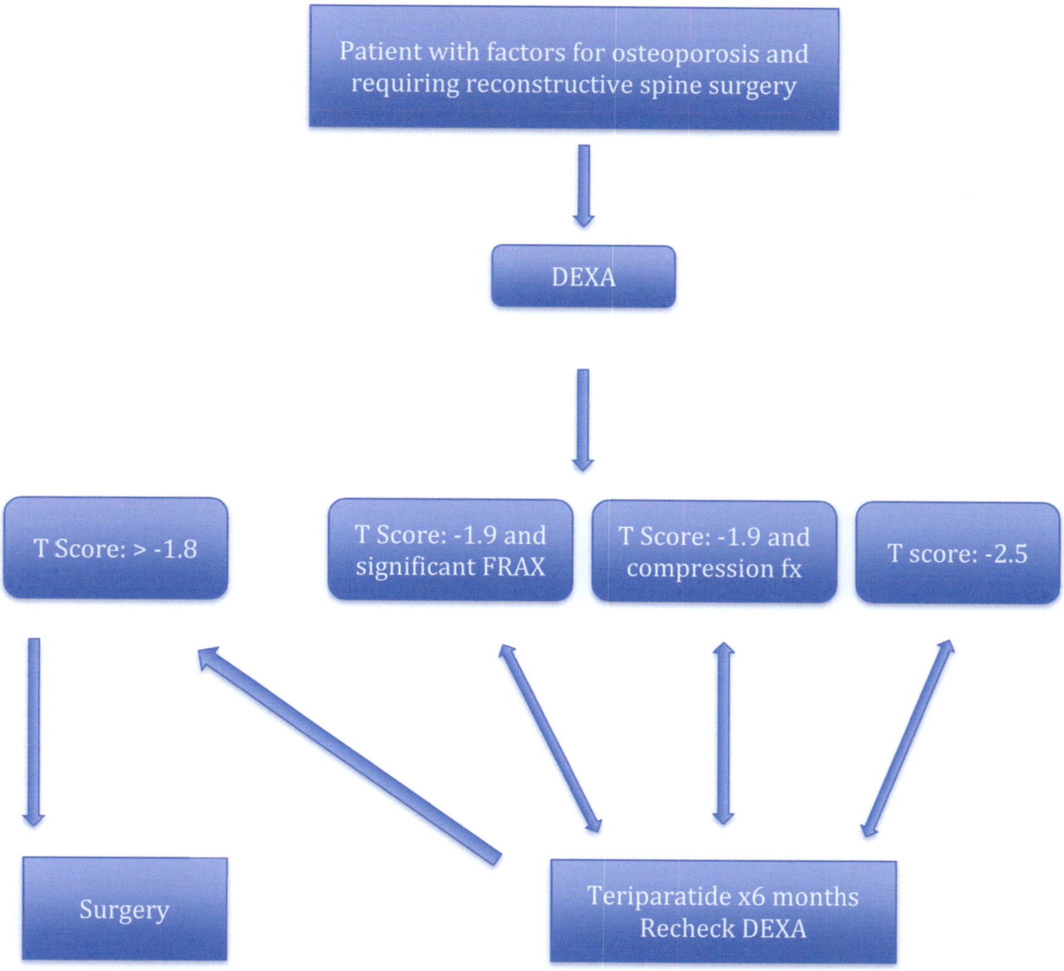

Fig. 32.1 Suggested guideline on perioperative management of the osteoporotic patient

Cross-Links, Hooks, and Wires

Cross-links distribute compressive and rotational forces across the entire implant. They are most useful in increasing torsional stiffness in pedicle screw and hook constructs but not in lateral flexion mode, allowing for increased stiffness of the entire construct [28, 30]. Since cancellous bone loss occurs primarily in osteoporosis, instrumentation constructs that utilize more cortical bone surface area are biomechanically stronger. Laminar hooks or sublaminar wires are good stabilization options but should be left as a last resort in case other methods fail and the patient requires revision surgery. They are however biomechanically superior in pullout strength and can be used at the ends of a kyphosis construct to prevent instrumentation pullout and progression of kyphosis [28].

Implants Designed for Osteoporotic Patient

Hollow cannulated screws for insertion of cement and expandable pedicle screws increase the pull-out strength, and a recent systematic review of literature has shown their ability to improve fusion rates more than traditional pedicle screws [26, 31]. However, there are no good clinical studies showing improved clinical outcomes with these implants [2]. Allograft such as osteopromoting osteoprogenitor cells, stem cells, and mesenchymal cellular bone matrix may increase the fusion rates and minimize the time to achieve a solid fusion [32, 33].

Interbody Fusion, Osteotomies, Mismatch Correction, and Spinal Balance

There is increasing clear evidence that maintenance of sagittal balance, spine neutrality, and harmony decreases late complications such adjacent segment disease, PJK, and PJF [34–38]. When operating on a patient with osteoporosis, it is even more crucial to maintain proper spinal biomechanics and restore normal spinal balance. Anterior hyperlordotic interbody implants can correct much of cervical kyphosis, especially in a non-fixed deformity. If necessary, posterior facetectomies or Ponte osteotomies may be utilized to release the posterior spinal elements and achieve even greater correction of cervical kyphosis. If posterior osteotomies are necessary, correction can be achieved by releasing posteriorly first, followed by anterior interbody cages, followed by posterior instrumentation and arthrodesis. Alternatively, stand-alone hyperlordotic anterior cages secured to only one endplate superiorly can be inserted first, followed by posterior osteotomies, dorsal instrumentation, and fusion. This allows the anterior column to open even further as necessary after posterior osteotomies are finished. Again, distraction with Caspar pins or compression of pedicle screws should be avoided to minimize chances of screw pullout. All necessary correction can be achieved with hyperlordotic cages, ALL release, PLL release, and posterior osteotomies as necessary.

Conclusion

Bone mineral density is increasingly thought of as one of the most important risk factors for instrumentation failure, PJK, non-fusion, and other short- and long-term postoperative complications in the osteoporotic patient. A plethora of surgical techniques for osteoporotic bone have been previously described over the past two decades without any major advances in improvement of clinical outcomes. While there are no current guidelines as to the management of patients with osteoporosis who require reconstructive spine surgery, new studies suggest that perhaps not operating on these patients until improvement of BMD is accomplished may be a better course of action. Perioperative pharmacological therapy with new class of bisphosphonates or recombinant human parathyroid hormone has been shown to not only improve BMD and increase DEXA T scores but also accomplish it in a relatively quick fashion. Most reconstructive spine surgery in an osteoporotic patient is not done on urgent or emergent basis but electively, and most of the time surgery can be easily postponed until correction of severe osteoporosis. Revision surgery in a patient with osteoporosis can be quite substantial and complicated, with a higher risk of a poor outcome. Reducing this risk with perioperative pharmacotherapy has already shown to be feasible. We recommend teriparatide treatment for approximately 6 months prior to reconstructive spine surgery and repeating a DEXA scan to confirm improvement in T scores. Teriparatide continues to have a lasting effect on BMD for up to 18 months after discontinuation of treatment, therefore allowing for adequate time for a solid fusion. Continuation of therapy postoperatively with zoledronic acid may further minimize osteoclast-mediated bone resorption and maintain the mineral bone density.

Key Recommendations

- The perioperative use of osteoblast activators (teriparatide/Forteo) should be used for 6 months prior to major reconstructive spine surgery to improve bone density and facilitate fusion postoperatively. This may be followed by postoperative bisphosphonate therapy with zoledronic acid for proper bone density maintenance.
- Surgical techniques should be used to maximize cortical purchase of implants such as the use of intraoperative fluoroscopy to facilitate bicortical anterior cervical screw purchase and neuronavigation for placement of cervical pedicle screws for more rigid dorsal instrumentation.
- Spinal deformity correction, realignment, and maintenance of spinal balance are even more important in patients with osteoporosis to reduce abnormal excessive forces on fusion construct and prevent complications.

Case Presentation

A 77-year-old Caucasian female presented to our hospital emergency room after a fall with central cord syndrome. The patient admitted to a recent history of increasing frequency of falling down but denied other symptoms of myelopathy prior to this. On examination, she was weaker in upper extremities more so than in lowers. She had very brisk Hoffman's reflexes, sustained clonus, and positive Babinski in bilateral feet. MRI cervical spine (Fig. 32.2a) revealed severe anterior and posterior spinal cord stenosis most severe from C3 to C6 with spinal cord compression, T2 signal changes, and myelomalacia. She had loss of cervical lordosis with mild to moderate kyphosis and cervical deformity. CT cervical spine (Fig. 32.2b) revealed a calcified C5/6 disc with a posterior osteophyte and loss of bone mineral density. Her DEXA scan revealed moderate osteoporosis. Because of patient's severe myelopathy, she was taken to the operating room for anterior/posterior cervical decompression and fusion. The patient had C3/4, C4/5 ACDF with C6 corpectomy, interbody cage with osteopromoting

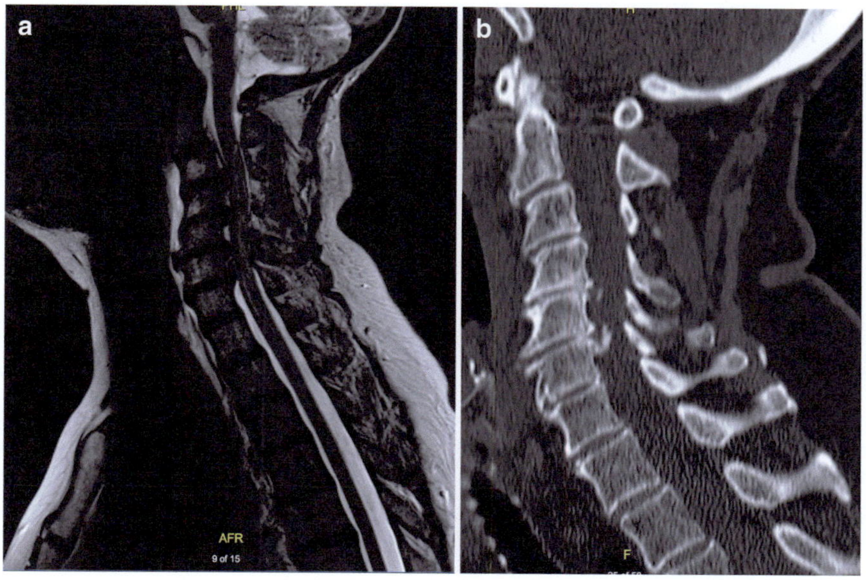

Fig. 32.2 Sagittal C-spine MRI without contrast (**a**) shows severe spondylosis and stenosis C3–C7, with anterior and posterior spinal cord compression especially at C5/6 with myelomalacia. Cervical spine CT (**b**) shows a large disc/osteophyte complex at C5/6, as well as reversal of cervical lordosis with mild-moderate kyphotic deformity

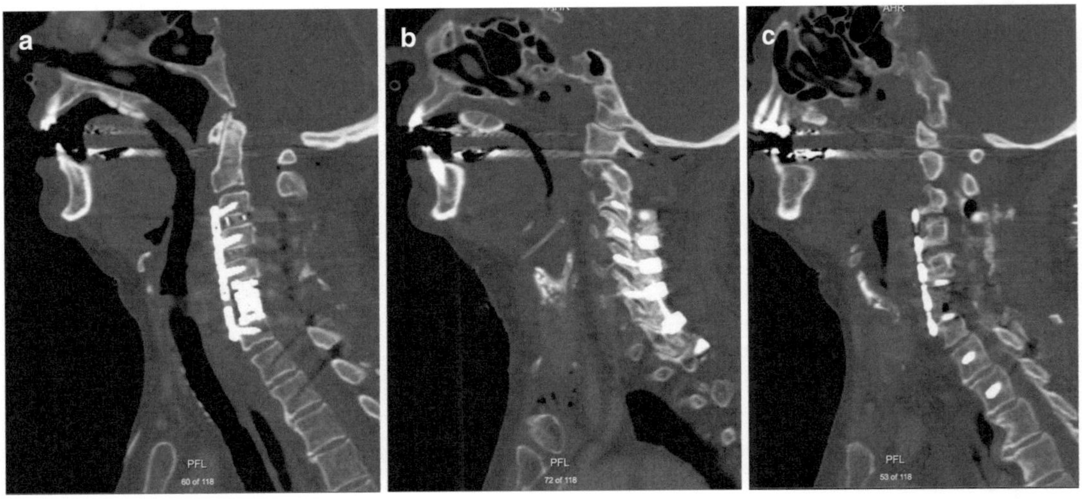

Fig. 32.3 Postoperative C-spine CT after C3/4, C4/5 ACDF, and C6 corpectomy with C3–T2 lateral mass and pedicle screw fusion showing C6 corpectomy cage in good position with excellent decompression of the spinal cord (**a**), restoration of cervical lordosis (**b**) with good posterior spinal cord decompression (**c**)

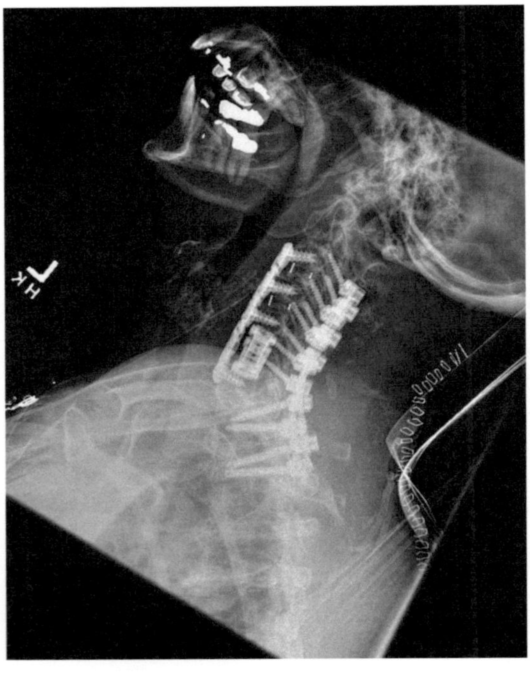

Fig. 32.4 A 12-month postoperative upright C-spine x-ray lateral view showing a 360° fusion construct with full restoration of cervical deformity and stable fusion

allograft, and C3–C7 anterior cervical translational plate. The patient's cervical deformity was easily corrected with positioning, and the translational cervical plate had interlocks removed prior to insertion to allow for more correction with posterior decompression. C3–C7 laminectomy was performed with C3-T2 lateral mass and thoracic pedicle screw fixation (Fig. 32.3). Both lateral mass and thoracic pedicle screws had bicortical purchase to increase the pullout strength due to the patient's osteoporosis and poor bone quality. The patient was placed on Forteo in the postoperative period to increase bone mineral density and facilitate fusion. On a 12-month follow-up, the patient's imaging showed excellent fusion without instrumentation failure or subsidence with good cervical deformity correction (Fig. 32.4).

References

1. Kanis JA, McCloskey EV, Johansson H, et al. A reference standard for the description of osteoporosis. Bone. 2008;42:467–75.
2. Steinmetz MP, Benzel EC. Benzel's spine surgery: techniques, complication avoidance, and management. 4th ed. Philadelphia: Elsevier; 2016.
3. Siris ES, Chen YT, Abbott TA, et al. Bone mineral density thresholds for pharmacological intervention to prevent fractures. Arch Intern Med. 2004;164:1108–12.
4. Cosman F, de Beur SJ, LeBoff MS, et al. Clinician's guide to prevention and treatment of osteoporosis. Osteoporos Int. 2014;25:2359–81.

5. Crandall CJ, Newberry SJ, Diamant A, et al. Comparative effectiveness of pharmacologic treatments to prevent fractures: an updated systematic review. Ann Intern Med. 2014;161:711–23.
6. Kim DK, Kim JY, Kim DY, et al. Risk factors of proximal junctional kyphosis after multilevel fusion surgery: more than 2 years follow-up data. J Korean Neurosurg Soc. 2017;60:174–80.
7. Liu FY, Wang T, Yang SD, et al. Incidence and risk factors for proximal junctional kyphosis: a meta-analysis. European spine J. 2016;25:2376–83.
8. Park SJ, Lee CS, Chung SS, et al. Different risk factors of proximal junctional kyphosis and proximal junctional failure following long instrumented fusion to the sacrum for adult spinal deformity: survivorship analysis of 160 patients. Neurosurgery. 2017;80:279–86.
9. Yagi M, King AB, Boachie-Adjei O. Incidence, risk factors, and natural course of proximal junctional kyphosis: surgical outcomes review of adult idiopathic scoliosis. Minimum 5 years of follow-up. Spine. 2012;37:1479–89.
10. Yagi M, Rahm M, Gaines R, et al. Characterization and surgical outcomes of proximal junctional failure in surgically treated patients with adult spinal deformity. Spine. 2014;39:E607–14.
11. Mauck KF, Clarke BL. Diagnosis, screening, prevention, and treatment of osteoporosis. Mayo Clin Proc. 2006;81:662–72.
12. El Maghraoui A, Roux C. DXA scanning in clinical practice. QJM. 2008;101:605–17.
13. Nelson HD, Haney EM, Chou R, et al. U.S. preventive services task force evidence syntheses, formerly systematic evidence reviews. Screening for osteoporosis: systematic review to update the 2002 U.S. preventive services task force recommendation. Rockville: Agency for Healthcare Research and Quality (US); 2010.
14. Cranney A, Tugwell P, Adachi J, et al. Meta-analyses of therapies for postmenopausal osteoporosis. III. Meta-analysis of risedronate for the treatment of postmenopausal osteoporosis. Endocr Rev. 2002;23:517–23.
15. Kanis JA, Borgstrom F, Johnell O, et al. Cost-effectiveness of risedronate for the treatment of osteoporosis and prevention of fractures in postmenopausal women. Osteoporos Int. 2004;15:862–71.
16. Bone HG, Chapurlat R, Brandi ML, et al. The effect of three or six years of denosumab exposure in women with postmenopausal osteoporosis: results from the FREEDOM extension. J Clin Endocrinol Metab. 2013;98:4483–92.
17. Cummings SR, San Martin J, McClung MR, et al. Denosumab for prevention of fractures in postmenopausal women with osteoporosis. N Engl J Med. 2009;361:756–65.
18. Chen F, Dai Z, Kang Y, et al. Effects of zoledronic acid on bone fusion in osteoporotic patients after lumbar fusion. Osteoporos Int. 2016;27:1469–76.
19. Schilcher J, Koeppen V, Aspenberg P, et al. Risk of atypical femoral fracture during and after bisphosphonate use. N Engl J Med. 2014;371:974–6.
20. Neer RM, Arnaud CD, Zanchetta JR, et al. Effect of parathyroid hormone (1-34) on fractures and bone mineral density in postmenopausal women with osteoporosis. N Engl J Med. 2001;344:1434–41.
21. Ebata S, Takahashi J, Hasegawa T, et al. Role of weekly Teriparatide Administration in Osseous Union Enhancement within six months after posterior or Transforaminal lumbar interbody fusion for osteoporosis-associated lumbar degenerative disorders: a multicenter, prospective randomized study. J Bone Joint Surg Am. 2017;99:365–72.
22. Kaliya-Perumal AK, Lu ML, Luo CA, et al. Retrospective radiological outcome analysis following teriparatide use in elderly patients undergoing multilevel instrumented lumbar fusion surgery. Medicine (Baltimore). 2017;96:e5996.
23. Cho PG, Ji GY, Shin DA, et al. An effect comparison of teriparatide and bisphosphonate on posterior lumbar interbody fusion in patients with osteoporosis: a prospective cohort study and preliminary data. European spine J. 2017;26:691–7.
24. Seki S, Hirano N, Kawaguchi Y, et al. Teriparatide versus low-dose bisphosphonates before and after surgery for adult spinal deformity in female Japanese patients with osteoporosis. Eur Spine J. 2017;26:2121.
25. Chaudhary N, Lee JS, Wu JY, et al. Evidence for use of Teriparatide in spinal fusion surgery in osteoporotic patients. World Neurosurg. 2017;100:551–6.
26. Fischer CR, Hanson G, Eller M, et al. A systematic review of treatment strategies for degenerative lumbar spine fusion surgery in patients with osteoporosis. Geriatr Orthop Surg Rehabil. 2016;7:188–96.
27. Cho SK, Bridwell KH, Lenke LG, et al. Major complications in revision adult deformity surgery: risk factors and clinical outcomes with 2- to 7-year follow-up. Spine. 2012;37:489–500.
28. Brodke DS, Bachus KN, Mohr RA, et al. Segmental pedicle screw fixation or cross-links in multilevel lumbar constructs. A biomechanical analysis. Spine J. 2001;1:373–9.
29. Mattei TA, Rehman AA, Issawi A, et al. Surgical challenges in the management of cervical kyphotic deformity in patients with severe osteoporosis: an illustrative case of a patient with Hajdu-Cheney syndrome. Eur Spine J. 2015;24:2746–53.
30. Dick JC, Zdeblick TA, Bartel BD, et al. Mechanical evaluation of cross-link designs in rigid pedicle screw systems. Spine. 1997;22:370–5.
31. Chen LH, Tai CL, Lee DM, et al. Pullout strength of pedicle screws with cement augmentation in severe osteoporosis: a comparative study between cannulated screws with cement injection and solid screws with cement pre-filling. BMC Musculoskelet Disord. 2011;12:33.
32. Divi SN, Mikhael MM. Use of allogenic mesenchymal cellular bone matrix in anterior and posterior cervical spinal fusion: a case series of 21 patients. Asian spine J. 2017;11:454–62.
33. Hansraj KK. Stem Cells in Spine Surgery. Surg Technol Int. 2016;XXIX:348–58.

34. Ames CP, Smith JS, Scheer JK, et al. Impact of spinopelvic alignment on decision making in deformity surgery in adults: a review. J Neurosurg Spine. 2012;16:547–64.
35. Hasegawa K, Okamoto M, Hatsushikano S, et al. Normative values of spino-pelvic sagittal alignment, balance, age, and health-related quality of life in a cohort of healthy adult subjects. Eur Spine J. 2016;25:3675–86.
36. Lafage R, Schwab F, Challier V, et al. Defining Spino-pelvic alignment thresholds: should operative goals in adult spinal deformity surgery account for age? Spine. 2016;41:62–8.
37. Maciejczak A, Jablonska-Sudol K. Correlation between correction of pelvic balance and clinical outcomes in mid- and low-grade adult isthmic spondylolisthesis. Eur Spine J. 2016;26(12):3112–21.
38. Yagi M, Kaneko S, Yato Y, et al. Standing balance and compensatory mechanisms in patients with adult spinal deformity. Spine. 2016;42(10):E584–91.

The Cervicothoracic Junction

33

Anthony M. DiGiorgio, Michael S. Virk,
Ming-Hsiao Hu, Mohanad Alazzeh,
Santan Thottempudi, and Praveen V. Mummaneni

Pearls and Pitfalls

- The cervicothoracic junction (CTJ) is an anatomically unique area and offers several options for fixation.
- Fixation at C3–C6 is typically performed with lateral mass screws, due to the presence of the vertebral artery and the small size of the pedicles.
- C7 may be fixated with either lateral mass screws or pedicle screws since usually the foramen transversarium at that level does not contain the vertebral artery.
- T1 and below is fixated with pedicle screws.
- Due to biomechanical concerns, posterior cervical stabilization terminating at C7 may be problematic.
- Anterior approaches to the CTJ are possible but the manubrium height must be assessed preoperatively. If a line drawn parallel to the most caudal operative end plate intersects the manubrium, it is recommended that an approach surgeon be utilized to perform manubriotomy.
- Other anatomic considerations for the anterior approach include the position of the aortic arch and brachiocephalic vessels.

A. M. DiGiorgio
Department of Neurological Surgery, University of California, San Francisco, CA, USA

Department of Neurological Surgery, Louisiana State University Health Sciences Center, New Orleans, LA, USA

M. S. Virk
Department of Neurosurgery, University of California, San Francisco, CA, USA

M.-H. Hu
Institute of Biomedical Engineering, College of Medicine and College of Engineering, National Taiwan University, Taipei, Taiwan

Department of Orthopedics, National Taiwan University College of Medicine and National Taiwan University Hospital, Taipei, Taiwan

M. Alazzeh · S. Thottempudi
University of California, San Francisco, CA, USA

P. V. Mummaneni (✉)
Department of Neurological Surgery, University of California, San Francisco, CA, USA
e-mail: Praveen.Mummaneni@ucsf.edu

M. G. Kaiser et al. (eds.), *Degenerative Cervical Myelopathy and Radiculopathy*,
https://doi.org/10.1007/978-3-319-97952-6_33

Introduction

The cervicothoracic junction (CTJ) serves as the interface between the flexible, lordotic cervical spine and the more rigid, kyphotic thoracic spine. It is comprised of the C7 and T1 vertebrae and the intervening discs, ribs, and spanning ligaments. The varying anatomy and load-bearing properties of these two spine regions require careful consideration. The transition from the mobile cervical spine to immobile thoracic spine exposes the CTJ to large forces, making it susceptible to trauma and requiring unique biomechanical considerations when planning stabilization constructs.

The cervical vertebrae have coronally aligned facets, thin laminae, and small, medially angled pedicles. Additionally, the vertebral artery runs through the foramen transversarium from C2 to C6. The thoracic vertebrae have larger pedicles, laminae, and spinous processes, but no lateral mass. The thoracic spine has complex articulations with the rib cage, and these joints contribute to the rigidity of this segment. Below T2, the nerve roots innervate the intercostal muscles and may be sacrificed if needed.

Because of the anatomic constraints, early fusions across the CTJ were performed using spinous process wiring and laminar hooks [1]. However, these constructs were not very rigid and fusion failure was common [2]. In addition, if an extensive laminectomy had been performed, these options were precluded at the operative level, necessitating extension of the fusion above and below the decompression. Extensive decompressions thus lacked intervening points of fixation, which further predisposed such constructs to failed arthrodesis.

Both anterior and posterior approaches are options to manage central and foraminal degenerative pathology. The need for an anterior approach for pure degenerative cases, as opposed to deformity or tumor cases, is not common. If it is needed, anterior approaches must consider the manubrium, sternum, and great vessels to achieve safe access. When planning for an anterior cervical decompression and fusion, there are various radiographic assessments [3–5] to determine if a more extensive approach is needed.

The posterior cervical decompression and fusion is a common neurosurgical procedure to treat myeloradiculopathy. With respect to instrumentation, however, there is no consensus on the ideal caudal stopping point of such constructs. Terminating a posterior fusion construct at C7 creates a long lever arm that pivots over a single mobile disc space, C7–T1. This isolates the load-bearing stresses and focuses motion across the CTJ. Theoretically, accelerated degeneration and adjacent segment disease can develop at this point [6, 7]. This may result in progressive spondylosis, facet arthrosis, deformity, and, ultimately, morbidity for the patient.

Main Ideas Supported by Relevant Literature

Dynamic instability at the CTJ leads to poor health-related quality of life (HRQOL) measures. Liu et al. found that C7 sagittal slip in flexion and extension has been shown to correlate with worse modified Japanese Orthopaedic Association (mJOA) scores than at other levels [8]. They postulate that because this level is biomechanically critical to the dynamic motion of the spine, degeneration leads to worse myelopathy.

When performing posterior surgical decompression of the cervical spine, it is common that an instrumented fusion may be done concomitantly [9]. Decompressions without instrumentation or failed arthrodesis across the CTJ are particularly prone to kyphotic deformity [10]. Yet there remains controversy regarding the caudal terminus of a cervical fusion, specifically whether or not to cross the CTJ. There are no large trials or consensus statements that address this controversy directly. It is suggested that fusions terminating at C7 are prone to deforming forces and high failure rates [6, 7]. An article by Steinmetz et al. [11] studied 593 fusions across the CTJ and found 14 cases of fusion failure. They found that stand-alone dorsal fixation that stopped at C7 trended toward failure, yet this finding wasn't statistically significant. They did find that multilevel corpectomies spanning the CTJ, uninstrumented laminectomy, and tobacco use were significantly associated with CTJ failure [11]. Conversely, extending a posterior fusion to the upper thoracic spine likely does not significantly affect recovery time or worsen outcomes, as shown in a study by Bechara et al. in 2012 [12]. Thoracic screws have a relatively low complication rate. Mazel et al. [13] had no neurovascular complications from posterior cervicothoracic screw placement in their series of 330 screws placed in patients fused across the CTJ for a variety of pathologies using lateral mass screws from C4 to C7 and pedicle screws in the thoracic spine [13].

Degenerative pathology necessitating an anterior approach is less common. However, ACDF at C7–T1 has good results [14]. In order to assess accessibility from an anterior approach, the manubrium has to be identified on imaging. Various authors suggest using CT, MRI, or X-ray [3–5]. The "surgeon's view line" can be drawn on MRI to determine if the CTJ can be accessed from an anterior approach (Fig. 33.1). It is a line drawn parallel to the end plate of C7 and needs to not intersect manubrium on the sagittal image [5]. If the manubrium obstructs the approach, there are a variety of manubrium splitting techniques, and the assistance of a thoracic surgeon is likely necessary [10, 15].

When performing posterior stabilization across CTJ, the literature does not identify an ideal caudal terminus. An in vitro biomechanical study by Chang et al. (2015) suggested fusing to T2 if crossing the CTJ [16]. If laminoplasty is performed and the intraspinous ligament at C7–T1 is maintained, the instrumentation need not cross the CTJ, as the posterior tension band prevents further deformity [17]. The authors of this chapter typically stop at T1 and have had few failures with that end point.

In addition to being off-label in this application, the use of BMP in instrumented fusion at the posterior CTJ is controversial [18] and may be associated with complications in the cervical spine, such as seroma formation postoperatively [19]. Some authors do use BMP for multilevel posterior cervical fusions to treat patients at high risk for pseudoarthrosis, but they leave subfascial drains for several days post-op to avoid the seroma issue [20]. The use of BMP for use in posterior fusions across the CTJ has not been evaluated by the FDA.

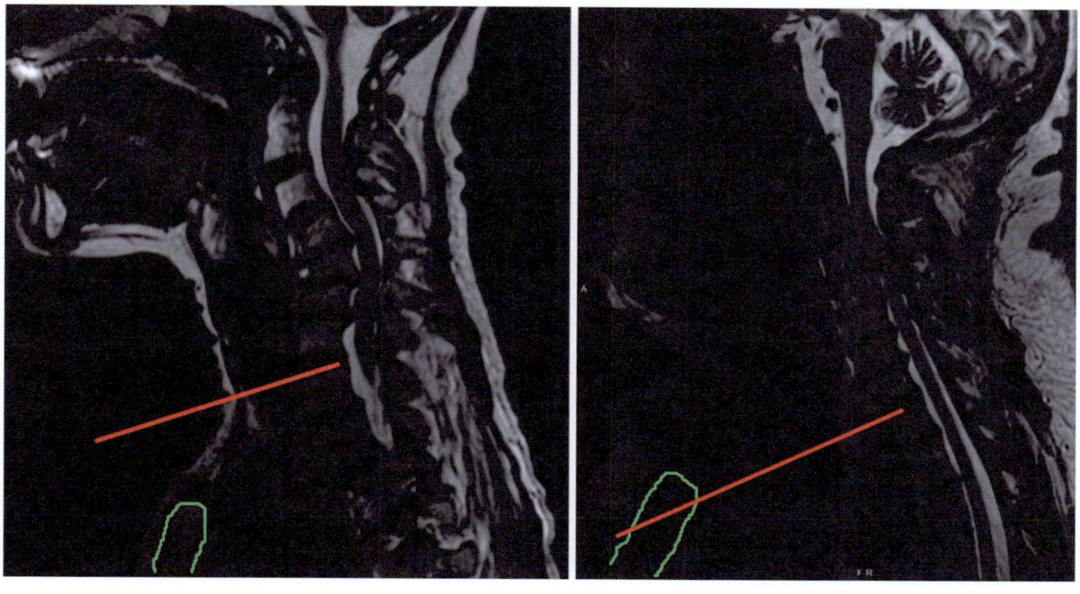

Fig. 33.1 The surgeon's view line. To determine if a C7–T1 discectomy can be performed from a traditional anterior approach, a line is drawn parallel to the end plate of C7 (red line). If this passes above the manubrium (outlined in green), a standard approach will be adequate, as seen on the right image. If this passes through the manubrium, a transsternal approach will be required

The transition from the smaller, medially located lateral mass screws in the cervical spine to the larger, more laterally placed thoracic pedicle screws also poses a technical challenge. Standard placement of C7 lateral mass screws and T1 pedicle screws typically results in screw tulip heads that do not align for rod placement. Additionally, thoracic screw tulip heads may not accommodate the same size rod as the cervical screws.

Multiple techniques have been developed to address this, but none has been shown to be superior. The most commonly used options are using a transitional rod that goes from a 3.5 mm diameter for the cervical screws to a 5.5 mm diameter for the thoracic screws, using a 3.5 mm titanium or cobalt chrome rod for the entire construct with smaller thoracic screws, or using two separate rods connected by side-to-side connectors. Tatsumi et al. [21] and Eleraky et al. [22] both directly compared the three in vitro. Tatsumi found that the 3.5 mm rod fails at a lower force than the other two constructs [21]. However, Eleraky did not duplicate these results in cadavers, finding no difference between the three [22]. Finally, Yang et al. [23] found that, in practice, there were no differences in failure rates between the smaller and transitional rods, but use of the transitional rods did add to operative time and blood loss. They did not compare the side-to-side construct [23].

The findings by Yang et al. reflect the difficulty in seating the transition rod. If the C7 lateral mass screws do not align with the T1 pedicle screws, bending the transitional rod at the C7–T1 can be a challenge. Clinically, we have successfully used single-diameter 3.5 mm cobalt-chromium rods, which have been found to be robust and stiff in cadavers [24].

When instrumenting C7, either pedicle screws or lateral mass screws can be utilized. This is due to the relatively larger pedicles at C7 along with the absence of the vertebral artery at that level. If C7 is the cranial-most segment instrumented, pedicle screws are stronger than lateral mass screws [25]. However, if including levels above C7, the screw types are equivalent [25]. Cervical pedicle screws at C3–C6 are problematic as they traverse a very narrow corridor between the vertebral artery and the neural structures. Their malposition rate is relatively high with or without navigation [26]. For placing cervical [27] and upper thoracic pedicle screws, navigation has been shown to be safe and effective, but it adds time and expense to the case. However, in the upper thoracic spine, it hasn't been shown to be superior to the freehand technique [28, 29]. This is likely due to the large diameter of the average T1–T3 pedicle.

Technique

Indications/Contraindications for a Posterior Approach Crossing the CTJ

Indications

- Cervical stenosis that requires posterior decompression or foraminal stenosis that requires extensive foraminotomies at the C6 or C7 level necessitates extension of the fusion across the CTJ.
- Cases of continued multisegmental OPLL should generally be addressed from a posterior approach.

Contraindications (relative)

- Loss of cervical lordosis (unless osteotomies are planned)

Indications/Contraindications for an Anterior Approach Crossing the CTJ

Indications

- Significant anterior pathology (tumor, infection, fracture) requiring anterior decompression
- Deformity correction that cannot be sufficiently addressed from a posterior approach

Contraindications

- High-riding manubrium or aortic arch blocking anterior access (unless an approach surgeon is to be considered for manubriotomy)

Preop Planning

- Preop MRI delineates the amount of stenosis requiring decompression.
- Preop CT is helpful for preop planning. The width, length, and angles of the cervical lateral masses and thoracic pedicles can be measured on CT to assist in screw starting points, trajectories, and sizing. Any anatomic abnormalities should also be noted.
- Standing 36" long cassette X-rays should be used for cases with suspected preexisting deformity [10].
- Intraoperative adjuncts:
  - Electrophysiological monitoring can be used to monitor SSEP, MEP, and free-running EMG.
    - Triggered EMG has little use at the cervicothoracic junction.
    - MEP has been shown to be useful in detecting neurologic deficits intraoperatively [30]. See Fig. 33.2 for our neuromonitoring alert checklist.
  - Intraoperative image guidance is an option, with most surgeons using fluoroscopy vs intraoperative CT with navigation.
- Anesthetic considerations: Efforts should be made for preoperative optimization, including cardiopulmonary clearance, blood pressure control, smoking cessation, and nutrition. Communication between anesthesiology and electrophysiology is essential for reliable SSEP and MEP. In case of a change in neuromonitoring signals, a checklist may be followed [31]. Intraoperatively, mean arterial blood pressure should be maintained above 85–90, if tolerated, to ensure adequate spinal cord perfusion.

Operative Technique

The patient is taken to the operating room and intubated by anesthesia services. Careful attention must be paid to avoid excessive extension by anesthesia during intubation. A fiber-optic intubation may be required. In cases of severe central stenosis, pre- and postpositioning intraoperative neuromonitoring baselines should be obtained.

A cranial fixation device is placed. Options include a Mayfield head holder, Gardner Wells tongs, or a Jackson table with traction. The patient is carefully turned prone on to a reversed OR bed with chest rolls. Care must be taken when turning a patient prone in order to keep from exacerbating spinal cord compression in the anesthetized patient. A careful log roll with full attention and coordination among the operating team is employed. The body should be parallel to the floor, and the chin should not be touching anything.

Careful attention needs to be paid to the positioning of the head. The patient's neck should be neutral. This can be confirmed by visualizing the patient's entire posture on the OR table and with intraoperative fluoroscopy. If correcting kyphosis, mild undercorrection is preferred to overcorrection, as this will still allow the patient to look at the ground while walking. Once adequate positioning is obtained, the head should be fixed to the table with the cranial fixation device.

Fluoroscopy is used to mark upper thoracic vertebrae. Lateral fluoroscopy is likely to be obscured by the shoulders, but anterior-posterior fluoroscopy may prove useful.

Preoperative antibiotics and steroids are given.

The cervical decompression and fusion is covered elsewhere and won't be described extensively. Mean arterial pressures should be maintained or elevated to 90 mm Hg during the decompression to ensure adequate spinal cord perfusion at this critical point.

A subperiosteal dissection of paraspinal muscles off posterior elements is performed. This is extended lateral to reveal transverse processes at thoracic vertebrae and lateral masses at cervical vertebrae. Care is taken to preserve facet capsules of cranial- and caudal-most levels.

C7 can be instrumented with either lateral mass or pedicle screws. The lateral masses tend to be smaller than those of the more cranial levels, but the starting points and trajectories are the same. For pedicle screw placement, the starting point is at the midpoint of the lateral mass with a 30–40° medial angulation. A laminotomy can be

Checklist for Neuromonitoring (MEP) Alert in Patients with Myelopathy or Deformity

***Spine Surgeon*:**

- ☐ Stop current manipulation
- ☐ Assess field for structural cord compression (misplaced hardware or bone graft, osteophytes, or hematoma)
  - ☐ Perform further decompression if stenosis is present
- ☐ Consider reversing correction of a spinal deformity

Neurophysiologist:

- ☐ Repeat trials of MEPs and SSEPs to rule out potential false positive
- ☐ Check all leads to make sure no pull-out, may add leads in proximal muscle groups if possible
- ☐ Assess the pattern of changes
  - ☐ Asymmetric changes (associated with cord or nerve root injury)
  - ☐ Symmetric changes (associated with anesthetic or hypotension issues)
- ☐ Quantify improvement and communicate to the surgical team

Anesthesiologist:

- ☐ Check if neuromuscular blockade (muscle relaxant) given
  - If yes, ☐ Check train of four (TOF)
- ☐ Verify that no change in anesthetic administration occurred
- ☐ Assess anesthetic depth
  - ☐ BP ☐ RR ☐ HR ☐ BIS monitor (If available)
- ☐ Restore or maintain blood pressure (goal mean arterial pressure of 90-100)
- ☐ Check Hemoglobin/Hematocrit (goal hemoglobin >9-10)
- ☐ Check temperature and I/O's for adequate resuscitation
- ☐ Check extremity position in case of plexus palsy
- ☐ Lighten depth of anesthesia
  - ☐ Reduce to 1/3 MAC or temporarily eliminate inhaled agents (i.e. desflurane)
  - ☐ Reduce intravenous anesthetics such as propofol (which may accumulate systemically during the case and blunt MEPs)
  - ☐ Add adjuvant agents such as Ketamine to permit reduction of MEP suppressive agents (i.e. propofol and inhalational anesthetics)

IF No Change:

- ☐ Increase MAP >100
- ☐ Consider Steroid Administration
- ☐ Consider Wake-up test
- ☐ Consider Aborting surgery
- ☐ Consider Calcium Channel Blocker (topical to cord or iv)

Fig. 33.2 Checklist for response to a neuromonitoring alert. This assumes the baseline anesthetic regimen is 1/3 – 1/2 MAC halogenated anesthetic and total intravenous anesthesia with propofol ± ketamine. BIS bispectral index, BP blood pressure, HR heart rate, I/O input/output, MAC minimum alveolar concentratio, MAP mean arterial pressure, MEP motor evoked potential, RR respiration rate, SSEP somatosensory evoked potential. (Adopted from Ziewacz et al. [31])

performed to palpate the medial edge of the pedicle and help guide trajectory [32]. Alternatively, C7 can be skipped to better align the tulip heads from the cervical to thoracic screws and make rod placement easier.

The entry point for upper thoracic screws is just caudal to the superior articulating process at the junction with the transverse process (Fig. 33.3). Adequate starting placement can be confirmed with AP fluoroscopy. Navigation can also be used. Similar to the technique described for C7, the medial pedicle of T1 can often be palpated via a laminotomy to assist in screw placement. Creating small laminotomies to palpate the superior and inferior borders of the pedicles is an alternative approach used to ensure accuracy.

The cortical bone over the starting point can be canulated with the high-speed drill, and a thoracic gearshift can be used to advance into the pedicle. A "pedicle blush" or bleeding cancellous bone of the pedicle often confirms accuracy of the starting point.

Medial angulation of the pedicle is approximately 30° at T1–2. Cranial-caudal angulation should be parallel to the end plate. A sharp, curved gearshift probe is used to enter the pedicle. The curve of the probe is turned laterally for the first 15 mm, which is the depth of the pedicle. This keeps the gearshift angled away from the spinal canal. At this point, the probe is removed and the hole is palpated with a ball-tip feeler. If no breach is felt, the probe can be reinserted with the curve pointed medial to a depth determined by preoperative imaging, usually 24–28 mm.

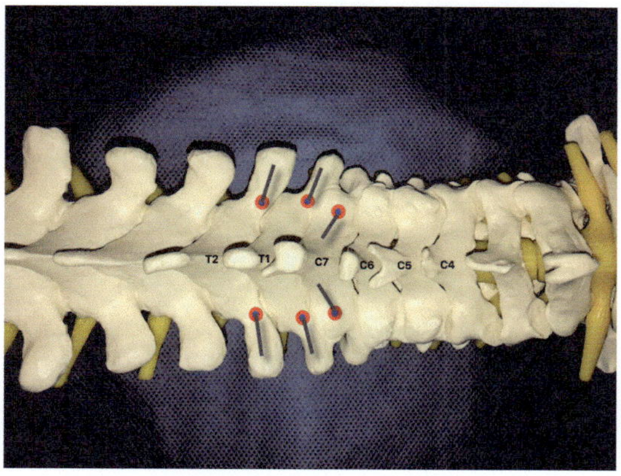

Fig. 33.3 Starting points for C7 lateral mass screws and T1–T2 pedicle screws. The starting point for the lateral mass screws is 1 mm medial and inferior to the midpoint of the lateral mass, although for C7 the entry point can be placed slightly more superior to allow for easy alignment of the rod as it transitions to the thoracic pedicle screws. The starting point for the thoracic screws is at the intersection of the transverse process to the superior articulating process. The thoracic screws are angled 30° lateral to medial in the axial plane and orthogonal to the curvature of the thoracic spine in the sagittal plane

The hole is then tapped 1 mm smaller than the intended screw diameter. A polyaxial screw is then inserted utilizing the same trajectories. This is repeated for the remaining levels. Adequate screw placement can be confirmed with intraoperative CT or AP fluoroscopy.

Thoracic screw heads can accommodate 3.5, 4.5, and 5.5 mm rods. Selection of thoracic screws will determine the eventual rod construct. If thoracic screw heads are larger than cervical screw heads, a transitional rod or side-to-side domino construct must be used.

The thoracic pedicle screw heads will likely be more lateral than the cervical lateral mass screws. This can create difficulty in aligning a rod across the CTJ. As previously mentioned, the C7 screws can be skipped to help with rod placement. The C7 lateral mass screw can also be placed slightly more superior to the midpoint of the lateral mass, to allow a more gradual transition and allow the rod to more easily capture the C7 screw head. Lateral offsets are also available and can be used as another option to help capture the rod.

Extensive decortication of facet joints and bony surfaces should be performed before rod placement. Autograft from the prior laminectomy can be morselized and placed posterolaterally. Allograft can be supplemented as well. BMP may be considered; however it is an off-label FDA application [19], with some surgeons using it for salvage of prior pseudoarthrosis cases.

The rods are then measured, cut, and contoured before placement. If using a transitional rod, careful marking of the length on either side of the taper is required. Each side must be separately cut to the appropriate size and contoured to the appropriate shape.

Some surgeons use 3.5 mm cobalt chromium rods to span the CTJ. Domino connectors can also be used to connect a 3.5 mm to 5.5 mm rod. These are equally strong as the transition rod; however they can be cumbersome and bulky. Care must be taken when working with hardware over an exposed cervical dura. Domino connectors can also take up valuable graft space.

After the rods are locked into place, vancomycin powder may be placed, along with local anesthetic in the muscle. The wound is closed in a standard layered closure over a subfascial drain.

Post-op Care

- Patients can typically be sent to the floor. However, it is not uncommon to send a patient to the ICU for close neuromonitoring or blood pressure control.
- Intraop or post-op CT may be used to confirm adequate hardware placement, but this is not mandatory. Many surgeons use intraoperative fluoroscopy and post-op X-rays.
- Patients may stay on IV antibiotics for 24 h post-op or while the drain is in place. The drain is typically removed when output declines.
- 36" standing long cassette X-rays can be obtained to assess new sagittal and coronal balance. This can be done at follow up as well.
- Bracing with a collar is typical for poor bone quality or significant deformity.
- Mobilize patients on post-op day 1 unless there was a CSF leak.
- Pain control with IV and oral narcotics. Avoid NSAID use to promote fusion.

Complication Management

- If a medial breach is detected, a new pilot hole will need to be placed using the gearshift. This should be tapped to ensure the screw doesn't follow the old path.
- Vascular injury is rare, and we would seek consultation to vascular surgery or interventional radiology. The contralateral side should not be cannulated if a vertebral artery injury is suspected.
- If a CSF leak occurs, then primary repair should be attempted. Dural sealants are also available to supplement a primary closure. A watertight fascial closure is essential, and we usually order that the head of the bed be elevated to 30° postoperatively. A soft tissue drain may be placed and connected to gravity bag to decrease potential for a pseudomeningocele. Lumbar drainage may be necessary for persistent leaks (Table 33.1).

Table 33.1 CSF leak management

Dura repair
Primary repair
Dural sealant – Supplement
Wound closure
Watertight fascial closure
Postoperative care
Head of bed elevated to 30°
Soft tissue drain connected to a gravity bag
Persistent leak
Lumbar drainage

Case Presentation

A 62-year-old female presented with 4 years of neck pain that radiates down the entirety of the right upper extremity. She also endorsed bilateral hand numbness and wasting of the muscles in both hands. She had difficulty with fine motor skills, had been dropping things, and noted a change in her handwriting. She had mild gait difficulty and denied any bowel or bladder symptoms. She had a history of osteoporosis, and despite a 2-year course of teriparatide, her T score remained a –2.5.

On physical exam, she had bilateral grip and intraosseous weakness with obvious bilateral muscle atrophy. She was diffusely hyperreflexic. She did not exhibit a Hoffman's or clonus. She could ambulate with an unsteady gait. Her mJOA score was 12/18.

Her preoperative imaging (Fig. 33.4) demonstrated a swan-neck cervical deformity, C3–C4 spondylolisthesis, and central canal stenosis. Her

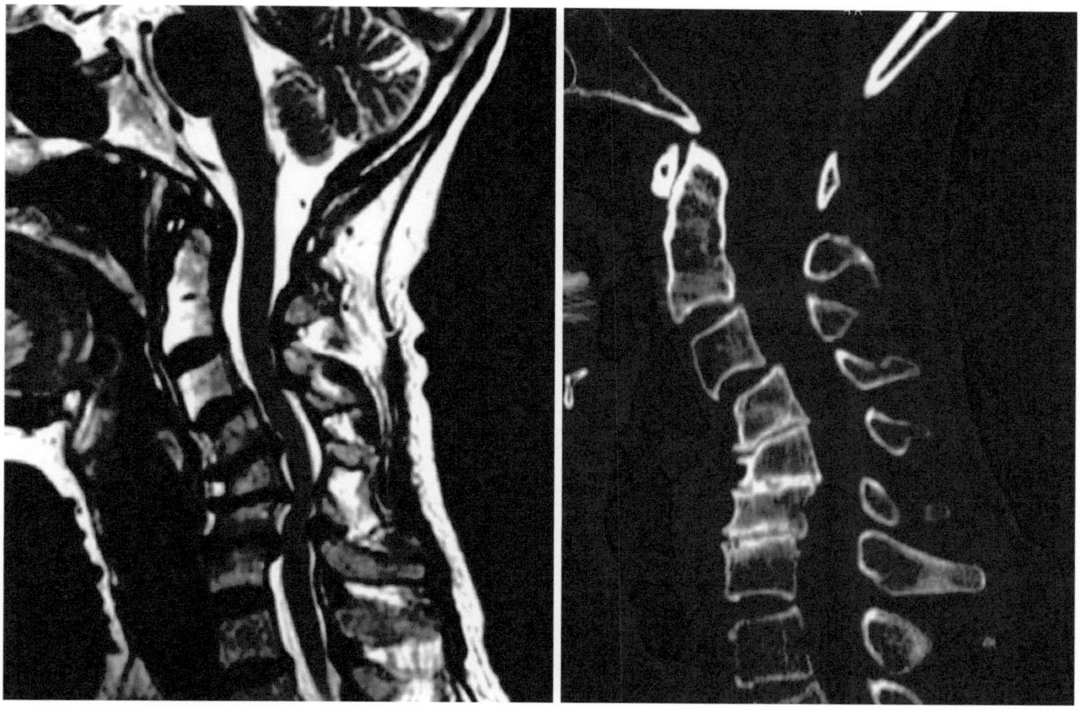

Fig. 33.4 Preoperative sagittal MRI and CT scan of the cervical spine. MRI shows disc bulges compressing the spinal cord anteriorly at C4–C5, C5–C6, and C6–C7. There is ligamentous buckling posteriorly at C6–C7 causing additional spinal cord compression. CT shows extensive disc osteophytes and C3–C4 spondylolisthesis

exam and imaging findings confirmed the diagnosis of cervical spondylotic myelopathy. The patient underwent a staged anterior and posterior decompression and fusion.

For the anterior stage, done first, the patient was positioned supine. A Mayfield clamp was placed and a 3 liter bag of saline attached to provide gentle traction. Anterior cervical discectomies were performed at C4–C5, C5–C6, and C6–C7; 6 mm allograft implants filled with autograft from osteophytes were used at each level. A plate and anterior drain were placed. Although C7/T1 could be accessed in this case, the anterior correction achieved from C4 to C7 was adequate. Inclusion of the additional level would increase the risk of postoperative swallowing difficulties, and thus it was addressed in the posterior stage.

The posterior stage was completed the following day. She was positioned prone in a Mayfield clamp. A midline incision was made, and a subperiosteal dissection was performed to expose the spinous processes of C2–T1. This was extended laterally to expose the lateral masses of C2–C7 along with the transverse processes of T1. Lateral mass screws were placed bilaterally at C4–C7. A left C3 lateral mass screw was placed, but the right C3 screw was left out due to an atretic lateral mass. Bilateral C2 pars screws were placed. A right C3–C4 allograft intrafacet spacer was placed for additional fusion mass and to distract the foramen. A C7 laminectomy was then performed.

Starting holes for bilateral C7 lateral mass screws and T1 pedicle screws were placed. The superior and medial borders of the T1 pedicles could be palpated because of the C7 laminectomy. Using this to guide trajectory, the pedicles were cannulated with a curved probe and tapped, and screws were placed (Fig. 33.5). C7 lateral mass screws were placed last, using a mildly superior starting position, 1 mm cranial to the center of the lateral mass, to allow easier alignment of the screw heads (Fig. 33.6). See Figs. 33.7 and 33.8 for the finished construct.

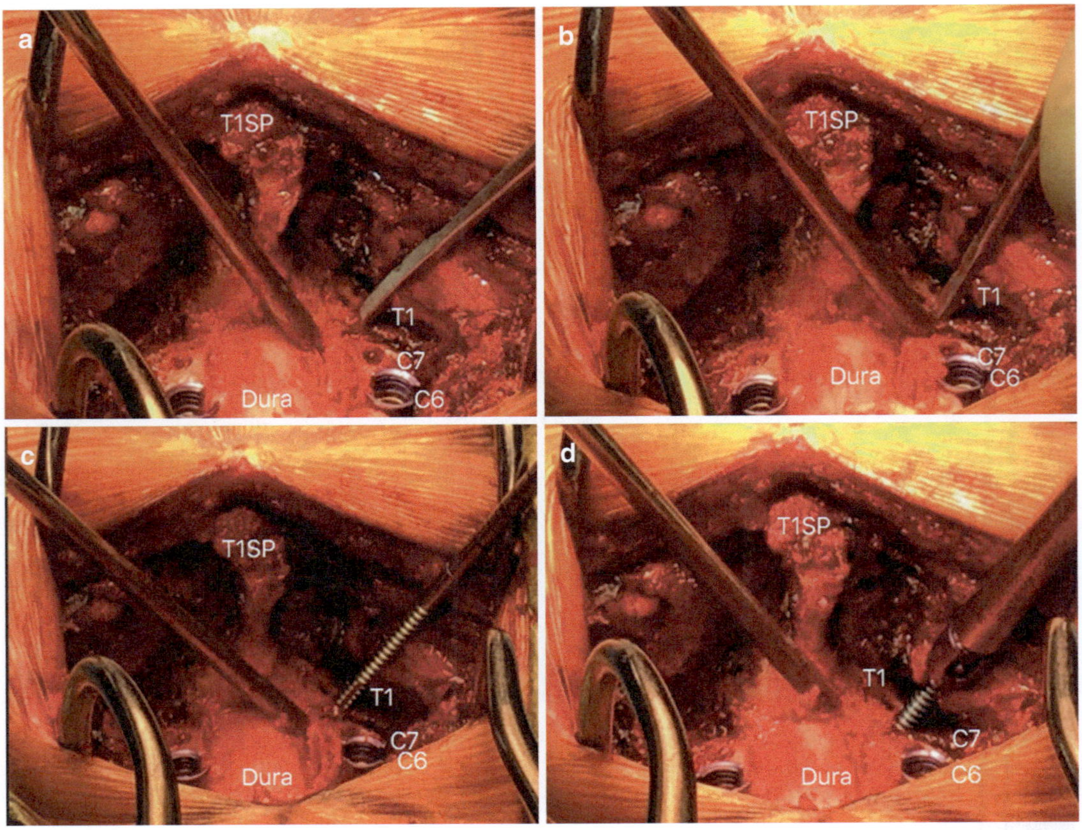

Fig. 33.5 Placement of the left T1 screw. The cortical bone over the starting point was drilled with the high-speed burr. (**a**) the curved gearshift is placed with the point facing lateral to direct it away from the medial neural structures. The medial and superior borders of the pedicle can be palpated due to the prior C7 laminectomy. (**b**) The probe is withdrawn after 15 mm, and the hole is palpated before reinserting the gearshift with the point facing medially. (**c**) The hole is palpated and tapped. (**d**) The screw is inserted. T1SP T1 spinous process

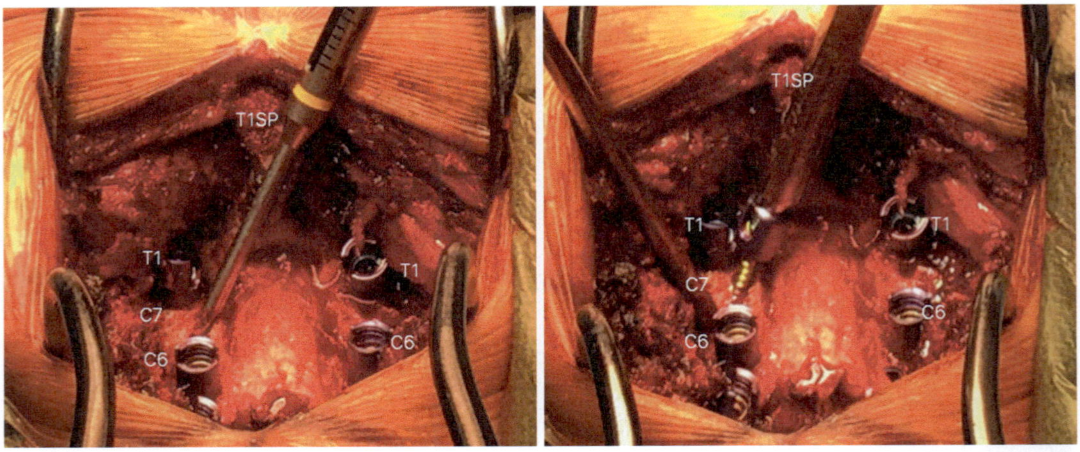

Fig. 33.6 Placement of right C7 lateral mass screw. A more cranial starting point was chosen (1 mm superior to the midpoint of the lateral mass). This provides more room between the screw heads of C7 and T1, facilitating easier rod placement. T1SP T1 spinous process

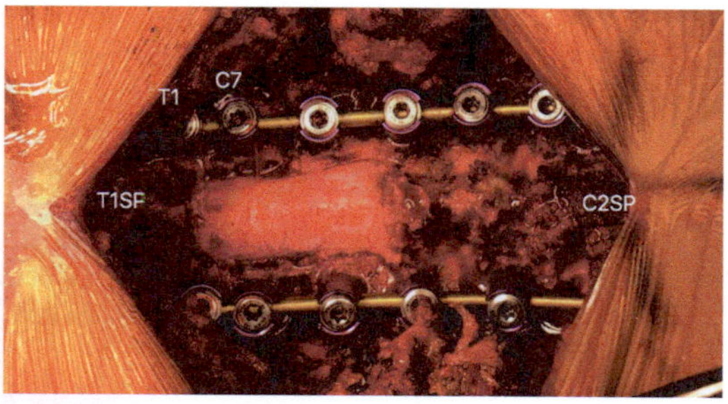

Fig. 33.7 The finished construct. The more cranial C7 lateral mass screw with polyaxial head allowed the rod to be placed with minimal manipulation, decreasing the chance that the exposed cervical cord would be inadvertently damaged. C2SP spinous process of C2, T1SP spinous process of T1

The patient was able to ambulate the next day. She was kept in a rigid collar for 6 weeks and has had no complications thus far.

Conclusion

The anatomically unique CTJ can present a challenge. Decompressions have a high likelihood of destabilizing the region, making it susceptible to deformity. Fusions that stop at C7, likewise, add stress to the junction and can predispose to increased degeneration.

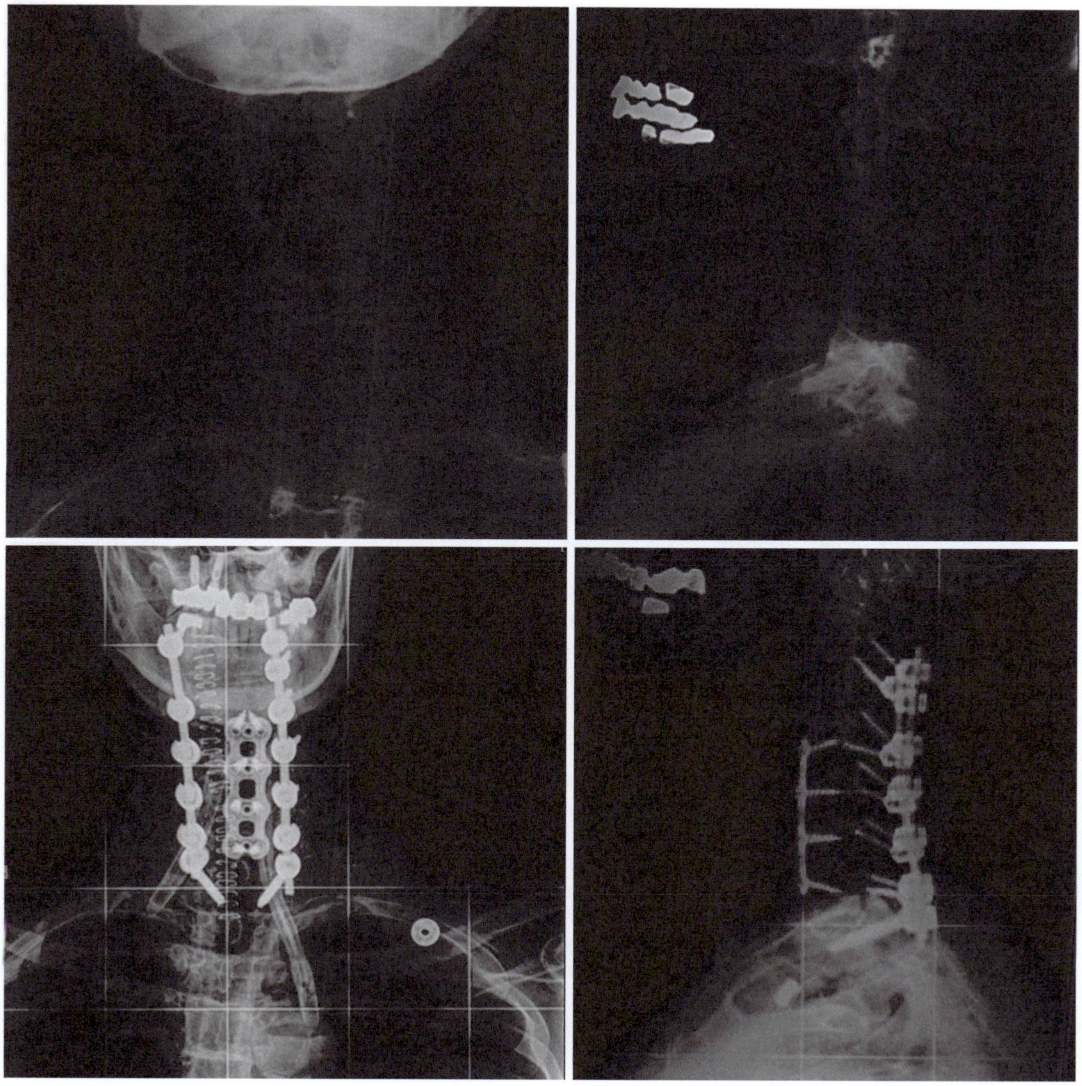

Fig. 33.8 Pre- and postoperative AP and lateral C spine X-rays showing correction of the deformity

In the case we presented, the deformity extending to the CT junction made the decision to fuse across it an easy one. However, this is not always the case, and some surgeons will stop a posterior fusion at C6 or C7. We do not recommend stopping at the junction, choosing a caudal fixation point of C6 or T1 instead of stopping at C7, as this does not lead to significantly greater disability and likely reduces the rate of deformity and fusion failure.

References

1. Jeanneret B, et al. Posterior stabilization of the cervical spine with hook plates. Spine (Phila Pa 1976). 1991;16(3 Suppl):S56–63.
2. Espinoza-Larios A, et al. Biomechanical comparison of two-level cervical locking posterior screw/rod and hook/rod techniques. Spine J. 2007;7(2):194–204.
3. Mihir B, et al. Anterior instrumentation of the cervicothoracic vertebrae: approach based on clinical and radiologic criteria. Spine (Phila Pa 1976). 2006;31(9):E244–9.
4. Mai HT, et al. Accessibility of the cervicothoracic junction through an anterior approach: an MRI-based algorithm. Spine (Phila Pa 1976). 2016;41(1):69–73.
5. Falavigna A, Righesso O, Teles AR. Anterior approach to the cervicothoracic junction: proposed indication for manubriotomy based on preoperative computed tomography findings. J Neurosurg Spine. 2011;15(1):38–47.
6. Schlenk RP, Kowalski RJ, Benzel EC. Biomechanics of spinal deformity. Neurosurg Focus. 2003;14(1):e2.
7. Lapsiwala S, Benzel E. Surgical management of cervical myelopathy dealing with the cervical-thoracic junction. Spine J. 2006;6(6 Suppl):268S–73S.
8. Liu S, et al. Impact of dynamic alignment, motion, and center of rotation on myelopathy grade and regional disability in cervical spondylotic myelopathy. J Neurosurg Spine. 2015;23(6):690–700.
9. Anderson PA, et al. Laminectomy and fusion for the treatment of cervical degenerative myelopathy. J Neurosurg Spine. 2009;11(2):150–6.
10. Mummaneni PV, Deutsch H, Mummaneni VP. Cervicothoracic kyphosis. Neurosurg Clin N Am. 2006;17(3):277–87. vi.
11. Steinmetz MP, et al. Regional instability following cervicothoracic junction surgery. J Neurosurg Spine. 2006;4(4):278–84.
12. Bechara BP, et al. In vivo analysis of cervical range of motion after 4- and 5-level subaxial cervical spine fusion. Spine (Phila Pa 1976). 2012;37(1):E23–9.
13. Mazel C, et al. Posterior cervicothoracic instrumentation in spine tumors. Spine (Phila Pa 1976). 2004;29(11):1246–53.
14. Post NH, et al. Unique features of herniated discs at the cervicothoracic junction: clinical presentation, imaging, operative management, and outcome after anterior decompressive operation in 10 patients. Neurosurgery. 2006;58(3):497–501. discussion 497-501.
15. Kaya RA, et al. A perspective for the selection of surgical approaches in patients with upper thoracic and cervicothoracic junction instabilities. Surg Neurol. 2006;65(5):454–63. discussion 463.
16. Cheng I, et al. Biomechanical determination of distal level for fusions across the cervicothoracic junction. Global Spine J. 2015;5(4):282–6.
17. Highsmith JM, et al. Treatment of cervical stenotic myelopathy: a cost and outcome comparison of laminoplasty versus laminectomy and lateral mass fusion. J Neurosurg Spine. 2011;14(5):619–25.
18. Guppy KH, et al. Reoperation rates for symptomatic nonunions in posterior cervicothoracic fusions with and without bone morphogenetic protein in a cohort of 450 patients. J Neurosurg Spine. 2016;25(3):309–17.
19. Goode AP, et al. Complications, revision fusions, readmissions, and utilization over a 1-year period after bone morphogenetic protein use during primary cervical spine fusions. Spine J. 2014;14(9):2051–9.
20. Hamilton DK, et al. Safety, efficacy, and dosing of recombinant human bone morphogenetic protein-2 for posterior cervical and cervicothoracic instrumented fusion with a minimum 2-year follow-up. Neurosurgery. 2011;69(1):103–11. discussion 111.
21. Tatsumi RL, et al. Mechanical comparison of posterior instrumentation constructs for spinal fixation across the cervicothoracic junction. Spine (Phila Pa 1976). 2007;32(10):1072–6.
22. Eleraky M, et al. Biomechanical comparison of posterior cervicothoracic instrumentation techniques after one-level laminectomy and facetectomy. J Neurosurg Spine. 2010;13(5):622–9.
23. Yang JS, Buchowski JM, Verma V. Construct type and risk factors for pseudarthrosis at the cervicothoracic junction. Spine (Phila Pa 1976). 2015;40(11):E613–7.
24. Scheer JK, et al. Biomechanical analysis of cervicothoracic junction osteotomy in cadaveric model of ankylosing spondylitis: effect of rod material and diameter. J Neurosurg Spine. 2011;14(3):330–5.
25. Rhee JM, Kraiwattanapong C, Hutton WC. A comparison of pedicle and lateral mass screw construct stiffnesses at the cervicothoracic junction: a biomechanical study. Spine (Phila Pa 1976). 2005;30(21):E636–40.
26. Hojo Y, et al. A multicenter study on accuracy and complications of freehand placement of cervical pedicle screws under lateral fluoroscopy in different pathological conditions: CT-based evaluation of more than 1,000 screws. Eur Spine J. 2014;23(10):2166–74.
27. Singh PK, et al. Computed tomography-guided C2 pedicle screw placement for treatment of unstable hangman fractures. Spine (Phila Pa 1976). 2014;39(18):E1058–65.

28. Nottmeier EW, Pirris SM. Placement of thoracic transvertebral pedicle screws using 3D image guidance. J Neurosurg Spine. 2013;18(5):479–83.
29. Hart RA, et al. Pedicle screw placement in the thoracic spine: a comparison of image-guided and manual techniques in cadavers. Spine (Phila Pa 1976). 2005;30(12):E326–31.
30. Clark AJ, et al. Comparative sensitivity of intraoperative motor evoked potential monitoring in predicting postoperative neurologic deficits: nondegenerative versus degenerative myelopathy. Global Spine J. 2016;6(5):452–8.
31. Ziewacz JE, et al. The design, development, and implementation of a checklist for intraoperative neuromonitoring changes. Neurosurg Focus. 2012;33(5):E11.
32. Jeanneret B, Gebhard JS, Magerl F. Transpedicular screw fixation of articular mass fracture-separation: results of an anatomical study and operative technique. J Spinal Disord. 1994;7(3):222–9.

Osteotomy for Cervical Kyphosis

34

Joseph A. Osorio, Justin K. Scheer,
Derek G. Southwell, and Christopher P. Ames

Pitfalls/Pearls Outline

1. Intraoperative neuromonitoring and imaging guidance systems can help prevent complications related to the cervical osteotomy.
2. All posterior approaches may reduce but do not eliminate swallowing dysfunction.
3. Given complexities of the regional anatomy, osteotomy techniques which are common in the thoracic and lumbar spine must be adapted to the cervical region.
4. Smith-Petersen osteotomy is ideal for subaxial flexible deformity.
5. C7 PSO is best for correction of mid to low subaxial rigid deformity for correction of cervical sagittal imbalance.

J. A. Osorio · J. K. Scheer
D. G. Southwell · C. P. Ames (✉)
Department of Neurological Surgery,
University of California, San Francisco, CA, USA
e-mail: Amesc@neurosurg.ucsf.edu

Introduction

Etiologies of cervical kyphosis are diverse and may include neuromuscular, degenerative, post-traumatic, neoplastic, and iatrogenic conditions as well as systemic conditions such as ankylosing spondylitis and rheumatoid arthritis [1].

Surgical correction should be considered if the patient does not respond to a nonoperative treatment or demonstrates evidence of progressive myelopathy, radiculopathy, or functional disability, such as inability to achieve horizontal gaze, tension-/kyphosis-induced myelopathy, neck pain due to head imbalance, or swallowing dysfunction related to head position [2–6]. The spinal cord may be decompressed effectively by an anterior, posterior, or combined approach, but full decompression may require deformity correction as in cases of kyphosis. Supplemental posterior fixation minimizes the risk of anterior dislodgement of the graft even in the presence of solid anterior fixation [7]. Surgical correction of cervical kyphosis is challenging and requires a clear understanding of the disease and the patient. The surgeon must be very comfortable with remobilizing the spinal column anteriorly and posteriorly, with vertebral artery anatomy and with methods of anterior and posterior correction.

Significant, irreducible deformity of the cervical spine may be sufficient to require corrective osteotomy. Rigid deformities of the cervical

M. G. Kaiser et al. (eds.), *Degenerative Cervical Myelopathy and Radiculopathy*,
https://doi.org/10.1007/978-3-319-97952-6_34

spine below the craniocervical junction are more likely to require some kind of osteotomy in order to correct the deformity and restore horizontal gaze. This chapter details the preoperative considerations and surgical procedures of two of the most common cervical osteotomies for cervical kyphosis: [1] Smith-Petersen osteotomy and the C7 subtraction osteotomy (PSO).

Main Ideas Supported by Relevant Literature and References

2013 Cervical SVA Matters

Cervical deformity can occur in both the sagittal and coronal planes, but the sagittal plane deformities arise more frequently. Correction of the sagittal plane deformity has been shown to have an important and positive impact on clinical outcomes. There are two broad categories that cervical deformities can be categorized into: primary or secondary deformity. Primary cervical deformities are congenital in etiology, whereas secondary deformities are a result of iatrogenic sequelae or ankylosing spondylitis.

The goal of cervical deformity surgery is an attempt to restore horizontal gaze, decompress any known compression upon the neural elements, and restore cervical spine alignment. Cervical spinal alignment is focally assessed by evaluating the cervical SVA, which has been shown that larger C2 SVA relates to poorer HRQOL.

2010: T1 Angle -> Proportional to Cervical Sagittal Balance

Cervical alignment parameters were studied to have a better understanding of how the measurement of SVA is differed when it was measured from C2 as opposed from C7. The 2010 study demonstrated that when SVA was measured from C2, the value was on average farther than when the measurement was taken from C7. Furthermore, when evaluating the usefulness of a T1 sagittal angle, there was a strong correlation with the SVA as it is measured using C2 and the T1 sagittal angle. This was suggestive that the T1 sagittal angle was very useful in evaluating sagittal balance, and this gave particular importance to the importance of the T1 angle and the particular significance to the role it holds when evaluating cervical deformity. In patients who are candidates for cervical deformity operations, the common indication being severe cervical kyphosis, these parameters become the keystone to correction of the regional spinal deformity.

2012: Standing Cervical Films Are Not Only Superior but a Requirement for Cervical Deformity

The radiographs used to calculate global alignment are known to be different in the standing versus the recumbent position, and the same holds true for cervical radiographs. Cervical sagittal alignment is affected by global alignment variables, and the impact of the global parameters upon the cervical region can be shown through the 2012 study. This study determined that a value of 40 mm was the upper limit of the normal range when evaluating the C2–C7 SVA parameter as it correlates to the impact upon HRQOL. Similar correlations were found between C2–C7 SVA and NDI scores.

CBVA: Chin-Brow Vertical Angle

The chin-brow vertical angle (CBVA) is a measurement that is made to give a numerical representation of the horizontal gaze of the patient. It should be included in all evaluations where cervical deformity is being considered, and the amount of correction that is planned could take into account the starting CBVA and the desired goal. After a patient has successfully completed surgery, it is imperative to have adequate follow-up care. Addressing the CBVA appropriately has shown to be valuable, with improvements having been associated with improved gaze, ambulation, and activities of daily living.

Cervical Alignment Is Proportional to HRQOL (2015)

Improvements in regional cervical alignment and cervical lordosis have demonstrated a relationship with HRQOL improvements in the thoracolumbar deformity patient. This impact upon the regional disability and health status of patients may be a direct or reciprocal effect of the global alignment and the importance of cervical alignment.

You Have to Be Mindful of Thoracolumbar Deformity Prior to Treating Cervical Deformity Because the T/L Deformity Correction May Also Complimentary Correct the Cervical Deformity

When evaluating cervical parameters, a complete evaluation should include films where the entire global balance can be assessed including any imbalance in the thoracolumbar region. These changes are important to note because of the potential implications that could have a causative effect from a separate, downstream problem. This was shown in a 2014 study by Ha et al., where cervical lordosis changes were noted in patients that had a thoracolumbar operation and correction of SVA imbalance.

Classification System of Cervical Deformity Exists and Should Be Used (2015 Ames)

A cervical spine deformity (CSD) classification system was generated to provide a mechanism to assess the CSD patient within a framework of global spinopelvic malalignment and clinically relevant parameters. This classification system included a deformity descriptor to describe the apex of the curve location, and it also included five modifiers (both radiographically measured parameters and a clinical score to characterize the degree of myelopathy). All of the five modifiers that were used as parameters that were used in this classification had been previously shown to have clinical impact. It is important to consider a common language for discussing these cases, and using this classification system provides a method for doing so.

Scoli Films in Fact Should Be Used Not Just Cervical Films (2015)

When addressing a cervical kyphosis primary problem, it still is important to consider global balance. As was previously discussed in the CSD classification, the Schwab classification system in characterizing global balance is integrated to provide a full assessment of alignment. Long-cassette standing X-rays are suggested when planning for cervical spine surgery to have a better understanding of both the current implications of global spinopelvic alignment and also to determine if there is a primary or additional thoracolumbar misalignment.

Management Is Quite Important, Different, and Delicate

In the decision and assessment prior to surgery, the flexibility of the kyphosis is an integral component to understanding the nature of the curve and how modifiable it is with an operation. Any curvature in the spine can be categorized into three separate categories, which include curves that are flexible, fixed, or fused. There are times when differentiating between a fixed and a fused curve can be challenging. A fixed curve is categorized in between a flexible and fused curve because although it has the ability to be mobile, this characteristic may not be easily apparent. There are times when placing a patient in traction will elicit the mobility of a kyphotic curve. Determining this additional information may change one's understanding of a kyphotic deformity from feeling as though a deformity is fused to one that is mobile. The importance here lies in that a fused curve will certainly require additional maneuvers and releasing maneuvers to manipulate and correct the curvature deformity. It is in the setting of a fused curve, that the most invasive osteotomies are often required.

Traction Could Give You Insight to the Kind of Deformity

Spinal traction is a useful intervention for the cervical deformity patient that can be an adjunct that could be utilized in the preoperative assessment and the perioperative and intraoperative management. Assessment of the kyphotic curve flexibility is not always straightforward, and there are curves that are in fact fixed, but they could appear to be fused. The value in appropriately classifying the flexibility of the curve in the preoperative stage could provide insight to an operative plan that would otherwise be quite different if it is believed that a curve is fused. It is in these settings that spinal traction will provide an assessment that will become a facet of the treatment and operative plan.

Osteotomies of the Cervical Spine

Indications/Contraindications

Cervical osteotomy could be considered as a surgical intervention if the patient does not respond to conservative treatment or shows evidence of deteriorating myelopathy, radiculopathy, or functional impairment, such as inability to achieve horizontal gaze, swallowing dysfunction related to head position, tension-/kyphosis-induced myelopathy, or neck pain due to head imbalance [2–5, 8]. Additionally the spinal cord may be decompressed effectively by the posterior approach, but full decompression may require deformity correction to allow cord migration and decrease cord tension as in cases of kyphosis. Supplemental posterior fixation minimizes the risk of anterior dislodgement of the graft even in the presence of solid anterior fixation [7]. Treatment of cervical kyphosis is challenging and requires a clear understanding of the regional and global balance (Fig. 34.4).

It is important when planning surgery for cervical kyphosis to consider whether the deformity is rigid or fixed and whether there is presence of neurological symptoms. In the flexible subaxial deformity, a posterior stabilization (usually C2–T2) is advocated, and when the deformity is semirigid, SPO with anterior osteoclasis should be considered. In the setting of a rigid cervical kyphosis with an apex in the low cervical spine with cervical sagittal imbalance or angle of gaze issues, a C7 or T1 PSO or SPO with a classic opening wedge osteotomy may be required. We typically perform PSO on all patients as we consider the closure to be more controlled and no anterior gap is created that may require subsequent grafting. Cervical PSO is biomechanically more stable than SPO [9].

Preoperative Planning

History

The patient's history may include past trauma and include concurrent illness of ankylosing spondylitis or rheumatoid arthritis as well as previous cervical spine surgery, degenerative, and neoplastic disorders.

Signs and Symptoms

Symptoms may include suboccipital headache and neck stiffness, occipital neuralgia, symptoms of myelopathy, or progressive deformity leading to functional impairment, such as difficulty with looking forward or with eating and drinking. Patients may complain of low back pain and standing fatigue due to use of compensatory muscles to elevate pelvic tilt to alter gaze angle.

Physical Examination

It is critical to obtain 3 foot X-rays and to examine patients while standing. Occasionally, lumbar sagittal deformities will need to be corrected first. Correction of lumbar imbalance will alter head position substantially especially in rigid deformities like ankylosing spondylitis. However, all corrective lumbar osteotomies will change T1 slope angle to some extent and therefore will change cervical alignment and often cervical C2 SVA. Signs of myelopathy may be evident due to past injury, compression, or cord tension due to stretch induced by kyphosis.

Imaging

The deformity should be evaluated by anterior/posterior and lateral cervical radiographs along with dynamic lateral flexion/extension views. The deformity is then accurately measured and any other abnormalities noted [2, 10, 11]. It is important to obtain full-length posteroanterior and lateral 36-inch scoliosis radiographs to examine overall sagittal and coronal balance in these patients [2, 11, 12]. It is recommended to assess cervical, thoracic, and lumbar sagittal alignment individually and globally and define the effect of regional imbalance on cervical balance and determine if it is a primary, secondary, or compensatory cervical deformity. The degree of required surgical sagittal correction depends on the angle of the cervical deformity (the chin-brow vertical angle), the C2 plumb line, and the desired final lordosis [6, 11, 13–15]. The goal of correction is to obtain sagittal alignment, horizontal gaze, cord decompression, and normalize cord tension. Dynamic (i.e., flexion/extension) radiographs permit an assessment of the overall flexibility of the cervical spine, which is paramount for preoperative planning. Computed tomographic (CT) scans of the cervical spine are also useful in determining the presence of fusion or ankylosis of the facet joints and discs and allow assessment of fixation points such as C2 and upper thoracic pedicles. All patients should be evaluated with preoperative magnetic resonance imaging or computed tomography myelography. These image modalities permit the evaluation of compressive pathology. If significant ventral compressive pathology (disc, osteophyte) is present, a ventral decompressive procedure may first be performed before the correction of the deformity.

Decision for Planning of Osteotomy

It is important when planning deformity surgery for cervical kyphosis to consider whether the deformity is rigid or fixed and whether there are neurological symptoms. In the flexible subaxial deformity, a posterior stabilization (usually C2–T2) is advocated; when deformity is semirigid, Smith-Petersen osteotomy should be considered. In the setting of a rigid cervical kyphosis in mid to low cervical spine with cervical sagittal imbalance, a C7 or T1 PSO may be sufficient.

Surgical Techniques

SPO with Controlled Anterior Osteoclasis

The patient is positioned in the prone position in a halo ring. The kyphotic head position is accommodated by additional rolls and pads as needed to elevate the patient's thorax. Additionally, transcortical motor evoked potential (MEP), somatosensory evoked potential (SSEP), and electromyography (EMG) are utilized and recommended.

A midline posterior incision is made, and the paraspinous muscles are dissected in a subperiosteal fashion, exposing the spinous processes, laminar facets, and lateral processes of C4–T2. Of note, if the bone is very soft, fixation can be extended to include bicortical C2 screws. Preoperative standing films allow for determination of the apex of the upper thoracic kyphosis, and the fixation is extended below this apex as needed.

Once the exposure is completed, the osteotomy is completed. A complete C7 laminectomy and partial C6 and T1 laminectomies are performed. The resection is then expanded laterally to include the removal of the C7 pedicle with the use of rongeurs. All resected bone is saved for bone graft (see Figs. 34.1 and 34.2). It's important that the remaining portions of the C6 and T1 laminae are carefully beveled and undercut to avoid any impingement or kinking of the spinal cord upon closure. Furthermore, all of the area near the C8 nerve root is carefully decompressed and exposed to provide ample room for the nerve root upon closure of the osteotomy.

The surgeon grasps the halo and extends the neck gradually with closure of the osteotomy posteriorly as the osteoclasis across C7–T1 occurs anteriorly. An audible snap and sensation of the osteoclasis is usually heard. The rotational malalignment and lateral tilt is also corrected at this time.

It's recommended that a temporary pre-bent rod is placed and locked down prior to closure of the osteotomy in order to decrease the risk of a sudden shift to an unstable spine. The C8 foramen is inspected to make sure the nerve is free after complete closure. At the C6–T1 area, the posterior aspects of the spine may then be decorticated. The autologous bone graft from the resection is packed bilaterally onto the decorticated areas. Since this is typically performed in patients with ankylosing spondylitis, anterior grafting is seldom required as the osteobiologic substrate is quite favorable.

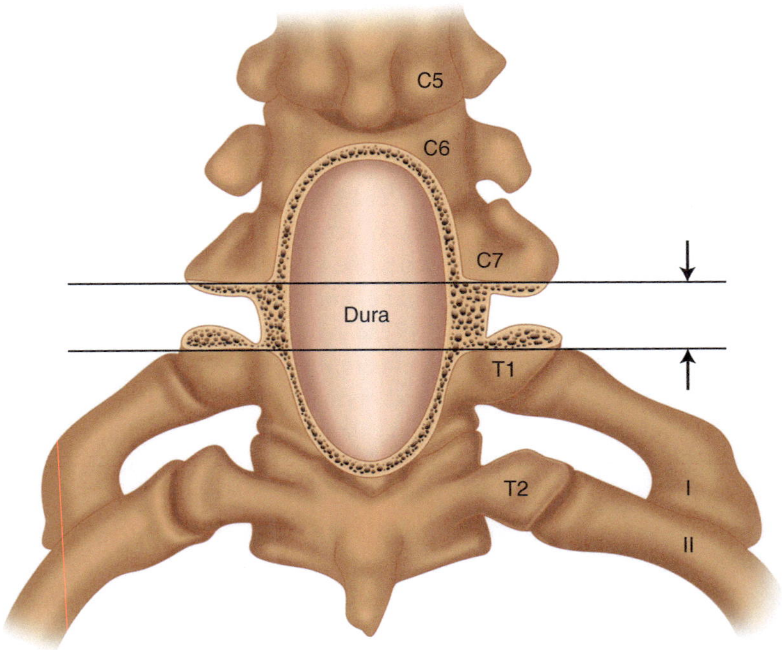

Fig. 34.1 Schematic diagram of the posterior surgical view of the area of SPO on C7. Subtotal laminectomy C6 and T1, total laminectomy C7, and total facetectomy on C7/T1 facet joints are performed

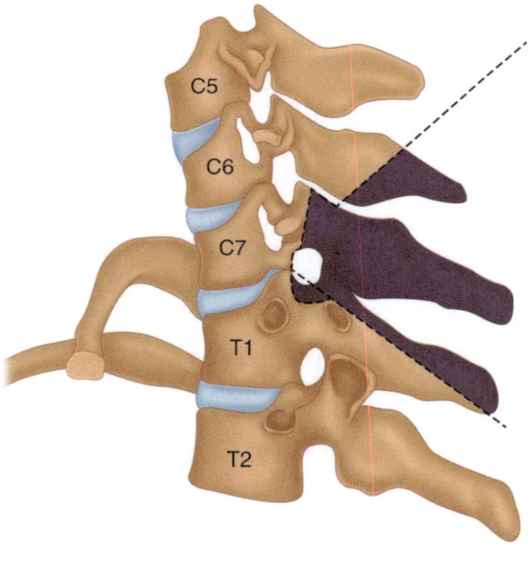

Fig. 34.2 Schematic diagram of the lateral surgical view of the area of SPO. Wedge-shaped osteotomy is performed to have more open space in posterior column. Majority of C7 pedicles are resected

Cervical PSO

The patient is placed prone in a halo ring and TC-MEP, SSEP, as well as EMG neuromonitoring is used. A standard posterior surgical approach is made to the cervical spine creating an incision from C2 to T3/T5 depending on the location of the kyphotic apex from preoperative imaging. The paraspinous muscles are dissected in a usual subperiosteal fashion, exposing the spinous processes, laminar facets, and lateral processes of the cervical spine and transverse processes in the thoracic spine.

After exposure is complete, the spine is instrumented accordingly using C2 bicortical pedicle screws, cervical lateral mass screws, and thoracic pedicle screws. Of note, it is preferable to extend the fixation to C2 in order to obtain bicortical screw placement for a stronger fixation point than at the lateral masses of the inferior vertebrae. Furthermore, it is preferable to have the caudal extent of the fusion terminate at either T3 or T5 depending on the extent of thoracic kyphosis to ensure the apex is within the fusion. Again, despite the fact that this is a cervical procedure, standing preoperative 3 foot films are critical to analyze regional and global alignment patterns prior to the procedure.

The osteotomy begins with performing facet release and removal of the facets of C6–C7 as well as C7–T1 (Fig. 34.3I). The nerve roots at C7 and C8 are then identified and followed out the foramen. The dissection is carried out completely laterally isolating the C7 pedicle (Fig. 34.4).

After the bilateral facetectomies and isolation of the C7 pedicle, the C7 pedicle is skeletonized and removed with Lempert rongeurs. Sequential lumbar or custom wedge-shaped spinal taps are used to decancellate the C7 vertebral body (Fig. 34.5) combined with osteotomes and downpushing curettes to create as wide a wedge as possible (Fig. 34.3II, III). The limiting factor is usually the proximity of the C7 and C8 roots.

The lateral wall of the C7 vertebral body is then dissected out with a Penfield 1 dissector and visualized (Figs. 34.3III and 34.6). The C7 lateral wall is

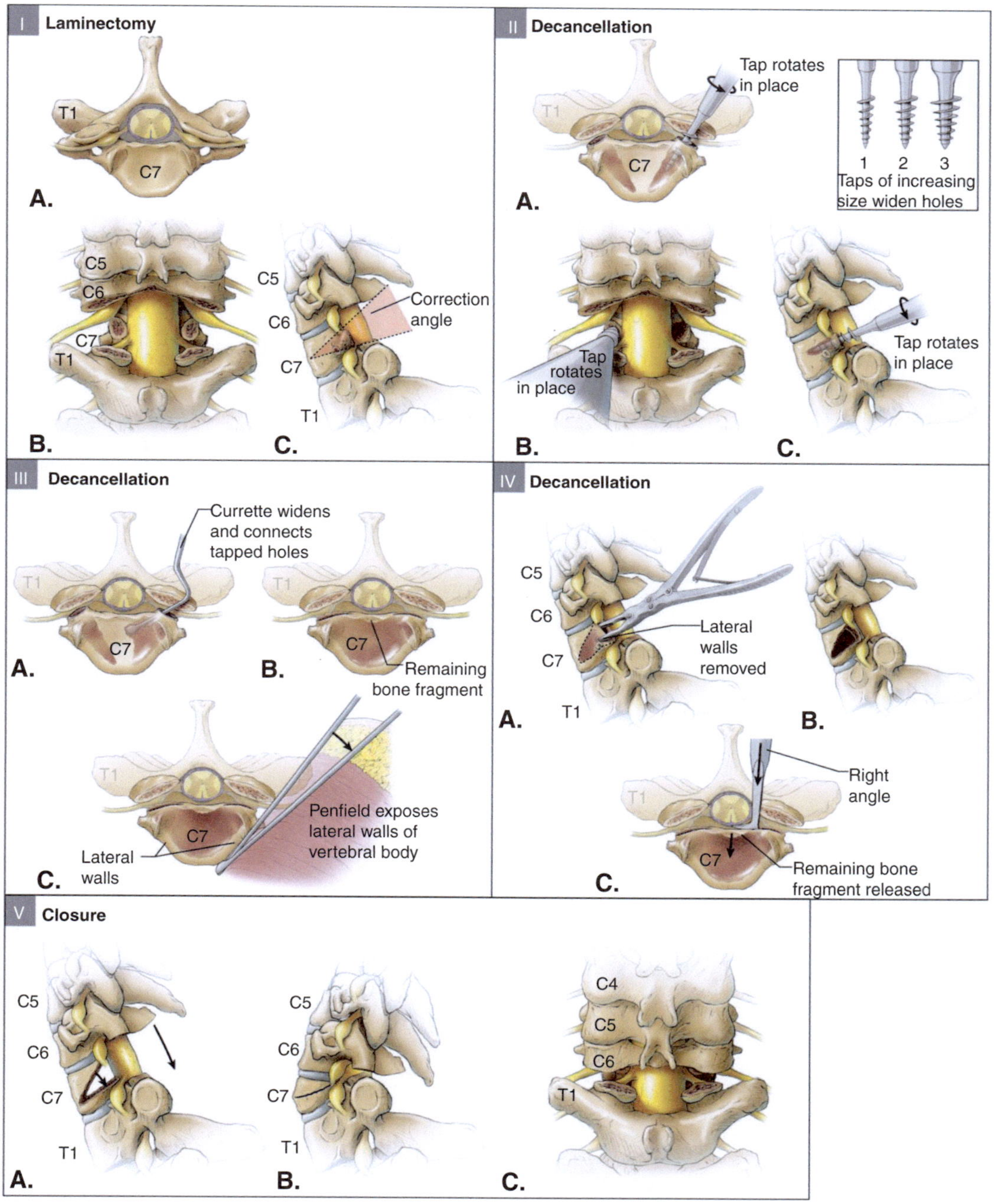

Fig. 34.3 C7 PSO technique. Schematic diagram demonstrating the five major operative steps involved in performing a cervical PSO. Step I is the laminectomy, step II is the decancelation through the pedicle corridor using taps that increase sequentially in size, step III is decancelation of the vertebral body through the pedicular corridor, step IV is decancelation of the posterior vertebral body cortex, and step V is the closure of the PSO

removed with needle nose rongeurs and osteotomes via the pedicle hole reamed out by the taps, followed by removal of the posterior vertebral body (Fig. 34.3IV) with a custom central impactor.

After completion of the osteotomy, the head is then loosened from the table, and the halo ring is used to extend the head and close the osteotomy (Figs. 34.3V and 34.7).

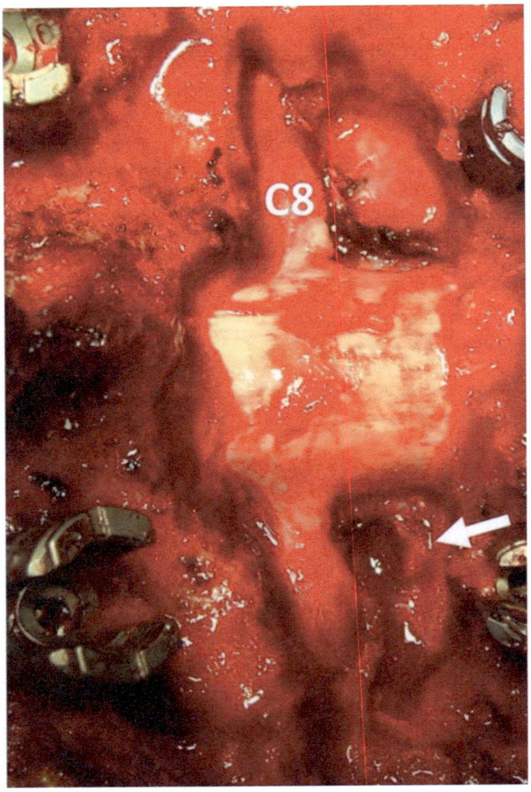

Fig. 34.4 Intraoperative photograph during C7 PSO showing isolation of the C7 pedicle and C8 nerve root

Postoperative Care/Concerns and Complication Management/Avoidance

The cervical PSO has two key benefits compared with the traditional cervical SPO. First, the PSO results in a mechanically stiffer result (greater biomechanical stability) than the SPO. [6, 9] The SPO generally results in disc disruption or, in cases of

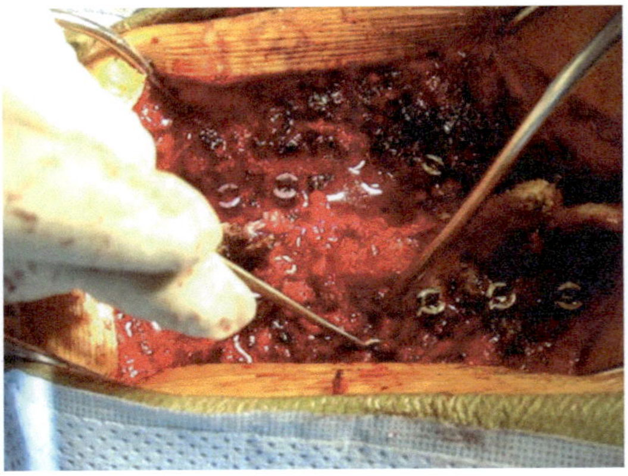

Fig. 34.6 Intraoperative photograph during C7 PSO showing the use of a Penfield retractor to expose the lateral wall of C7

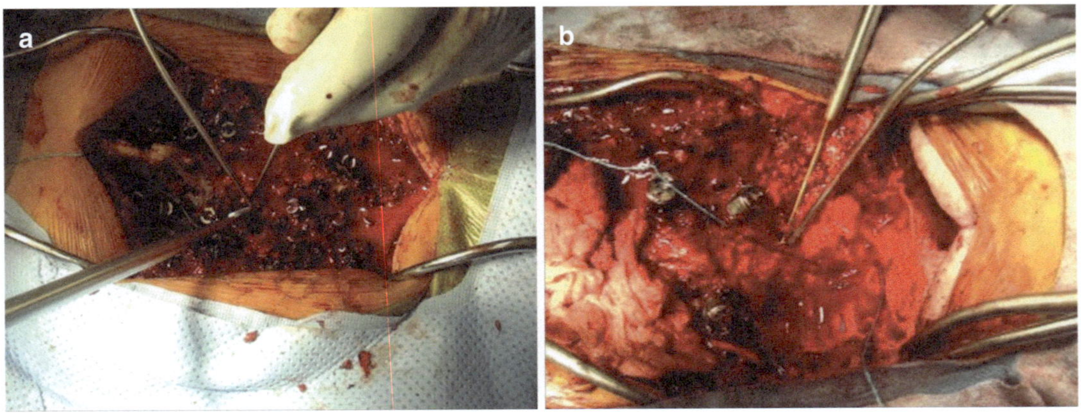

Fig. 34.5 Intraoperative photograph during C7 PSO showing two different views (**a, b**) of using lumbar taps to decancellate the C7 vertebral body

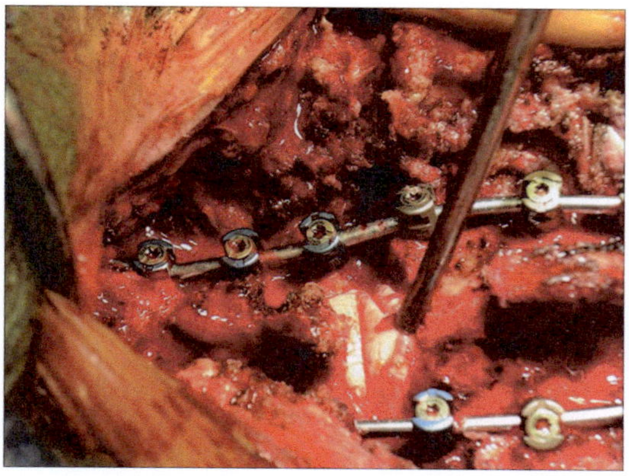

Fig. 34.7 Intraoperative photograph during C7 PSO showing closure of the osteotomy

ankylosing spondylitis, osteoclasis through a fused disc space or the anterior cortex of the vertebral body, causing a significant anterior gap in which the anterior longitudinal ligament is completely torn or the autofused anterior bridging osteophyte has been fractured. The PSO leaves the anterior longitudinal ligament intact. In addition, the PSO has a wedge component that cleaves the vertebral body creating a larger bone-on-bone load-bearing interface even when compared with a SPO that is fully closed posteriorly. This greater bone-on-bone contact significantly increases stiffness, especially in compression, and may provide better fusion rates in patients who do not have ankylosing spondylitis, as the PSO provides a substantial load-bearing surface area in the uniting of the anterior and posterior columns upon closure [6, 9]. No secondary anterior grafting is required. Second, the PSO results in a more controlled closure than the SPO because no sudden osteoclastic fracture is necessary.

Due to the recent advance in surgical technique, anesthesia and intraoperative neuromonitoring, CTJ PSO has been considered a safe, reproducible, and effective procedure for the management of cervical kyphotic deformities [8]. Daubs et al. [16] found that increasing age was a significant factor in predicting a complication for patients over the age of 60. However, in the authors' series, 8 of 11 patients were over the age of 60 years, and there were no perioperative neurological deficits, and there were perioperative medical complications in only 2 of 11 cases [8]. The lower medical complication rate and decreased incidence of dysphagia may be due to the all-posterior nature of this technique. Posterior-only deformity corrections have also been associated with lower complication rates in thoracolumbar surgery compared with staged anterior-posterior procedures.

Case Presentations

Case 1, Fig. 34.8

A 63-year-old woman presented with neck pain, a sensation of heaviness to her head, and change in posture for over 9 months. She was noted on exam that her head would fall forward during standing, and she had difficulty maintaining horizontal gaze. She was full strength on neurological exam. Her standing X-ray films showed a cervical kyphosis that was measured at 4 cm, and her cervical kyphosis was flexible to a neutral position. Her MRI demonstrated no stenosis. She had a posterior spine instrumentation and spinal fusion at C2 to T3. Type 1 posterior spine osteotomies were performed at C2–C3, C3–C4, C4–C5, C5–C6, C6–C7, and C7–T1. The postoperative films are shown demonstrating resolution of her cervical sagittal imbalance and kyphosis.

Case 2, Fig. 34.9

A 58-year-old woman with a history of prior laminectomy for urgent spinal cord compression and severe myelopathy developed postoperative kyphosis and recurrent progressive myelopathy with upper and lower extremity weakness. She failed nonoperative treatment. She had a posterior spine instrumentation and spinal fusion at C2 to T3, with a revision of the laminectomy (C3 to C7). Smith-Petersen osteotomies were performed at C2–C3, C3–C4, and C6–C7. Sublaminar wiring at C2. The postoperative films are shown demonstrating resolution of her cervical sagittal imbalance and kyphosis.

Case 3, Fig. 34.10

A 68-year-old man with a history of a prior cervical fusion presented with neck pain, bilateral

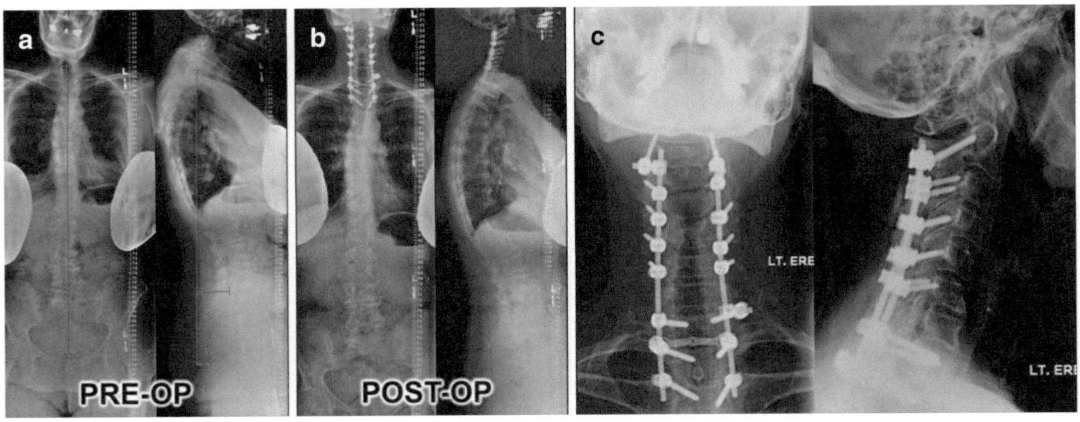

Fig. 34.8 (**a, b**) are preoperative and post-op, respectively, for Case 1. (**c**) represents close-ups of postoperative construct

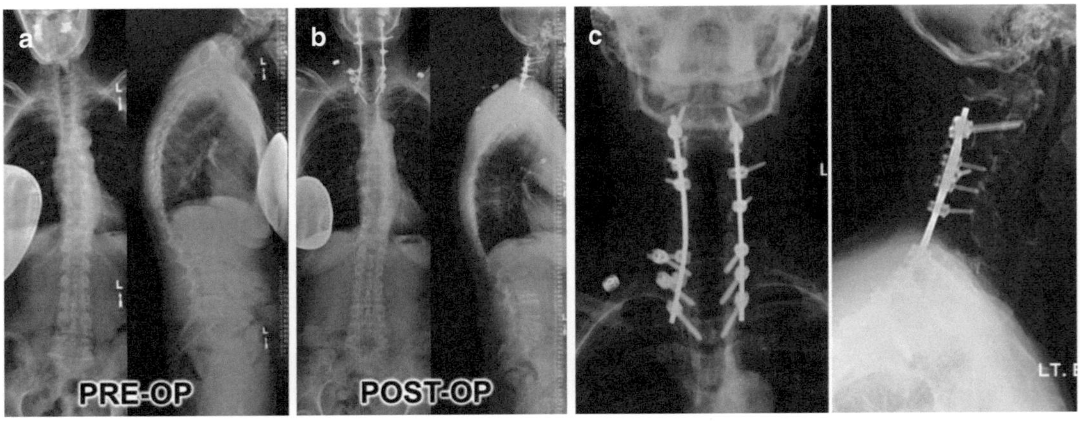

Fig. 34.9 (**a, b**) are preoperative and post-op, respectively, for Case 3. (**c**) represents close-ups of postoperative construct

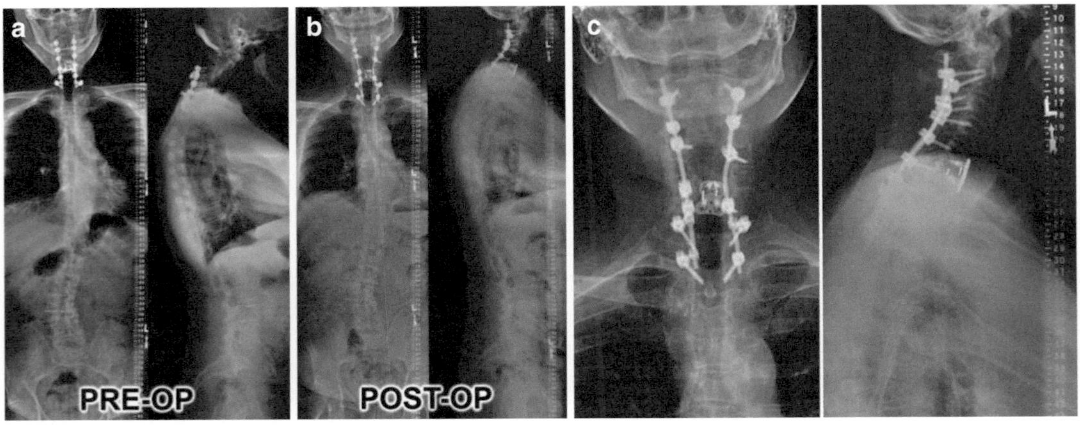

Fig. 34.10 (**a, b**) are preoperative and post-op, respectively, for Case 3. (**c**) represents close-ups of postoperative construct

arm pain down to his elbows, and decrease in strength in both the arms and legs. He was noted on imaging to have developed hardware failure and proximal junctional kyphosis. His cervical sagittal deformity was noted on studies to be reducible. He underwent a revision operation that included a decompression laminectomy from C2 to C5. Smith-Petersen osteotomies were performed at C3–C4 and C4–C5. The fusion was revised, and the upper instrumented level was extended to C2. The posterior spine instrumentation and spinal fusion was from C2 to T2. The postoperative films are shown demonstrating resolution of his cervical sagittal imbalance and kyphosis.

Discussion/Conclusions

This chapter focuses on correction of cervical kyphosis with either cervical SPO or PSO. A recent study by Tang et al. [17] showed the clinical effect of increased cervical SVA on health-related quality-of-life (HRQOL) scores. The authors found significant correlations of increased cervical SVA with worse HRQOL, specifically with the neck disability index (NDI) and PCS component of the SF36 (Figs. 34.9 and 34.10). They also determined a cervical SVA threshold of 4.1 cm in which significant clinical disability may be seen [17]. This outlines the importance of correcting the cervical kyphosis to below a value of 4 cm, similar to the value of 5 cm in the lumbar spine.

Although the cervical SPO can offer sagittal correction, we feel the C7 PSO is beneficial over it. The PSO is more mechanically stiff than the SPO resulting in increased biomechanical stability [18]. This is mostly due to anatomical differences between the two osteotomy types. The SPO generally results in disc disruption or, in cases of ankylosing spondylitis, osteoclasis through a fused disc space or the anterior cortex of the vertebral body causing a significant anterior gap in which the anterior longitudinal ligament (ALL) or autofused anterior bridging osteophyte has been fractured. The PSO leaves the ALL intact. In addition, the PSO intersects the vertebral body creating a larger bone-on-bone load-bearing interface even when compared to an SPO that is fully closed posteriorly. This greater bone-on-bone contact significantly increases stiffness [18], especially in compression, and may provide better fusion rates to the non-ankylosing spondylitis patient population as the PSO provides a substantial load-bearing surface area by having the anterior, middle, and posterior columns unite upon closure. No secondary anterior grafting is required. Second, the PSO results in a more controlled closure than the SPO because no sudden osteoclastic fracture is necessary. It is important to note that other cervical extension osteotomy reports have reported complications that include neurological deficits, sudden subluxation, and even death [19–23]. The cervical PSO has similar risks, and given it's more complex nature, it should be performed by very experienced spinal deformity surgeons.

Key Recommendations

1. SPO osteotomy is used for subaxial flexible deformity.
2. Classic SPO may be used in cases of chin-on-chest deformity for patients with ankylosing spondylitis or DISH.
3. PSO is our preferred technique for cervical sagittal imbalance and chin-on-chest deformity.
4. Intraoperative imaging guidance systems and intraoperative neuromonitoring can help prevent complications related to the osteotomy closure, translation, and dural buckling.
5. All posterior approaches may reduce but do not eliminate swallowing dysfunction.
6. Cervical sagittal balance is a complex issue as cervical alignment depends in large part on global T/L alignment, pelvic tilt, and T1 slope.
7. Standing 3 foot films are mandatory prior to any deformity correction including deformities of the cervical spine.

References

1. Steinmetz MP, Stewart TJ, Kager CD, Benzel EC, Vaccaro AR. Cervical deformity correction. Neurosurgery. 2007;60(1 Suppl 1):S90–7.
2. Chi JH, Tay B, Stahl D, Lee R. Complex deformities of the cervical spine. Neurosurg Clin N Am. 2007;18(2):295–304.
3. Epstein NE. Evaluation and treatment of clinical instability associated with pseudoarthrosis after anterior cervical surgery for ossification of the posterior longitudinal ligament. Surg Neurol. 1998;49(3):246–52.
4. Hilibrand AS, Carlson GD, Palumbo MA, Jones PK, Bohlman HH. Radiculopathy and myelopathy at segments adjacent to the site of a previous anterior cervical arthrodesis. J Bone Joint Surg Am. 1999;81(4):519–28.
5. Mason C, Cozen L, Adelstein L. Surgical correction of flexion deformity of the cervical spine. Calif Med. 1953;79(3):244–6.
6. Scheer JK, Tang JA, Deviren V, Acosta F, Buckley JM, Pekmezci M, et al. Biomechanical analysis of cervicothoracic junction osteotomy in cadaveric model of ankylosing spondylitis: effect of rod material and diameter. J Neurosurg Spine. 2011;14(3):330–5.
7. Chapman JR, Anderson PA, Pepin C, Toomey S, Newell DW, Grady MS. Posterior instrumentation of the unstable cervicothoracic spine. J Neurosurg. 1996;84(4):552–8.
8. Deviren V, Scheer JK, Ames CP. Technique of cervicothoracic junction pedicle subtraction osteotomy for cervical sagittal imbalance: report of 11 cases. J Neurosurg Spine. 2011;15(2):174–81.
9. Scheer JK, Tang JA, Buckley JM, Deviren V, Pekmezci M, McClellan RT, et al. Biomechanical analysis of osteotomy type and rod diameter for treatment of cervicothoracic kyphosis. Spine. 2011;36(8):E519–23.
10. Edwards CC 2nd, Riew KD, Anderson PA, Hilibrand AS, Vaccaro AF. Cervical myelopathy. Current diagnostic and treatment strategies. Spine J. 2003;3(1):68–81.
11. Mummaneni PV, Deutsch H, Mummaneni VP. Cervicothoracic kyphosis. Neurosurg Clin N Am. 2006;17(3):277–87. vi.
12. Mummaneni PV, Mummaneni VP, Haid RW Jr, Rodts GE Jr, Sasso RC. Cervical osteotomy for the correction of chin-on-chest deformity in ankylosing spondylitis. Technical note. Neurosurg Focus. 2003;14(1):e9.
13. Belanger TA, Milam RA, Roh JS, Bohlman HH. Cervicothoracic extension osteotomy for chin-on-chest deformity in ankylosing spondylitis. J Bone Joint Surg Am. 2005;87(8):1732–8.
14. Simmons ED, DiStefano RJ, Zheng Y, Simmons EH. Thirty-six years experience of cervical extension osteotomy in ankylosing spondylitis: techniques and outcomes. Spine. 2006;31(26):3006–12.
15. Suk KS, Kim KT, Lee SH, Kim JM. Significance of chin-brow vertical angle in correction of kyphotic deformity of ankylosing spondylitis patients. Spine. 2003;28(17):2001–5.
16. Daubs MD, Lenke LG, Cheh G, Stobbs G, Bridwell KH. Adult spinal deformity surgery: complications and outcomes in patients over age 60. Spine. 2007;32(20):2238–44.
17. Tang JA, Scheer JK, Smith JS, Deviren V, Bess S, Hart RA, et al. The impact of standing regional cervical sagittal alignment on outcomes in posterior cervical fusion surgery. Neurosurgery. 2012;71(3):662–9. discussion 9.
18. Scheer JK, Tang JA, Buckley JM, Pekmezci M, McClellan RT, Ames CP. Biomechanical analysis of osteotomy type (OWO, CWO) and rod diameter for treatment of cervicothoracic kyphosis. 17th Annual International Meeting on Advanced Spine Techniques, Toronto, Canada; 2010.
19. Sansur CA, Fu KM, Oskouian RJ Jr, Jagannathan J, Kuntz C, Shaffrey CI. Surgical management of global sagittal deformity in ankylosing spondylitis. Neurosurg Focus. 2008;24(1):E8.
20. Etame AB, Than KD, Wang AC, La Marca F, Park P. Surgical management of symptomatic cervical or cervicothoracic kyphosis due to ankylosing spondylitis. Spine. 2008;33(16):E559–64.
21. Etame AB, Wang AC, Than KD, La Marca F, Park P. Outcomes after surgery for cervical spine deformity: review of the literature. Neurosurg Focus. 2010;28(3):E14.
22. Hoh DJ, Khoueir P, Wang MY. Management of cervical deformity in ankylosing spondylitis. Neurosurg Focus. 2008;24(1):E9.
23. Nottmeier EW, Deen HG, Patel N, Birch B. Cervical kyphotic deformity correction using 360-degree reconstruction. J Spinal Disord Tech. 2009;22(6):385–91.

Index

M. G. Kaiser et al. (eds.), *Degenerative Cervical Myelopathy and Radiculopathy*,
https://doi.org/10.1007/978-3-319-97952-6

D

N

MIX
Papier aus verantwortungsvollen Quellen
Paper from responsible sources
FSC® C105338

If you have any concerns about our products,
you can contact us on
ProductSafety@springernature.com

In case Publisher is established outside the EU,
the EU authorized representative is:
Springer Nature Customer Service Center GmbH
Europaplatz 3, 69115 Heidelberg, Germany

Printed by Libri Plureos GmbH
in Hamburg, Germany